Eye Infections: Essentials in Ophthalmology

Eye Infections: Essentials in Ophthalmology

Edited by Anastasia Maddox

hayle
medical

New York

Hayle Medical,
750 Third Avenue, 9th Floor,
New York, NY 10017, USA

Visit us on the World Wide Web at:
www.haylemedical.com

ISBN: 978-1-63241-708-4

Cataloging-in-Publication Data

Eye infections : essentials in ophthalmology / edited by Anastasia Maddox.
    p. cm.
Includes bibliographical references and index.
ISBN 978-1-63241-708-4
1. Eye--Infections. 2. Eye--Diseases. 3. Ophthalmology. I. Maddox, Anastasia.
RE96 .E94 2019
617.7--dc23

Table of Contents

Preface

The human eye and its associated structures are susceptible to several diseases and disorders, and age-related changes. Eye infections, such as conjunctivitis are characterized by inflammation, pain, scratchiness, burning and itchiness. It is a fairly common infection occurring in children, people wearing contact lenses and people infected with chlamydia or gonorrhea. It is primarily caused by a viral or bacterial infection. Keratitis is another infection of the eye in which the cornea of the eye becomes inflamed. It is characterized by photophobia, impaired eyesight, red eye and pain. It can be acute or chronic. Such infections can be caused due to bacterial, fungal, viral and parasitic agents. Endophthalmitis is another eye infection in which the interior of the eye gets inflamed. It can potentially lead to a loss of vision and the eye itself. Although it is triggered by a viral or fungal infection, it can occur due to a penetrating trauma, intravitreal injections and retained intraocular foreign bodies. Antibiotic and steroid eye drops are used to treat eye infections or to prevent them from occurring after eye surgeries. The branch of medicine and surgery that is concerned with the diagnosis and treatment of eye infections is known as ophthalmology. Some of the diverse topics covered in this book address the various infections of the eye. The various advancements in ophthalmology, in relation to eye infection diagnosis and management, are glanced at and their applications as well as ramifications are looked at in detail. It will provide comprehensive knowledge to the readers.

The researches compiled throughout the book are authentic and of high quality, combining several disciplines and from very diverse regions from around the world. Drawing on the contributions of many researchers from diverse countries, the book's objective is to provide the readers with the latest achievements in the area of research. This book will surely be a source of knowledge to all interested and researching the field.

In the end, I would like to express my deep sense of gratitude to all the authors for meeting the set deadlines in completing and submitting their research chapters. I would also like to thank the publisher for the support offered to us throughout the course of the book. Finally, I extend my sincere thanks to my family for being a constant source of inspiration and encouragement.

Editor

IL-2 Suppression of IL-12p70 by a Recombinant HSV-1 Expressing IL-2 Induces T-Cell Auto-Reactivity and CNS Demyelination

Mandana Zandian[1], Kevin R. Mott[1], Sariah J. Allen[1], Shuang Chen[2], Moshe Arditi[2,3], Homayon Ghiasi[1]*

1 Department of Surgery, Center for Neurobiology and Vaccine Development, Ophthalmology Research, Cedars-Sinai Medical Center, Los Angeles, California, United States of America, 2 Division of Pediatric Infectious Diseases and Immunology, Cedars-Sinai Medical Center, Los Angeles, California, United States of America, 3 Department of Medicine, David Geffen School of Medicine at UCLA, Los Angeles, California, United States of America

Abstract

To evaluate the role of cellular infiltrates in CNS demyelination in immunocompetent mice, we have used a model of multiple sclerosis (MS) in which different strains of mice are infected with a recombinant HSV-1 expressing IL-2. Histologic examination of the mice infected with HSV-IL-2 demonstrates that natural killer cells, dendritic cells, B cells, and CD25 (IL-2rα) do not play any role in the HSV-IL-2-induced demyelination. T cell depletion, T cell knockout and T cell adoptive transfer experiments suggest that both CD8[+] and CD4[+] T cells contribute to HSV-IL-2-induced CNS demyelination with CD8[+] T cells being the primary inducers. In the adoptive transfer studies, all of the transferred T cells irrespective of their CD25 status at the time of transfer were positive for expression of FoxP3 and depletion of FoxP3 blocked CNS demyelination by HSV-IL-2. The expression levels of IL-12p35 relative to IL-12p40 differed in BM-derived macrophages infected with HSV-IL-2 from those infected with wild-type HSV-1. HSV-IL-2-induced demyelination was blocked by injecting HSV-IL-2-infected mice with IL-12p70 DNA. This study demonstrates that suppression of the IL-12p70 function of macrophages by IL-2 causes T cells to become auto-aggressive. Interruption of this immunoregulatory axis results in demyelination of the optic nerve, the spinal cord and the brain by autoreactive T cells in the HSV-IL-2 mouse model of MS.

Editor: Maria Castro, University of California, Los Angeles, and Cedars-Sinai Medical Center, United States of America

Funding: This work was supported by Public Health Service grant EY15557 from the National Eye Institute. The funders had no role in study design, data collection and analysis, decision to publish, or preparation of the manuscript.

Competing Interests: The authors have declared that no competing interests exist.

* E-mail: ghiasih@cshs.org

Introduction

Epidemiologic studies have implicated genetic, as well as environmental factors, in the development of multiple sclerosis (MS) [1,2]. The possibility that infectious agents, particularly viruses, are involved [3,4] remains controversial [5,6,7] and the evidence suggests that if an infectious agent is involved, it alone may not be sufficient to initiate the observed pathology [5,6,7]. There are several lines of evidence implicating the cytokine, interleukin-2 (IL-2) in the pathology of MS [8,9,10,11]. Patients with MS have elevated levels of IL-2 in their cerebrospinal fluid (CSF) and sera and IL-2-deficient mice are more resistant to experimental autoimmune encephalitis (EAE) than their heterozygote and wild-type counterparts [12]. To explore the possibility that IL-2 may play a role in the pathology of MS in conjunction with viral infection, we constructed a recombinant herpes simplex virus type 1 (HSV-1) that expresses murine IL-2 constitutively [13] as well as a panel of control recombinant viruses that express murine IL-4, interferon (IFN)-γ, IL-12p35, or IL-12p40 continuously [14,15,16]. We have shown previously that ocular infection of different strains of mice (i.e., BALB/c, C57BL/6, SJL/6, and 129SVE) with the HSV-IL-2 virus results in demyelination of the optic nerves (ON), the spinal cords (SC) and the brains of infected mice as determined by histologic examination of tissues

obtained at necropsy [17,18]. The demyelinated lesions involved the periventricular white matter, brain stem, and SC white matter, and had striking similarities to the plaques seen in patients with MS [17]. Demyelination was detected in the CNS of infected mice up to 75 days (the longest time point tested) post HSV-IL-2 infection. However, the severity of demyelination did not increase from 14 days to 75 days post infection. In addition, the HSV-IL-2 infected mice developed optic neuropathy as determined by changes in the visual-evoked cortical potentials (VECPs) [18]. In contrast, demyelination was not detectable after infection of the mice with wild-type (wt) HSV-1 alone or infection of the mice with the HSV-IL-4 or HSV-IFN-γ viruses, which are identical to HSV-IL-2 except that they express IL-4 or IFN-γ instead of IL-2 [17,18].

The pathogenic processes that underlie demyelination in MS have not yet been elucidated. One hypothesis is that autoimmunity to CNS antigens is triggered by environmental factors in genetically susceptible individuals and that the activated immune response leads to destruction of the myelin [1,2]. Our published studies suggest that HSV plays an important role in initiating destruction of the myelin in the presence of elevated levels of IL-2. Thus, the HSV-IL-2-induced demyelination could be associated with the innate or the adaptive arms of the immune response in the infected mice. Therefore, we undertook the current studies to determine the role of NK-cells, dendritic cells (DCs), B-cells, IL-2rα (CD25), CD4$^+$ T cells, and CD8$^+$ T cells in the HSV-IL2-induced CNS demyelination. The results indicate that the demyelinated lesions observed after infection with HSV-IL-2 are associated with both CD4$^+$ and CD8$^+$ T cells, with CD8$^+$ T cells playing the more prominent role. Furthermore, the demyelination was found to be associated with IL-2-mediated suppression of IL-12p70 expression by macrophages. The expression of IL-12p70 in the macrophages in the presence of IL-2 was restored by co-infection of mice with recombinant HSV-IL-12p70 virus, which also prevented demyelination. Thus, IL-12p70 expression by macrophages can act to regulate induction of T-cell autoimmune disease. Our results suggest a potential mechanism for the association of higher levels of IL-2 expression with susceptibility to MS, in which the IL-2 inhibits the ability of the macrophages to suppress an autoimmune T-cell response to infection with neurotropic viruses.

Results

Role of B cells, DCs, and NK cells in HSV-IL-2 induced demyelination in infected mice

To determine the possible involvement of innate immunity in the regulation of HSV-IL-2-induced demyelination in the present study, we used B-cell deficient mice (BALB/c-CD19$^{-/-}$), BALB/c-DTR transgenic mice (CD11c-diphtheria toxin receptor-GFP) that were depleted of DCs using DT, and C57BL/6 mice that were depleted of NK cells using anti-asialo GM1 monoclonal antibodies. All of the mice, including the female BALB/c-CD19$^{-/-}$, control BALB/c, BALB/c-DTR transgenic mice with and without DC depletion, and C57BL/6 mice with and without NK depletion, were infected ocularly with either HSV-IL-2 or HSV-IL-4. At day 14 PI, the mice were sacrificed and the ONs collected post-fixed and stained with the myelin stain, LFB. Representative photomicrographs of the ON sections from mice infected with HSV-IL-2 or HSV-IL-4 are shown in Figure 1.

Demyelination was observed in the HSV-IL-2-infected BALB/c-DTR mice that had been depleted of their DCs (Fig. 1A) but not in the HSV-IL-4-infected BALB/c-DTR mice that had been depleted of their DCs (Fig. 1B). Similarly, demyelination of the ON was observed in HSV-IL-2-infected mice that had been depleted of their NK cells (Fig. 1C) but not in NK-depleted mice following ocular infection with HSV-IL-4 (Fig. 1D).

Finally, demyelination of the ON was observed in the HSV-IL-2-infected BALB/c-CD19$^{-/-}$ mice (Fig. 1E), but not in the HSV-IL-4-infected BALB/c-CD19$^{-/-}$ mice (Fig. 1F). The patterns of demyelination of the ON in the absence of DCs, NK cells, or B cells were similar to the patterns of demyelination observed in wt mice infected with HSV-IL-2 (data not shown). Similar results were obtained with regards to demyelination in the SC and brains of the infected mice (data not shown). The failure of depletion of the cells to block the HSV-IL-2-induced demyelination suggests that B cells, NK cells, and DCs do not contribute to the demyelination of the ON in this mouse model. As the depletion did not result in exacerbation of the demyelination, the results also suggest that these components of the innate immune response do not act to suppress the autoimmune response. We have observed that the absence of macrophages exacerbates HSV-IL-2-induced demyelination and that even wt HSV-1 induces demyelination in infected BALB/c or C57BL/6 mice in the absence of macrophages (data not shown), which suggests that macrophages are not required for the development of the autoreactive demyelinating response, but may act to suppress it, as discussed in detail below.

Role of T cells in HSV-IL-2-induced demyelination

To determine whether T cells contribute to the HSV-IL-2-induced demyelination, BALB/c mice were depleted of CD4$^+$ and CD8$^+$ cells and infected ocularly with HSV-IL-2 or control HSV-IL-4. Demyelination was not detectable in ON, brain, or SC of BALB/c mice depleted of both CD4$^+$ and CD8$^+$ T cells and infected ocularly with HSV-IL-2 (Fig. 2, Panels A, B, C). Similarly, demyelination was not detectable in C57BL/6 mice depleted of

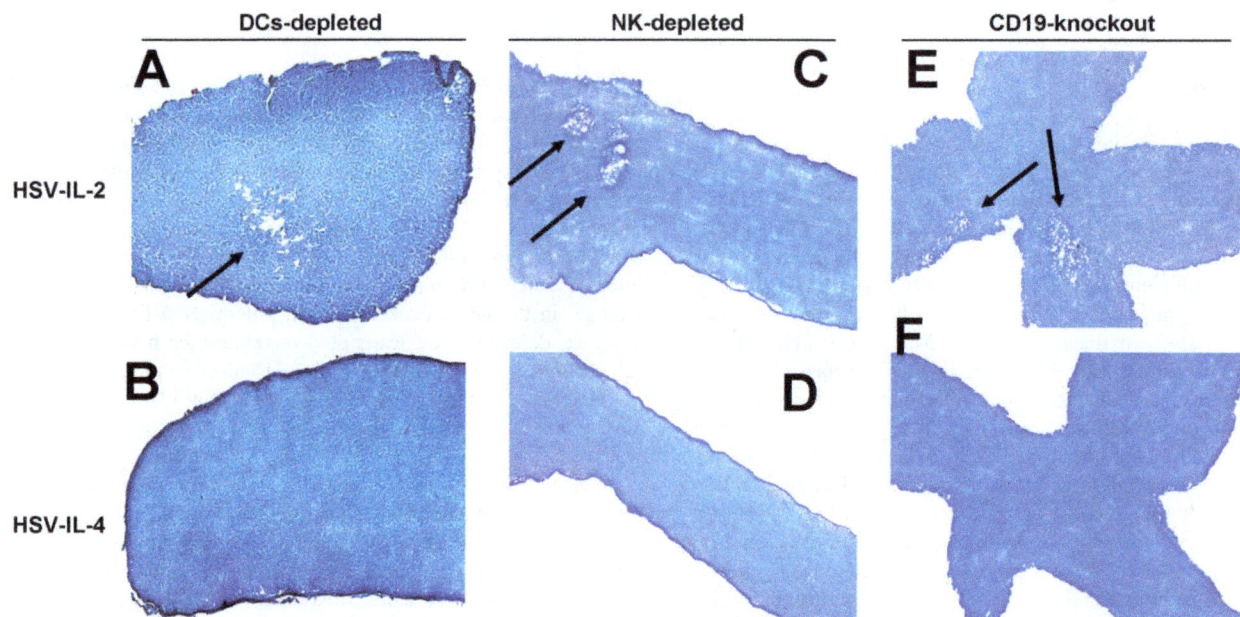

Figure 1. Role of innate immunity in HSV-IL-2 induced CNS demyelination. Female BALB/c-CD19$^{-/-}$, BALB/c-DTR transgenic mice, and NK-depleted C57BL/6 mice were infected ocularly with HSV-IL-2 or HSV-IL-4 as described in Materials and Methods. On day 14 PI, ON were collected, fixed, sectioned, and stained with LFB. Representative photomicrographs are shown. Arrows indicate areas of demyelination.

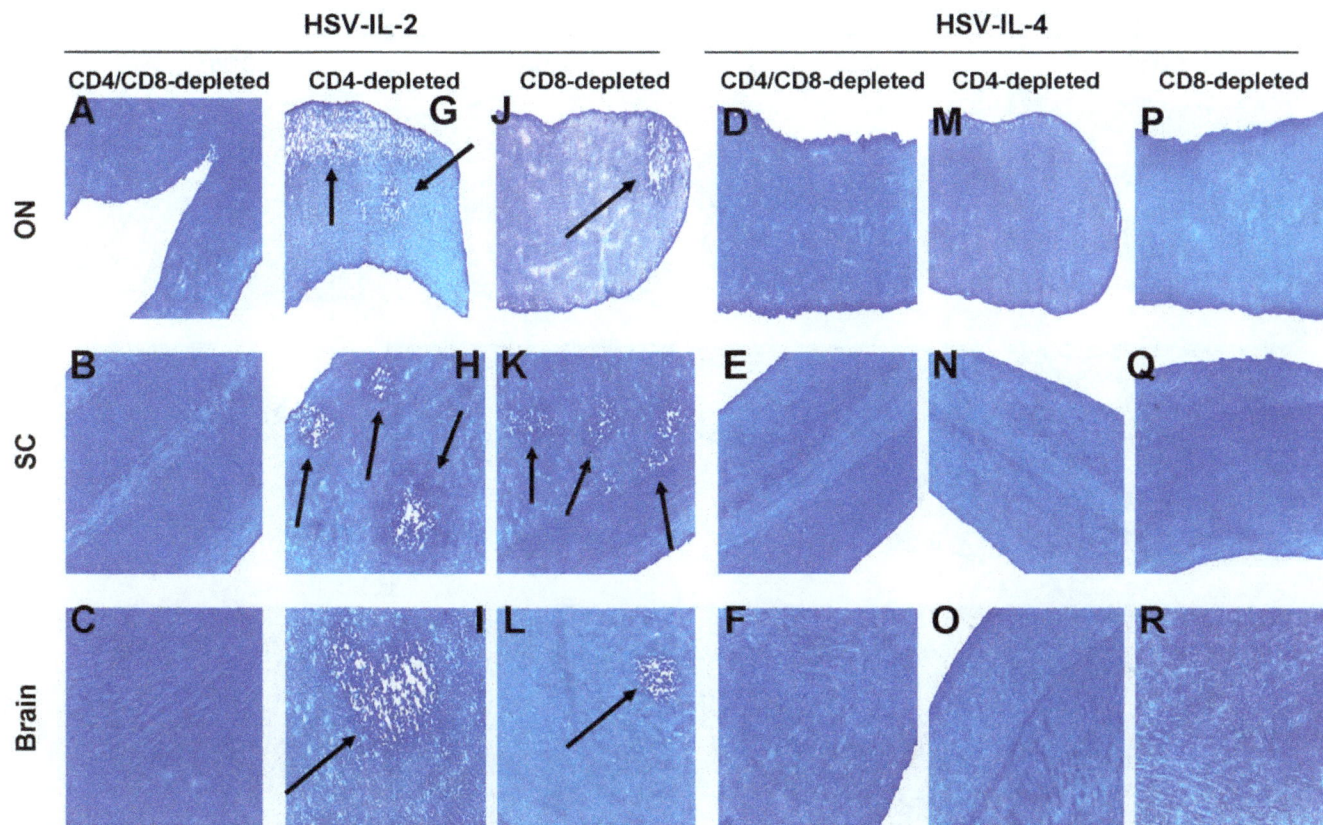

Figure 2. Demyelination in T cells-depleted mice. Mice were infected ocularly with HSV-IL-2 or HSV-IL-4. Forty-eight hr prior to infection, and on days 1, 5, and 9 days PI mice were depleted of CD4$^+$ T cell, CD8$^+$ T cell, or both T cell populations as described in Materials and Methods. After 14 days, brains, SC, and ON were removed, sectioned, and stained for LFB. Arrows indicate areas of demyelination in ON, SC, and brains of HSV-IL-2 infected mice.

both CD4$^+$ and CD8$^+$ cells and infected ocularly with HSV-IL-2 (data not shown). As expected mice of either strain that were depleted of CD4$^+$ and CD8$^+$ T cells and infected with HSV-IL-4 rather than HSV-IL-2 showed no sign of demyelination in ON (Fig. 2, Panels D, E, and F). These results suggested that, as has been described in MS and other models of MS [19,20,21], T cells do contribute to the HSV-IL-2-induced demyelination.

HSV-IL-2-infection of the BALB/c mice that had been depleted of their CD4$^+$ T cells, but not their CD8$^+$ cells, resulted in demyelination in the ON, SC, and brain, which was detected as the pale blue area in LFB staining (Fig. 2, Arrows, Panels G, H, and I). Similarly, HSV-IL-2 infection of mice that had been depleted of their CD8$^+$ T cells but not their CD4$^+$ cells, resulted in demyelination in their ON, SC, and brain (Fig. 2, arrows; Panels J, K, and L). As expected neither CD4-depleted nor CD8-depleted mice infected with HSV-IL-4 showed any signs of demyelination (Fig. 2, Panels M-R). Similar results were obtained when C57BL/6 mice were depleted of their CD4$^+$ T cells alone or CD8$^+$ T cells alone and infected ocularly with HSV-IL-2 or control HSV-IL-4 (data not shown). As depletion of both CD4$^+$ and CD8$^+$ T cells prevented the HSV-IL-2-induced demyelination, these results suggest that both CD4$^+$ and CD8$^+$ T cells contribute to the CNS demyelination. To verify these results, we analyzed demyelination in CD4 (C57BL/6-CD4$^{-/-}$) and CD8 (C57BL/6-CD8$^{-/-}$) knockout mice. Demyelination was observed in the ON, SC, and brain of the CD4 knockout mice infected with HSV-IL-2 (Fig. 3, CD4$^{-/-}$) and the ON, SC, and brain of the CD8 knockout mice infected with HSV-IL-2 (Fig. 3, CD8$^{-/-}$). No demyelination

was observed in ON, SC, and brain of CD4 knockout mice (Fig. 3, CD4$^{-/-}$) or CD8 knockout mice infected with HSV-IL-4 (Fig. 3, CD4$^{-/-}$). Collectively, these data strongly implicate both CD4$^+$ and CD8$^+$ T cells in HSV-IL-2-induced CNS demyelination.

We noted that the severity of the HSV-IL-2-induced demyelination appeared to be greater in the presence of CD8$^+$ T cells (in the CD4 knockout mice) than in the presence of CD4$^+$ T cells (in the CD8 knockout mice) (Fig. 3). Thus, to determine if more plaques are present in the CNS of CD4-knockout mice as compared with their CD8-knockout counterparts or wt C57BL/6 mice, we counted the number of observed plaques in the ON, SC and brain of CD4$^{-/-}$, CD8$^{-/-}$, and wt control mice. The data are shown as the number of sections showing demyelination plaques per total stained sections counted in Figure S1. More plaques were detected in the brains of both the HSV-IL-2-infected CD4- and CD8-knockout mice than in the brains of the HSV-IL-2-infected wt mice, but these differences were only significant when the numbers of plaques in the brains of the CD4-knockout mice were compared with the numbers in the brains of the wt mice (Figure S1-A; Brain; p<0.05). The number of HSV-IL-2-induced plaques detected in the SC were significantly higher in both the CD4- and CD8- knockout mice as compared with the numbers of plaques in the SC of wt mice (Figure S1-A, SC). In contrast, No significant differences were observed in the number of HSV-IL-2-induced plaques detected in ON of the knockout mice and the wt control mice (Figure S1-A, ON). Overall, more HSV-IL-2-induced demyelination plaques were detected in the SC of the knockout mice than their ON or brain

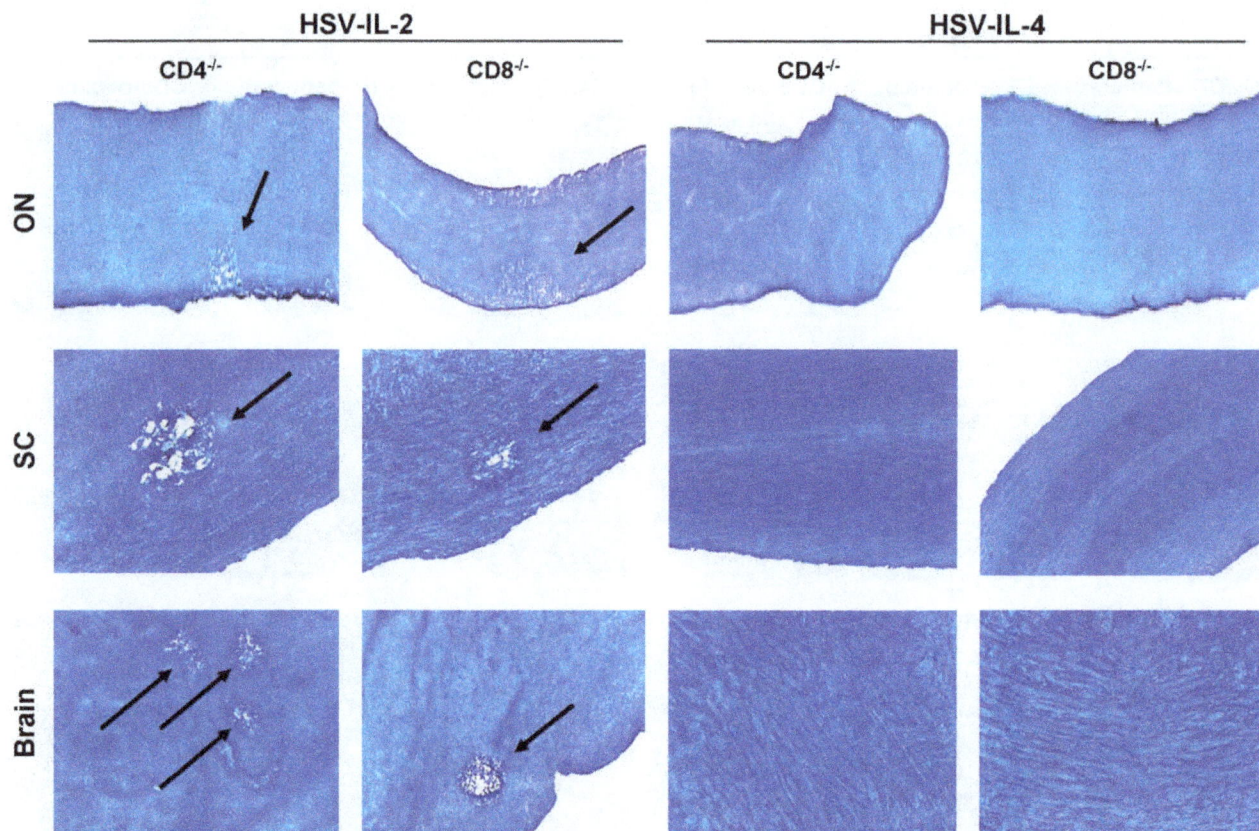

Figure 3. Demyelination in T cells-knockout mice. CD4$^{-/-}$ and CD8$^{-/-}$ mice were infected ocularly with HSV-IL-2 or HSV-IL-4 as described in Materials and Methods. After 14 days, ON, SC, and brains were removed, sectioned, and stained for LFB. Arrows indicate areas of demyelination in ON, SC, and brain of HSV-IL-2 infected mice.

(Figure S1-A). The number of plaques detected in brain, SC, and ON of depleted and mock-depleted BALB/c mice are presented in Figure 1B (Figure S1-B). Similar to knockout mice, more plaques were present in the CNS of CD4-depleted mice compare with their CD8-depleted counterparts but these differences did not reach statistical significance compared with the number of plaques in the mock-depleted control mice (Figure S1-B). As anticipated, the CD4-, CD8-, or mock-depleted groups of mice had significantly higher number of plaques than mice that were depleted of both CD4$^+$ and CD8$^+$ T cells (Figure S1-B) Thus, our CD4 and CD8 knockout studies suggest that both CD4 and CD8 T cells contribute to CNS demyelination and in the absence of the missing T cell subset the level of demyelination is increased in HSV-IL-2 infected mice.

Role of natural and HSV-IL-2-induced T cells in CNS demyelination

As the above results suggested that not only are both CD4$^+$ and CD8$^+$ T cells are involved in CNS demyelination but that CD8$^+$ T cells play a more prominent role (Figures 2, 3), we extended the studies to differentiate between responses of CD4$^+$ or CD8$^+$ naive T cells verses effectors T cells in CNS demyelination. CD4$^+$CD25$^+$, CD4$^+$CD25$^-$, CD8$^+$CD25$^+$, and CD8$^+$CD25$^-$ T cells were isolated using magnetic beads from naive BALB/c mice (naive T cell, nT cell) or BALB/c mice infected ocularly with HSV-IL-2 (effector T cell, effT cell) and the cells injected intraperitoneally into BALB/c-SCID recipient mice. Four hours after adoptive transfer, all of the SCID

recipient mice were infected ocularly with HSV-IL-2 or HSV-1 strain KOS. Control SCID mice that received tissue culture media only also were infected ocularly with HSV-IL-2 or KOS. Fourteen days after infection, the mice were sacrificed and the SC removed, post-fixed and stained with LFB. Representative photomicrographs are shown in Figure 4 and a summary of the data concerning the demyelination of the SC sections from mice infected with HSV-IL-2 or HSV-1 KOS is shown in Table 1.

We found that demyelination was undetectable in the mice that received nCD4$^+$CD25$^+$ T cells prior to infection with HSV-IL-2 (Fig. 4, HSV-IL-2), whereas demyelination occurred in the mice that received nCD4$^+$CD25$^-$ T cells prior to infection (Fig. 4, HSV-IL-2, arrow). Demyelination was detectable in mice that received either nCD8$^+$CD25$^+$ or nCD8$^+$CD25$^-$ prior to infection with HSV-IL-2 virus (Fig. 4, HSV-IL-2, arrows). There were no signs of demyelination in KOS-infected mice that received nCD4$^+$CD25$^+$, nCD4$^+$CD25$^-$, nCD8$^+$CD25$^+$, or nCD8$^+$CD25$^-$ T cells (Fig. 4, KOS).

In contrast, demyelination in the SC was observed in all SCID mice that received effCD4$^+$CD25$^+$, effCD4$^+$CD25$^-$, effCD8$^+$CD25$^+$, or effCD8$^+$CD25$^-$ T cells and were infected with HSV-IL-2 (Fig. 4, HSV-IL-2, arrows). Demyelination was not observed in mice that received effCD4$^+$CD25$^+$ T cells and were infected with KOS (Fig. 4, KOS), although mice that received effCD4$^+$CD25$^-$, effCD8$^+$CD25$^+$, or effCD8$^+$CD25$^-$ T cells and were infected with KOS developed demyelination (Fig. 4, KOS, arrows). As expected SCID mice that received induced T cells but

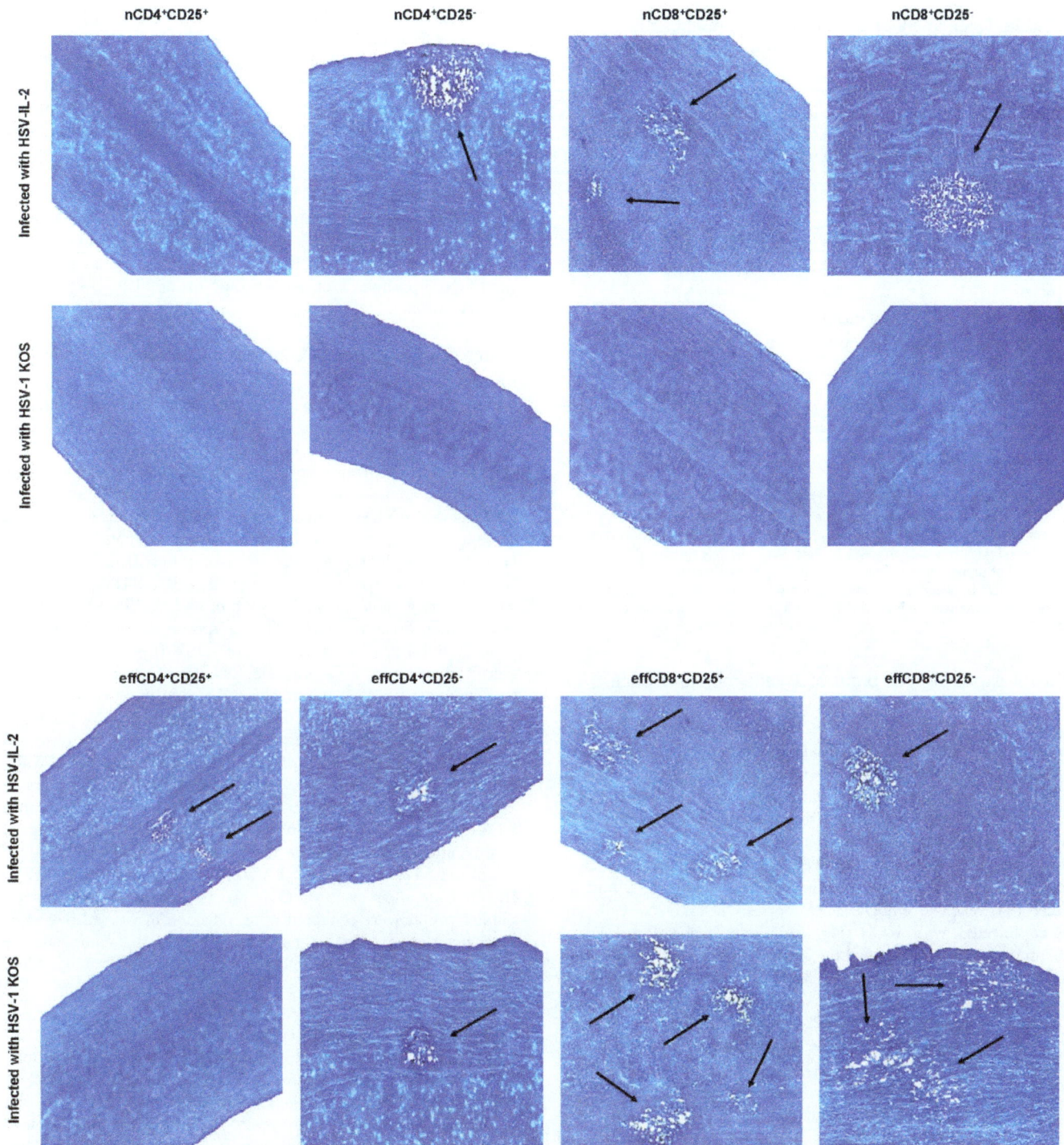

Figure 4. Adoptive transfer of naive and effector T cells to SCID mice. Naive T cells (nCD8⁺CD25⁺, nCD8⁺CD25⁻, nCD4⁺CD25⁺, and nCD4⁺CD25⁻) were isolated from naive mice, while the effector T cells (effCD8⁺CD25⁺, effCD8⁺CD25⁻, effCD4⁺CD25⁺, and effCD4⁺CD25⁻) were isolated from mice infected with HSV-IL-2 on day 5 PI. Magnetically isolated cells were transferred IP into recipient SCID mice and 4hr post-adoptive transfer, recipient SCID mice were infected ocularly with HSV-IL-2 or WT HSV-1 strain KOS. Representative ON sections on day 14 PI from infected mice are shown. Arrows indicate areas of demyelination.

were not subsequently infected did not show any sign of demyelination (data not shown). Furthermore, SCID mice that received media without T cells prior to infection with HSV-IL-2 or KOS did not develop any demyelination (Table 1). The patterns of demyelination in the brain and ON of the different groups of infected mice were similar to the patterns of demyelination in the SC described above (data not shown). The results of these studies provide further evidence that both CD4⁺ and CD8⁺ T cells contribute to CNS demyelination with CD8⁺ T cells playing a more prominent role than CD4⁺ T cells.

Table 1. Summary of LFB staining for presence of demyelination in ON, SC, and brain of SCID mice following adoptive transfer.[a]

	Number of mice with CNS demyelination following infection with[c]	
Adoptive transfer[b]	HSV-IL-2	WT KOS
nCD4+CD25+	0/5 (0%)	0/5 (0%)
nCD4+CD25−	5/5 (100%)	0/5 (0%)
nCD8+CD25+	5/5 (100%)	0/5 (0%)
nCD8+CD25−	5/5 (100%)	0/5 (0%)
effCD8+CD25+	5/5 (100%)	5/5 (100%)
effCD8+CD25−	5/5 (100%)	5/5 (100%)
effCD4+CD25+	5/5 (100%)	0/5 (0%)
effCD4+CD25−	5/5 (100%)	5/5 (100%)
Media	0/5 (0%)	0/5 (0%)

[a]Presence of demyelination in ON, SC, and brain of 5 recipient mice per group were assessed on day 14 PI.
[b]Naive T cells (nCD8+CD25+, nCD8+CD25−, nCD4+CD25+, and nCD4+CD25−) were isolated from naive mice, while the effector T cells (effCD8+CD25+, effCD8+CD25−, effCD4+CD25+, and effCD4+CD25−) were isolated from mice infected with HSV-IL-2 on day 5 PI. Each SCID mice received 2×10^5 cells in 300 µl of tissue culture media or tissue culture media only.
[c]Differences between group with CNS demyelination versus group with no CNS demyelination were statistically significant (p = 0.008, n = 5, Fisher exact test).

FoxP3 expression in brain of T cells recipient mice

The results described above (Fig. 5) suggested that both CD25+ and CD25− T cells can induce CNS demyelination in SCID mice that are infected with HSV-IL-2. To determine if the transferred T cells are expressing FoxP3, we measured FoxP3 transcripts by qRT-PCR using total RNA isolated from the brains of the mice described above and in Figure 5 that were sacrificed on day 14 PI. FoxP3 transcripts were found in the brains of the mice that received nCD4+CD25+, nCD4+CD25−, effCD4+CD25+, or effCD4+CD25− cells and were infected with HSV-IL-2, and the mice that received effCD4+CD25+ or effCD4+CD25− cells and were infected with KOS (Fig. 5A). The levels of the Foxp3 transcripts were similar in all the groups of mice irrespective of the CD25 status of the transferred cells (Fig. 5A). No differences in the expression of the CD4 transcript were observed among the groups (data not shown). Similarly, FoxP3 transcripts were observed in the brains of the mice that received nCD8+CD25+, nCD8+CD25−, effCD8+CD25+, or effCD8+CD25− and were infected with HSV-IL-2, and the mice that received effCD8+CD25+ or effCD8+CD25− and were infected with KOS (Fig. 5B). The expression of CD8 transcript was similar among these groups and statistically significant differences were not observed (data not shown). Similar level of FoxP3 transcript was detected in the isolated T cell population before transfer (not shown). Collectively, these results suggest that both the CD25+ and CD25− T cells expressed FoxP3 transcripts and that the transferred T cells may have a Treg rather then a Teff phenotype. Previously it was reported that FoxP3 is a better indicator of Treg cell linage specification factor than CD25 [22,23].

Role of FoxP3 in HSV-IL-2-induced demyelination

Our qRT-PCR analyses described above (Fig. 5) suggested that all transferred T cells irrespective of presence or absence of CD25 had similar levels of FoxP3 transcript in the brain of recipient SCID mice suggesting that FoxP3 may play a role in HSV-IL-2-induced CNS demyelination. To determine whether FoxP3 contributed to the HSV-IL-2-induced demyelination, FoxP3[DTR] mice were depleted of FoxP3 using diphtheria toxin and infected ocularly with HSV-IL-2 or control HSV-IL-4. Demyelination was not detectable in ON, SC or brain of FoxP3 depleted mice infected ocularly with HSV-IL-2 (Fig. 6, Left Panels). However, demyelination was detected in CNS of mice that were mock-depleted and infected with HSV-IL-2 (Fig. 6, Middle Panels). As expected mice of that were mock-depleted and infected with HSV-IL-4 rather than HSV-IL-2 showed no sign of demyelination in ON, brain, or SC (Fig. 6, Right Panels). These results suggested that, FoxP3-positive T cells contribute to the HSV-IL-2-induced demyelination.

Effect of endogenous IL-2 on the outcome of HSV-IL-2 infection

Previously we have shown that splenocytes from mice infected with HSV-IL-2 induced a $T_H 0/T_C 0$ type of immune response during early phase of infection suggesting that the host IL-2 may contribute to demyelination [13,17]. Moreover, our confocal microscopic analyses of double-stained brain sections from HSV-IL-2-infected mice suggested the presence of both exogenous IL-2 (produced by HSV-IL-2) and endogenous IL-2 (produced by host) [17]. To assess the possible involvement of host IL-2 in the HSV-IL-2-induced demyelination, we used BALB/c-STAT4$^{-/-}$ mice, which do not mount a $T_H 1$ response, and BALB/c-STAT6$^{-/-}$ mice, which do not mount a $T_H 2$ response. Mice were infected ocularly with 2×10^5 PFU/eye of HSV-IL-2 or HSV-IL-4, sacrificed at day 14 PI and the ON, brain, and SC dissected and stained with LFB. Control wt BALB/c mice were infected similarly with HSV-IL-2 or HSV-IL-4. Representative photomicrographs of are shown in Figure 7. Demyelination was observed in the ON, SC, and brain of both STAT4$^{-/-}$ and STAT6$^{-/-}$ mice (Fig. 7, Left Panels, arrows). No such lesions or other signs of demyelination were observed in the ON, SC, and brain of either STAT4$^{-/-}$ or STAT6$^{-/-}$ mice infected with HSV-IL-4 (Fig. 7, Right Panels). Overall, more demyelination was detected in the SC of the STAT4$^{-/-}$ and STAT6$^{-/-}$ mice infected with HSV-IL-2 than in their brain or ON (Fig. 6, HSV-IL-2, Left panels). Similar results were obtained upon infection of wt BALB/c mice (data not shown). Thus, these results suggest that endogenously produced $T_H 1$ and $T_H 2$ cytokines did not contribute to CNS demyelination.

Role of CD25 (IL-2rα) in HSV-IL-2-induced demyelination

CD25, also known as IL-2rα, is a component of the high-affinity IL-2R, which increases the sensitivity of the receptor for IL-2 by more than 100-fold [24,25]. Our transfer studies suggest that CD25 does not play any role in the HSV-IL-2-induced demyelination. To further determine the lack of CD25 involvement in HSV-IL-2-induced demyelination, we used C57BL/6-IL-2rα$^{-/-}$ mice as well as depletion of CD25 in C57BL/6 mice using anti-CD25 mAb. Knockout mice and depleted mice were infected ocularly with HSV-IL-2 or HSV-IL-4. Fourteen days after infection, the mice were sacrificed and the ON, SC, and brain removed, post-fixed and stained with LFB. Representative photomicrographs of ON, SC, and brain sections from the knockout and depleted mice infected with HSV-IL-2 or HSV-IL-4 are shown in Figure 8. HSV-IL-2 virus induced demyelination in ON, SC, and brain of both CD25$^{-/-}$ and CD25-depleted mice (Fig. 8, Left Panels), while mice infected with HSV-IL-4 did not show any sign of demyelination in their ON, SC, or brain (Fig. 8, Right Panels). Overall, the number of plaques detected in ON,

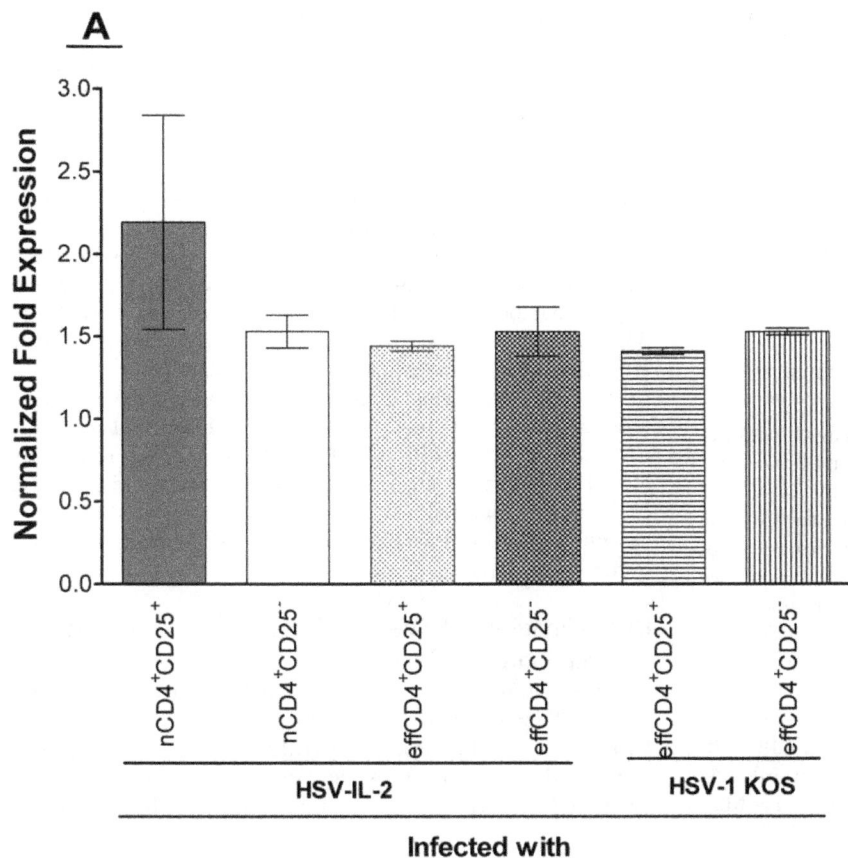

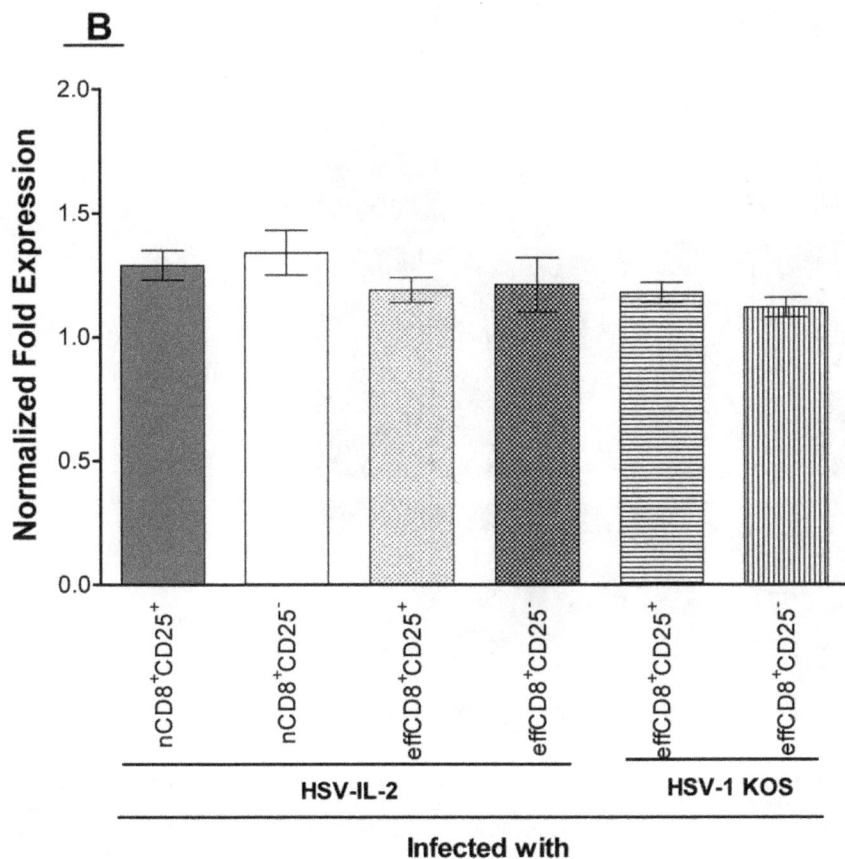

Figure. 5. qRT-PCR analyses of FoxP3 transcript in brain of recipient SCID mice. Total RNA from brains of SCID mice described in Fig. 4 and Table 1 was isolated on day 14 PI. FoxP3 expression in SCID mice infected with the virus and without T cells transfer was used to estimate the relative expression of FoxP3 transcript in brains of each group of recipient SCID mice. GAPDH expression was used to normalize the relative expression of each transcript in brain of each group of mice. Each point represents the mean ± SEM from 3 mice. Panels: A) FoxP3 transcript isolated from SCID mice received CD4[+] T cells; and B) FoxP3 transcript isolated from SCID mice received CD8[+] T cells.

SC, or brain of both knockout and depleted mice was similar to that of wt mice infected with HSV-IL-2 (not shown). These results were consistent with the results obtained in the adoptive transfer studies and confirm that HSV-IL-2-induced demyelination can occur independently of CD25 (IL-2rα).

HSV-IL-2 suppresses IL-12p35 and IL-12p40 transcripts in BM-derived macrophages

As we have detected an exacerbation of CNS demyelination in macrophage-depleted mice following ocular infection of mice with wt HSV-1 (unpublished results), we reasoned that the HSV-IL-2 induced demyelination could be due to suppression of the macrophages and an associated alteration in the expression of IL-12p35 and IL-12p40 transcripts. To test this possibility, we isolated macrophages from BALB/c and C57BL/6 mice and infected them with 10 PFU/cell of HSV-IL-2 or wt HSV-1, or mock infected them as we described previously [26]. Previously, we have shown that macrophages are infected with HSV-1 but the virus does not replicate in the infected cells [26]. The infected or mock-infected macrophages were harvested 12, 24, and 48 h PI, the total RNA was isolated, and IL-12p35 and IL-12p40 mRNAs levels were quantified by qRT-PCR. We performed TaqMan

qRT-PCR on isolated RNA to determine the amount of IL-12p35 and IL-12p40 mRNAs in infected macrophages relative to levels of each transcript in the mock-infected macrophages. Cellular GAPDH mRNA was used as an internal control. Our results suggest that between 12 h and 48 h PI, the levels of IL-12p35 (Fig. 9, BALB/c) and IL-12p40 (Fig. 9, BALB/c) transcripts in the HSV-IL-2 infected macrophages was significantly lower than the levels of these transcripts in the wt HSV-1-infected macrophages. Similar results were observed in macrophages isolated from C57BL/6 mice (Fig. 9, C57BL/6). These results suggest that HSV-IL-2 infection alters the ratio of IL-12p35 and IL-12p40 transcripts in infected macrophages and that this could be a contributing factor in the development of the T-cell autoimmunity in the infected mice.

Demyelination in HSV-IL-2-infected mice can be blocked by injection of IL-12p70 DNA

Our results described above in Figure 9 suggested that HSV-IL-2 induced demyelination may be associated with an imbalance of IL-12p70. Thus, the absence of IL-12 function of macrophages may be the main contributing factor to HSV-IL-2- induced demyelination and the IL-12p70 arm of macrophage responses

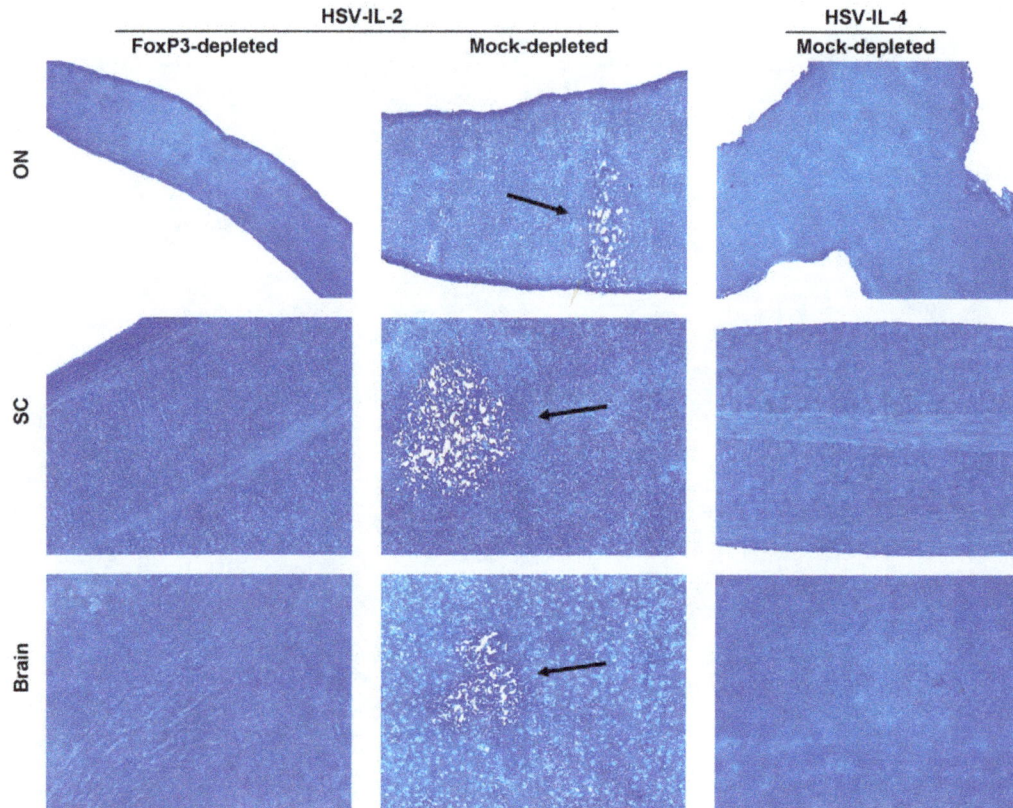

Figure 6. Demyelination in FoxP3^{DTR}-depleted mice. FoxP3^{DTR} mice were infected ocularly with HSV-IL-2 or HSV-IL-4. Seventy-two and 24 hrs prior to infection, and 1, 3, 5, 7, and 9 days PI mice were depleted of their FoxP3 using diphtheria toxin as described previously [69]. After 14 days, ON, SC and brain were removed, sectioned, and stained for LFB. Arrows indicate areas of demyelination in ON, SC, and brains of HSV-IL-2 infected mice.

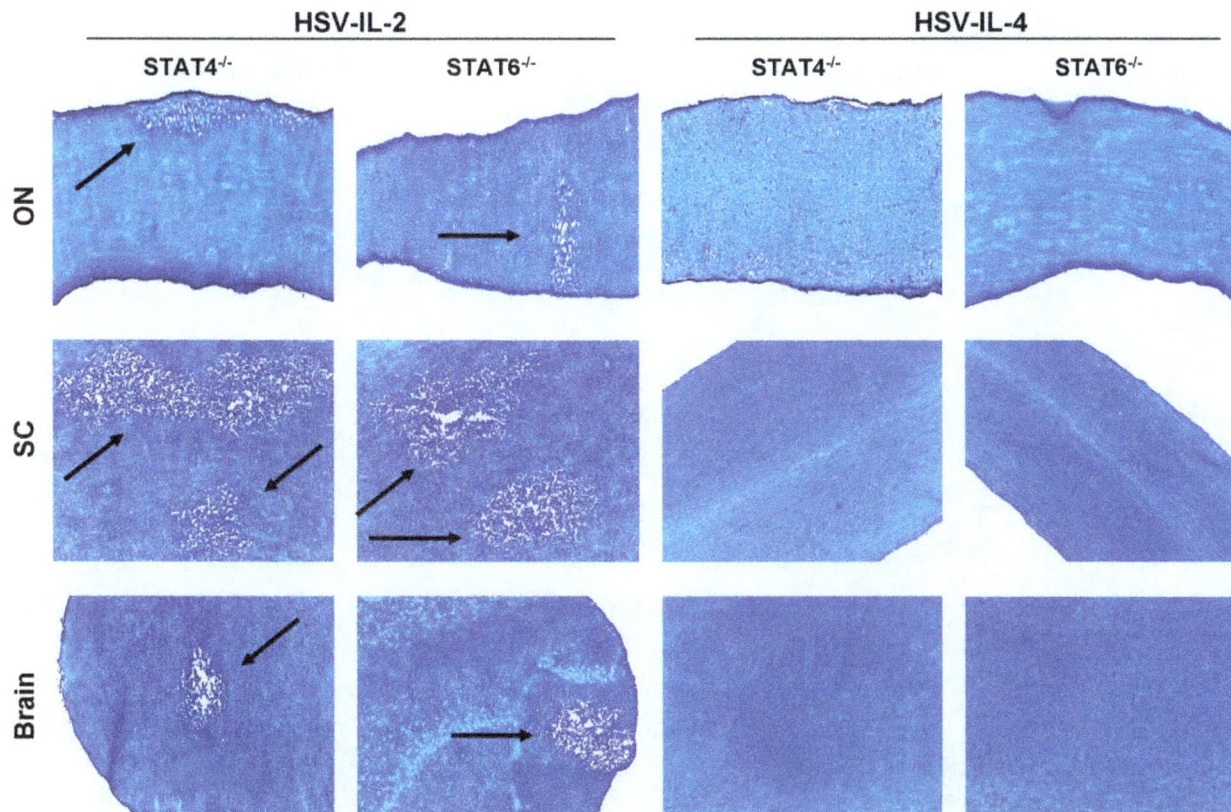

Figure 7. Demyelination in STAT4$^{-/-}$ and STAT6$^{-/-}$ mice. Female STAT4$^{-/-}$ and STAT6$^{-/-}$ mice were infected ocularly with HSV-IL-2 or HSV-IL-4 as described in Materials and Methods. After 14 days, ON, SC, and brains were removed, sectioned, and stained for LFB. Arrows indicate areas of demyelination in ON, SC, and brains of HSV-IL-2 infected mice.

may be essential for prevention of demyelination. To confirm this hypothesis, we looked at the possibility of whether IL-12p70 injection in HSV-IL-2 infected mice may compensate for the imbalance of IL-12p35 and IL-12p40 transcripts and thus prevent demyelination in infected mice. BALB/c mice were immunized with IL-12p70 DNA or vector DNA and infected 4hr later with HSV-IL-2. Demyelination in ON, SC, and brain of infected mice was measured on day 14 PI. Demyelination was not observed in the ON, SC, and brain of BALB/c mice injected with IL-12p70 DNA (Fig. 10, IL-12p70). However, mice injected with vector DNA, displayed demyelination in their ON, SC, and brain (Fig. 10, Vector). Similar result was observed in C57BL/6 mice injected with IL-12p70 DNA and infected with HSV-IL-2 (not shown). However, demyelination was not blocked when mice were injected with IL-23, IL-27, or IL-35 and infected with HSV-IL-2 (not shown). Thus, our results suggest that demyelination in the CNS of the HSV-IL-2 infected mice is due to the downregulation of IL-12p70 expression by the macrophages.

Discussion

In order to mimic the elevation of IL-2 expression that is typical of MS we have used the neurotropic potential of HSV-1 and the unique characteristics of the *LAT* (latency-associated transcript) promoter that is active in most cell types to extend expression of murine IL-2 [13]. This model of MS in which mice are infected with HSV-IL-2 differs from most animal models of MS that are based on either the autoimmune model [27] or the viral model [21] in that this model incorporates both viral and immune aspects

of the disease process. Recently, we reported that this recombinant virus causes CNS demyelination in four different strains of mice and that the demyelination is more severe in female then male mice [18]. A summary of the results obtained here with regards to the mechanism of HSV-IL-2-induced CNS demyelination and blocking CNS demyelination is presented schematically in Figure 11. The results of the present study, in which we used both the BALB/c and C57BL/6 mouse strains, indicate that B-cells, DCs, and NK cells do not play a role in the HSV-IL-2-induced demyelination. In contrast, evidence for involvement of both CD4$^+$ and CD8$^+$ T cells in the HSV-IL-2-induced demyelination was observed using knockout mice, depletion studies and transfer studies. Moreover, we show that the CD8$^+$ T cells played a more significant role in HSV-IL-2 induced demyelination than the CD4$^+$ T cells. These findings are consistent with the published data concerning histologic analyses of specimens obtained from patients with MS at autopsy, which have shown a possible correlation between the presence of CD4$^+$ and CD8$^+$ T cells and the development of demyelinating lesions [19,20]. The results are also consistent with the reports that demyelination induced by mouse hepatitis virus (MHV) is associated with both T cell types [21]. In the EAE model of MS, it was believed originally that only CD4$^+$ T cells were involved in the CNS demyelination [28], but later studies showed that CD8$^+$ T cells can also induce demyelination [19].

We extended the studies to evaluate the role of "naïve" and HSV-IL-2 "effector" T cells in CNS demyelination using SCID mice. Based on their constitutive expression of CD25 (the IL-2rα-chain), T cells can be divided into CD25$^+$ and CD25$^-$

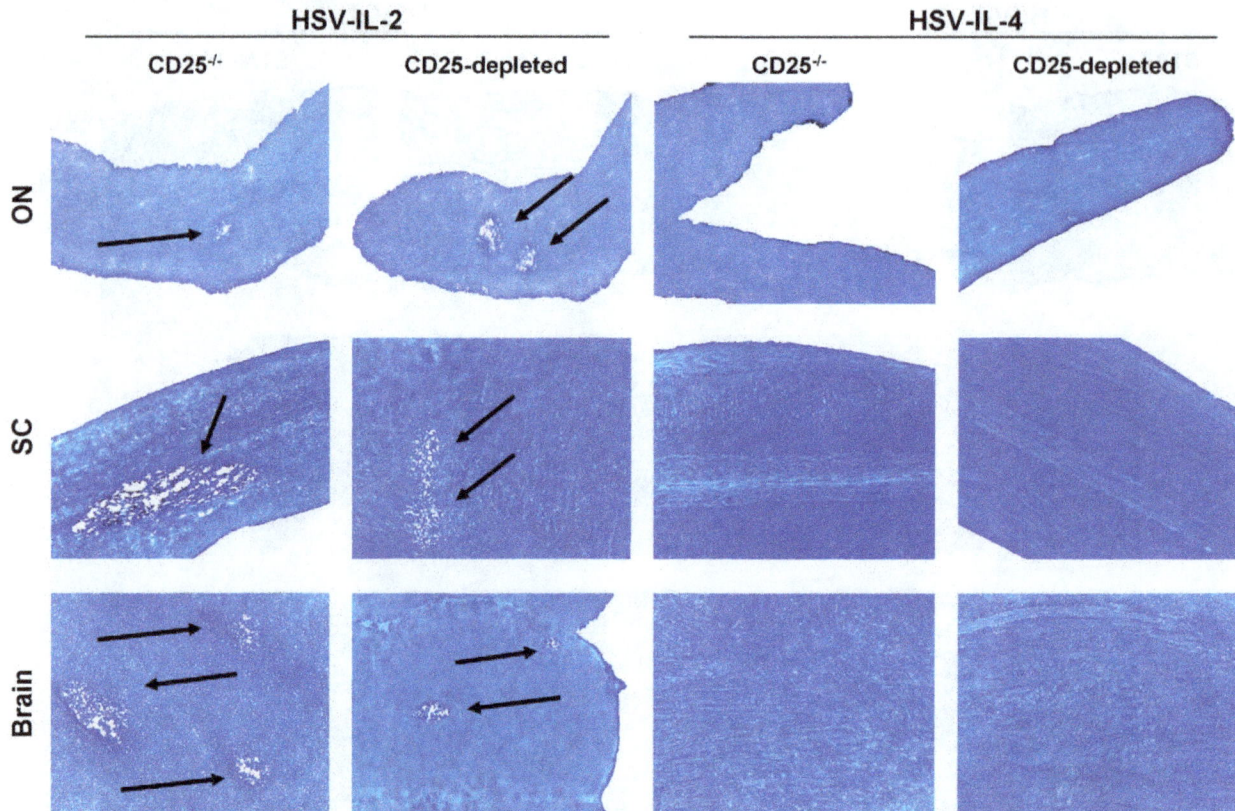

Figure 8. Role of CD25 (IL-2rα) in CNS demyelination. Female C57BL/6 IL-2rα$^{-/-}$ mice were infected ocularly with HSV-IL-2 or HSV-IL-4 as described in Materials and Methods. For CD25 depletion, female C57BL/6 mice were infected ocularly with HSV-IL-2 or HSV-IL-4. Forty-eight hr prior to infection, and 1, 5, and 9 days PI mice were depleted of CD25 population as described in Materials and Methods. After 14 days, ON, SC, and brains were removed, sectioned, and stained for LFB. Arrows indicate areas of demyelination.

subpopulations [29]. Although it has been reported that only CD25$^+$ T cells constitutively express forkhead/winged-helix transcription factor (Foxp3), recent studies have shown that CD25$^-$ T cells also can express FoxP3 [22,30,31]. In the present study, we show that both CD4$^+$ and CD8$^+$ T cells irrespective of their CD25 status express the FoxP3 gene at equal levels. In line with the detection of FoxP3 transcript in brain of recipient SCID mice, our FoxP3 depletion studies suggest that FoxP3 is contributing to CNS demyelination. Our results suggest that T cells, whether they express CD25 or not, contribute to the development of autoimmunity in this model and this could be due to the fact that both the CD25$^+$ and CD25$^-$ cells express similar levels of FoxP3. FoxP3 expression on Teff T cells is transient and its expression in Teff cells is not enough to convert them into Treg, although under repetitive in vitro stimulation this could occur [32]. FoxP3 expression in Teff cells and its maintenance in Treg cells are both dependent on IL-2 [33,34]. Consequently, in the presence of IL-2-expressing HSV-1 T cells irrespective of being regulatory or effector cells all expressing FoxP3 and HSV-IL-2-induced CNS demyelination is dependent on FoxP3. Thus, our result is similar to the results of previous studies that suggest that both CD8$^+$ Treg [35,36,37] and CD4$^+$ Treg [38,39,40,41,42] can cause autoimmunity.

In addition to T cells, macrophages have been implicated in CNS pathology and MS [43,44]; however, they may play only an indirect role. The macrophage plays a variety of roles in the immune defense system, including phagocytosis, tumor cytotoxicity, cytokine secretion and antigen presentation [45,46], as well as

cross-presentation of antigens to naive T cells in vivo [47,48,49]. A number of factors are known to "activate" or engage macrophages in these activities, including viral infection. In this study, we show that HSV-IL-2 infection of macrophages alters the balance of IL-12p35 and IL12p40 transcripts, which theoretically could favor the development of autoreactive T cell in the HSV-IL-2 infected mice. This possibility is supported by our results that showed that injection of mice with IL-12p70 DNA blocked HSV-IL-2-induced demyelination. Similar results were obtained when HSV-IL-2 infected mice were also infected with a recombinant HSV-1 expressing IL-12p70 (not shown). Co-infection of mice with HSV-IL-2 + HSV-IL-12p35, HSV-IL-2 + IL-12p40 alone, or a mixture did not block demyelination (not shown). Similarly injection of IL-12p35 DNA alone, IL-12p40 DNA alone, or a mixture did not block demyelination (not shown). Thus, the in vivo biological activity of IL-12p70 is dependent on the use of a heterodimer. Macrophages are the main source of IL-12 production [50,51]. IL-12 was considered to be a critical cytokine in the pathogenesis of EAE [52] and later studies showed that although the IL-12p40 component of IL-12 is involved in EAE-induced CNS pathology this effect is mediated by the binding of the IL-12p40 to IL-23p19 rather than its binding to IL-12p35 [53,54]. Thus, the imbalance of IL-12p40 and IL-12p35 in the HSV-IL-2 infected mice may be responsible for a shift in T_H1 and T_H2 pattern of cytokine responses as we reported previously [17], and this shift could be responsible for the development of the autoreactive T cells. This would be consistent with our detection of demyelination in both STAT4$^{-/-}$ (no T_H1 response) and STAT6$^{-/-}$ (no T_H2 response)

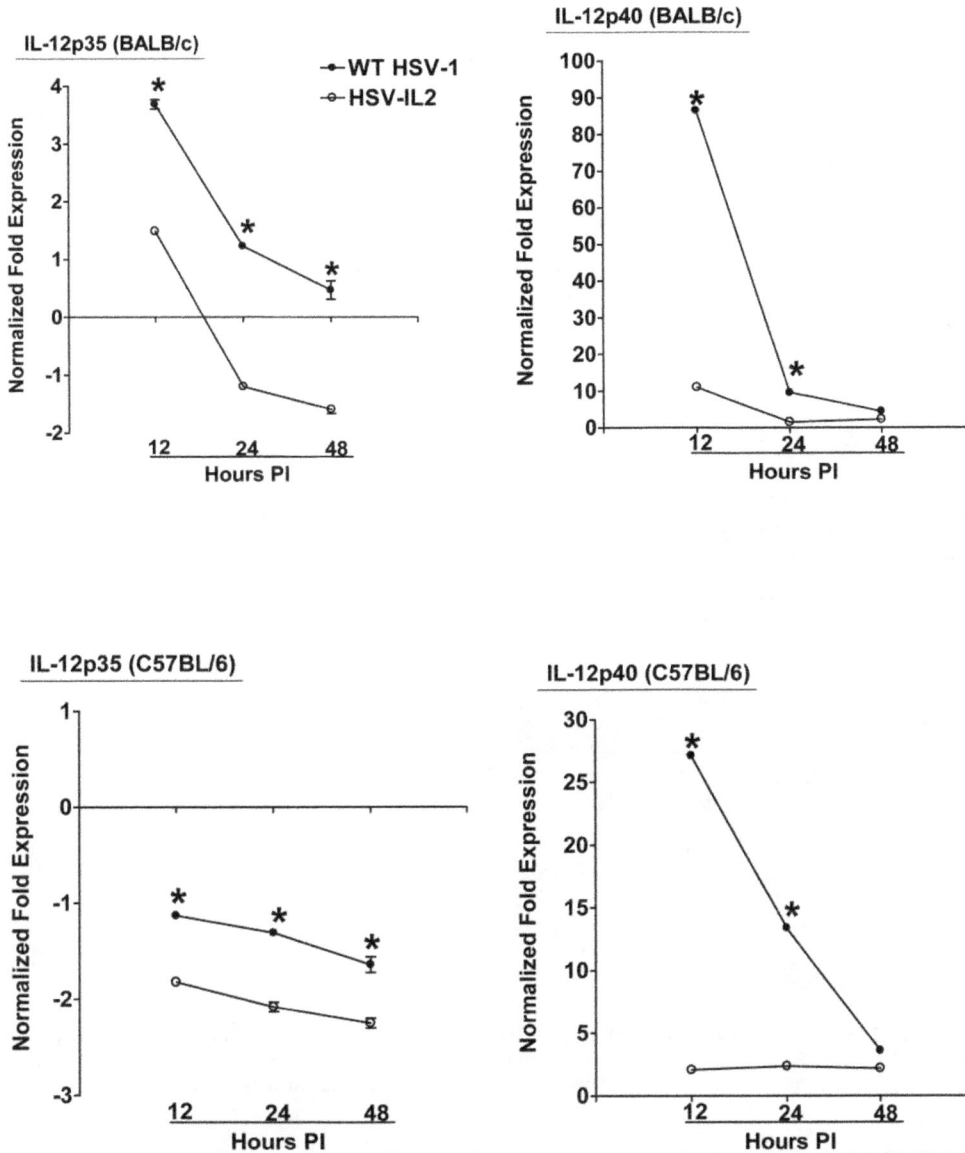

Figure 9. Level of IL-12p35 and IL-12p40 transcripts in macrophages infected with HSV-IL-2. Subconfluent monolayers of macrophages from BALB/c and C57BL/6 mice were infected with 10 PFU/cell of HSV-IL-2 or WT HSV-1. Total RNA was isolated 12, 24, and 48hr PI and TaqMan qRT-PCR was performed using IL-12p35- and IL-12p40-specific primers as described in Materials and Methods. IL-12p35 and IL-12p40 mRNA levels were normalized in comparison to each transcript in mock-infected macrophages. GAPDH was used as internal control. Each point represents the mean ± SEM (n = 6) from two separate experiments.

mice infected with HSV-IL-2 virus. Previously, it was shown that STAT6-deficient mice develop a more severe clinical course of EAE as compared with wild-type or STAT4 knockout mice [55], while it was reported that IL-2-knockout mice developed less demyelination compare with their wt counterparts [12]. Thus, some studies suggest that T_H1 cells are protective while other studies suggest they are pathogenic. These discrepancies could be due to the use of different antigen, mouse strain, or the methods of measurement of autoreactivity.

Previously it was shown that IL-2 was essential for the survival of T regs *in vivo* [56,57], and exogenous administration of IL-2 can boost antigen-specific T cell responses and delay the death of superantigen-reactive T cells [58,59,60]. Furthermore, IL-2/IL-2 mAb complexes also was shown to increase biological activity of preexisting IL-2 leading to expansion of CD8+ T cells as well as

CD4+ T regs in vivo [61]. Our results suggest that constitutive expression of IL-2 by HSV-IL-2 may prolong the survival of autoreactive T cells in addition to enhancing the homing of activated T cells to the CNS. Previously it was shown that nTreg cells suppress IL-2 mRNA transcription and proliferation of CD4+ and CD8+ Teff cells [62]. This could be the reason that in the present study we did not detect CNS demyelination in SCID mice that received nCD4+CD25+ T cells following ocular infection with HSV-IL-2. In MS a functional defect of nTreg cells has been reported [63], despite a frequency of nTrg cells that is similar in patients and in healthy individuals [64]. Similarly to MS, a normal number of nTreg cells but with decreased function had been described in type I diabetes (TID) [65] and in autoimmune polyglandular syndrome type II [66]. In contrast to CD4+ T cell transfer, both naive and effector CD8+ T cells caused CNS

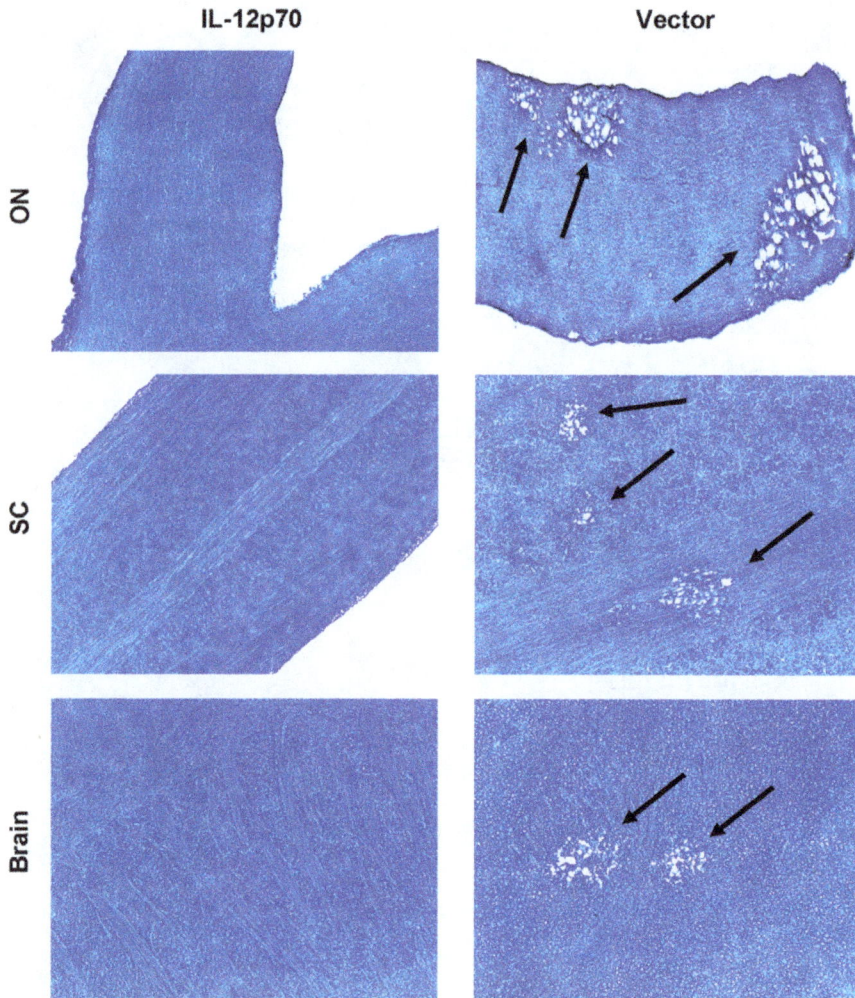

Figure 10. Blocking demyelination in HSV-IL-2 infected mice by IL-12p70 DNA injection. BALB/c mice were injected IM with IL-12p70 DNA or vector DNA as described in Materials and Methods. Four hours after the third DNA injected, mice were infected ocularly with HSV-IL-2. Representative ON, SC and brain sections on day 14 PI from infected mice are shown. The arrows indicate areas of demyelination.

demyelination in HSV-IL-2 infected mice, whereas in KOS-infected mice only effector $CD8^+$ T cells caused demyelination. This is similar to the results of previous studies that suggest that $CD8^+$ Treg cells can cause autoimmunity [35,36,37].

In addition to the expression of the IL-2 increasing T cell survival, we find that it also causes an alteration in the IL-12p70 production by macrophages. This alteration in the IL-12p70 component of the macrophage response and increase in T cell survival in the presence of IL-2 may lead to the development of autoimmune T cells. In line with the inhibitory effects of HSV-IL-2 on IL-12p70 function of macrophages, we have shown that depletion of macrophages also causes CNS demyelination following ocular infection of depleted mice by wild-type HSV-1. Similar to this study, demyelination in macrophage depleted mice can be blocked by IL-12p70 DNA injection (manuscript in preparation). Thus, our results suggest that communication between macrophages and T cells *via* the production of IL-12p70 by the macrophages acts as a critical suppressor of T-cell autoreactivity. This inter-relationship between the macrophages and T cells can be affected by elevated expression of IL-2, which leads to loss of the suppressive effect; however, the inhibitory effects of the IL-2 can be restored by IL-12p70 supplementation.

Materials and Methods

Ethics Statement

All animal care and experimental protocols were conducted in accordance with the regulations of the institutional care and use committee at the Cedars-Sinai Medical center and the NIH *Guide for the Care and Use of Laboratory Animals* (ISBN 0-309-05377-3).

Mice, viruses, and cells

Female BALB/c, BALB/c-STAT4$^{-/-}$, BALB/c-STAT6$^{-/-}$, BALB/c-CD19$^{-/-}$ (B cell-deficient), BALB/c-SCID, C57BL/6, C57BL/6-CD4$^{-/-}$, C57BL/6-CD8$^{-/-}$, and C57BL/6-IL-12r$\alpha^{-/-}$ (CD25-deficient) mice 6-weeks of age were purchased from the Jackson Laboratory (Bar Harbor, ME). Female CD19$^{-/-}$ (B cell-deficient) and hemizygous C.FVB-Tg (Itgax-DTR/GFP) 57Lan/J mice on a BALB/c background were obtained from The Jackson Laboratory, while FoxP3^{DTR} mice in C57BL/6 background were a gift from Alexander Y Rudensky. CD19$^{-/-}$, C.FVB-Tg (Itgax-DTR/GFP) 57Lan/J, and FoxP3^{DTR} mice were bred at Cedars-Sinai Medical Center.

Six-week-old female BALB/c or C57BL/6 (The Jackson Laboratory) mice were used as a source of bone marrow (BM)

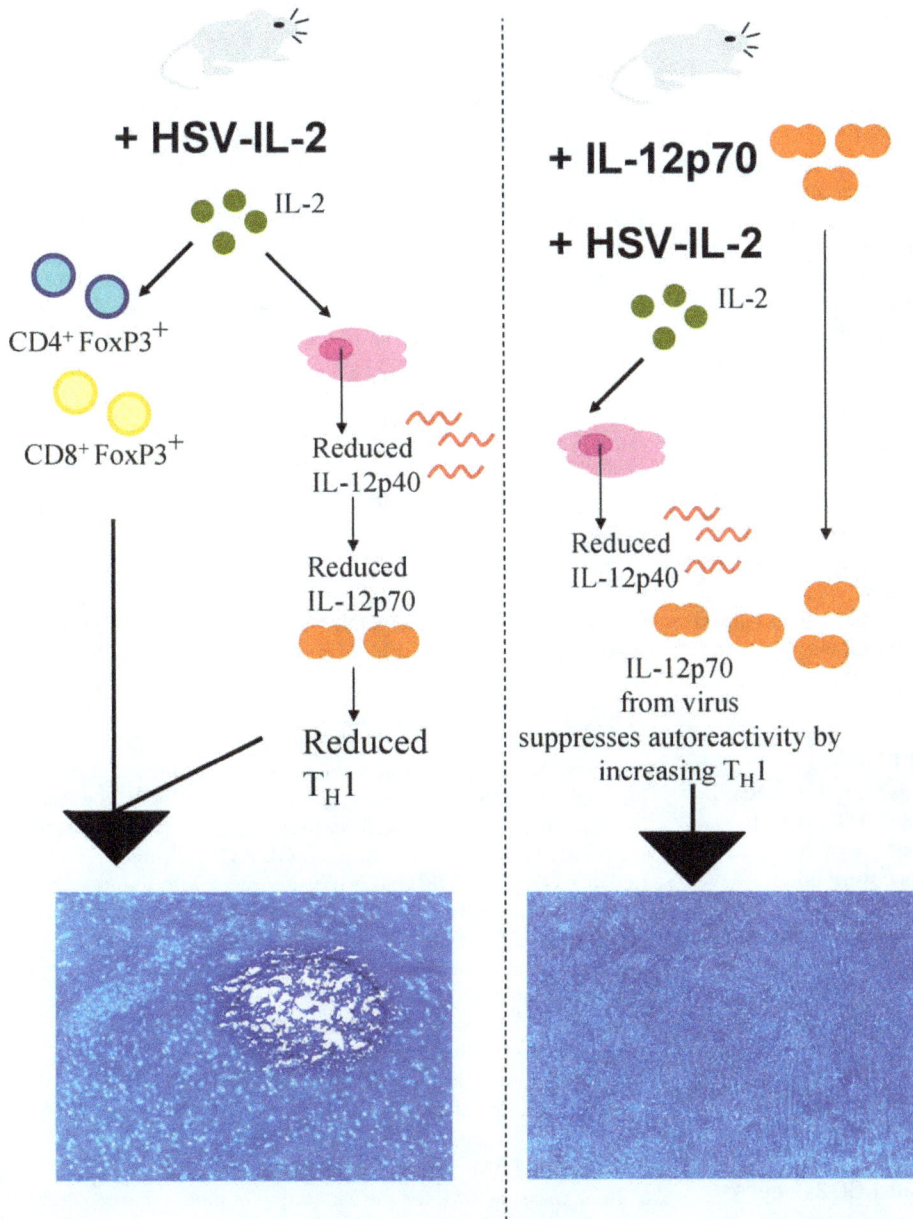

Figure 11. Proposed mechanism for HSV-IL-2 induced CNS demyelination. The cartoon demonstrates that when mice are infected with HSV-IL-2 they develop CNS demyelination but when they are co-infected with HSV-IL-2 and IL-12p70 this demyelination is blocked. We propose that this is caused via the effect of IL-2 on reducing the expression of IL-12p40 in macrophages. Less IL-12p40 means less of the heterodimer IL-12p70 leads to imbalance T_H1 response and favors the production of more autoreactive CD4$^+$FoxP3$^+$ and CD8$^+$ FoxP3$^+$ T cells. Constitutive expression of IL-2 by HSV-IL-2 sustains an active autoreactive CD4$^+$FoxP3$^+$ and CD8$^+$ FoxP3$^+$ populations. The combination of FoxP3$^+$ T cells and reduced T_H1 leads to CNS demyelination (left side). In contrast, co-infection of IL-12p70 with HSV-IL2 compensates for the reduction in IL-12p70 caused by IL-2 leading to functional T_H1 populations and reduced demyelination (right side).

cells that were used to generate macrophages in culture as we described previously [26]. Briefly, BM cells were collected by flushing the femurs with PBS. The cells were pelleted and resuspended briefly in water to lyse red blood cells then stabilized by adding complete medium (RPMI 1640, 10% fetal bovine serum, 100 U/ml penicillin, 100 μg/ml streptomycin, 2 mM L-glutamine). After centrifugation and resuspension in complete medium supplemented with macrophage-colony stimulator factor (M-CSF) (100 ng/ml; Peprotech, NJ), the cells were plated in non-tissue culture plastic Petri dishes (cells from 1 bone per 10 cm dish) and incubated for 5 days at 37°C with CO_2. After 5 days, the media was removed and the adherent cells were recovered by incubating the cells with Versene (Invitrogen, San Diego, CA) for 5 min. at 37°C. The cells were washed, counted, and plated onto tissue-culture dishes for use the following day.

Plaque-purified HSV-1 strains, McKrae (wild type) or KOS and HSV-1 recombinant viruses expressing IL-2 and IL-4 (HSV-IL-2, HSV-IL-4) were grown in rabbit skin (RS) cell monolayers in minimal essential medium (MEM) containing 5% fetal calf serum (FCS), as described previously [13,14,16]. McKrae virus is virulent at an infectious dose of 2×10^5 plaque forming units (PFU)/eye, whereas the KOS, HSV-IL-2, HSV-IL12p70 (M002), and HSV-

IL-4 viruses are attenuated. Previously we have shown that the recombinant HSV-IL-2 is expressing IL-2 at high levels in different tissues [13].

Ocular infection

Mice were infected ocularly with 2×10^5 PFU of McKrae, KOS, recombinant HSV-IL-2, or HSV-IL-4 per eye. Each virus was suspended in 5 μl of tissue culture media and administered as an eye drop. In contrast to mice with the C57BL/6 background that are refractory to McKrae infection, mice with the BALB/c background are highly susceptible to McKrae infection. Thus, mice with BALB/c background were infected with KOS rather then McKrae virus. Corneal scarification was not used.

DNA immunization

The complete open-reading frame (ORF) for IL-12p70 (pORF-mIL12) was purchased from InvivoGen (San Diego, CA). Plasmid DNA was purified using cesium chloride gradient. In each experiment, five mice per group were injected intramuscularly (IM) (into each of the quadriceps) using a 27 gauge needle with 100 μg of cesium chloride-purified DNA in a total volume of 50 μl of PBS 3 times. DNA injections were done 14 days, 7 days, and 4 hrs before ocular infection. As a negative control, we used mock-treated vaccinated mice that were similarly injected with vector DNA alone.

Depletion of dendritic cells (DCs) and FOxP3

Female BALB/c-DTR mice were depleted of their DCs by treatment with 100 ng of diphtheria toxin (DT), which was administered in 100 μl of PBS and injected intraperitoneally as we described previously [67,68]. Briefly, the mice were administered DT 24 h before ocular infection, followed by four additional treatments on days +1, +4, +7, and +10 post infection (PI). FoxP3^{DTR} mice were depleted of their FoxP3 by treatment with DT as described previously [69]. Briefly, the mice were administered DT 72 and 24 h before ocular infection, followed by 5 additional treatments on days +1, +3, +5, +7, and +9 PI. This regimen of treatments reduced each population by more than 97% as confirmed by FACS analysis of spleen cells 24 hours after the second depletion as described previously [69].

Depletion of CD4$^+$ and CD8$^+$ T cells, and CD25$^+$ cells

Each mouse received an intraperitoneal injection of 100 μg of purified GK1.5 (anti-CD4$^+$), or 2.43 (anti-CD8$^+$), or both GK1.5 and 2.43, or PC61.5.3 (anti-CD25) monoclonal antibodies (NCCC, Minneapolis, MN) in 100 μl of PBS, -5 and -2 days before ocular infection. The injections were then repeated on days +1, +4, +7, and +10 relative to ocular infection. Control mice were depleted with an irrelevant mAb of the same isotype. The efficiency of CD4$^+$, CD8$^+$, and CD25$^+$ depletion was monitored by FACS analysis of splenocytes 24 h after the second depletion and before ocular infection. After the second depletion, more than 95% of CD4+ T cells, CD8+ T cells, or CD25+ T cells were depleted from the spleens as we described previously [72]. However, based on our results these residual of T cells did not have any effect on inducing demyelination when both CD4+ and CD8+ T cells were depleted.

Depletion of NK cells with anti-asialo GM1

One mg of rabbit anti-asialo GM$_1$ antibody (Wako Chemicals, Dallas, TX) was dissolved in 1 ml of PBS and each mouse received multiple intraperitoneal injections of 100 μg of antibody in 100 μl of PBS. The first depletion was done -5 days before ocular infection and this was followed by five additional depletions on days −2, +1, +4, +7, and +10 PI as we described previously [70]. After the second depletion, more than 93% of NK cells were depleted from the spleens as we described previously [70]. Control mice were treated with an equal concentration of freeze-dried normal rabbit serum in PBS.

Preparation of ON, SC, and brain for pathologic analysis

The ON, SC, and brain of infected mice were removed at necropsy on day 14 PI. ON, SC, and brain were collected from experimental and control mice, then placed in Tissue-TeK OCT embedding medium (SaKura Fintek, Torrence, CA) and then stored at −80°C. Transverse sections of each tissue, 8-10 μm thick, were cut, air-dried overnight, and fixed in acetone for 3 min at 25°C [71]. Demyelination in each section was confirmed by monitoring adjacent sections.

Analysis of demyelination using Luxol Fast Blue (LFB) staining

The presence or absence of demyelination in ON, SC, and brain of infected mice was evaluated using LFB staining of formalin-fixed sections of ON, SC, and brain as we described previously [17]. Every 4th section of ON, SC, and brain was stained with LFB.

Adoptive transfer of T cells

Donor BALB/c mice that were either mock-infected or ocularly infected with HSV-IL-2 were sacrificed on day 5 PI, the spleens were pooled, and single-cell suspensions prepared as described previously [72]. Naive T cells (i.e., nCD4$^+$CD25$^+$, nCD4$^+$CD25$^-$, nCD8$^+$CD25$^+$, nCD8$^+$CD25$^-$) from mock-infected mice, and effector T cells from HSV-IL-2-infected mice (i.e., effCD4$^+$CD25$^+$, effCD4$^+$CD25$^-$, effCD8$^+$CD25$^+$, effCD8$^+$CD25$^-$) were isolated using magnetic beads as described by the manufacturer (Miltenyi Biotec, Auburn, CA). Each recipient SCID mouse was injected once with 2×10^5 cells in 300 μl of MEM intraperitoneally. The control mice received 300 μl MEM alone. The recipient and control mice were infected ocularly with KOS or HSV-IL-2 virus 4 h after transfer of the cells.

Infection of BM-derived macrophages in vitro

Bone marrow (BM) for the generation of mouse macrophages in cultures were isolated by flushing femurs and tibiae with PBS as we described previously [26]. Monolayers of macrophages isolated from BALB/c or C57BL/6 mice were infected with 10 PFU/cell of HSV-1 strain KOS or HSV-IL-2 or mock-infected. One hour after infection at 37°C, virus was removed and the infected cells were washed three times with fresh media and fresh media was added to each well. The monolayers including media were harvested at 12, 24, and 48 h PI. RNA preparation was done as we described previously [26]. Briefly, frozen cells were resuspended in TRIzol and homogenized, followed by addition of chloroform, and subsequent precipitation using isopropanol. The RNA was then treated with DNase I to degrade any contaminating genomic DNA followed by clean-up using a Qiagen RNeasy column as described in the manufacturer's instructions. The RNA yield from all samples was determined by spectroscopy (NanoDrop ND-1000, NanoDrop Technologies, Inc., Wilmington, Delaware). Finally, 1000 ng of total RNA was reverse-transcribed using random hexamer primers and Murine Leukemia Virus (MuLV) Reverse Transcriptase from the High Capacity cDNA Reverse Transcription Kit (Applied Biosystems, Foster City, CA), in accordance with the manufacturer's recommendations.

TaqMan Real-Time PCR (qRT-PCR)

The expression levels of IL-12p35 and IL-12p40 genes in BM-derived macrophages and expression of CD4, CD8, and FoxP3 in brain of recipient SCID mice were evaluated using commercially available TaqMan Gene Expression Assays (Applied Biosystems, Foster City, CA) with optimized primer and probe concentrations as we described previously [73,74]. Cellular GAPDH gene expression was used as an internal control. Primer-probe sets consisted of two unlabeled PCR primers and the FAM^{TM} dye-labeled TaqMan MGB probe formulated into a single mixture. The primers and probe used were as follows: 1) IL-12p35 (ABI ASSAY I.D. Mm00434165_m1 – Amplicon length = 68 bp); 2) IL-12p40 (ABI ASSAY I.D. Mm 01288992_m1 – Amplcon length = 109 bp); 3) GAPDH (ABI ASSAY I.D. m999999.15_G1 - Amplicon Length = 107 bp); and 4) FoxP3 (ABI ASSAY I.D. Mm00475164_m1 – Amplicon length = 80bp).

Quantitative real-time PCR was performed as we described previously [73]. Real-time PCR was performed in triplicate for each sample from each time point. Relative gene expression levels were normalized to the expression of the GAPDH housekeeping gene (endogenous loading control).

Statistical analysis

Fisher's exact tests were performed using the computer program Instat (GraphPad, San Diego) to compare demyelination in infected mice with the absence of demyelination in control groups. Results were considered statistically significant when the P value was <0.05.

Supporting Information

Figure S1 Severity of CNS demyelination in knockout and depleted mice infected with HSV-IL-2. The entire brain, SC and ON of each of the 5 animals described in Figs. 2 and 3 were sectioned and every 4 slides of each tissues were stained. The numbers of demyelination plaques in the entire sections of ON, SC and brain were counted. Data are presented as percent of sections with plaques per total sections stained (number on each bar graph shows the number of section showing plaques/total stained section). Panels: A) Percent of plaque/section in C57BL/6-CD4$^{-/-}$, C57BL/6-CD8$^{-/-}$, and WT C57BL/6 mice; and B) Percent of plaque/section in CD4-depleted, CD8-depleted, both CD4- and CD8-depleted, and WT mock depleted C57BL/6 mice.

Author Contributions

Conceived and designed the experiments: HG. Performed the experiments: MZ KM. Analyzed the data: SA HG. Contributed reagents/materials/analysis tools: SC MA. Wrote the paper: HG.

References

1. Hafler DA (2004) Multiple sclerosis. J Clin Invest 113: 788–794.
2. Hemmer B, Cepok S, Nessler S, Sommer N (2002) Pathogenesis of multiple sclerosis: an update on immunology. Curr Opin Neurol 15: 227–231.
3. Challoner PB, Smith KT, Parker JD, MacLeod DL, Coulter SN, et al. (1995) Plaque-associated expression of human herpesvirus 6 in multiple sclerosis. Proc Natl Acad Sci U S A 92: 7440–7444.
4. Friedman JE, Lyons MJ, Cu G, Ablashl DV, Whitman JE, et al. (1999) The association of the human herpesvirus-6 and MS. Mult Scler 5: 355–362.
5. Boman J, Roblin PM, Sundstrom P, Sandstrom M, Hammerschlag MR (2000) Failure to detect Chlamydia pneumoniae in the central nervous system of patients with MS. Neurology 54: 265.
6. Martin C, Enbom M, Soderstrom M, Fredrikson S, Dahl H, et al. (1997) Absence of seven human herpesviruses, including HHV-6, by polymerase chain reaction in CSF and blood from patients with multiple sclerosis and optic neuritis. Acta Neurol Scand 95: 280–283.
7. Mirandola P, Stefan A, Brambilla E, Campadelli-Fiume G, Grimaldi LM (1999) Absence of human herpesvirus 6 and 7 from spinal fluid and serum of multiple sclerosis patients. Neurology 53: 1367–1368.
8. Lu CZ, Fredrikson S, Xiao BG, Link H (1993) Interleukin-2 secreting cells in multiple sclerosis and controls. J Neurol Sci 120: 99–106.
9. Gallo P, Piccinno M, Pagni S, Tavolato B (1988) Interleukin-2 levels in serum and cerebrospinal fluid of multiple sclerosis patients. Ann Neurol 24: 795–797.
10. Gallo P, Piccinno MG, Pagni S, Argentiero V, Giometto B, et al. (1989) Immune activation in multiple sclerosis: study of IL-2, sIL-2R, and gamma-IFN levels in serum and cerebrospinal fluid. J Neurol Sci 92: 9–15.
11. Trotter JL, Clifford DB, McInnis JE, Griffeth RC, Bruns KA, et al. (1989) Correlation of immunological studies and disease progression in chronic progressive multiple sclerosis. Ann Neurol 25: 172–178.
12. Petitto JM, Streit WJ, Huang Z, Butfiloski E, Schiffenbauer J (2000) Interleukin-2 gene deletion produces a robust reduction in susceptibility to experimental autoimmune encephalomyelitis in C57BL/6 mice. Neurosci Lett 285: 66–70.
13. Ghiasi H, Osorio Y, Perng GC, Nesburn AB, Wechsler SL (2002) Overexpression of interleukin-2 by a recombinant herpes simplex virus type 1 attenuates pathogenicity and enhances antiviral immunity. J Virol 76: 9069–9078.
14. Ghiasi H, Osorio Y, Hedvat Y, Perng GC, Nesburn AB, et al. (2002) Infection of BALB/c mice with a herpes simplex virus type 1 recombinant virus expressing IFN-g driven by the LAT promoter. Virology 302: 144–154.
15. Osorio Y, Sharifi BG, Perng G, Ghiasi NS, Ghiasi H (2002) The role of T(H)1 and T(H)2 cytokines in HSV-1-induced corneal scarring. Ocular Immunol Inflamm 10: 105–116.
16. Ghiasi H, Osorio Y, Perng GC, Nesburn AB, Wechsler SL (2001) Recombinant herpes simplex virus type 1 expressing murine interleukin-4 is less virulent than wild-type virus in mice. J Virol 75: 9029–9036.
17. Osorio Y, La Point SF, Nusinowitz S, Hofman FM, Ghiasi H (2005) CD8+-dependent CNS demyelination following ocular infection of mice with a recombinant HSV-1 expressing murine IL-2. Exp Neurol 193: 1–18.
18. Zandian M, Belisle R, Mott KR, Nusinowitz S, Hofman FM, et al. (2009) Optic neuritis in different strains of mice by a recombinant HSV-1 expressing murine interleukin-2. Invest Ophthalmol Vis Sci 50: 3275–3282.
19. Steinman L (2001) Myelin-specific CD8 T cells in the pathogenesis of experimental allergic encephalitis and multiple sclerosis. J Exp Med 194: F27–30.
20. Traugott U, Reinherz EL, Raine CS (1983) Multiple sclerosis. Distribution of T cells, T cell subsets and Ia- positive macrophages in lesions of different ages. J Neuroimmunol 4: 201–221.
21. Wu GF, Dandekar AA, Pewe L, Perlman S (2000) CD4 and CD8 T cells have redundant but not identical roles in virus- induced demyelination. J Immunol 165: 2278–2286.
22. Fontenot JD, Rudensky AY (2005) A well adapted regulatory contrivance: regulatory T cell development and the forkhead family transcription factor Foxp3. Nat Immunol 6: 331–337.
23. Fontenot JD, Rasmussen JP, Williams LM, Dooley JL, Farr AG, et al. (2005) Regulatory T cell lineage specification by the forkhead transcription factor foxp3. Immunity 22: 329–341.
24. Nelson BH (2004) IL-2, regulatory T cells, and tolerance. J Immunol 172: 3983–3988.
25. Antony PA, Restifo NP (2005) CD4+CD25+ T regulatory cells, immunotherapy of cancer, and interleukin-2. J Immunother 28: 120–128.
26. Mott KR, Underhill D, Wechsler SL, Town T, Ghiasi H (2009) A role for the JAK-STAT1 pathway in blocking replication of HSV-1 in dendritic cells and macrophages. Virol J 6: 56.
27. Cua DJ, Groux H, Hinton DR, Stohlman SA, Coffman RL (1999) Transgenic interleukin 10 prevents induction of experimental autoimmune encephalomyelitis. J Exp Med 189: 1005–1010.
28. Zamvil S, Nelson P, Trotter J, Mitchell D, Knobler R, et al. (1985) T-cell clones specific for myelin basic protein induce chronic relapsing paralysis and demyelination. Nature 317: 355–358.
29. Maloy KJ, Powrie F (2001) Regulatory T cells in the control of immune pathology. Nat Immunol 2: 816–822.
30. Khattri R, Cox T, Yasayko SA, Ramsdell F (2003) An essential role for Scurfin in CD4+CD25+ T regulatory cells. Nat Immunol 4: 337–342.
31. Nishioka T, Shimizu J, Iida R, Yamazaki S, Sakaguchi S (2006) CD4+CD25+Foxp3+ T cells and CD4+CD25-Foxp3+ T cells in aged mice. J Immunol 176: 6586–6593.
32. Walker MR, Carson BD, Nepom GT, Ziegler SF, Buckner JH (2005) De novo generation of antigen-specific CD4+CD25+ regulatory T cells from human CD4+CD25- cells. Proc Natl Acad Sci U S A 102: 4103–4108.
33. Zorn E, Nelson EA, Mohseni M, Porcheray F, Kim H, et al. (2006) IL-2 regulates FOXP3 expression in human CD4+CD25+ regulatory T cells through a STAT-dependent mechanism and induces the expansion of these cells in vivo. Blood 108: 1571–1579.
34. Wang J, Ioan-Facsinay A, van der Voort EI, Huizinga TW, Toes RE (2007) Transient expression of FOXP3 in human activated nonregulatory CD4+ T cells. Eur J Immunol 37: 129–138.

35. Lin HH, Faunce DE, Stacey M, Terajewicz A, Nakamura T, et al. (2005) The macrophage F4/80 receptor is required for the induction of antigen-specific efferent regulatory T cells in peripheral tolerance. J Exp Med 201: 1615–1625.

36. Chen Y, Inobe J, Weiner HL (1995) Induction of oral tolerance to myelin basic protein in CD8-depleted mice: both CD4+ and CD8+ cells mediate active suppression. J Immunol 155: 910–916.

37. Kohlmann WM, Urban W, Sterry W, Foerster J (2004) Correlation of psoriasis activity with abundance of CD25+CD8+ T cells: conditions for cloning T cells from psoriatic plaques. Exp Dermatol 13: 607–612.

38. Mendez S, Reckling SK, Piccirillo CA, Sacks D, Belkaid Y (2004) Role for CD4(+) CD25(+) regulatory T cells in reactivation of persistent leishmaniasis and control of concomitant immunity. J Exp Med 200: 201–210.

39. Suffia IJ, Reckling SK, Piccirillo CA, Goldszmid RS, Belkaid Y (2006) Infected site-restricted Foxp3+ natural regulatory T cells are specific for microbial antigens. J Exp Med 203: 777–788.

40. Lundgren A, Stromberg E, Sjoling A, Lindholm C, Enarsson K, et al. (2005) Mucosal FOXP3-expressing CD4+ CD25high regulatory T cells in Helicobacter pylori-infected patients. Infect Immun 73: 523–531.

41. Kursar M, Koch M, Mittrucker HW, Nouailles G, Bonhagen K, et al. (2007) Cutting Edge: Regulatory T cells prevent efficient clearance of Mycobacterium tuberculosis. J Immunol 178: 2661–2665.

42. Scott-Browne JP, Shafiani S, Tucker-Heard G, Ishida-Tsubota K, Fontenot JD, et al. (2007) Expansion and function of Foxp3-expressing T regulatory cells during tuberculosis. J Exp Med 204: 2159–2169.

43. Prineas JW, Wright RG (1978) Macrophages, lymphocytes, and plasma cells in the perivascular compartment in chronic multiple sclerosis. Lab Invest 38: 409–421.

44. Tran EH, Hoekstra K, van Rooijen N, Dijkstra CD, Owens T (1998) Immune invasion of the central nervous system parenchyma and experimental allergic encephalomyelitis, but not leukocyte extravasation from blood, are prevented in macrophage-depleted mice. J Immunol 161: 3767–3775.

45. Young HA, Hardy KJ (1995) Role of interferon-gamma in immune cell regulation. J Leukoc Biol 58: 373–381.

46. Peters JH, Gieseler R, Thiele B, Steinbach F (1996) Dendritic cells: from ontogenetic orphans to myelomonocytic descendants. Immunol Today 17: 273–278.

47. Pozzi LA, Maciaszek JW, Rock KL (2005) Both dendritic cells and macrophages can stimulate naive CD8 T cells in vivo to proliferate, develop effector function, and differentiate into memory cells. J Immunol 175: 2071–2081.

48. Ramirez MC, Sigal LJ (2004) The multiple routes of MHC-I cross-presentation. Trends Microbiol 12: 204–207.

49. Ramirez MC, Sigal LJ (2002) Macrophages and dendritic cells use the cytosolic pathway to rapidly cross-present antigen from live, vaccinia-infected cells. J Immunol 169: 6733–6742.

50. D'Andrea A, Rengaraju M, Valiante NM, Chehimi J, Kubin M, et al. (1992) Production of natural killer cell stimulatory factor (interleukin 12) by peripheral blood mononuclear cells. J Exp Med 176: 1387–1398.

51. Schwarz T (1995) Interleukin-12 and its role in cutaneous sensitization. Res Immunol 146: 494–499.

52. Karp CL, van Boxel-Dezaire AH, Byrnes AA, Nagelkerken L (2001) Interferon-beta in multiple sclerosis: altering the balance of interleukin-12 and interleukin-10? Curr Opin Neurol 14: 361–368.

53. Gran B, Zhang GX, Yu S, Li J, Chen XH, et al. (2002) IL-12p35-Deficient Mice Are Susceptible to Experimental Autoimmune Encephalomyelitis: Evidence for Redundancy in the IL-12 System in the Induction of Central Nervous System Autoimmune Demyelination. J Immunol 169: 7104–7110.

54. Cua DJ, Sherlock J, Chen Y, Murphy CA, Joyce B, et al. (2003) Interleukin-23 rather than interleukin-12 is the critical cytokine for autoimmune inflammation of the brain. Nature 421: 744–748.

55. Chitnis T, Najafian N, Benou C, Salama AD, Grusby MJ, et al. (2001) Effect of targeted disruption of STAT4 and STAT6 on the induction of experimental autoimmune encephalomyelitis. J Clin Invest 108: 739–747.

56. Webster KE, Walters S, Kohler RE, Mrkvan T, Boyman O, et al. (2009) In vivo expansion of T reg cells with IL-2-mAb complexes: induction of resistance to EAE and long-term acceptance of islet allografts without immunosuppression. J Exp Med 206: 751–760.

57. D'Cruz LM, Klein L (2005) Development and function of agonist-induced CD25+Foxp3+ regulatory T cells in the absence of interleukin 2 signaling. Nat Immunol 6: 1152–1159.

58. Kuroda K, Yagi J, Imanishi K, Yan XJ, Li XY, et al. (1996) Implantation of IL-2-containing osmotic pump prolongs the survival of superantigen-reactive T cells expanded in mice injected with bacterial superantigen. J Immunol 157: 1422–1431.

59. Kang BY, Lim YS, Chung SW, Kim EJ, Kim SH, et al. (1999) Antigen-specific cytotoxicity and cell number of adoptively transferred T cells are efficiently maintained in vivo by re-stimulation with an antigen/interleukin-2 fusion protein. Int J Cancer 82: 569–573.

60. Blattman JN, Grayson JM, Wherry EJ, Kaech SM, Smith KA, et al. (2003) Therapeutic use of IL-2 to enhance antiviral T-cell responses in vivo. Nat Med 9: 540–547.

61. Boyman O, Surh CD, Sprent J (2006) Potential use of IL-2/anti-IL-2 antibody immune complexes for the treatment of cancer and autoimmune disease. Expert Opin Biol Ther 6: 1323–1331.

62. Bacchetta R, Gambineri E, Roncarolo MG (2007) Role of regulatory T cells and FOXP3 in human diseases. J Allergy Clin Immunol 120: 227–235.

63. Viglietta V, Baecher-Allan C, Weiner HL, Hafler DA (2004) Loss of functional suppression by CD4+CD25+ regulatory T cells in patients with multiple sclerosis. J Exp Med 199: 971–979.

64. Putheti P, Pettersson A, Soderstrom M, Link H, Huang YM (2004) Circulating CD4+CD25+ T regulatory cells are not altered in multiple sclerosis and unaffected by disease-modulating drugs. J Clin Immunol 24: 155–161.

65. Battaglia M, Stabilini A, Migliavacca B, Horejs-Hoeck J, Kaupper T, et al. (2006) Rapamycin promotes expansion of functional CD4+CD25+FOXP3+ regulatory T cells of both healthy subjects and type 1 diabetic patients. J Immunol 177: 8338–8347.

66. Kriegel MA, Lohmann T, Gabler C, Blank N, Kalden JR, et al. (2004) Defective suppressor function of human CD4+ CD25+ regulatory T cells in autoimmune polyglandular syndrome type II. J Exp Med 199: 1285–1291.

67. Mott KR, Ghiasi H (2008) Role of dendritic cells in enhancement of herpes simplex virus type 1 latency and reactivation in vaccinated mice. Clin Vaccine Immunol 15: 1859–1867.

68. Mott KR, UnderHill D, Wechsler SL, Ghiasi H (2008) Lymphoid-related CD11c+CD8a+ dendritic cells are involved in enhancing HSV-1 latency. J Virol 82: 9870–9879.

69. Kim JM, Rasmussen JP, Rudensky AY (2007) Regulatory T cells prevent catastrophic autoimmunity throughout the lifespan of mice. Nat Immunol 8: 191–197.

70. Ghiasi H, Cai S, Perng GC, Nesburn AB, Wechsler SL (2000) The role of natural killer cells in protection of mice against death and corneal scarring following ocular HSV-1 infection. Antiviral Res 45: 33–45.

71. Ghiasi H, Wechsler SL, Kaiwar R, Nesburn AB, Hofman FM (1995) Local expression of tumor necrosis factor alpha and interleukin-2 correlates with protection against corneal scarring after ocular challenge of vaccinated mice with herpes simplex virus type 1. J Virol 69: 334–340.

72. Ahmed R, King CC, Oldstone MB (1987) Virus-lymphocyte interaction: T cells of the helper subset are infected with lymphocytic choriomeningitis virus during persistent infection in vivo. J Virol 61: 1571–1576.

73. Mott KR, Osorio Y, Brown DJ, Morishige N, Wahlert A, et al. (2007) The corneas of naive mice contain both CD4+ and CD8+ T cells. Mol Vis 13: 1802–1812.

74. Mott KR, Perng GC, Osorio Y, Kousoulas KG, Ghiasi H (2007) A recombinant herpes simplex virus type 1 expressing two additional copies of gK is more pathogenic than wild-type virus in two different strains of mice. J Virol 81: 12962–12972.

2

Effect of the H1N1 Influenza Pandemic on the Incidence of Epidemic Keratoconjunctivitis and on Hygiene Behavior

Hyun Su Kim[1], Ho Chun Choi[1], Belong Cho[1]*, Joon Yong Lee[2], Min Jeong Kwon[3]

1 Department of Family Medicine, Seoul National University Hospital, Seoul, Republic of Korea, **2** Department of Family Medicine, Korea University Guro Hospital, Seoul, Republic of Korea, **3** Division of Infectious Disease Surveillance, Korea Centers for Disease Control and Prevention, Chungcheongbuk-Do, Republic of Korea

Abstract

Background: EKC is transmitted chiefly by direct hand contact. It is suspected that the 2009/2010 influenza pandemic influenced hand washing. This study aims to examine the relationship between the 2009/2010 H1N1 influenza pandemic and hygiene behavior.

Methods: We compared the EKC prevalence trends before, during and after the 2009/2010 influenza pandemic by using a t-test comparison of EKC sentinel surveillance.

Results: During the pre-pandemic period, the incidence of EKC increased from the 21st to the 44th week each year. However, during the pandemic period in 2009, there was no epidemic peak. In the post-pandemic period, the epidemic curve was similar to that in the pre-pandemic period. Compared to the pre-pandemic period, the total number of EKC patients during the pandemic period showed a decrease of 44.9% (t value = −7.23, p = 0.002). Comparing the pre-pandemic and pandemic periods by age group, we found there to be a significant decrease in the number of EKC patients for all age groups (−4.12 ≤ t value ≤ −7.23, all P<0.05). This finding was most evident in the teenage group (62%) compared to the other age groups (decreases of 29 to 44%).

Conclusions: A continuing effort should be made to educate the public on basic infection prevention behaviors in the aftermath of the pandemic, particularly to teenagers.

Editor: Abdisalan Mohamed Noor, Kenya Medical Research Institute - Wellcome Trust Research Programme, Kenya

Funding: These authors have no support or funding to report.

Competing Interests: The authors have declared that no competing interests exist.

* E-mail: Belong@snu.ac.kr

Introduction

While the World Health Organization (WHO) declared on August 10, 2010 that the influenza A (H1N1) pandemic was over, the Korean Government had already changed the National Infectious Disease Crisis Level to its lowest grading on April 1, 2010 [1,2]. In Korea, from the time the first case of influenza A was confirmed on May 3, 2009, until late January, 2010, a total of 740,835 patients were confirmed, with 225 of these reported to have died [3]. During the pandemic in Korea, before an effective vaccine was made available, mitigation strategies were aimed at identifying, isolating and treating individual patients, in addition to educating the public about preventive behaviors that could reduce the spread of infection. These messages emphasized covering the mouth and nose when coughing and sneezing, washing hands frequently with soap and water, and avoiding crowded places [4].

It is suspected that the 2009/2010 influenza pandemic influenced hygiene-related behavior such as hand washing. However, previous studies were mainly interested in the association between these behaviors and disease anxiety, flu severity, information reliability and effectiveness of control measures [5–11]. While some studies show that these behaviors can be improved transiently [11–14], we

have little information on how long these improved behaviors will continue or what kind of groups could be most motivated.

Among the various infectious diseases, we considered those that can be transmitted by direct hand contact. As a result, EKC was selected for evaluation. This condition is transmitted chiefly by direct hand contact rather than other pathways, and cannot be prevented by vaccination [15–18]. In the present study, we assessed the effect of the 2009/2010 influenza pandemic on these behaviors by analyzing the incidence of this disease before, during and after the influenza pandemic.

Methods

We analyzed the EKC data of the Korean National Infectious Disease Surveillance System. The system in place to report EKC cases was not affected by the 2009 pandemic season because ophthalmology clinics were not busy managing patients who were infected with influenza. In addition, there were sufficient cases of EKC for analysis.

The sentinel surveillance of EKC is supported by the Korean Ophthalmologists Association and Korean Ophthalmological Society. 80 private ophthalmological clinics voluntarily report

Table 1. EKC[*] cases reported from 2004 to 2010 according to age group.

	Number of EKC cases						
	2004	2005	2006	2007	2008	2009	2010
0–9yr	10,329	9,937	9,422	10,101	6,997	5,558	12,689
10–19yr	12,379	10,678	14,871	19,242	13,365	5,406	13,435
20–29yr	7,725	6,700	6,702	6,503	4,420	3,792	6,407
30–39yr	10,601	9,873	9,452	9,051	6,066	5,109	9,492
40–49yr	6,597	6,424	7,017	7,300	4,695	3,720	7,184
50–59yr	4,701	4,830	4,701	4,854	3,522	3,225	6,144
60yr or more	4,950	5,687	5,282	5,424	3,471	3,349	6,494
All ages	57,282	54,129	57,447	62,475	42,222	30,159	61,845

*Epidemic keratoconjunctivitis.

cases of patients with EKC on a weekly basis. We used the diagnostic criteria for EKC that were defined for the National Infectious Disease Surveillance. The criteria has been defined as a clinically compatible illness that was observed to have subcorneal opacity or one of several symptoms such as excessive tearing, soreness, eyelid swelling and preauricular lymphadenopathy with tenderness as observed by an ophthalmologist.

Based on the Korean National Disaster Level and Influenza-Like Illness surveillance, the study period was divided into three phases: 2004–2008 as 'pre-pandemic,' 2009 as 'pandemic,' and 2010 as 'post-pandemic' [4]. According to this classification, we assessed the change in the weekly number of EKC cases for each of the three phases. For the pre-pandemic period we estimated the mean weekly number of cases (and 95% confidence interval) of EKC reported. After separating the total number of EKC cases into the epidemic season (weeks 21 to 44) and non-epidemic season (week 0 to 20 and 45 to 52), we investigated whether there was significant variation among the pre-pandemic, pandemic and post-pandemic periods for each season. For assessing the decrease of EKC patients during influenza pandemic, we performed t-test between mean of total EKC numbers in pre-pandemic period and those in pandemic period. As the same way, we assessed the increase of EKC patients after influenza pandemic by using a t-test between pre-pandemic and post-pandemic period. These tests were performed on the assumption that annual EKC epidemic is independent each other. Patients were grouped into ten year age

Table 2. Comparison of EKC patients among pre-pandemic, pandemic and post-pandemic periods.

Age	Weeks[*]	Periods[†]			t-value of t-test between pre-pandemic & pandemic[‡]	t-value of t-test between pre & post-pandemic[‡]
		Pre-pandemic cases mean [CI]	Pandemic cases	Post-pandemic cases		
Total age	Total	54711 [45282–64140]	30159	61845	t value = −7.23 (p = 0.002)	t value = 2.10 (p = 0.104)
	Epidemic	36608 [27092–46124]	17188	43095	t value = −5.67 (p = 0.005)	t value = 1.89 (p = 0.131)
	Non-epidemic	18103 [15415–20791]	12971	18750	t value = −5.30 (p = 0.006)	t value = 0.67 (p = 0.541)
0–9yr	Total	9357 [7667–11047]	5558	12689	t value = −6.24 (p = 0.003)	t value = 5.47 (p = 0.005)
	Epidemic	6223 [4859–7588]	3243	9173	t value = −6.06 (p = 0.004)	t value = 6.02 (p = 0.004)
	Non-epidemic	3134 [2590–3678]	2315	3516	t value = −4.18 (p = 0.014)	t value = 1.95 (p = 0.123)
10–19yr	Total	14107 [10072–18142]	5406	13435	t value = −5.99 (p = 0.004)	t value = −0.46 (p = 0.668)
	Epidemic	10943 [6425–15461]	3426	9869	t value = −4.62 (p = 0.010)	t value = −0.66 (p = 0.545)
	Non-epidemic	3164 [2528–3800]	1980	3566	t value = −5.17 (p = 0.007)	t value = 1.75 (p = 0.154)
20–29yr	Total	6410 [4906–7914]	3792	6407	t value = −4.83 (p = 0.008)	t value = −0.01 (p = 0.996)
	Epidemic	4071 [2950–5192]	2194	4516	t value = −4.65 (p = 0.010)	t value = 1.10 (p = 0.332)
	Non-epidemic	2339 [1827–2852]	1598	1891	t value = −4.02 (p = 0.016)	t value = −2.43 (p = 0.072)
30–39yr	Total	9009 [6845–11172]	5109	9492	t value = −5.01 (p = 0.008)	t value = 0.62 (p = 0.569)
	Epidemic	5590 [4073–7107]	2854	6627	t value = −5.01 (p = 0.007)	t value = 1.90 (p = 0.131)
	Non-epidemic	3419 [2609–4229]	2255	2865	t value = −3.99 (p = 0.016)	t value = −1.90 (p = 0.131)
40–49yr	Total	6407 [5144–7669]	3720	7184	t value = −5.91 (p = 0.004)	t value = 1.71 (p = 0.163)
	Epidemic	4035 [2749–5322]	1969	4792	t value = −4.46 (p = 0.011)	t value = 1.63 (p = 0.178)
	Non-epidemic	2371 [2004–2738]	1751	2392	t value = −4.69 (p = 0.009)	t value = 0.16 (p = 0.883)
50–59yr	Total	4522 [3822–5221]	3225	6144	t value = −5.15 (p = 0.007)	t value = 6.44 (p = 0.003)
	Epidemic	2694 [2042–3346]	1671	3897	t value = −4.36 (p = 0.012)	t value = 5.12 (p = 0.007)
	Non-epidemic	1827 [1585–2071]	1554	2247	t value = −3.11 (p = 0.036)	t value = 4.79 (p = 0.009)
≥60yr	Total	4963 [3876–6050]	3349	6494	t value = −4.12 (p = 0.015)	t value = 3.91 (p = 0.174)
	Epidemic	3115 [2220–4009]	1831	4221	t value = −3.98 (p = 0.016)	t value = 3.43 (p = 0.026)
	Non-epidemic	1848 [1608–2088]	1518	2273	t value = −3.82 (p = 0.019)	t value = 4.92 (p = 0.008)

*Total, epidemic, and non-epidemic seasons are weeks 1 to 52, weeks 21 to 44, and weeks 1 to 20 and 45 to 52, respectively.
†Pre-pandemic mean cases from 2004 to 2008, Pandemic cases in 2009, Post-pandemic cases in 2010.
‡Degrees of freedom of all values = 4.

brackets, and analyses carried out with a view to identifying those age groups exhibiting the greatest overall change. All analyses were carried out with the use of STATA 10.0.

Results

The number of reported EKC cases from 2004 to 2010 is shown in Table 1. The mean number of total EKC patients during the pre-pandemic period was 54,711 (95% Confidence Interval [CI],

45,499 to 64,344). By comparison with pre-pandemic period, the total number of EKC patients during pandemic period showed a significant decrease of 44.9% (t value = −7.23, p = 0.002) and those during the post-pandemic period increased to 113.0% (t value = 2.10, p = 0.104) (Table 2).

With respect to changes in the weekly EKC incidence, while an increase was observed from the 21st through to the 44th week (epidemic season) during both the pre- and post-pandemic periods, there was no epidemic peak during the pandemic period (Figure 1).

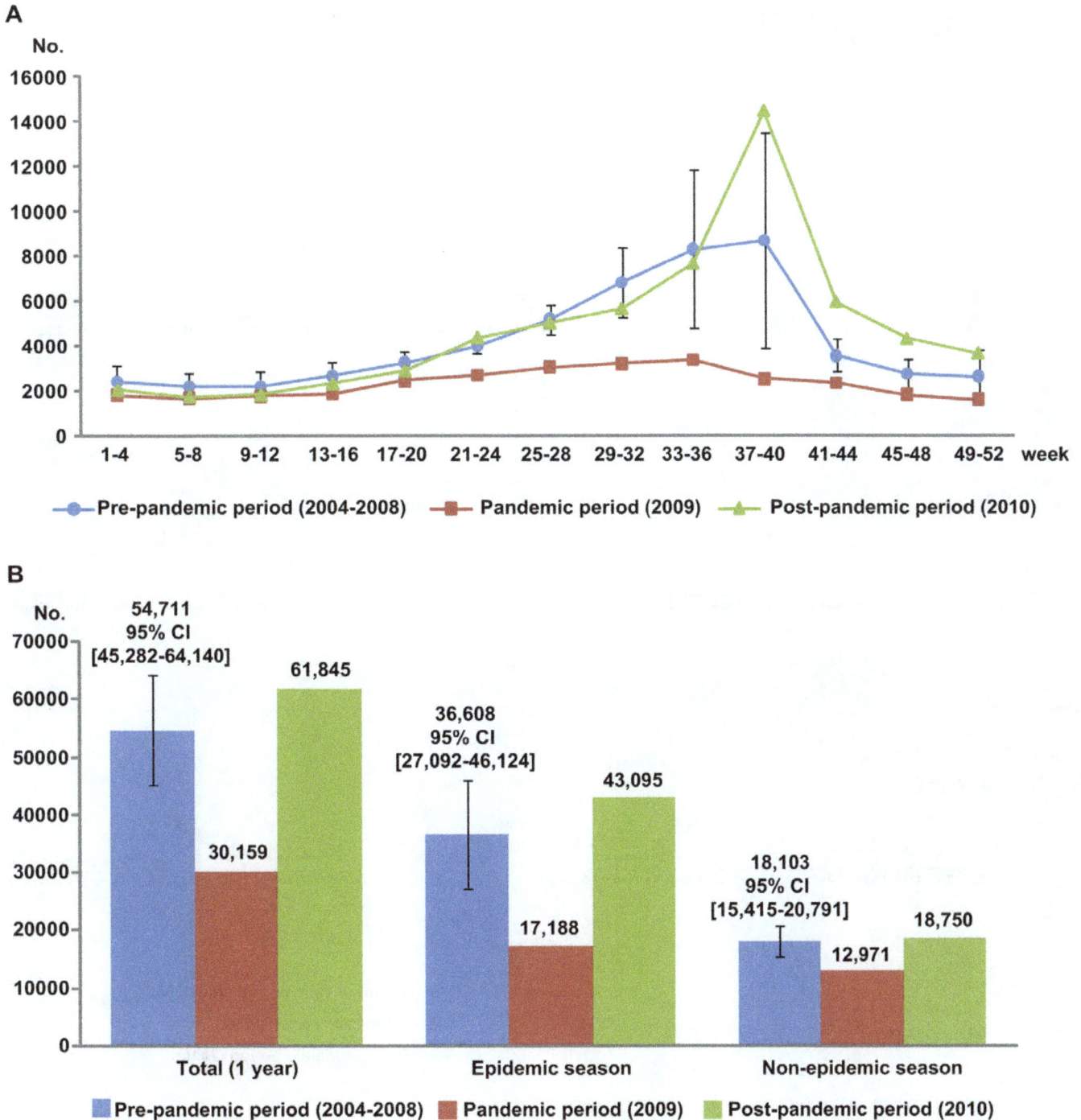

A

B

Figure 1. Comparison of the EKC incidence among pre-pandemic, pandemic and post-pandemic periods. A. Trends of the number of patients on a monthly basis. B. EKC incidence according to total, epidemic and non-epidemic season.

In addition, there was also a significant decrease in the number of EKC patients during pandemic period in both the epidemic (t value = −5.67, p = 0.005) and non-epidemic seasons (t value = −5.30, p = 0.006) compared to the pre-pandemic period (Table 2). Moreover this result was more prominent in the epidemic season (from 36,608 to 17,188, 53.0% decrease) than in the non-epidemic season (from 18,103 to 12,971, 28.3% decrease).

Comparing the pre-pandemic and pandemic periods by age group, we found there to be a significant decrease in the number of EKC patients for all age groups (Figure 2, Table 2). This finding was most evident in the teenage group (decreased of 62%) compared to the other age groups (decreases of 29 to 44%)

Discussion

This study attempted to evaluate the effect of the H1N1pandemic influenza on the incidence of epidemic keratoconjunctivitis (EKC) and hygiene behavior in Korea. Although we did not carry out a questionnaire-based study to investigate whether the public complied with recommended hygiene behavior such as hand washing, we utilized the incidence of EKC as an indirect indicator of hand washing on the assumption that hand washing is one of the most effective ways to prevent EKC infection [15–18].

Regarding the absence of an EKC epidemic peak during the pandemic period, it is assumed that the influenza pandemic helped

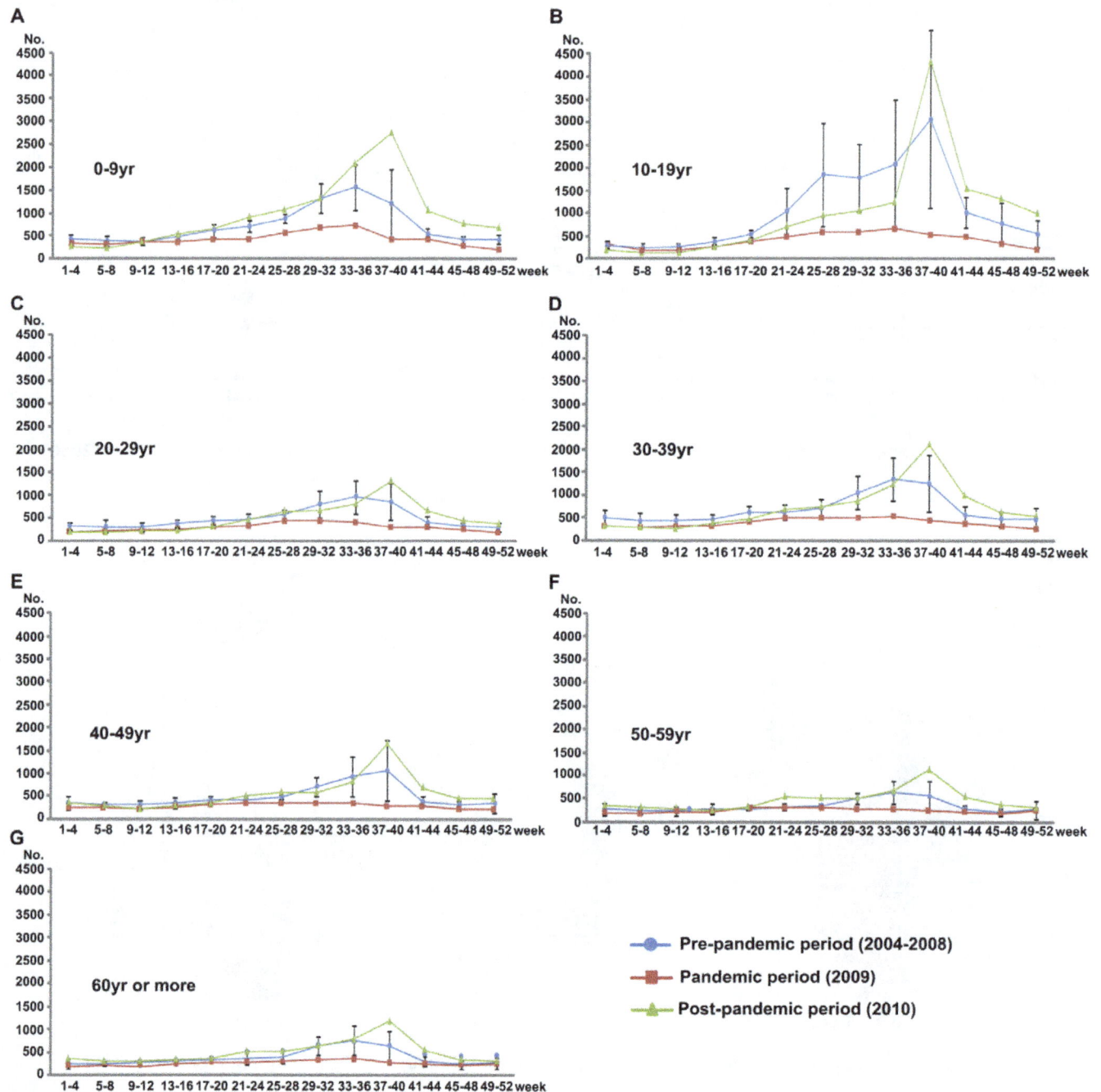

Figure 2. EKC cases among pre-pandemic, pandemic and post-pandemic periods according to age group.

to reinforce preventive behavior. This result is supported by data from a cross-sectional web-based survey of 75,000 Korean middle and high school students which reported on the percentage of students performing frequent hand washing with soap before a meal and after using the toilet; values increased dramatically to 56.5% and 72.3% respectively in October 2009 (peak pandemic season) compared to 32.8% and 47.9% in October 2008 (pre-pandemic season) [19]. However, considering that the number of EKC patients increased again just after the pandemic period, we postulate that the positive hygiene effect was maintained only during the pandemic period. These results are consistent with data suggesting that preventive behavior declined as the frequency of reports of influenza-related deaths or the intensity of influenza spread also declined [11,14].

In addition, the number of EKC patients during the pandemic period compared to the pre-pandemic period was significantly reduced in the teenage group. The reason for this is that wide publicity and education encouraging preventive behavior may have been more effective in this age group. We recommend that health authorities may need to intensify and sustain hygiene messages to the public throughout a pandemic, especially with respect to teenagers because their incidence of EKC is returned to its high levels in the post-epidemic period.

As the influenza virus is known to compete with other respiratory viruses, the influenza pandemic could have suppressed an adenovirus epidemic, this being the main cause of EKC. However, the typical epidemic season for EKC is different from that for influenza. In North East Asia, while influenza activity tends to peak in winter or spring, seasonal epidemics of adenoviral conjunctivitis occur in the summer in association with higher temperatures and humidity [20,21]. Therefore, an adenovirus epidemic would not have been influenced by the pandemic influenza.

We have demonstrated an association between pandemic influenza and hygiene behavior by analyzing the incidence of another infectious disease (EKC) over several years.

Our study has several limitations. First, because it had a cross-sectional design format, we cannot definitively infer a causal relationship between the increase of hand washing and the decrease of EKC. Second, the diagnosis of EKC is based on clinical symptoms, so it is possible that some forms of non-infectious conjunctivitis which are not related to hand washing, such as allergic conjunctivitis, were included in our data. However, such cases would only contribute to a very small proportion of the total number of cases of EKC. The reason for this is that epidemic season of EKC is different from that of allergic conjunctivitis and EKC has more severe symptoms that could discriminate from allergic conjunctivitis. Lastly, given the lack of specific sociodemographic informations such as sex and detailed age, we couldn't analyze the epidemic trends according to those.

In conclusion, we postulate that hygiene behaviors improved during the pandemic period, which lead to a reduction in the number of EKC cases during this period. However, this behavioral change did not persist into the post-pandemic period in Korea. This relationship was most marked in teenagers. WHO and Public Health Service of governments should do to sustain hygiene behaviors in the post-pandemic period.

Acknowledgments

We acknowledge 80 private ophthalmology clinics which have participated in the Sentinel Surveillance of epidemic keratoconjunctivitis.

Author Contributions

Conceived and designed the experiments: HSK HCC. Performed the experiments: HSK HCC BC JYL MJK. Analyzed the data: HSK HCC BC JYL MJK. Contributed reagents/materials/analysis tools: HSK HCC BC. Wrote the paper: HSK HCC.

References

1. World Health Organization (2010) H1N1 in post-pandemic period. Available: www.who.int/mediacentre/news/statements/2010/h1n1_vpc_20100810/en/index.html. Accessed 23 January 2011.
2. Korea Centers for Disease Control and Prevention (2010) Pandemic alert status downgraded to "interest (Blue)". Available: www.cdc.go.kr/flu/WebContent. Accessed 23 January 2011.
3. Kim JH, Yoo HS, Lee JS, Lee EG, Park HK, et al. (2010) The spread of pandemic H1N1 2009 by age and region and the comparison among monitoring tools. J Korean Med Sci 25: 709–12.
4. Lee DH, Shin SS, Jun BY, Lee JK (2010) National level response to pandemic (H1N1) 2009. J Prev Med Public Health 43: 99–104.
5. Akan H, Gurol Y, Izbirak G, Ozdatli S, Yilmaz G, et al. (2010) Knowledge and attitudes of university students toward pandemic influenza: a cross-sectional study from Turkey. BMC Public Health 10: 413.
6. Cowling BJ, Ng DM, Ip DK, Liao Q, Lam WW, et al. (2010) Community psychological and behavioral responses through the first wave of the 2009 influenza A(H1N1) pandemic in Hong Kong. J Infect Dis 202: 867–76.
7. Lau JT, Griffiths S, Choi KC, Lin C (2010) Prevalence of preventive behaviors and associated factors during early phase of the H1N1 influenza epidemic. Am J Infect Control 38: 374–80.
8. Liao Q, Cowling B, Lam WT, Ng MW, Fielding R (2010) Situational awareness and health protective responses to pandemic influenza A (H1N1) in Hong Kong: a cross-sectional study. PLoS One 5: e13350.
9. Park JH, Cheong HK, Son DY, Kim SU, Ha CM (2010) Perceptions and behaviors related to hand hygiene for the prevention of H1N1 influenza transmission among Korean university students during the peak pandemic period. BMC Infect Dis 10: 222.
10. Rubin GJ, Amlot R, Page L, Wessely S (2009) Public perceptions, anxiety, and behaviour change in relation to the swine flu outbreak: cross sectional telephone survey. BMJ 339: b2651.
11. Wong LP, Sam IC (2010) Temporal changes in psychobehavioral responses during the 2009 H1N1 influenza pandemic. Prev Med 51: 92–3.
12. Schmidt WP, Wloch C, Biran A, Curtis V, Mangtani P (2009) Formative research on the feasibility of hygiene interventions for influenza control in UK primary schools. BMC Public Health 9: 390.
13. Yuan J, Zhang L, Xu W, Shen J, Zhang P, et al. (2009) Reported changes in health-related behaviours in Chinese urban residents in response to an influenza pandemic. Epidemiol Infect 137: 988–93.
14. Manning S, Barry T, Wilson N, Baker M (2010) Update: follow-up study showing post-pandemic decline in hand sanitiser use, New Zealand, December 2009. Euro Surveill : 15: pii = 19466.
15. Chaberny IE, Schnitzler P, Geiss HK, Wendt C (2003) An outbreak of epidemic keratoconjunctivitis in a pediatric unit due to adenovirus type 8. Infect Control Hosp Epidemiol 24: 514–9.
16. Gottsch JD, Froggatt JW 3rd, Smith DM, Dwyer DM, Borenstein P, et al. (1999) Prevention and control of epidemic keratoconjunctivitis in a teaching eye institute. Opthalmic Epidemiol 6: 29–39.
17. Azar MJ, Dhaliwal DK, Bower KS, Kowalski RP, Gordon YJ (1996) Possible consequences of shaking hands with your patients with epidemic keratoconjunctivitis. Am J Ophthalmol 121: 711–2.
18. Stefkovicová M, Sokolik J, Vicianová V, Madar R (2005) Outbreaks of epidemic kerato-conjunctivitis in two hospital wards. Cent Eur J Public Health 13: 29–31.
19. Jung SH, Kim YJ, Park SM, Jeon CM, Kim YT (2010) Personal hygiene behaviors among adolescents in South Korea. Available at: http://yhs.go.kr/application/situation_view.asp?seq = 55&page = 1. Accessed at 23 January 2011.
20. Kang S, Yang IS, Lee JY, Park Y, Oh HB, et al. (2010) Epidemiologic study of human influenza virus infection in South Korea from 1999 to 2007: origin and evolution of A/Fujian/411/2002-like strains. J Clin Microbiol 48: 2177–85.
21. Aoki K, Tagawa Y (2002) A twenty-one year surveillance of adenoviral conjunctivitis in Sapporo, Japan. Int ophthalmol clin 42: 49–54.

3

Pseudomonas aeruginosa Keratitis in Mice: Effects of Topical Bacteriophage KPP12 Administration

Ken Fukuda[1]*, Waka Ishida[1], Jumpei Uchiyama[2], Mohammad Rashel[2], Shin-ichiro Kato[3], Tamae Morita[4], Asako Muraoka[5], Tamaki Sumi[1], Shigenobu Matsuzaki[2], Masanori Daibata[2], Atsuki Fukushima[1]

1 Department of Ophthalmology and Visual Science, Kochi Medical School, Kochi, Japan, 2 Department of Microbiology and Infection, Kochi Medical School, Kochi, Japan, 3 Research Institute of Molecular Genetics, Kochi University, Kochi, Japan, 4 Kochi Medical School Hospital, Kochi, Japan, 5 Kochi Gakuen Junior College, Kochi, Japan

Abstract

The therapeutic effects of bacteriophage (phage) KPP12 in Pseudomonas aeruginosa keratitis were investigated in mice. Morphological analysis showed that phage KPP12 is a member of the family Myoviridae, morphotype A1, and DNA sequence analysis revealed that phage KPP12 is similar to PB1-like viruses. Analysis of the phage KPP12 genome did not identify any genes related to drug resistance, pathogenicity or lysogenicity, and so phage KPP12 may be a good candidate for therapeutic. KPP12 showed a broad host range for P. aeruginosa strains isolated from clinical ophthalmic infections. Inoculation of the scarified cornea with P. aeruginosa caused severe keratitis and eventual corneal perforation. Subsequent single-dose administration of KPP12 eye-drops significantly improved disease outcome, and preserved the structural integrity and transparency of the infected cornea. KPP12 treatment resulted in the suppression of neutrophil infiltration and greatly enhanced bacterial clearance in the infected cornea. These results indicate that bacteriophage eye-drops may be a novel adjunctive or alternative therapeutic agent for the treatment of infectious keratitis secondary to antibiotic-resistant bacteria.

Editor: Markus M. Heimesaat, Charité, Campus Benjamin Franklin, Germany

Funding: No current external funding sources for this study.

Competing Interests: The authors have declared that no competing interests exist.

* E-mail: k.fukuda@kochi-u.ac.jp

Introduction

Bacteriophages (phages) are viruses that are omnipresent in the environment (including water, soil, food, and the gastrointestinal tract) and which were discovered more than 80 years ago [1,2]. Phages infect, lyse, and kill bacteria without damage to mammalian cells. Thus, phage therapy was immediately considered a potential treatment for bacterial infectious diseases. However, the introduction of antibiotic therapy meant that phage therapy was restricted to countries in Eastern Europe and the former Soviet Union. Since the 1980s, phage therapy has been re-evaluated in Western countries due to the emergence of antibiotic resistance [3]. The therapeutic efficacy of phage therapy in vivo has been demonstrated in several murine models of antibiotic-resistant bacterial infection, including methicillin-resistant Staphylococcus aureus (MRSA), vancomycin-resistant Enterococcus (VRE), and multidrug-resistant Pseudomonas aeruginosa (P. aeruginosa) and Escherichia coli [4,5,6,7]. In addition, results from clinical studies into bacteriophage treatment in humans, which have been performed mainly in Eastern Europe, have been reported [8,9,10]. Few studies have investigated phage therapy for ocular diseases, and these have mainly focused on conjunctivitis [8,11].

The cornea is an avascular and transparent tissue that acts as a lens. Its transparency is primarily attributable to the architecture of corneal stromal collagen. Infectious keratitis is a sight-threatening disease that requires prompt diagnosis and appropriate treatment if tissue damage and scarring are to be prevented. P. aeruginosa is an important cause of destructive ocular infection, especially in contact lens wearers [12]. P. aeruginosa keratitis progresses rapidly and is characterized by the infiltration of inflammatory cells and tissue destruction, which can result in corneal perforation. Standard treatment is the administration of antibiotics to eliminate the infectious organisms. In recent years, however, antibiotic-resistant bacterial infections such as MRSA, multidrug-resistant P. aeruginosa, and VRE have emerged as a major clinical problem. The ocular surface is a common site of infection for multidrug-resistant bacteria such as MRSA [13,14]. The development of new adjunctive or alternative therapies for the treatment of bacterial keratitis is therefore warranted.

The aim of the present study was to characterize P. aeruginosa-specific bacteriophage KPP12 and investigate the effects of single-dose administration of KPP12 eye-drops on P. aeruginosa keratitis in mice.

Materials and Methods

Ethical Treatment of Animals

This study was approved by the Committee for Care and Use of Laboratory Animals at Kochi University (Permit Number: H23-070/E-00058) and was carried out in strict accordance with the Association for Research in Vision and Ophthalmology Statement on the Use of Animals in Ophthalmic and Vision Research. The animals were treated humanely and all efforts were made to minimize suffering.

Bacterial Strains, Reagents and Culture Media

All bacterial strains used in the present study are listed in Table 1. The *P. aeruginosa* strains PA21 and PA33 were used for phage preparation and the infection experiments, respectively. All chemicals and reagents were purchased from Nacalai (Kyoto, Japan) and Sigma-Aldrich (St. Louis, MO), unless otherwise stated. Luria-Bertani (LB) medium was used for bacteria or phage culture. M9 medium was used for phage dilution. Difco *Pseudomonas* isolation agar (Becton, Dickinson and Co., Sparks, MD) was used for counting colony forming units (CFU) of *P. aeruginosa* harvested from eye tissue. Culture media for phage preparation were purchased from Becton, Dickinson and Co. During phage-plaque formation, a LB medium containing 1.5% or 0.5% agar was used for the lower and the upper layer, respectively.

Isolation and Host Specificity of Phage KPP12

Phage KPP12 was isolated from a water sample using a *P. aeruginosa* strain (strain PA21) as the host. The water sample had been collected from a river in Kochi prefecture, Japan. An inoculation loop was used to streak a drop of phage (ca. 10 μl) onto double-layer agar containing a *P. aeruginosa* strain. This was then incubated at 37°C overnight. After incubation, the presence of a plaque or broad diffusible translucent areas indicated sensitivity to phage KPP12 (lysis from within). No plaques/traces or a semi-translucent trace that disappeared gradually indicated no sensitivity to phage KPP12 or lysis from without, respectively.

Large-scale Culture and Purification of *P. aeruginosa* Phages

Phage was cultured with *P. aeruginosa* strain PA21 in 300 ml of LB. After complete bacterial lysis, the phage lysate was collected by centrifugation, and polyethylene glycol 6000 and NaCl were added to final concentrations of 10% and 0.5 M, respectively. The mixture was stored at 4°C overnight, and the phage pellet was obtained by centrifugation ($10,000 \times g$, 20 min, 4°C). The phage pellet was dissolved in TM buffer (10 mM Tris-HCl [pH 7.2], 5 mM MgCl$_2$) containing 50 μg/ml of DNase I and RNase A and then incubated at 37°C for 1 h. The phage was then purified by density gradient ultracentrifugation using either CsCl or iodixanol as the centrifugal medium.

For the non-animal experiments, the phage suspension was placed on top of a discontinuous CsCl gradient ($\rho = 1.3$, 1.5, and 1.7) and centrifuged ($100,000 \times g$, 1 h, 4°C). After phage band collection, the phage band was again purified by CsCl density gradient ultracentrifugation. The phage band was collected and dialyzed against 0.1 M ammonium acetate, 10 mM NaCl, 1 mM CaCl$_2$, and 1 mM MgCl$_2$ (pH 7.2; AAS) for 1 h at 4°C. The phage concentration was measured by plaque assay.

For the animal experiments, phages were purified by iodixanol density gradient ultracentrifugation. Iodixanol ultracentrifugation medium was purchased from AXIS-SHIELD PoC AS (Opti-Prep™, Oslo, Norway). Iodixanol was diluted to the appropriate concentration using saline. The phage suspension was then placed on top of a discontinuous iodixanol gradient (30%, 35%, and 40%) and centrifuged ($200,000 \times g$, 2 h, 4°C). After collection of the phage band, iodixanol density gradient ultracentrifugation was repeated. The phage band was collected and stored at 4°C until use. The concentration of the purified phage was measured by plaque assay.

Genome Sequence Analysis

The phage in AAS was pelleted by ultracentrifugation ($100,000 \times g$, 1 h, 4°C). The phage pellet was then treated with

Table 1. *P. aeruginosa* strains used in the present study and their sensitivity to phage KPP12.

Strain*	Sensitivity to KPP12**	Department of Origin	Material
PA1	+	Neurosurgery	Sputum
PA2	+	Surgery	Pus
PA3	−	Internal Medicine	Sputum
PA4	−	Internal Medicine	Sputum
PA5	L	Surgery	Pus
PA6	+	Internal Medicine	Sputum
PA7	+	Otolaryngology	Pus
PA8	+	Internal Medicine	Sputum
PA9	L	Otolaryngology	Pus
PA10	+	Internal Medicine	Other
PA11	−	Pediatrics	Other
PA12	L	Pediatrics	Pharynx
PA13	+	Otolaryngology	Pus
PA14	−	Urology	Urine
PA15	−	Urology	Catheter
PA16	−	Surgery	Intestine
PA17	+	Surgery	Pus
PA18	+	Surgery	Pus
PA19	+	Urology	Sputum
PA20	−	Internal Medicine	Urine
PA21	+	Dermatology	Pus
PA22	L	Pediatrics	Sputum
PA23	−	Pediatrics	Pharynx
PA24	+	Otolaryngology	Sputum
PA25	−	Surgery	Sputum
PA26	+	Internal Medicine	Sputum
PA27	−	Otolaryngology	Pus
PA28	−	Dermatology	Pus
PA29	−	Internal Medicine	Blood
PA30	+	Internal Medicine	Sputum
PA31	+	Ophthalmology	Pus
PA32	+	Ophthalmology	Pus
PA33	+	Ophthalmology	Pus
PA34	+	Ophthalmology	Pus
PA35	L	Ophthalmology	Pus
PAO1	+		
D4	+		
S10	L		

*PA1 to PA35, Kochi Medical School Hospital; PAO1, D4, and S10, Dr. Matsumoto, Tokyo Medical University.
**+, plaque formation; −, no plaque formation; L, lysis from without.

1% SDS for 10 min at 37°C, and phage DNA was extracted with water-saturated phenol. The DNA was washed twice in 70% ethanol prior to preparation. Finally, the phage DNA was dissolved in sterile distilled water. The genome was digested by EcoRI (Takara Bio, Shiga, Japan), and shotgun clones were prepared using plasmid pUC18. Primers were designed on the basis of the clone sequences, and the genome sequence was determined by genome direct sequencing using the primer walking method. Both strands were sequenced (at least 2-fold redundancy). Assembly of the determined sequences was performed manually by comparing overlapping regions. All sequencing was performed using a BigDye Terminator v1.1 Cycle Sequencing Kit (Applied Biosystems, Foster City, CA, USA) according to the manufacturer's instructions, and an ABI PRISM 3100-Avant Genetic Analyzer (Applied Biosystems). Putative open reading frames (ORFs) were determined manually, using the automatic prediction provided by the microbial gene-finding program Prodigal as a reference (http://prodigal.ornl.gov/) [15]. Putative tRNA genes were screened using tRNAscan-SE 1.21 (http://selab.janelia.org/tRNAscan-SE/) [16]. The genome sequence of phage KPP12 was deposited into Genbank (accession: AB560486). Amino acid sequences were compared using the protein Basic Local Alignment Search Tool (BLASTp) of the National Center for Biotechnology Information (NCBI). The protein domain was predicted from a Conserved Domain Database (CDD) search using the NCBI website (http://www.ncbi.nlm.nih.gov/Structure/cdd/wrpsb.cgi). The results of the CDD search and BLASTp were used to predict the function of the ORF.

Structural Protein Analysis of Phage KPP12

After dissolving the purified phage pellet into AAS and adding an equal volume of 2× Laemmli sample buffer, the sample was boiled for 5 min. The phage proteins were separated using a 12.5% SDS-polyacrylamide gel electrophoresis (PAGE) gel. After electrophoresis, the gel was stained with Coomassie brilliant blue R-250.

After SDS-PAGE, the phage proteins were blotted onto a polyvinylidene difluoride (PVDF) membrane (Sequi-Blot PVDF Membrane, Bio-Rad Laboratories) using a blotting solution (10 mM CHAPS [pH 11], 10% methanol), and a Hoefer TE70 semi-dry transfer unit (Hoefer, San Francisco, CA) at 1.2 cm^2/mA for 90 min at 4°C. The blotted membrane was stained with Coomassie brilliant blue R-250. The target protein band was excised from the membrane and analyzed using a protein sequencer PPSQ-31A/33A (Shimadzu Biotech, Kyoto, Japan).

Electron Microscopy

The purified phage sample in AAS was loaded onto a formvar-carbon coated copper membrane and negatively stained with 2% uranyl acetate (pH 4.0). Electron micrograph images were obtained with a Hitachi H-7100 transmission electron microscope (Hitachi) at 100 kV.

Mouse Model of *P. aeruginosa* Keratitis

Specific-pathogen-free female C57BL/6 mice were purchased from Japan SLC Inc. (Shizuoka, Japan) and housed under pathogen-free conditions at the animal facility of Kochi Medical School. *P. aeruginosa* PA33 cells were grown in 30 ml LB medium at 37°C, and then centrifuged at 7,000 *g* for 5 min at the logarithmic growth phase (ca.100 Klett units). The cell pellet was washed with 30 ml saline, re-centrifuged under the same conditions, and then resuspended in ca. 3 ml saline. After appropriate dilution, turbidity (in Klett units) was measured to determine bacterial cell numbers. One Klett unit was assumed to be equivalent to 6.2×10^6 *P. aeruginosa* cells/ml. This assumption was based on a previously standardized correlation between turbidity and bacterial cell numbers counted directly with a Petroff-Hausser counting chamber (Hausser Scientific, Suite C Horsham, PA).

The present mouse model of *P. aeruginosa* keratitis is described elsewhere 17]. Briefly, the cornea of the left eye in eight-week-old female C57BL/6 mice was then visualized under a stereoscopic microscope, and three 1 mm scratches were made using a sterile 25 gauge needle. A 5 µl aliquot containing 5×10^6 cells of *P. aeruginosa* (PA33) was applied to the corneal surface. Thirty minutes after infection, 5×10^8 plaque forming units (PFU) of phage in 5 µl or vehicle was applied to the corneal surface. The eyes were examined at 1, 3, and 5 days post-infection (p.i.) to grade disease severity according to an established scale, as described previously 18]. Strain PA33 was derived from a specimen obtained from a patient with *Pseudomonas* keratitis at the Kochi Medical School Hospital, Kochi, Japan.

Determination of the Number of Viable Bacteria in the Infected Cornea

Mice were euthanized by inhalation of ether on day 5 p.i. and the corneas were harvested. Individual corneas were homogenized with a tissue homogenizer in sterile saline. Portions of the homogenized tissue samples were plated onto Difco *Pseudomonas* isolation agar after dilution in saline (either 1:1, 1:100, or 1:10,000) and cultured at 37°C for 48 h to detect *P. aeruginosa* challenge. Results are reported as CFU per ml.

Myeloperoxidase (MPO) Assay

A MPO assay was used to quantitate PMN number in the cornea, as described previously with slight modification [19]. Infected corneas were excised on day 5 p.i. and homogenized in 1.0 ml of 50 mM potassium phosphate (pH 6.0). The samples were then centrifuged. Pellets were resuspended in 0.03 ml of 50 mM phosphate buffer and 50 mM hexadecyltrimethylammonium bromide (Sigma-Aldrich), and 0.07 ml of 50 mM potassium phosphate was added. Then samples were freeze-thawed three times and centrifuged at 10,000 rpm for 10 min, and 0.02 ml of the supernatant was added to 0.05 ml substrate reagent (R&D systems, Minneapolis, MN) for 20 min at room temperature. Then $2N H_2SO_4$ was added to the samples. Absorption was assessed by measuring the optical density at 450 nm.

Histology and Immunostaining of PMN, *P. aeruuginosa*, and Collagen Fibrils

Eyes were harvested on day 5 p.i. and fixed in 4% formalin and embedded in paraffin. Sections were stained with hematoxylin/eosin, picrosirius red, and with the antibodies for granulocytes and *P. aeruginosa*. The antigen unmasking procedures involved heating with 10 mM citrate buffer, pH 6.0, for 15 min. Endogenous peroxidase activity was inhibited by adding 0.1% H_2O_2 in methanol for 15 min at room temperature. Sections were incubated with a rat anti-mouse Ly-6G and Ly6C antibody (1:200; Becton, Dickinson and Co.) overnight at 4 °C. This was followed by incubation with a biotinylated rabbit anti-rat IgG antibody (1:200; Dako Cytomation, Glostrup, Denmark) for 1 h. Sections were icubated using an Avidin-Biotin-Complex kit (Vector Laboratories, Burlingame, CA). *P. aeruginosa* was stained using mouse anti-*Pseudomonas aeruginosa* antibody (1:50; Abcam, Cambridge, United Kingdom) and the Histofine mouse stain kit (Nichirei Biosciences Inc., Tokyo, Japan). Counterstaining was performed using Mayer's Hematoxylin (Wako Pure Chemical Industries, Osaka, Japan). Control sections were processed in a similar manner but with the omission of the primary antibody. Staining of collagen type I and type III was performed using picrosirius red stain kit (Polysciences, Inc., Warrington, PA). Sections were photographed under a microscope (Biorevo; Keyence Corporation, Osaka, Japan).

Statistical Analysis

The difference in the clinical scores between the two groups at each time point and the results of the MPO assays were tested using an unpaired, two-tailed Student's t-test. The Mann-Whitney U test was used to determine the significance of viable bacterial counts. Data were considered significant at $p < 0.05$.

Results

Characterization of Phage KPP12

Morphological analysis showed that phage KPP12 was classified into the family *Myoviridae* morphotype A1 (Fig. 1A). Genome sequencing of phage KPP12 revealed the presence of 64,144 bp, which corresponded approximately to the 64 kbp estimated by pulsed-field gel electrophoresis. The sequencing of the genome was circularly connected, implying that phage KPP12 genome is a linear form with terminal redundancy. Eighty-eight ORFs were predicted but no tRNA gene (Table S1). Analysis of the ORF by BLASTp revealed that the ORFs of phage KPP12 frequently showed high similarity to those of PB1-like viruses, including *Pseudomonas* phages LMA2, LBL3, SN, JG024, 14-1, F8, and PB1. Phage KPP12 and these PB1-like viruses also showed high similarity in terms of whole genomic DNA sequence (Fig. S1). BLASTp analysis of the phage KPP12 ORFs against the phage PB1 ORFs with an e-value cut-off of 0.1 revealed that 93.2% (82 out of 88 ORFs) of phage KPP12 ORFs were similar to those of phage PB1. Thus, phage KPP12 was considered to be a member of the PB1-like viruses. Moreover, structural protein analysis (Fig. 1B) showed that the major structural protein was ORF23, which is considered to be a major capsid protein. Since major capsid proteins can generally be used for phylogenetic analysis [20], the relationship between phage KPP12 and PB1-like viruses was investigated. Phage KPP12 showed the closest relationship to phage LMP2 (Fig. 1C). PB1-like viruses have been used in phage therapy [21] and are considered to be lytic phages.

Next, the therapeutic eligibility of KPP12 against *P. aeruginosa* infections was examined *in vitro*. This was achieved by the following: (i) determination of the *in vitro* activity of the phage against clinical strains, (ii) *in silico* examination of therapeutic phage eligibility, and (iii) assessment of the stability of the phage during storage. Firstly, KPP12 showed a host spectrum of 52.6% (20/38) against various clinical isolates and seemed to have a broader host range (80%, 4/5) for *P. aeruginosa* strains isolated from ophthalmic infections (Table 1). Genomic analysis of phage KPP12 identified no genes related to drug resistance, pathogenicity or lysogenicity (Table S1). In addition, phage KPP12 was categorized into the PB1-like phage group, which includes the therapeutic phage 14-1 (Fig. S1, Table S2, and Fig. 1C) [21]. Thirdly, although the infectivity of some phages decreased over time during storage, phage KPP12 was stable at 4°C for one month, even after iodixanol density gradient ultracentrifugation (Fig. 1D).

On the basis of the characteristics described above, KPP12 was considered to be a possible candidate phage for therapeutic and was used in the following experiments.

Effects of Bacteriophage on Disease Course, Bacterial load, and PMN Infiltration in *P. aeruginosa* Keratitis

Firstly, the effects of bacteriophage on non-infected corneal tissue were examined. The application of bacteriophage KPP12 or vehicle to the scarified cornea without prior inoculation induced no inflammatory responses, such as corneal opacity or inflammatory cell infiltrations (Fig. 2).

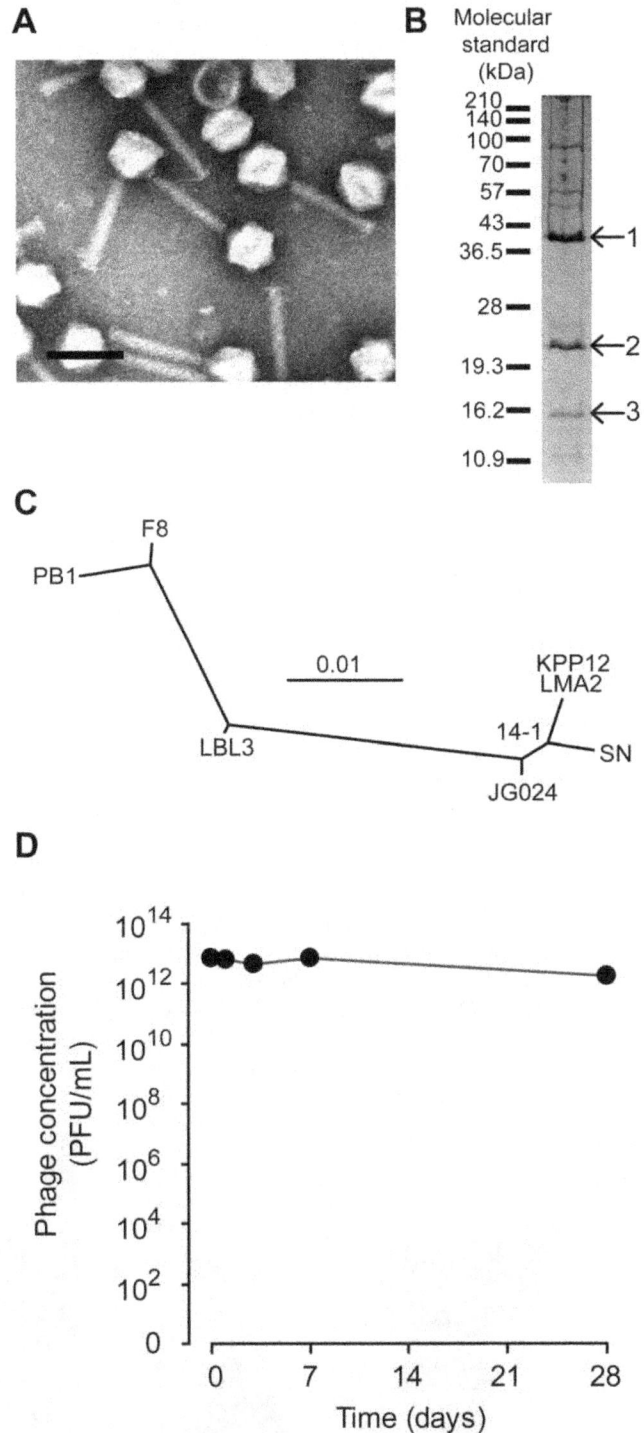

Figure 1. Characteristics of *P. aeruginosa* phage KPP12. (A) Morphology. The bar indicates 100 nm. The head diameter and tail length were 62.5±2.5 nm and 124.2±3.4 nm (mean ± SD nm; n = 12), respectively. (B) Structural proteins. The structural proteins were separated using a 12.5% SDS-PAGE gel. The N-terminal of the structural proteins (indicated by arrows and numbers) were sequenced. The protein sequences (numbered from 1 to 3) were SNFTAPVTTPSIPT-PIQFLQ, MFQKQVYRQYTPGFPGDLIE, and MINISAFGSIVQFTASRTFP, respectively. The proteins numbered from 1 to 3 were identified as ORF23, ORF22, and ORF30, respectively. (C) Phylogenetic analysis based on the major structural proteins of PB1-like phage. Phage KPP12 was closely related to phage LMA2 of the PB1-like viruses. (D) Stability. After iodixanol density gradient ultra-centrifugal purification, phage KPP12

was stored in the dark at 4°C for one month. Data are shown as mean values with SD (n = 3). The phage was fairly stable during the experimental period.

Secondly, a mouse model of keratitis was used to assess the ability of phage KPP12 eye-drops to kill *P. aeruginosa in vivo*. After infection of the cornea with *P. aeruginosa* PA33, the mice were treated with bacteriophage KPP12 eye-drops. Infected control mice received mock-treatment in the form of buffer without phages. A very severe clinical course was observed in mock-treated mice. A ring abscess was observed on day 1 p.i., and opacities had spread across the entire cornea by day 3 p.i. Most of the corneas perforated on day 5 p.i. (Fig. 2A). In contrast, PA33-infected mice treated with single-dose KPP12 eye-drops showed only slight or focal corneal opacities on day 1 p.i., and the corneal opacities gradually faded by day 5 p.i. (Fig. 2B). Treatment with KPP12 eye-drops resulted in a significantly improved disease outcome at days 1, 3, and 5 p.i., as indicated by the clinical scores (Fig. 2C).

Corneas from vehicle- and phage-treated mice were subjected to histopathological examination on day 5 p.i. The corneas of vehicle-treated mice exhibited denuded epithelium, central thinning and edema of the corneal stroma, and large neutrophilic abscesses. In mock-treated mice, picrosirius red staining revealed that the stromal structure of cornea was destroyed and that very few stromal collagen fibrils remained at the center of the cornea (Fig. 3B, C). In contrast, phage-treated mice showed an almost normal corneal structure (Fig. 3D, E, F). Examination of mAb-labeled histological sections revealed that *P. aeruginosa* was present within the abscess in mock-treated mice, whereas bacteria were barely detectable in phage-treated corneas. The bacterial load in the vehicle-treated mouse cornea was significantly higher at day 5 p.i. than in bacteriophage-treated mice (Fig. 4).

Immunostaining of neutrophils revealed the presence of numerous inflammatory cells in the cornea and the anterior chamber. An MPO assay to quantify PMN infiltration/persistence in the infected cornea revealed that the corneas of mock-treated mice contained significantly more PMN than those of bacteriophage-treated mice on day 5 p.i. (Fig. 5).

Discussion

The present study demonstrated that the administration of a single-dose of bacteriophage KPP12 in the form of eye-drops efficiently eliminated bacteria from the infected cornea in a mouse model of *P. aeruginosa* keratitis. This resulted in improved disease outcome, preservation of the structural integrity and transparency of the cornea, and the suppression of neutrophils. These results suggest that bacteriophage eye-drops may represent a novel adjunctive or alternative therapy for antibiotic-resistant bacterial keratitis. To our knowledge, the present paper is the first to describe basic science research into bacteriophage therapy for ocular disease.

In terms of potential future clinical application, KPP12 appears to offer several important advantages. Firstly, KPP12 showed a broad host range for *P. aeruginosa* strains isolated from ophthalmic infections. Secondly, among the 88 predicted genes of phage KPP12, no genes related to drug resistance or pathogenicity were identified, and the genome does not contain a recognizable integrase gene, suggesting that this bacteriophage is lytic in nature. Thirdly, phage KPP12 was genetically related to the PB1-like phage group. DNA sequence analysis and structural protein analysis showed that KPP12 is a PB1-like virus (Fig. 1). Research suggests that PB-1 like viruses are lytic phages. In fact, a PB1-like virus (14-1) was selected for the treatment of burn-wounds in human clinical trials [21]. Fourthly, KPP12 could be stored at 4 °C for a period of one month with no decrease in infectivity, even after iodixanol density gradient ultracentrifugation. Finally, the phage can be administered in the form of eye-drops. The route of phage delivery appears to be a critical determinant of successful therapy [22]. In an acute respiratory infection model, phages were more effective when administered via intraperitoneal injection than via intranasal inhalation. This suggests that the phages may have been unable to penetrate the respiratory epithelium and encounter bacteria [22,23]. The cornea is the outermost region of the eyeball, and the corneal epithelium is usually damaged at the site of infection in bacterial keratitis. Administration of the phage in the form of eye-drops may thus facilitate contact and infection of the bacteria present in the diseased cornea.

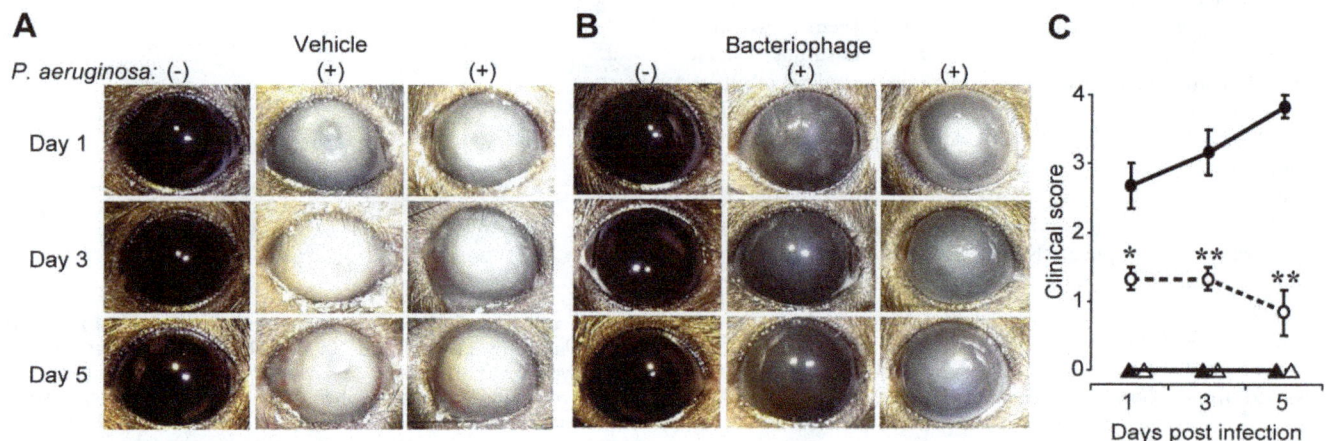

Figure 2. Effects of single-dose administration of topical phage KPP12 on the clinical signs of keratitis in infected mice. The scarified corneas were applied with 5.0×10^6 CFU of *P. aeruginosa* or PBS as a control condition. Thirty minutes post-infection, 5 μl of vehicle (**A**) or bacteriophage (**B**) was administered topically. Representative photographs of vehicle- and bacteriophage-treated cornea on days 1, 3, and 5 p.i. (**C**) Clinical scores for corneal response in the vehicle-treated (closed circles) and bacteriophage-treated (open circles) mice assigned on days 1, 3, and 5 p.i. Clinical scores in vehicle- (closed triangles) and phage-treated (open triangles) mice without prior inoculation are shown. Data represent the mean +/− SEM of three experiments. *p<0.05, **P<0.01 (unpaired *t*-test) vs vehicle-treated mice.

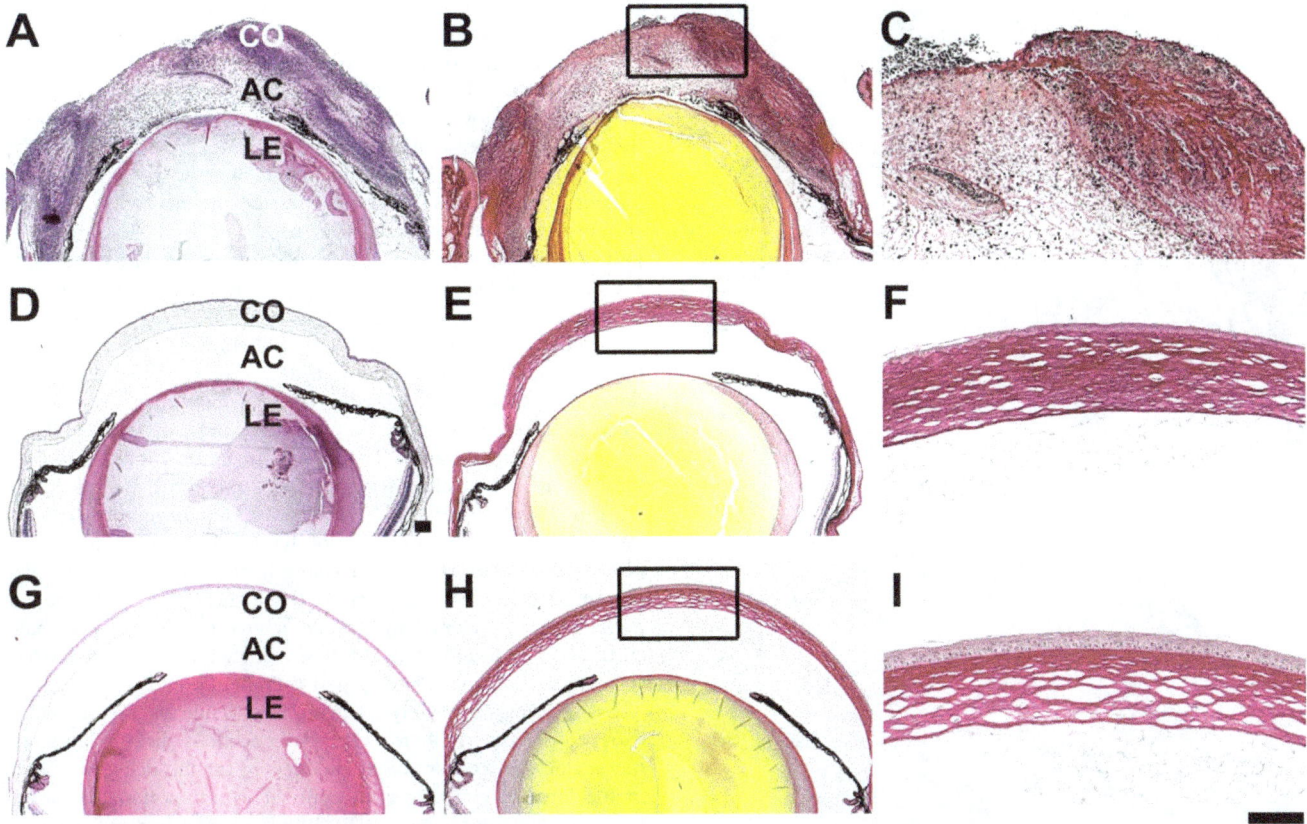

Figure 3. Histopathology of infected corneas treated with vehicle or bacteriophage. Representative photomicrographs of sections of the infected cornea on day 5 p.i. that were stained with H&E (A, D) or picrosirius red (B-C, E-F). Uninfected corneal sections stained with H&E (G) or picrosirius red (H-I) are shown as a control. In vehicle-treated mice (A-C), stromal collagen fibrils were severely damaged, resulting in central thinning and corneal stromal edema, and numerous inflammatory cells were observed. In phage-treated mice (D-F), normal corneal structure was maintained and no inflammatory cells were present. Bars: 100 μm. Co: cornea, AC: anterior chamber, L: lens.

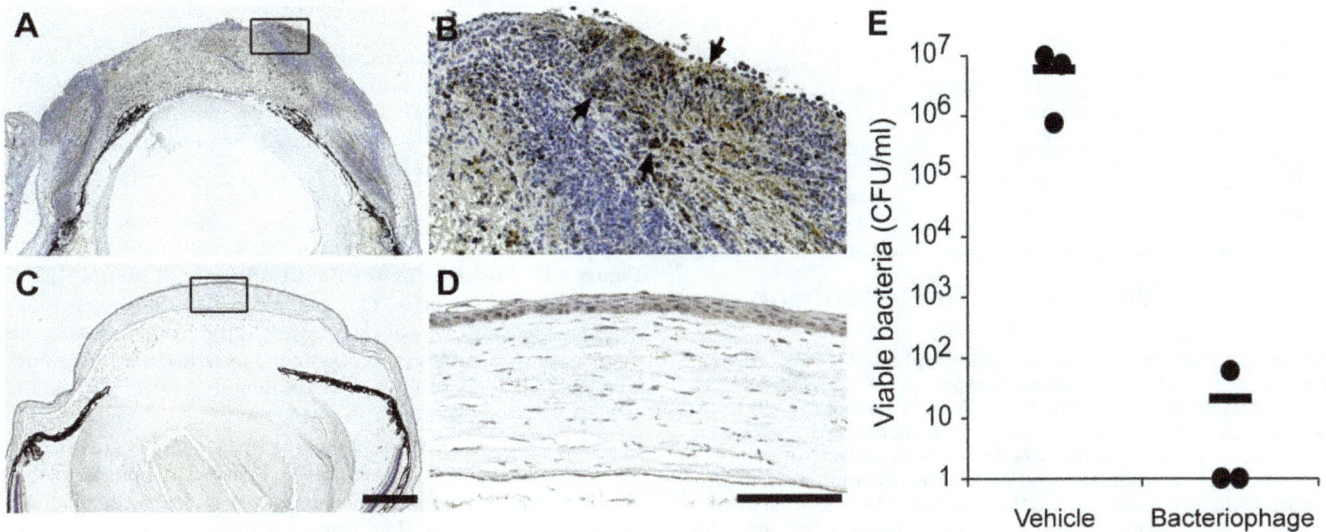

Figure 4. Bacterial clearance in bacteriophage-treated corneas. Representative photomicrographs of sections of infected cornea that were treated with vehicle (**A–B**) or bacteriophage KPP12 (**C–D**) at day 5 p.i. and stained with anti-P. aeruginosa Ab. P. *aeruginosa* within the abscess was stained brown (arrows) in mock-treated mice (**B**). **E**, on day 5 p.i., the corneas were excised and subjected to plate bacterial counting. Circles represent the data obtained from each mouse; horizontal bars represent mean values calculated from all mice in each group. *P<0.05 (Mann-Whitney *U* test) vs vehicle-treated mice. Bars: 100 μm.

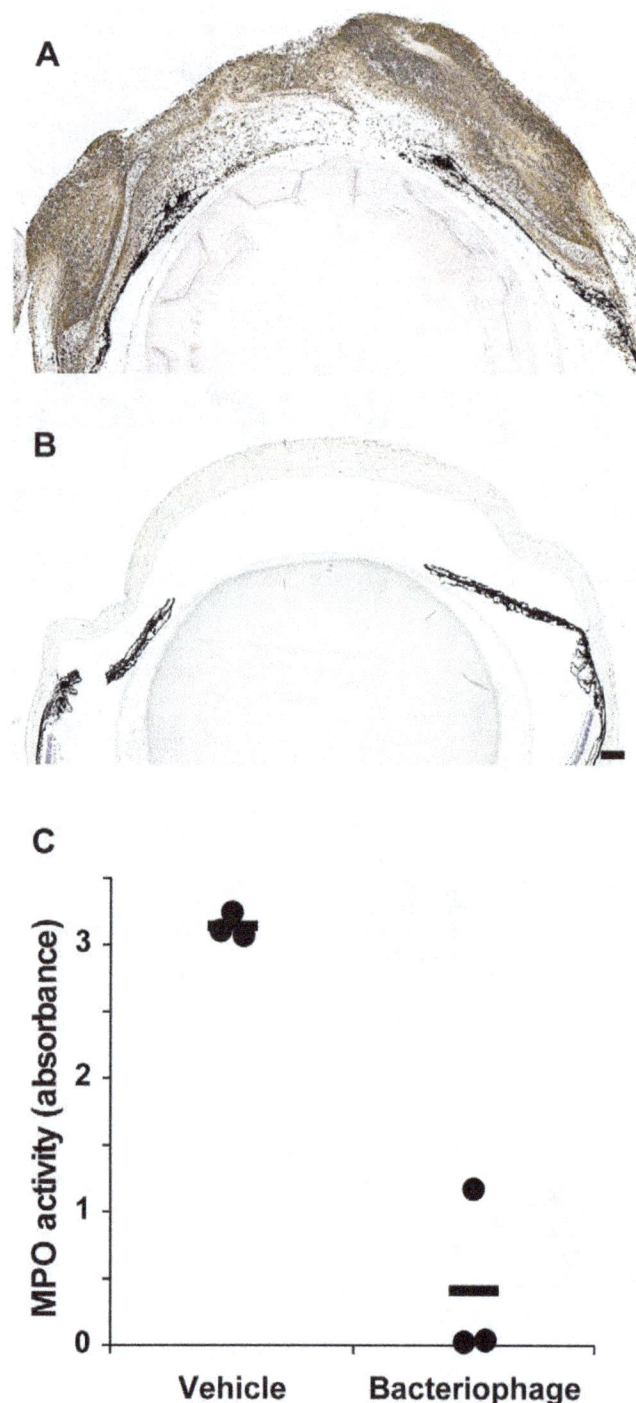

Figure 5. PMN infiltration in bacteriophage-treated corneal tissue. Representative photomicrographs of sections of infected cornea that were treated with vehicle (**A**) or bacteriophage KPP12 (**B**) on day 5 p.i. and stained with anti-Gr-1 Ab. C, on day 5 p.i., the corneas were excised and MPO activity was determined as a parameter of PMN infiltration. Circles represent the data obtained from each mouse; horizontal bars represent mean values calculated from all mice in each group. **P<0.01 (unpaired t-test) versus the corresponding value for vehicle-treated mice. Bar: 100 μm.

Although no basic science research into phage application in ocular disease has been published to date, two clinical studies have been reported [8,11]. In 1970, Proskurov reported a good clinical outcome in 17 patients with conjunctivitis and blepharitis who were treated with anti-staphylococcal phage eye-drops [11]. However, no specific details concerning clinical course were reported. More recently, Slopek et al. reported the results of phage therapy in 550 patients with suppurative bacterial infection who presented at their institute between 1981 and 1986 [8]. Of these, good clinical outcome was reported in 16 patients with ocular infection, seven patients with purulent conjunctivitis, three patients with recurrent hordeolum, and one patient with dacryocystitis who had all been treated with phage eye-drops. Neither study reported any side effects to this treatment.

Another possible phage-related therapeutic agent is the bacterial cell-wall peptidoglycan-degrading enzyme lysin (endolysin), which is produced by the bacteriophage at the end stage of infection to allow the release of progeny virions. Phage endolysin is particularly effective against Gram-positive bacteria, because it specifically degrades the outermost peptidoglycan layer of these bacteria [24]. Recent studies have revealed that the exogenous administration of lysins extracted from certain phages was highly efficient in killing bacteria [25,26,27,28]. The present authors previously reported the successful purification of a cloned lysin encoded by the *Staphylococcus aureus* bacteriophage φMR11. We found that this lysin efficiently lysed multidrug-resistant *S. aureus in vitro* and had therapeutic effects *in vivo* [29]. These findings strongly suggest the clinical usefulness of exogenous phage lysin for bacterial infectious diseases and that the ocular surface may be a suitable site for the delivery of lysin in the form of eye drops. In contrast to antibiotics, the cloned lysin, as with the phage itself, is highly specific to target bacteria but not to other members of the indigenous bacterial flora. The high specificity of lysin is an advantage in the clinical setting, since no substituted microbism can occur. Phage-related side-effects per se are uncommon, as neither phages nor their products (such as lysin) affect eukaryotic cells.

In conclusion, the present study has shown that KPP12 eye-drops may be a viable alternative therapy for *P. aeruginosa* keratitis in clinical practice. Since the incidence of bacterial keratitis is increasing due to inappropriate soft contact lens use and infection with multidrug-resistant bacteria, our results provide important fundamental data for future clinical studies into the use of phages on the ocular surface. As pointed out by Gorski et al, clinical trials are warranted to assess the therapeutic potential of phages in ocular disease, in particular in antibiotic-resistant cases [30].

Supporting Information

Figure S1 Multiple genomic alignments of phage KPP12 with PB1-like viruses. The multiple genomic alignments were generated using Mauve software (http://gel.ahabs.wisc.edu/mauve/) and a progressive alignment with the default settings. The horizontal axis indicates the location of the genomes, and the vertical axis indicates the degree of DNA sequence similarity. The degree of similarity level is shown as percentage length (i.e., the higher bar indicates closer similarity). Phages are indicated on the right. A high degree of similarity was detected throughout the genomes of all phages. The degree of similarity declined around middle and terminal parts of the genome. The middle parts of the genomes showing lower similarity (i.e., 32–33.5 and 35–36.5 kbp in phage KPP) were considered to contain ORFs for tail proteins and DNA replication. The terminal parts of the genomes showing lower similarity were only seen sporadically and the function of their ORFs were not predictable. The genomic data of the PB1-

like viruses were retrieved from the GenBank (phage 14-1, FM897211; phage F8, DQ163917; phage SN, FM887021; phage PB1, EU716414; phage LMA2, FM201282; phage LBL3, FM201281; phage JG024, GU815091).

Table S1   Annotation of phage KPP12.

Table S2   Phages hit by BLASTp search based on the major capsid protein.

Author Contributions

Conceived and designed the experiments: KF WI JU SM MD AF. Performed the experiments: KF WI JU MR SK TS AM SM. Analyzed the data: KF WI JU MR SK AM TS SM MD AF. Contributed reagents/materials/analysis tools: TM. Wrote the paper: KF SM.

References

1. D'Herelle F (1917) Sur un microbe invisible antagoniste des bacilles dysentériques. CR Acad Sci Paris 165: 373–375.
2. Duckworth DH (1976) "Who discovered bacteriophage?". Bacteriological reviews 40: 793–802.
3. Merril CR, Scholl D, Adhya SL (2003) The prospect for bacteriophage therapy in Western medicine. Nat Rev Drug Discov 2: 489–497.
4. Matsuzaki S, Yasuda M, Nishikawa H, Kuroda M, Ujihara T, et al. (2003) Experimental protection of mice against lethal *Staphylococcus aureus* infection by novel bacteriophage phi MR11. J Infect Dis 187: 613–624.
5. Wang J, Hu B, Xu M, Yan Q, Liu S, et al. (2006) Use of bacteriophage in the treatment of experimental animal bacteremia from imipenem-resistant *Pseudomonas aeruginosa*. Int J Mol Med 17: 309–317.
6. Wang J, Hu B, Xu M, Yan Q, Liu S, et al. (2006) Therapeutic effectiveness of bacteriophages in the rescue of mice with extended spectrum beta-lactamase-producing *Escherichia coli* bacteremia. Int J Mol Med 17: 347–355.
7. Biswas B, Adhya S, Washart P, Paul B, Trostel AN, et al. (2002) Bacteriophage therapy rescues mice bacteremic from a clinical isolate of vancomycin-resistant *Enterococcus faecium*. Infect Immun 70: 204–210.
8. Slopek S, Weber-Dabrowska B, Dabrowski M, Kucharewicz-Krukowska A (1987) Results of bacteriophage treatment of suppurative bacterial infections in the years 1981–1986. Arch Immunol Ther Exp (Warsz) 35: 569–583.
9. Sulakvelidze A, Kutte E (2004) Bacteriophage therapy in humans. In: Kutter E, Sulakvelidze A, editors. Bacteriophages: Biology and Application: CRC Press. 381–436.
10. Weber-Dabrowska B, Mulczyk M, Gorski A (2000) Bacteriophage therapy of bacterial infections: an update of our institute's experience. Arch Immunol Ther Exp (Warsz) 48: 547–551.
11. Proskurov VA (1970) [Treatment of staphylococcal diseases of the eye]. Vestn Oftalmol 6: 82–83.
12. Willcox MD (2007) *Pseudomonas aeruginosa* infection and inflammation during contact lens wear: a review. Optom Vis Sci 84: 273–278.
13. Khosravi AD, Mehdinejad M, Heidari M (2007) Bacteriological findings in patients with ocular infection and antibiotic susceptibility patterns of isolated pathogens. Singapore Med J 48: 741–743.
14. Willcox MD (2011) Review of resistance of ocular isolates of *Pseudomonas aeruginosa* and staphylococci from keratitis to ciprofloxacin, gentamicin and cephalosporins. Clin Exp Optom 94: 161–168.
15. Hyatt D, Chen GL, Locascio PF, Land ML, Larimer FW, et al. (2010) Prodigal: prokaryotic gene recognition and translation initiation site identification. BMC Bioinformatics 11: 119.
16. Lowe TM, Eddy SR (1997) tRNAscan-SE: a program for improved detection of transfer RNA genes in genomic sequence. Nucleic Acids Res 25: 955–964.
17. Wu M, McClellan SA, Barrett RP, Hazlett LD (2009) Beta-defensin-2 promotes resistance against infection with *P. aeruginosa*. J Immunol 182: 1609–1616.
18. Hazlett LD, McClellan S, Kwon B, Barrett R (2000) Increased severity of *Pseudomonas aeruginosa* corneal infection in strains of mice designated as Th1 versus Th2 responsive. Invest Ophthalmol Vis Sci 41: 805–810.
19. Williams RN, Paterson CA, Eakins KE, Bhattacherjee P (1982) Quantification of ocular inflammation: evaluation of polymorphonuclear leucocyte infiltration by measuring myeloperoxidase activity. Curr Eye Res 2: 465–470.
20. Comeau AM, Krisch HM (2008) The capsid of the T4 phage superfamily: the evolution, diversity, and structure of some of the most prevalent proteins in the biosphere. Mol Biol Evol 25: 1321–1332.
21. Merabishvili M, Pirnay JP, Verbeken G, Chanishvili N, Tediashvili M, et al. (2009) Quality-controlled small-scale production of a well-defined bacteriophage cocktail for use in human clinical trials. PloS one 4: e4944.
22. Carmody LA, Gill JJ, Summer EJ, Sajjan US, Gonzalez CF, et al. (2010) Efficacy of bacteriophage therapy in a model of *Burkholderia cenocepacia* pulmonary infection. J Infect Dis 201: 264–271.
23. Dabrowska K, Switala-Jelen K, Opolski A, Weber-Dabrowska B, Gorski A (2005) Bacteriophage penetration in vertebrates. J Appl Microbiol 98: 7–13.
24. Fischetti VA (2010) Bacteriophage endolysins: a novel anti-infective to control Gram-positive pathogens. International journal of medical microbiology : IJMM 300: 357–362.
25. Loeffler JM, Nelson D, Fischetti VA (2001) Rapid killing of *Streptococcus pneumoniae* with a bacteriophage cell wall hydrolase. Science 294: 2170–2172.
26. Nelson D, Loomis L, Fischetti VA (2001) Prevention and elimination of upper respiratory colonization of mice by group A streptococci by using a bacteriophage lytic enzyme. Proc Natl Acad Sci U S A 98: 4107–4112.
27. Sheehan MM, Garcia JL, Lopez R, Garcia P (1997) The lytic enzyme of the pneumococcal phage Dp-1: a chimeric lysin of intergeneric origin. Mol Microbiol 25: 717–725.
28. Schuch R, Nelson D, Fischetti VA (2002) A bacteriolytic agent that detects and kills *Bacillus anthracis*. Nature 418: 884–889.
29. Rashel M, Uchiyama J, Ujihara T, Uehara Y, Kuramoto S, et al. (2007) Efficient elimination of multidrug-resistant *Staphylococcus aureus* by cloned lysin derived from bacteriophage phi MR11. J Infect Dis 196: 1237–1247.
30. Gorski A, Targonska M, Borysowski J, Weber-Dabrowska B (2009) The potential of phage therapy in bacterial infections of the eye. Ophthalmologica 223: 162–165.

4

Dynamics of an Infectious Keratoconjunctivitis Outbreak by *Mycoplasma conjunctivae* on Pyrenean Chamois *Rupicapra p. pyrenaica*

MaríaCruz Arnal[1*⑨], **Juan Herrero**[2⑨], **Christian de la Fe**[3], **Miguel Revilla**[1], **Carlos Prada**[4], **David Martínez-Durán**[1], **Ángel Gómez-Martín**[3], **Olatz Fernández-Arberas**[4], **Joaquín Amores**[3], **Antonio Contreras**[3], **Alicia García-Serrano**[4], **Daniel Fernández de Luco**[1]

1 Departamento de Patología Animal, Facultad de Veterinaria, Universidad de Zaragoza, Zaragoza, Spain, 2 Área de Ecología, Departamento de Ciencias Agrarias y Medio Natural, Escuela Politécnica Superior de Huesca, Universidad de Zaragoza, Huesca, Spain, 3 Departamento de Sanidad Animal, Facultad de Veterinaria, Universidad de Murcia, Murcia, Spain, 4 Ega Wildlife Consultants, Zaragoza, Spain

Abstract

Between 2006 and 2008, an outbreak of Infectious Keratoconjunctivitis (IKC) affected Pyrenean chamois *Rupicapra p. pyrenaica*, an endemic subspecies of mountain ungulate that lives in the Pyrenees. The study focused on 14 mountain massifs (180,000 ha) where the species' population is stable. Cases of IKC were detected in ten of the massifs and, in five of them, mortality was substantial. The outbreak spread quickly from the first location detected, with two peaks in mortality that affected one (2007) and three (2008) massifs. In the latter, the peak was seasonal (spring to autumn) and, in the former, the outbreak persisted through winter. To identify the outbreak's aetiology, we examined 105 Pyrenean chamois clinically affected with IKC. TaqMan rt-PCR identified *Mycoplasma conjunctivae* in 93 (88.5%) of the chamois. Another rt-PCR detected *Chlamydophila spp.* in 14 of chamois, and 12 of those had mixed infections with mycoplasmas. In the period 2000–2007, the chamois population increased slightly (λ 1.026) but decreased significantly during the IKC outbreak (λ 0.8, 2007–2008; λ 0.85, 2008–2009) before increasing significantly after the outbreak (λ 1.1, 2009–2010). Sex-biased mortality shifted the adult sex ratio toward males (from 0.6 to 0.7 males per female) and reduced productivity slightly. Hunting was practically banned in the massifs where chamois experienced significant mortality and allowed again after the outbreak ended. Long-term monitoring of wild populations provides a basis for understanding the impacts of disease outbreaks and improves management decisions, particularly when species are subject to extractive exploitation.

Editor: Marco Festa-Bianchet, Université de Sherbrooke, Canada

Funding: The study was funded by Departamento de Agricultura, Ganadería y Medio Ambiente, Gobierno de Aragón and Departamento de Desarrollo Rural, Medio Ambiente y Administración Local, Gobierno de Navarra. The funders had no role in study design, data collection and analysis, decision to publish, or preparation of the manuscript.

Competing Interests: The authors have declared that no competing interests exist.

* E-mail: maricruz@unizar.es

⑨ These authors contributed equally to this work.

Introduction

Infectious keratoconjunctivitis (IKC) is a contagious disease that is common in domestic ruminants and wild *Caprinae*. Domestic sheep can act as reservoir hosts and are the probable source of infections in wildlife, for which the impact of IKC is comparatively higher [1], [2].

Several microorganisms including *Chlamydophila* and *Mycoplasma* species are suspected IKC aetiological agents [3], [1]. *Mycoplasma conjunctivae* occurs in wild ruminants, and is known to affect Alpine ibex *Capra ibex*, Alpine chamois *Rupicapra r. rupicapra* [4], [5], [6], Pyrenean chamois *Rupicapra p. pyrenaica* [7], European mouflon *Ovis aries* [8], and Himalayan thar *Hemitragus jemlaicus* [9]. *Chlamydophila spp.* was the causative organism in outbreaks of IKC in bighorn sheep *Ovis canadensis* [10], and was isolated in IKC-affected mule deer *Odocoileus hemionus* [11]. Other bacteria such as *Moraxella ovis*, *Corynebacterium pyogenes*, *Rickettsia conjunctivae*, and *Staphyloccocus aureus* have been isolated from animals that were affected with IKC [12], [5]. However, *Mycoplasma conjunctivae* is considered the primary cause of IKC in wild *Caprinae* [5].

Multiple outbreaks of IKC in Alpine ibex and Alpine chamois populations have been described in the literature [4], [5], [6], [13]. In Spain, the first reported cases of IKC in wild *Caprinae* occurred in 1952 in Pyrenean chamois and in 1979 in Cantabrian chamois *Rupicapra pyrenaica parva*. Other outbreaks of IKC occurred in the Pyrenees in 1982 and 1992 [14], [15]. In the 1982 outbreak, the pathogen *Chlamydia psittaci* was isolated from a single affected animal [16]; however, the principal etiological agent was never identified. In that outbreak, most of the subpopulations of Pyrenean chamois were affected. Considering that there was no population monitoring, approximate estimations considered a decrease in 50% of total animals. Almost 30 yr later, a new outbreak of IKC affected populations of Pyrenean chamois, which have been subjected to long-term monitoring [17], [18], [19], and has provided an opportunity to quantify the effects of the outbreak on Pyrenean chamois.

The aims of the study were (i) to describe the spread of IKC in the 2006–2008 outbreak and its effects on the population of Pyrenean chamois, (ii) to determine whether the aetiology of the IKC outbreak was associated with the presence of mycoplasmas or *Chlamydophila spp.*, (iii) to assess the occurrence of *M. conjunctivae* in domestic and other wild ruminants in the area, and (iv) to describe the lesions associated with the infection.

Materials and Methods

Study Area

The study area comprised the entire distribution area of the subspecies in Aragon and Navarre (Spanish Pyrenees), which is divided into 14 natural management units (massifs); 10 in the Pyrenees (North) and 4 in the Pre-Pyrenees (South). Among the massifs (180,000 ha) there are 50 hunting grounds (which are managed by local hunters), a National Park and a Nature Reserve (where hunting is forbidden) and five Game Reserves (GR) that are managed by the Government of Aragon (Figure 1). Massifs are the planimetrical surfaces above 1,600 m in mountains that are >2,000 m high, which is the area of biological significance for the species that has seasonal vertical migrations in the Pyrenees [20], [21]. The highest elevation is 3,404 m. The climate is influenced by the relief. Mean annual T is <12°C, average T is <0°C at 3,000 m and 11°C at 600 m. In the high western valleys, where there is an Atlantic influence, annual precipitation is >2,000 mm;

in the east, precipitation is <1,000 mm, and a significant proportion falls as snow. Biogeographically, the area is within the Eurosiberian region, with some areas that are transitional to the Mediterranean. Subalpine pastures occur between 1,600–2,000 m, in areas that are dominated by forests of Scots pine *Pinus sylvatica* and mountain pine *Pinus uncinata*. In the montane habitats below 1,600 m, European beech *Fagus sylvatica* and silver fir *Abies alba* predominate. In the lowest forests, holm oak *Quercus ilex* and white oak *Quercus humilis* predominate, along with pastures.

Other important wild ungulates in the area include wild boar *Sus scrofa*, roe deer *Capreolus capreolus*, and red deer *Cervus elaphus* (in order of density and distribution) [22], [23]. Golden eagle *Aquila chrysaetos* and red fox *Vulpes vulpes* are the most important predators. Hunting quotas are based on population estimates [18], and about 500 adult chamois (1:1 sex ratio, SR) are hunter-harvested each year. In the area, the human density is about 4 inhabitants km^{-2}. The main economic activities are tourism and livestock farming.

Ethics Statement

This study on free-ranging chamois was performed with the permission and support of local authorities (Aragon Government) to update information on the demographic and health status of current populations of game species in the Aragonese jurisdiction, the Hunting Law 5/2002. All samples were collected from legally hunted Pyrenean chamois during the hunting season (hunting

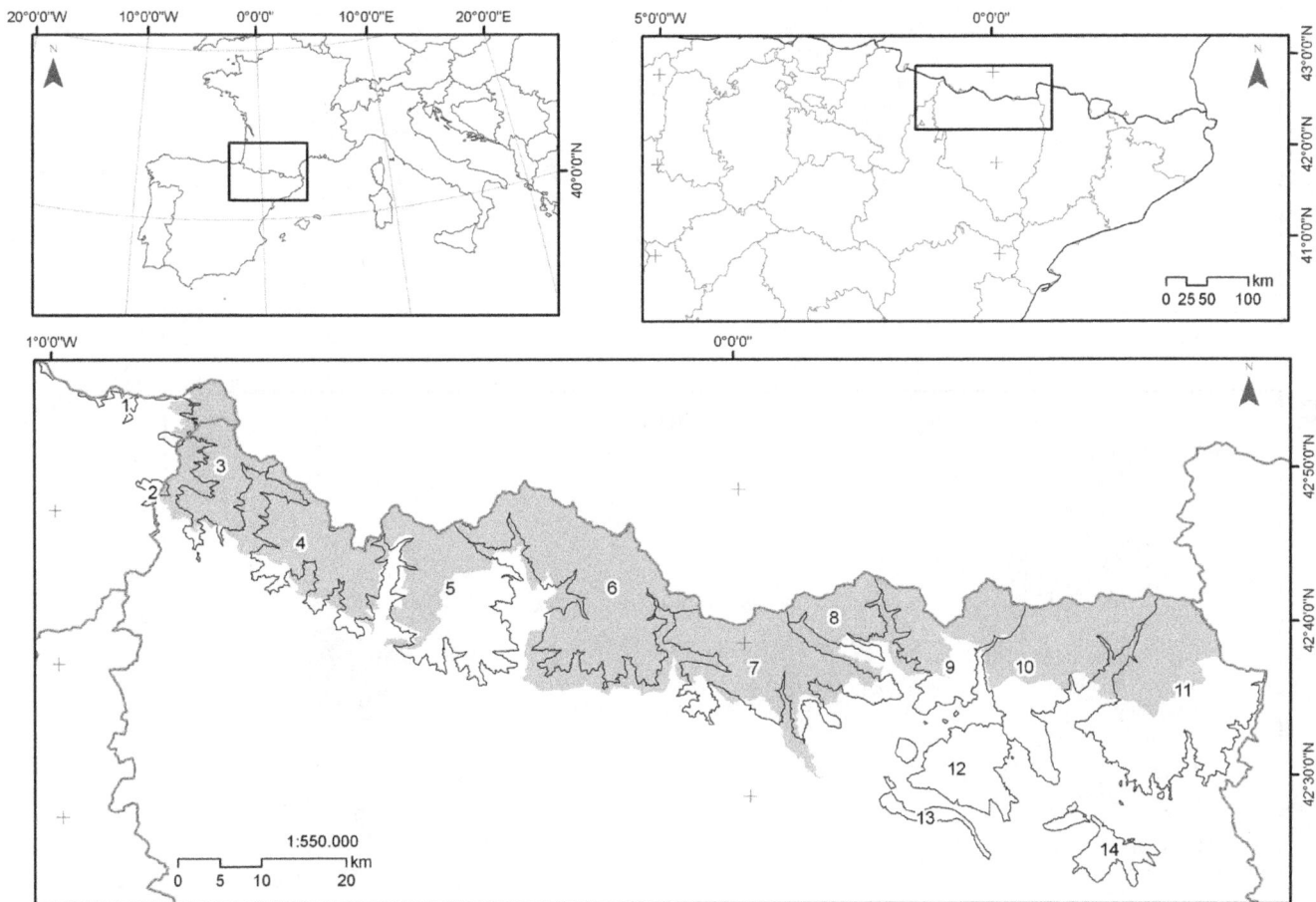

Figure 1. Study area. Mountain massifs in the study area within the Spanish Pyrenees. 1. Ori; 2. Ezkaurre; 3. Larra – Peña Forca; 4. Bixaurín; 5. Anayet; 6. Biñamala; 7. Monte Perdido; 8. Liena; 9. Punta Suelsa; 10. Posets; 11. Maladeta; 12. Cotiella; 13. Sierra Ferrera; 14. Turbón. Grey indicates the area directly managed by the regional administration in Aragon.

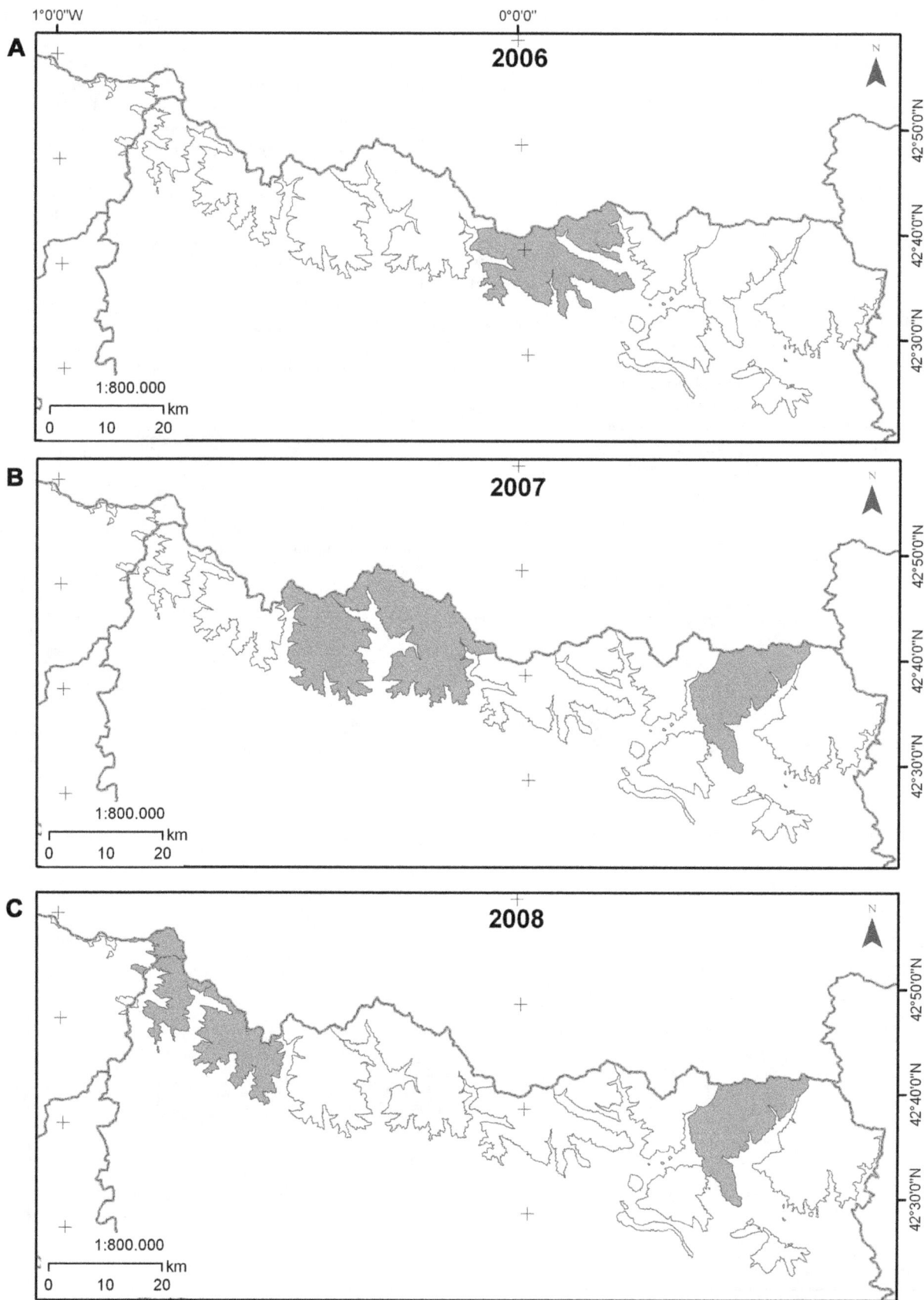

Figure 2. Spatial distribution over Pyrenean massifs of IKC-outbreak locations for years: A) 2006, B) 2007 and C) 2008.

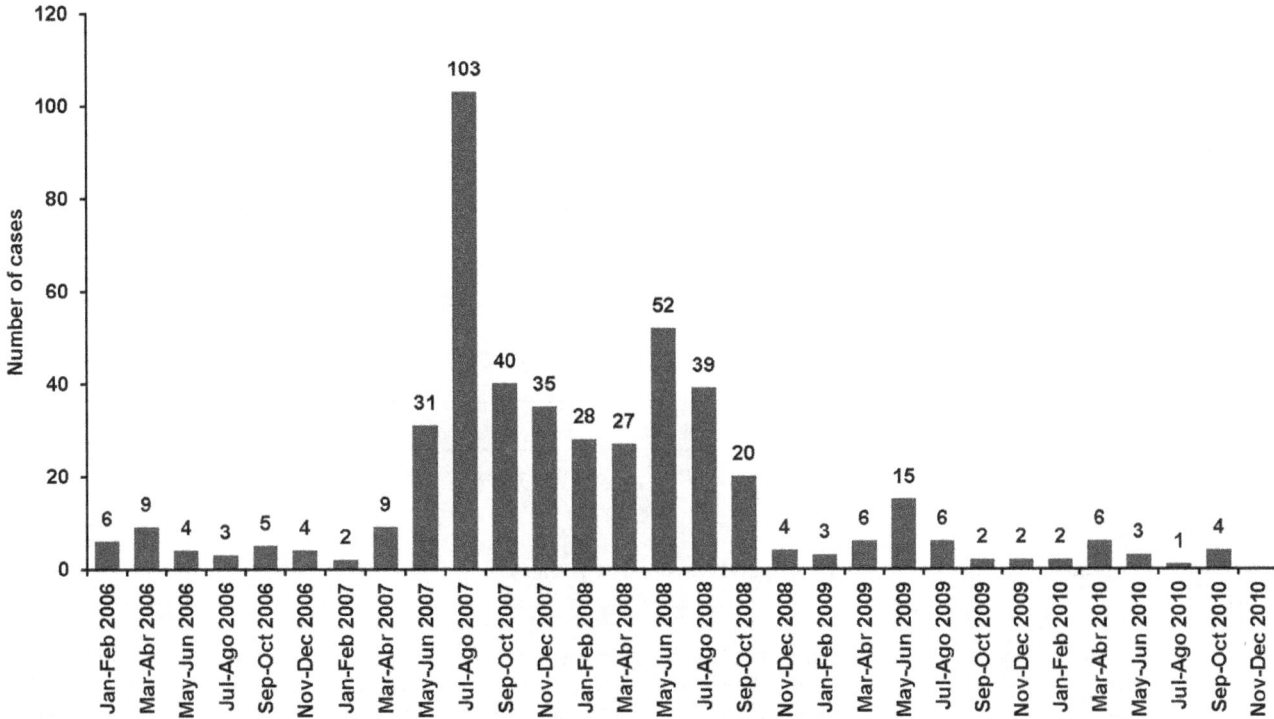

Figure 3. Pyrenean chamois found dead in the Aragonese and Navarrese Pyrenees.

Table 1. Age and sex of chamois found dead in the Aragonese Pyrenees (N = 471, 2006–2010).

Year	Sex	Age 0	1	<=2	Unknown	Total
2006	Female		1	3	3	7
	Male	2		7		9
	Unknown	4	4	1	6	15
		6	**5**	**11**	**9**	**31**
2007	Female		7	95	12	114
	Male	1	2	48	9	60
	Unknown	18	24		4	46
		19	**33**	**143**	**25**	**220**
2008	Female	1	11	45	9	66
	Male	1	4	21	6	32
	Unknown	12	14	12	34	72
		14	**29**	**78**	**49**	**170**
2009	Female		2	9	2	13
	Male		2	7	1	10
	Unknown	2	2	2	5	11
		2	**6**	**18**	**8**	**34**
2010	Female	2		3	1	6
	Male			5		5
	Unknown	1	1	1	2	5
		3	**1**	**9**	**3**	**16**
	Total	**44**	**74**	**259**	**94**	**471**

quotas are annually established by the Department of Agriculture, Livestock and Environment of the Aragon Government) and from animals that died or were ill and euthanized by intravenous injection of sodium pentobarbital. The collection of this material did not require the approval of the Ethics Committee for Animal Experimentation because they are considered routine veterinary practice without experimentation.

In Navarre, Pyrenean chamois are categorized as Vulnerable, and local authorities allow demographic and sanitary monitoring.

In coordination with the Department of Agriculture, Livestock and Environment of the Aragon Government, sheep samples were also collected in chamois areas in collaboration with sheep owners.

Demographic Procedures

In Aragon and Navarre (Spain), populations of Pyrenean chamois are monitored using total counts above the timberline based on itineraries [24] performed in June or July and November. The first is used to estimate productivity and the latter to estimate the adult SR. In one of the massifs, animals were counted in April because of the low elevations and scarce grasslands in areas where chamois occupy open areas. During surveys, individuals were identified as adult males, adult females, yearlings (1–2 yr of age), kids, or undetermined. Above 1,600 m, the area was divided into natural management units (massifs) (Figure 1). Above the timberline, total counts were performed each year in the small massifs and every five years in the large ones. In the latter, in years without a complete survey, an annual selection of fixed itineraries was made to provide representative estimates of the population's demographic parameters, structure, and trends, because they included at least 50% of the number of individuals seen in the complete counts. Adult SR was calculated dividing adult males per adult females and productivity dividing kids per female. Since 1995, when the first surveys were performed, the number of large massifs that were surveyed using global total counts, rather than

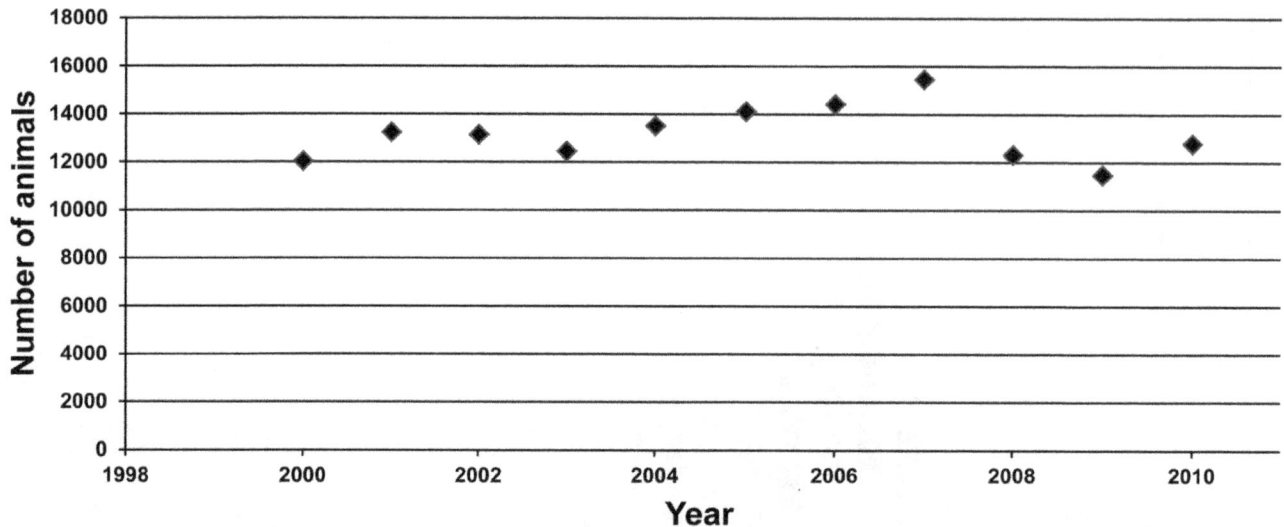

Figure 4. Trend of Pyrenean chamois in the Aragonese and Navarrese Pyrenees.

annual selected itineraries, increased gradually and, since 2008, all of the massifs were surveyed fully each year. Professional rangers performed most of the counts, with the assistance of hunters, technicians, local volunteers, and the authors, using binoculars, spotting scopes, and maps of the itineraries, upon which the locations of groups were recorded.

Since 2006, rangers at the GR and Ordesa and Monte Perdido National Park filed bi-monthly reports of the number of chamois found dead, some of which were collected for necropsy.

Animals and Sample Collection

IKC-affected chamois. Between 2006 and 2008, 105 Pyrenean chamois clinically affected with IKC were examined (1 in 2006, 32 in 2007, and 72 in 2008). Systematic necropsies were performed on 24 dead animals and 81 ill animals which were euthanized after inspection by a qualified veterinarian. Samples of the eye, the third eyelid, eyelids, lung, liver, spleen, kidney, and central nervous system were collected and fixed in 10% neutral buffered formalin and embedded in paraffin. Tissue sections (5 μm) were stained with Haematoxilin-Eosine (HE) for histopathological analyses.

Healthy wild ruminants. To assess the prevalence of *M. conjunctivae* from apparently (clinically) healthy chamois, 190 eye swabs were collected in the GR during the hunting season (April-

May and September-December) over a four-year period between 2006 and 2009. Consequently, we analyzed samples collected during (n = 108) and after (n = 82) the outbreak. In addition, in 2008, eye swabs were collected from 33 roe deer and 14 red deer hunter-harvested in GR, none of which had signs of IKC. Swabs samples from hunter-harvested animals were taken from behind the third eyelid of each eye, and immediately frozen at −20°C.

Sheep. In 2008 and 2009, respectively, livestock censuses indicated that there were 206 and 199 sheep owners in the study area. In those years, 67,163 and 70,577 domestic sheep spent the spring, summer, and autumn in Pyrenean meadows, some in mixed flocks (mixing of sheep between flocks). In the meadows, most (64.7%) of those flocks contained 20–850 small ruminants and the others (35.3%) had 1,200–2,700 animals. To verify the presence of *M. conjunctivae* in domestic sheep, in 2008 and 2009, respectively, 17 and 13 flocks from the study area were selected. In autumn, almost 20 apparently (clinically) healthy animals from each flock were sampled. A total of 617 animals were sampled, 349 in 2008 and 268 in 2009. Conjunctival eye swabs were collected from each eye, and immediately frozen at −20°C.

DNA Extraction

Conjunctival swabs were placed into microcentrifuge tubes that contained 0.5 ml of lysis buffer (100 mM Tris.HCl pH 8.5, 0.05% Tween 20, and 0.24 mg/ml proteinase K) and mixed using the vortex for 1 min at room temperature. The swabs were removed and, to obtain the lysates for the PCR reactions, the buffer was incubated at 60°C for 60 min and at 95°C for 15 min. The DNA from the tissue was extracted from 25 μg of each sample using the High Pure PCR Template Preparation Kit (Roche Diagnostics) in accordance with manufacturer's instructions.

PCR and Real-time PCR Techniques

Mycoplasma spp. To detect *M. conjunctivae*, an *lppS*-based TaqMan real-time PCR was initially performed [25] by using 2 μl of test sample, including 900 nM of primers LPPS-TM-L, LPPS-TM-R, and 300 nM of probe LPPS-TM-FT and TaqMan Universal PCR Master Mix No AmpErase UNG (Applied Biosystems) in 20 μl volume in the presence of an exogenous internal positive control (Applied Biosystems) that verified amplification. The PCR reactions were run on a 7500 Fast real-

Table 2. Age and sex of chamois analyzed in the Aragonese and Navarrese Pyrenees with infectious keratoconjunctivitis during the outbreak (N = 105, 2006–2008).

Age	Found dead Females	Males	Euthanized Females	Males	Total
Adults	16	8	54	13	91
Yearlings	0	0	5	2	7
Kids	0	0	4	3	7
Total	**16**	**8**	**63**	**18**	**105**
	24		81		

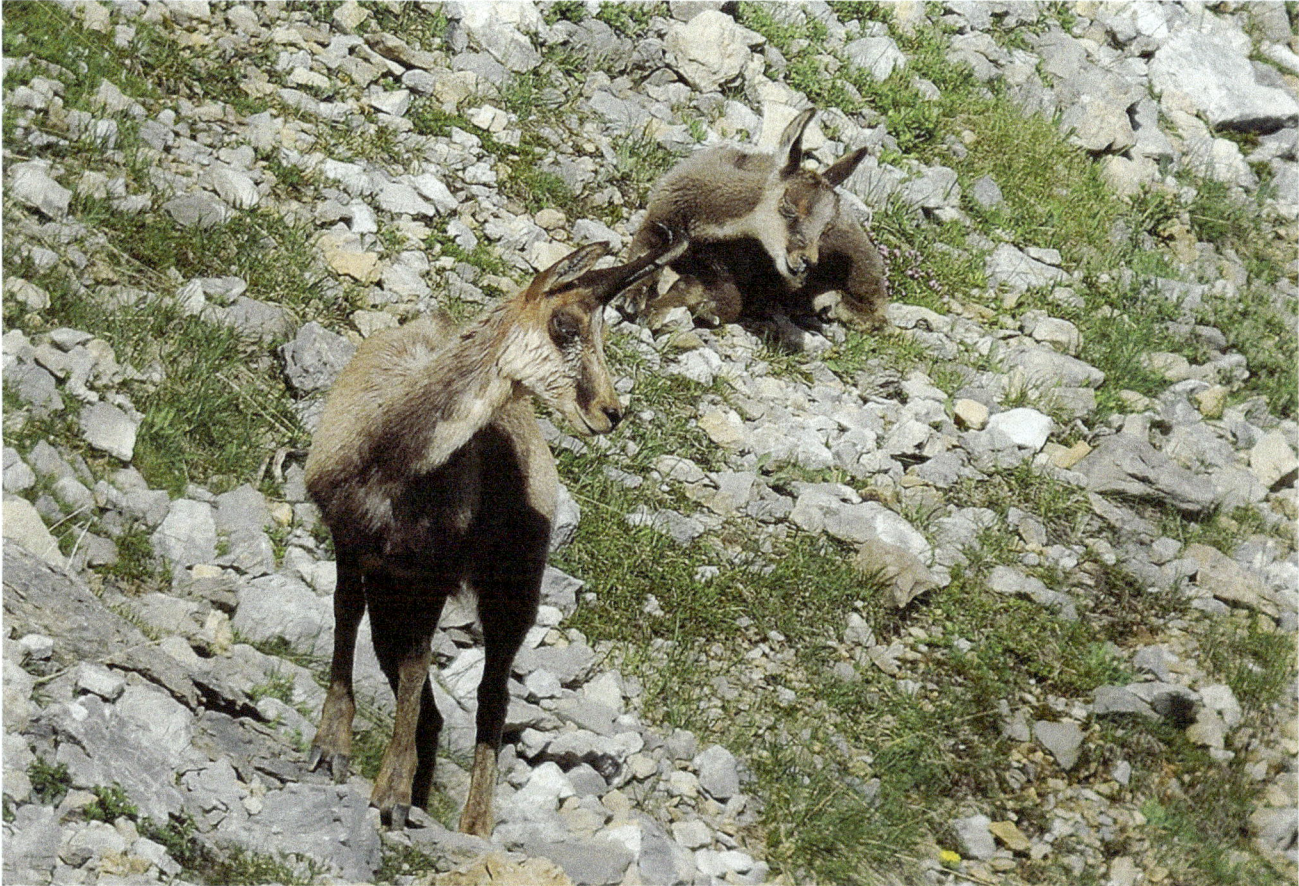

Figure 5. Adult female and kid affected with IKC.

time PCR system (Applied Biosystems) using the standardized parameters and the presence/absence endpoint assays. The amplification products were detected using the 7500 Software v2.0.3 Fast Systems (Applied Biosystems).

In addition, a conventional PCR for detecting *Mycoplasma* spp. [26] and specific detection assays for *M. agalactiae* [27] and *Mycoplasma mycoides* cluster members [28] were also performed in a total volume of 25 μl. Each amplification reaction mixture was prepared containing 200 mM of each deoxynucleoside triphosphate, 10 mM Tris-HCl, 2 mM MgCl2, 2 U Taq DNA polymerase (Bio Line, Barcelona, Spain), 0.2 mM of each corresponding primer pair, and 8 μl of template DNA. Amplification was performed in a DNA thermal I-cycler (Bio-Rad, Hercules, CA, USA). The PCR amplification products were run by gel electrophoresis on 1% (wt/vol) agarose gels and visualized using a UV transilluminator (Syngene, Frederick, MD, USA) after ethidium bromide staining.

Chlamydophila spp. We developed a *Chlamydophila* genus-specific real-time PCR that amplified a conserved region of 16S rRNA. All of the *Chlamydophila* 16S rRNA regions in the GenBank database were included in the design. We designed the primers Chl16S880F (5′-TATGCCGCCTGAGGAGTACAC; nucleotide (nt) 880–900) and Chl16S959R (5′-ACAAGCAGTGGAG-CATGTGG; nt 940–959), and the TaqMan MGB probe Chl16S904P (5′-FAM-CAAGGGTGAAACTC-MGB; nt 904–917) using the Primer Express software 3.0 (Applied Biosystems, Foster City, CA, USA). The primers amplify an 80 bp fragment of the conserved region of 16S rRNA. The specificity of the

oligonucleotides was confirmed using BLAST-N software (NCBI; www.ncbi.nlm.nih.gov). The assays used 2 μl of test sample, 900 nM of each primer, and 200 nM of probe in a 20 μl reaction mixture volume that contained Universal PCR Master Mix No AmpErase UNG (Applied Biosystems). An exogenous internal positive control (Applied Biosystems) was introduced into each reaction well. The DNA was amplified using the following cycling parameters: heating at 50°C for 2 min and at 95°C for 10 min, followed by 40 cycles of a two-stage temperature profile of 95°C for 15 s and 60°C for 1 min. The cycle threshold value (Ct) was calculated automatically.

The detection and quantification limits of the PCR assays were identified using genomic DNA isolated from the *Chlamydophila abortus* strain AB7. The standard curve (Ct values vs. log DNA copies) generated by eight serial dilutions of *C. abortus* was linear with an R^2 value of 0.9983, a slope of -3.5221, and the efficiency was very close to 2 (100% efficiency).

Statistical Analysis

Changes in the annual number of chamois as a function of time were analyzed using Poisson regression [29], [30], in which the dependent variable is a count that follows the Poisson distribution. We defined a generalized linear model fit with the GLM procedure of R [31] with the response variable given by the annual count of chamois, a Poisson error distribution, and a natural log link function for the exponential growth model for which the parameter b can be interpreted as r, the intrinsic rate of increase, and lambda λ comes from the r neperian antilog.

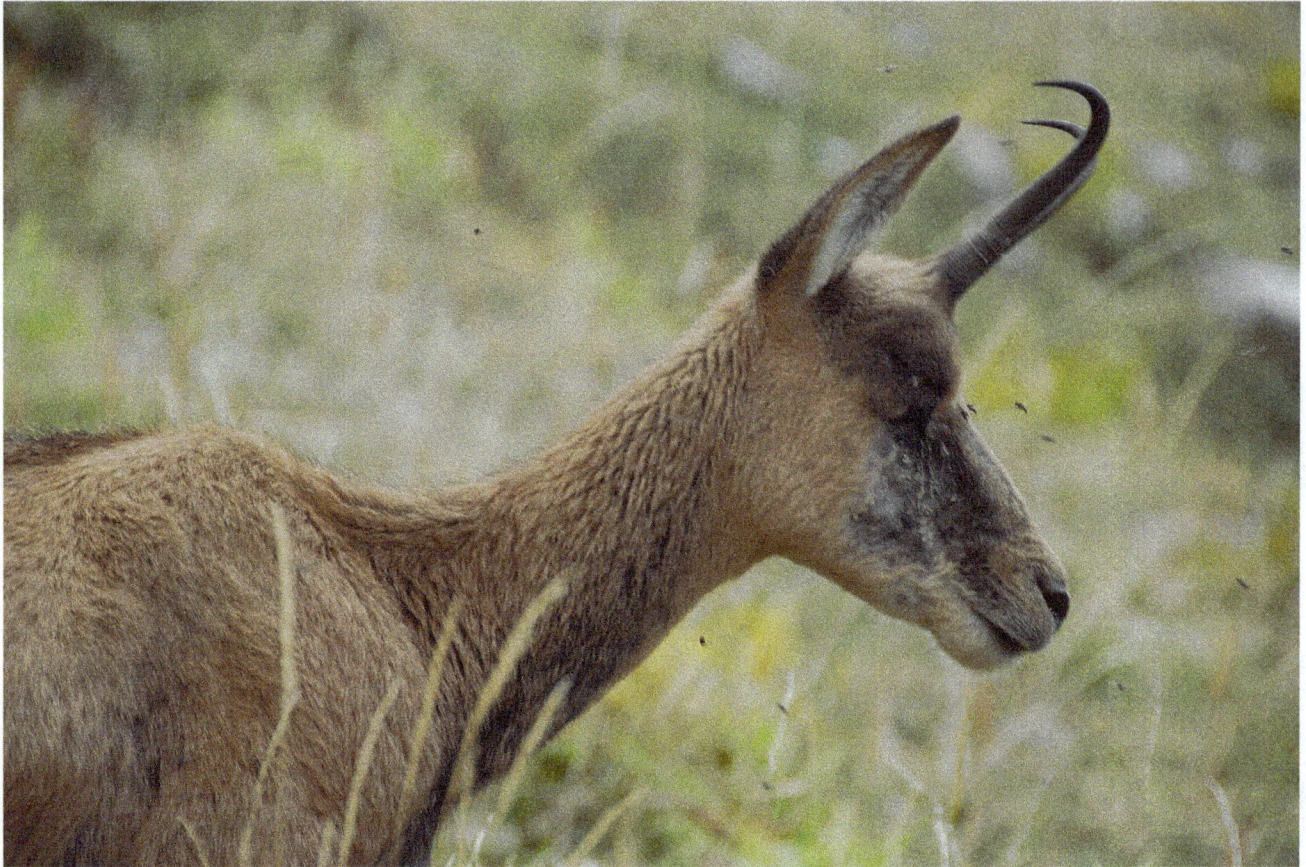

Figure 6. IKC-affected female whit many flies around the head.

We applied a logistic regression to data regarding presence or absence of *M. conjunctivae* in the sheep flocks in order to study the relation of this variable with the variables year, massif and flock. We used the Backward Stepwise method considering the likelihood ratio.

Means were compared using T test after the variables were tested for normality. We also used χ^2 test. These analyses were performed using SPSS (SPSS inc., Chicago, Illinois, USA).

Results

Outbreak Description

In summer 2006, an outbreak was detected in Ordesa and Monte Perdido National Park within Monte Perdido massif. By autumn 2006, it had spread eastward into Liena and, by summer 2007 reached Posets, where it persisted until autumn 2008. By spring 2007, the outbreak had spread westward to Biñamala. By summer 2007, the disease reached Anayet and, by spring 2008, chamois in Bixaurín and Larra-Peña Forca, the western limit of population, were affected. Stable populations in the Pre-Pyrenean massifs were not affected (Ezcaurre, Cotiella, Sierra Ferrera and Turbón) (Figure 2). Although sporadic cases were observed in the affected massifs, until autumn 2008, the outbreak did not recur in subsequent years and only lasted more than a year in Posets.

Population Trend

In the period 2000–2007, the chamois population increased slightly (λ 1.0301; 95% CI: 1.0275–1.0328; $p<0.001$) but it decreased significantly during the IKC outbreak (λ 0.8586; 95% CI: 0.8482–0.8691; $p<0.001$, 2007–2009), before increasing significantly after the outbreak (λ 1.1138; 95% CI: 1.0861–1.1422; $p<0.001$, 2009–2010) (Figure 3).

Changes in SR, Productivity, and Grouping

The average SR in the periods 2000–2007 (0.59; n = 8; SE = 0.00964; 95% CI: 0.5722–0.6178) and 2008–2010 (0.717; n = 3; SE = 0.00882; 95% CI: 0.6787–0.7546) differed significantly (t = −7.2; df = 9; $p<0.0001$) by 0.122 (SE = 0.017). The SR was between 0.08 and 0.16 higher after the outbreak.

Average productivity between 2000 and 2007 (0.708; n = 8; SE = 0.0144) was higher than it was between 2008 and 2010 (0.65; n = 3; SE = 0.03), and the difference was marginally statistically significant (t = 2, df = 9; $p = 0.082$). During the outbreak, individuals were observed as a singleton kid, kids with adult males only, and females with two or three kids.

Chamois Found Dead

Between 2006 and 2010, in the bi-monthly reports, 471 chamois were found dead within the study area (Figure 4). In 2010, only 16 chamois were found dead; however, in 2007 and 2008 mortality was substantial. About half of the deaths were recorded in 2007 (n = 220), particularly in summer (n = 103) and primarily in Biñamala (n = 93). In 2008 (n = 170), most of the dead animals were found in Larra-Peña Forca, Bixaurín, Anayet, and Posets. In Posets, the disease persisted between autumn 2007 and autumn 2008. Among the dead animals in these two years (2007–2008,

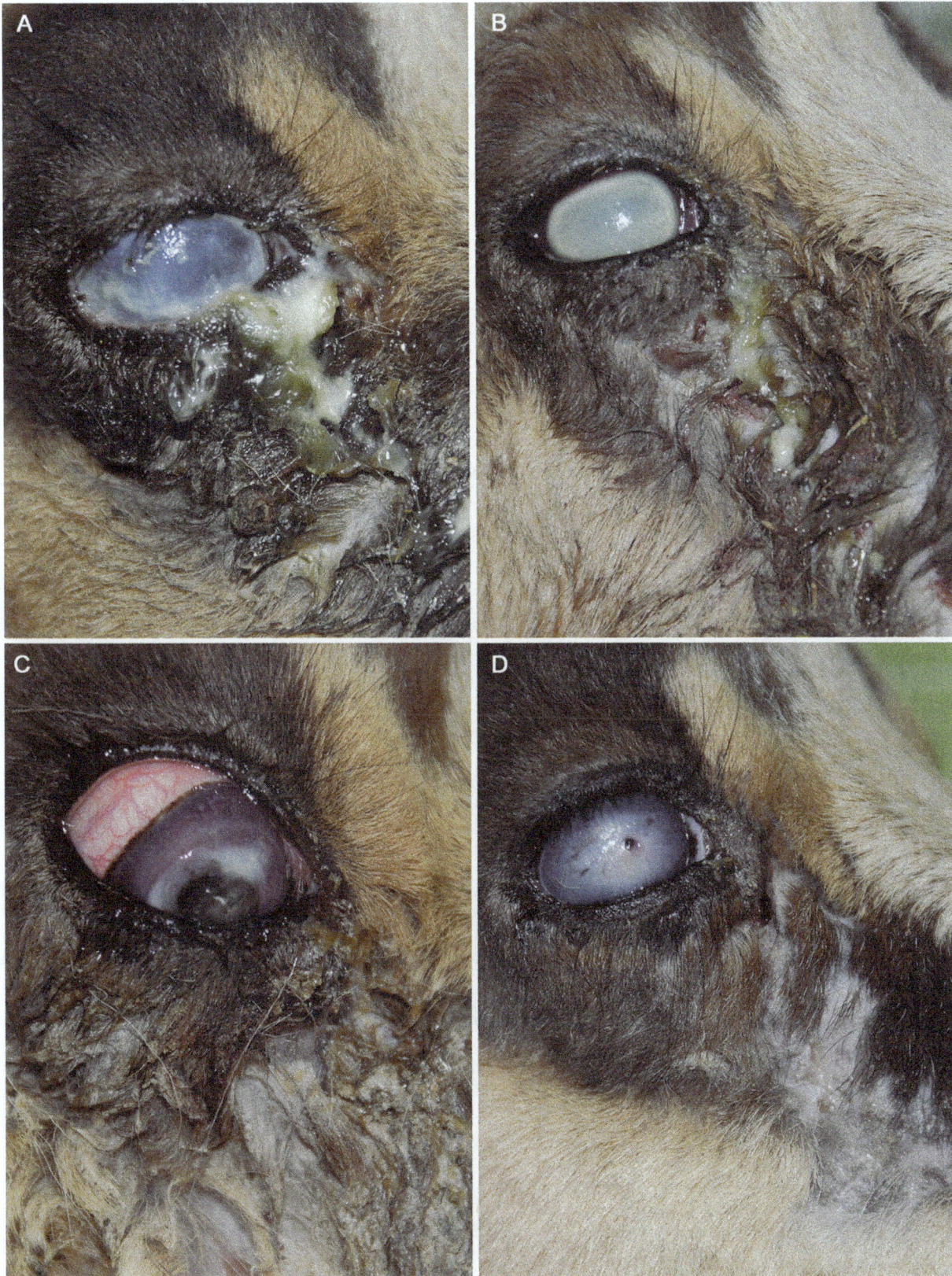

Figure 7. Stages lesion of IKC in Pyrenean chamois during 2006–2008 outbreak. Pictures show animals with different levels of disease severity. **A)** Purulent ocular lacrimation and mild corneal opacity (stage II). **B)** Corneal opacity (stage III). **C)** Late stage of IKC, with purulent exudation, evident conjunctivitis and corneal perforation (stage IV). **D)** Animal without lacrimation that had chronic corneal lesions showing the face without hair.

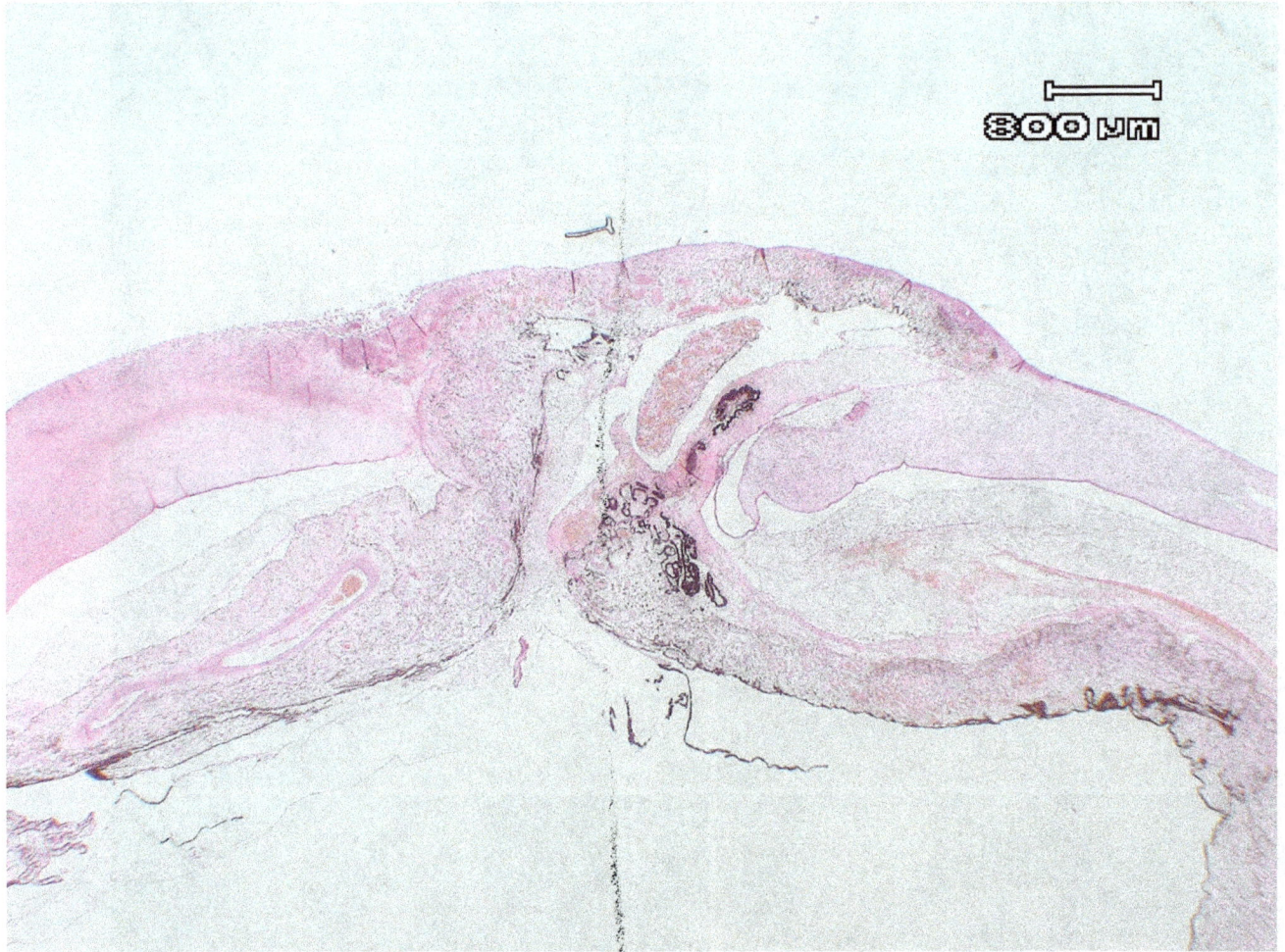

Figure 8. General view of the stage IV lesion of IKC in Pyrenean chamois. Note the ruptured Descemet's membrane and synechia with the incarcerated iris and severe keratitis.

n = 272), 66% were females and 34% were males, age was described by rangers in 316 animals, 70% were adults, 20% were yearlings, and 10% were kids (Table 1).

IKC-affected Chamois

Macroscopic and microscopic lesions. In this study, 105 Pyrenean chamois were analysed (Table 2). Eighty-one (77.1%) of them were euthanized after inspection and exhibited behavioural changes such as circling, disorientation, stumbling, and signs of

Table 3. Detection of *Mycoplasma conjunctivae* based on the ages and sexes of the animals checked (N = 105, 2006–2008).

Ages	Sex	Positive/tested (%)
Adults	Males	15/21 (71.5)
	Females	65/70 (92.9)
Yearlings/Kids	Males	4/5 (80)
	Females	9/9 (100)
Total		**93/105 (88.6)**

blindness (Figure 5–6). Another 24 chamois (22.8%) were found dead with signs of IKC. Among the dead animals, four were found drowned in mountain lakes, four had wounds consistent with dog bites, four had polytrauma, one had enterotoxaemia and three had been partially eaten after death. Eight of the 24 had no other injuries. The SR among the analysed animals (24.8% males, 75.2% females) was significantly more female-biased than the population before the outbreak (0.59, 2000–2007; χ^2 6.9; df = 1; $p = 0.009$). No IKC-affected animals were found in 2009 and 2010.

All the affected chamois had lacrimation which ranged from serous to purulent. Three animals exhibited alopecia under the eye, but without lacrimation, and 91.4% (96/105) of the animals had bilateral macroscopic lesions. Individuals exhibited conjunctivitis and corneal opacity at various stages of lesion development. Based on a classification of ocular lesions [32], 26% (25/96) were at stage II or III and 63.5% (61/96) were at stage IV (e.g., severe lesions in the cornea such as perforation with iris protrusion) (Figure 7).

Two animals had unilateral lesions with corneal opacity and ocular effusion; the other eye was normal, but there were crusts on the hair below the eye. Three animals had been partially eaten by predators had both eyeballs missing, and four had one eyeball. Among the eyes that were present, three had ocular perforations and one exhibited corneal opacity. Three animals without lacrimation had chronic corneal lesions; one had bilateral corneal opacity in the vertex, and the other two had lesions that were characterized by an incarcerated iris in the cornea, and one exhibited corneal retraction.

Animals in the early stages of the disease exhibited conjunctival hyperaemia, neutrophil and mononuclear cell infiltration, and lymphofollicular hyperplasia in the palpebral conjunctiva. Affected cornea exhibited inflammatory cells and vascular phenomena. In the advanced stages of the disease, the corneal epithelium was eroded, ulcerated, or perforated. Inflammatory cell infiltration and necrosis were present in the cornea. Most of the advanced cases exhibited ruptured Descemet's membrane and synechia with the incarcerated iris (Figure 8). No lesions associated with IKC were found in the lung, liver, heart, kidney, or central nervous system tissues.

Mycoplasma and *Chlamydophila spp*. Detection. *M. conjunctivae* was detected in 93 (88.6%) out of 105 affected chamois. The age and sex of the infected chamois are shown in Table 3. In addition, *Mycoplasma spp.* was detected in three samples that were negative for *M. conjunctivae* (25%, 3/12). All the specific PCR assays used to detect *M. agalactiae* or the members of the *M. mycoides* cluster were negative. Fourteen samples tested positive for *Chlamydophila spp.* and 12 were positive for both *Chlamydophila spp.* and *M. conjunctivae*.

IKC-non-affected Ruminants

Eight (4.2%) of the 190 chamois that did not have IKC signs, tested positive for *M. conjunctivae*. Among the animals sampled, prevalence was slightly, but not significantly higher during the outbreak (6.5%, 7/108) (95% CI: 2–11.15) than after (1.2%; 1/82) (95% CI: 0–3.6). None of the roe deer or red deer tested positive.

Sheep

In 2008, among a sample of 349 animals from 17 flocks, *M. conjunctivae* was identified 102 times (29.2%; 95% CI: 24.5–34.3) and 15 flocks (82.3%; 95% CI: 56.6–96.2) tested positive. In 2009, among 268 animals from 15 flocks it was identified 57 times (21.3%; 95% CI: 16.5–26.7) and 13 flocks (84.6%; 95% CI: 54.6–98.1) tested positive. No significant differences were detected in the prevalence between years and between massifs. However, significant differences were observed between flocks (R^2 Nagelkerke = 0.250; $p<0.01$).

Management Actions

In the most affected GR (3) and massifs (8), hunting was banned until new population estimation was performed after the end of the outbreak. A small hunting quota (<1% extraction) was given to hunting ground owners (municipalities and communal owners) in two of the GR because of the economic importance of hunting to local communities, until a new population estimation was performed in the following year.

Discussion

During the 2006–2008 IKC-outbreak, the spread of the disease was continuous and did not recur in the areas where it had already occurred, affecting a significant number of Pyrenean chamois and killing many animals. Recovery of the population was spontaneous. In most cases, reductions in infections and mortality paralleled the arrival of cold temperatures (a seasonal pattern), although a mild winter allowed the disease to persist until spring (no seasonality), as described in the Alps [5], [33].

In this outbreak, the distribution of dead animals among age classes did not differ significantly from the population at large, but adult females experienced significantly higher mortality than did adult males. Other studies have also found that mortality is biased toward adult females, but did not report the age-sex class structure of the population [5], [33].

The reduction of size of the population was similar to IKC responses in the Alps [5], [6], [13], [34]. It has been suggested that the mortality rates in subsequent outbreaks of IKC are lower than in the first outbreak [35]. We suspect that the 2006–2008 outbreak produced less mortality than the outbreaks in the late 1970s and the early 1980s in the Aragonese Pyrenees. The recovery after the outbreak showed an important annual increase, much larger than the pre-outbreak period.

In 2006–2008, *M. conjunctivae* was the main causal agent of the IKC outbreak, as reported in affected Pyrenean chamois in the Central Pyrenees, Spain [7]. The results also support the role of *M. conjunctivae* as the main aetiological agent of IKC in wild *Caprinae* [5], as previously reported in the Alps [4–6]. *M. conjunctivae* was common in all samples tested and despite the poor condition of some samples (e.g., partially eaten, frozen or in advanced stages of lesion), which underscored the benefits of the rt-PCR test for the routine diagnosis of *M. conjunctivae* [25]. However, the detection of this microorganism proved negative in 12 samples. It is possible that some or all of these were false-negatives because they were taken from animals in an advanced state of autolysis and, in three cases, with chronic corneal lesions. The lesion may suggest that the agent was no longer present, but other studies have demonstrated the temporary persistence of *M. conjunctivae* in the eyes of experimentally infected Alpine ibex [36]. Secondary bacterial infections of the conjunctiva and eye, contamination during sampling and extended period storage before analysis might have led to the absence of mycoplasma, which increases the difficulty of monitoring IKC in wild populations [7].

As in recent studies in Alpine chamois [37], in our study, mixed infections were associated with the outbreak of the Pyrenees. *Mycoplasma* and *Chlamydophila spp.* were found together in a significant number of animals, which indicated a possible occasional presence [38] or confirmed previous reports suggesting *Chlamydophila spp.* as a causal agent of IKC [10], [11]. *Chlamydophila spp.* was considered the most important species associated with IKC in the Pyrenees [16], although this might be because of the unusual difficulties involved in detecting a fastidious microorganism such as *M. conjunctivae*. Furthermore, in our study, *Chlamydophila spp.* was detected alone in two animals, which suggests either that it was an IKC infection caused by this bacterium only, or *M. conjunctivae* disappeared before the samples were analysed.

In addition, we detected non-identified mycoplasmas in conjunctiva samples, which had been found in Iberian wild goat *Capra pyrenaica* [39]. Other mycoplasma species such as *M. arginini*, which have been detected in the conjunctiva of other wild and domestic ruminants [39], [40], might have been present in the animals examined, usually associated with mixed infection.

Some mycoplasma species are known to cause keratoconjunctivitis in domestic small ruminant populations; such as *M. agalactiae*, and *M. mycoides* cluster members. Those species have been found in the conjunctiva of some wild ruminants such as the Iberian wild goat [39]. Other authors [41] have reported that many Iberian wild goats have been infected by *M. agalactiae* in southern Spain, which suggests that there is the potential for interspecific transmission between domestic and wild ruminants in that area. Those species were not agents of the IKC outbreak in Pyrenean chamois, which suggested a different epidemiological role of the various wild ruminants as carriers of contagious agalactia causing agents.

Some of the male samples were in poor condition or in advanced stages of lesion, which made it difficult to identify the agent. Field observations demonstrated that females and juveniles in herds were easier to detect by human observers than were male chamois, which are solitary for most of the year [42], [43]. In our study, most of the chamois examined were adults, and infections were biased toward females. In some cases, the largely solitary life of adult males might help them to eliminate the infection because the infection period in wild *Caprinae* appears to be temporary [6], [36], and does not exceed 6 months in sheep [44]. This behaviour could help avoid re-infections. As in populations of other wild Alpine *Caprinae*, the prevalence of *M. conjunctivae* in healthy Pyrenean chamois carried was low [45].

Early lesions were observed less frequently during the histopathological study. No animals were found at stage I because the game rangers documented only those animals that had evidence of blindness, which is apparent only when the ocular lesions are in an advanced stage [32]. No lesions associated with IKC were found in the histological sections of encephalon, which was previously described in Alpine chamois affected with IKC [46]. The histopathological lesions found in the eyes might not have been associated with a specific agent because *Chlamydophila spp.*- and *M. conjunctivae*-positive animals did not differ [1], [32].

Sheep farmers did not encounter more cases of IKC in the years of the outbreak (2006–2008); as also occurred in IKC-affected bighorn sheep foraged among domestic goats (Arizona, USA), which did not exhibit ocular signs [47], however, during outbreaks in mule deer in Utah, USA, and in chamois in the Central Pyrenees, Spain, cattle and, domestic sheep and goats, were affected, respectively [11], [15].

In the Suisse Alps, IKC persists in sheep, but not in chamois, being endemic in some areas. The transmission occurred in shared pastures between infected sheep and chamois, through flies and wind [2]. The specific dynamics in Pyrenean chamois outbreak might indicate that flies are more actives in warm season and probably imply more risk than wind to spread the disease.

IKC outbreaks in sheep [40] and wild ruminants have been linked to the introduction of new animals that did not have ocular

signs, but were carriers of *M. conjunctivae* [47]. In our study, livestock were not affected by *M. conjunctivae*, which might suggest their involvement in the outbreak as asymptomatic carriers and that other factors were involved at the onset of the outbreak [48].

Our study demonstrates that *M. conjunctivae* is widespread among grazing sheep in all of the GR of the Aragonese Pyrenees; however, the persistence of infection in chamois is sporadic. Interactions with domestic sheep and other factors might have initiated the infection in chamois and its spread to other areas by the movements of infected animals. Not all of *M. conjunctivae* strains carried by sheep are transmitted to chamois or cause IKC [49]; therefore it is necessary to determine which of these strains were responsible for the outbreak.

In the Pyrenees, despite the restrictions on hunting rights and the negative economic impact, local hunters and municipalities agreed on a hunting ban. This was possible because of the strong implication of these interest groups in the management of the Pyrenean chamois population, specifically, through their participation on the advisory boards of the GR.

Long-term monitoring of the Pyrenean chamois population provided a basis for understanding the effect of the outbreaks, which improved management decisions, particularly important in a species subjected to extractive exploitation.

Acknowledgments

The authors acknowledge the dedicated assistance of the game rangers. We thank Dr. E. Vilei (University of Berne, Switzerland) for providing *Mycoplasma conjunctivae* purified DNA, and Dr. N. Ortega (University of Murcia, Spain) for providing *Chlamydophila abortus* purified DNA. We also would like to thank Cristina Acín and Morris Villarroel for a critical review of a previous draft.

Author Contributions

Critically revised manuscript: MCA JH CF MR CP DMD AGM OFA JA AC AGS DFL. Conceived and designed the experiments: MCA JH CF AC DFL. Performed the experiments: MCA JH CF MR CP DMD AGM OFA JA AGS DFL. Analyzed the data: MCA JH CF AGS DFL. Contributed reagents/materials/analysis tools: MCA MR CP DMD AGM OFA JA. Wrote the paper: MCA JH CF DFL.

References

1. Hosie BD (2000) Ocular diseases. In: Martin WB, Aitken ID editors. Diseases of Sheep, 3rd Edition, Blackwell Science Ltd. 301–305.

2. Giacometti M, Janovsky M, Jenny H, Nicolet J, Belloy L, et al. (2002) *Mycoplasma conjunctivae* infection is not maintained in Alpine chamois in eastern Switzerland. J Wildl Dis 38: 297–304.

3. Egwu GO, Faull WB, Bradbury JM, Clarkson MJ (1989) Ovine infectious keratoconjunctivitis: A microbiological study of clinically unaffected and affected sheep's eyes with special reference to *Mycoplasma conjunctivae*. Vet Rec 125: 253–256.

4. Grattarola C, Frey J, Abdo EM, Orusa R, Nicolet J, et al. (1999) *Mycoplasma conjunctivae* infections in chamois and ibexes affected with infectious keratoconjunctivitis in the Italian Alps. Vet Rec 145: 588–589.

5. Giacometti M, Janovsky L, Belloy L, Frey J (2002) Infectious keratoconjunctivitis of ibex, chamois and other Caprinae. Rev Sci Tech Off Int Epiz 21: 335–345.

6. Tschopp R, Frey J, Zimmermann L, Giacometti M (2005) Outbreaks of infectious keratoconjunctivitis in alpine chamois and ibex in Switzerland between 2001 and 2003. Vet Rec 157: 13–18.

7. Marco I, Mentaberre G, Ballesteros C, Bischof D, Lavín S, et al. (2009) First report of Mycoplasma conjunctivae from wild caprinae with infectious keratoconjunctivits in the Pyrenees (NE Spain). J Wildl Dis 45: 238–241.

8. Cugnase JM (1997) L'enzootie de kérato-conjonctivite chez le mouflon méditerranéen (*Ovis gmelini musimon* x *Ovis* sp.) du massif du Caroux-Espinouse (Hérault) à l'automne 1993. Gibier faune sauvage, Game and Wildlife 14: 569–584.

9. Daniel MJ, Christie AHC (1963) Untersuchungen über Krankheiten der Gemse (*Rupicapra rupicapra* L.) und des Thars (*Hemitragus jemlaicus* Smith) in den Südalpen von Neuseeland. Schweiz Arch Tierh 105: 399–411.

10. Meagher M, Quinn WJ, Stackhouse L (1992) Chlamydial-caused infectious keratoconjunctivitis in bighorn sheep of Yellowstone National Park. J Wildl Dis. 28: 171–176.

11. Taylor SK, Vieira VG, Williams ES, Pilkington R, Fedorchak SL, et al. (1996) Infectious keratoconjunctivitis in free-ranging mule deer (*Odocoileus hemionus*) from Zion National Park, Utah. J Wildl Dis 32: 326–330.

12. Dubay SA, Williams EE, Mills K, Boerger-Fields AM (2000) Association of *Moraxella ovis* with keratoconjunctivitis in mule deer and moose in Wyoming. J Wildl Dis 36: 241–247.

13. Loison A, Gaillard JM, Jullien JM (1996) Demographic patterns after an epizootic of keratoconjunctivitis in a chamois population. J Wildl Manage 60 (3): 517–527.

14. Sánchez A, Martínez J (1985) Contribution au diagnostique de la kerato-conjonctivite du chamois (*Rupicapra rupicapra*) en Espagne. In: Balbo T, Lanfranchi P, Rossi L, Stero P editors. Atti del Simposio internazionale sulla cheratocongiuntivite infettiva del camoscio. University of Torino, Torino, Italy, 73–77.

15. Marco I, Lavín S, Gonzalo J, Viñas L (1992) Estudio de un brote de querato-conjuntivitis infecciosa en los rebecos (*Rupicapra pyrenaica*) del Pirineo leridano. Veterinaria en Praxis 6: 57–62.

16. Blanco A, Marcotegui MA, de Frutos I, de la Esperanza P, Sáez C (1982) Queratoconjuntivitis clamidial en el rebeco (*Rupicapra rupicapra* ssp. *pyrenaica*). INIA: Serie Ganadera 17: 79–85.

17. Herrero J, Garin I, Prada C, García-Serrano A (2010) Inter-agency coordination fosters the recovery of the Pyrenean chamois *Rupicapra pyrenaica pyrenaica* at its western limit. Oryx, 44(4): 529–532.

18. Herrero J, Escudero E, García JM, García-Serrano A, Prada C, et al. (2004) Management and survey of the Pyrenean chamois in the Aragonian Pyrenees.

In: Herrero J, Escudero E, Fernández de Luco D, García-González R editors. The Pyrenean Chamois *Rupicapra p. pyrenaica*: Biology, Pathology and Management. Publications of the Council for the Protection of Nature, Government of Aragon, Saragossa, Spain. 69–83.

19. Arnal MC, Fernández de Luco D (2004) Sanitary survey of Pyrenean chamois in the Aragonian Pyrenees (1997–2002). In: Herrero J, Escudero E, Fernández de Luco D, García-González R editors. The Pyrenean Chamois *Rupicapra p. pyrenaica*: Biology, Pathology and Management. Publications of the Council for the Protection of Nature, Government of Aragon, Saragossa, Spain. 125–132.

20. Herrero J, García-Serrano A, Garin I, García-González R (1996) Habitat use in a forest *Rupicapra pyrenaica pyrenaica* population. Forest Ecol Manag 88: 25–29.

21. García-González R, Hidalgo R, Ameztoy JM, Herrero J (1992). Census, population structure and habitat use of chamois population in Ordesa N.P. living in sympatry with the Pyrenean wild goat. In: Spitz F, Janeau G, Gonzalez G, Aulagnier S editors, Ongulés/Ungulates 91. SFEPMIRGM, Toulouse, 321–325.

22. Marco J, Herrero J, Escudero MA, Fernández-Arberas O, Ferreres J, et al. (2011) Veinte años de seguimiento poblacional de ungulados silvestres de Aragón. Pirineos. Revista de Ecología de Montaña 166: 135–153.

23. Gortázar C, Herrero J, Villafuerte R, Marco J (2000) Historical examination of the status of large mammals in Aragon, Spain. Mammalia 64 (4): 411–422.

24. Berducou C, JP Besson, Gardes Moniteurs du P.N.P.O. (1982) Dynamique des populations d'isards du Parc National des Pyrénées Occidentales de 1968–1981. Acta Biol Montana 1: 153–175.

25. Vilei EM, Bonvin-Klotz L, Zimmermann L, Degiorgis MP, Giacometti M, et al. (2007) Validation and diagnostic efficacy of a TaqMan real-time PCR for the detection of *Mycoplasma conjunctivae* in eyes of infected Caprinae. J Microbiol Methods 70: 384–386.

26. Van Kuppeveld FJ, Johansson KE, Galama JM, Kissing J, Bölske G, et al. (1994) Detection of mycoplasma contamination in cell cultures by a mycoplasma group-specific PCR. Appl Environ Microbiol 60: 149–152.

27. Marenda MS, Sagné E, Poumarat F, Citti C (2005) Suppression subtractive hybridization as a basis to assess *Mycoplasma agalactiae* and *Mycoplasma bovis* genomic diversity and species-specific sequences. Microbiol 151: 475–489.

28. Hotzel H, Sachse K, Pfützner H (1996) A PCR scheme for differentiation of organisms belonging to the *Mycoplasma mycoides* cluster. Vet Microbiol 49: 31–43.

29. Kleinbaum DG, Lawrence KL, Keith ME (1988) Applied regression analysis and other multivariable methods. 2nd edition. The Duxbury Series in Statistics and Decision Sciences. PWS-KENT Publishing Co., Boston, Mssachusetts, USA.

30. Domenech JM, Navarro JB (2005) Regresión logística binaria, multinomial y de Poisson. Signo, Barcelona, Spain.

31. R Development Core Team (2012) R: A language and environment for statistical computing. R Foundation for Statistical Computing, Vienna, Austria. ISBN 3-900051-07-0. Available: http://www.R-project.org. Accessed 2013 Feb 28.

32. Mayer D, Degiorgis MP, Meier W, Nicolet J, Giacometti M (1997) Lesions associated with infectious keratoconjunctivitis in alpine ibex. J Wildl Dis 33: 413–419.

33. Degiorgis MP, Frey J, Nicolet J, Abdo EM, Fatzer R, et al. (2000) An outbreak of infectious keratoconjunctivitis in Apine chamois, (*Rupicapra r.rupicapra*) in Simmental-Gruyères, Switzerland. Schweiz Arch Thierheilk 142 (9): 520–527.

34. Balbo T, Lanfranchi P, Rossi L (1985) Parasitological and Pathological Observations on the Chamois in the Western Alps. In: Lovari S editor. The

Biology and Management of Mountain Ungulates. Proceedings of the Fourth International Conference on Chamois and other Mountain Ungulates, held in Pescasseroli, Abruzzo National Park, Italy, June 17–19 1983. Editorial Croom Helm, London, UK.

35. Gauthier D (1991) La kérato-conjunctivitie infectieuse du chamois. Etude épidémiologique dans le départemente de la Savoie, 1983–1990. PhD Thesis. Université de Lyon, Lyon, France.

36. Giacometti M, Nicolet J, Frey J, Krawinkler M, Meier W, et al. (1998) Susceptibility of alpine ibex to conjunctivitis caused by instillation of a sheep-strain of *Mycoplasma conjunctivae*. Vet Microbiol 61: 279–288.

37. Holzwarth N, Pospischil A, Mavrot F, Vilei EM, Hilbe M, et al. (2011) Occurrence of *Chlamydiaceae, Mycoplasma conjunctivae*, and pestiviruses in Alpine chamois (*Rupicapra r. rupicapra*) of Grisons, Switzerland. J Vet Diagn Invest 23(2): 333–7.

38. Polkinghorne A, Borel N, Becker A, Lu ZH, Zimmermann DR, et al. (2009) Molecular evidence for chlamydial infections in the eyes of sheep. Vet Microbiol 135: 142–6.

39. González-Candela M, Verbisck-Buker G, Martín-Atance P, Cubero-Pablo MJ, León-Vizcaíno L (2007) Mycoplasmas isolated from Spanish ibex (*Capra pyrenaica hispanica*): frequency and risk factors. Vet Rec 161: 167–168.

40. Naglić T, Hajsig D, Frey J, Šeol B, Busch K, et al. (2000) Epidemiological and microbiological study of an outbreak of infectious keratoconjunctivitis in sheep. Vet Rec 147: 72–75.

41. Verbisck-Bucker G, González-Candela M, Galián J, Cubero-Pablo MJ, Martín-Atance P, et al. (2008) Epidemiology of *Mycoplasma agalactiae* infection in free-ranging Spanish ibex (*Capra pyrenaica*) in Andalusia, southern Spain. J Wildl Dis 44: 369–380.

42. Berducou C, Bousses P (1985) Social grouping patterns of a dense population of chamois in the western Pyrenees national Park, France. In: Lovari S editor. The biology and management of mountain ungulates. Editorial Croom Helm, London, UK, 166–175.

43. Herrero J, Garín I, García-Serrano A, García-González R, Aldezábal A (2002) Grouping patterns in a forest dwelling population of Pyrenean chamois. Pirineos 157: 89–101.

44. Janovsky M, Frey J, Nicolet J, Belloy L, Goldschmidt-Clermont E, et al. (2001) *Mycoplasma conjunctivae* infection is self-maintained in the Swiss domestic sheep population. Vet Microbiol 83: 11–22.

45. Mavrot F, Vilei EM, Marreros N, Signer C, Frey J, et al. (2012) Occurrence, quantification, and genotyping of Mycoplasma conjunctivae in wild Caprinae with and without infectious keratoconjunctivitis. J Wildl Dis 48(3): 619–31.

46. Bassano B, Bollo E, Peracino V, Guarda F (1994) Brain lesions associated with infectious keratoconjunctivitis in chamois and Alpine ibex. Ibex J Mount Ecol 2: 17–22.

47. Jansen BD, Heffelfinger JR, Noon TH, Krausman PR, deVos JC (1996) Infectious keratoconjunctivitis in Bighorn Sheep, Silver Bell Mountains, Arizona, USA. J Wildl Dis 42: 407–411.

48. Egwu GO (1991) Ovine infectious keratoconjunctivitis: an update. Vet Bull 61: 547–559.

49. Zimmermann L, Jambresic S, Giacometti M, Frey J (2008) Specificity of *Mycoplasma conjunctivae* strains for alpine *Rupicapra r.rupicapra*. Wildlife Biol 14: 118–124.

5

Trends in Patterns of Intermediate Uveitis in a Tertiary Institution

Helen Mi[1], Su L. Ho[2], Wee K. Lim[2,3], Elizabeth P. Y. Wong[2], Stephen C. Teoh[2,3]*

1 Yong Loo Lin School of Medicine, National University of Singapore, Singapore, Singapore, 2 National Healthcare Group Eye Institute, Tan Tock Seng Hospital, Singapore, Singapore, 3 Eagle Eye Centre, Singapore, Singapore

Abstract

Purpose: The study aims to describe the characteristics and etiologic causes of intermediate uveitis (IU) patients seen by a tertiary eye center in Singapore over 8 years.

Methods: This was a retrospective analysis of the clinical records of consecutive new cases of IU that presented to the uveitis subspecialty clinic from 2004–2011 at Tan Tock Seng Hospital. Data collected included demographics, clinical and laboratory findings. Diagnoses were based on standardized clinical history, ophthalmological examination and investigations.

Results: There were 66 new cases of IU, comprising 5.7% of 1168 new uveitis patients. The median age of diagnosis was 40 years (mean 39.4 ± 15.9), with largest subgroup of the patients in the age group of 41–60 years (36.4%). The majority was Chinese (57.6%), followed by Asian Indians (18.2%) and Malays (16.7%). The ethnicity distribution was dissimilar to our ethnic distribution in Singapore ($p<0.001$) with an increased incidence of IU in the Asian Indian population. Most were idiopathic (59.1%) in etiology, followed by tuberculosis (TB) (15.2%). Ocular complications developed in 21 patients (31.8%), with cystoid macular edema (CME) being the commonest (28.8%). Severe vitritis occurred in 9.1% of patients, and was significantly associated with TB-associated IU ($p<0.001$). There was a downward trend for the incidence of the proportion of IU patients over the total uveitis patients ($p=0.021$), with Spearman's rho of -0.786.

Conclusions: Despite the downward trend, TB-associated IU was still of higher prevalence compared to less endemic areas, emphasizing the need for increased TB surveillance. A high index of suspicion for TB-associated IU is required in patients with severe vitritis. Comparisons with other countries revealed disparities in the IU etiologies, indicating possible geographical differences. Prevalence of known immune-mediated etiologies of IU is less compared to the western population. Our study also suggests a probable predisposition of the Singapore local Indian population for IU.

Editor: James T. Rosenbaum, Oregon Health & Science University, United States of America

Funding: The authors have no support or funding to report.

Competing Interests: The authors have declared that no competing interests exist.

* E-mail: Stephen_Teoh@ttsh.com.sg

Introduction

Intermediate uveitis (IU) is the form of uveitis least commonly associated with a systemic disorder [1–2], with its etiological patterns not well-described in the literature [2–5], especially in an Asian multi-racial population. The anatomical classification of IU was based on the criteria of the International Uveitis Study Group (IUSG) [6]. This classification was affirmed by the Standardization of Uveitis Nomenclature (SUN) Working Group, which defined IU as a subset of uveitis where vitreous is the major site of inflammation, with or without peripheral vascular sheathing and macular edema [7].

IU can be associated with systemic infectious diseases, or known immune-mediated illness such as sarcoidosis and multiple sclerosis (MS) [8]. Geographical, demographic and ethnic factors may influence its pattern [3–4,9]. Improvement in diagnostic techniques may also change the apparent prevalence of etiological diagnoses [5]. Studies of the distribution of the various types and causes of uveitis are important in aiding the clinician in the appropriate and focused approach to investigation, diagnosis and management [10]. Comprehending the global variations in epidemiology of IU patterns is crucial for comparison of treatment practices, optimal assessment, management and complications of IU. By investigating trends of the etiologies of IU, patterns of various diseases in the population may also be identified and monitored.

We had previously described the clinical characteristics and changing trends in patterns of etiologies among anterior uveitis (AU) patients seen by the uveitis service of a tertiary eye care center in Singapore [11]. Currently, we aim to report the pattern of etiology trends and clinical characteristics in patients with IU seen similarly by the uveitis service at our center over an 8-year period.

Materials and Methods

We retrospectively analyzed the case records of all consecutive new cases seen at the Uveitis and Ocular Inflammation service of

Table 1. Comparison of demographic details of uveitis patients and the Singapore population.

Etiology	IU	AU	Posterior uveitis	Panuveitis	Singapore (Thousands)
Number of patients/people (n, %)	66 (5.7)	795 (68.1)	177 (15.2)	130 (11.1)	3789.3
Gender					
Male	30 (45.5)	484 (60.9)	97 (54.8)	71 (54.6)	1868.2 (49.3)
Female	36 (54.5)	311 (39.1)	80 (45.2)	59 (45.4)	1921.1 (50.7)
Laterality					
Bilateral	37 (56.1)	157 (19.7)	67 (37.9)	36 (27.7)	–
Race					
Chinese	38 (57.6)	564 (70.9)	98 (55.4)	90 (69.2)	2808.3 (74.1)
Malay	11 (16.7)	91 (11.4)	29 (16.4)	18 (13.8)	506.6 (13.4)
Asian Indians	12 (18.2)	73 (9.2)	21 (11.9)	8 (6.2)	349.0 (9.2)
Others	5 (7.6)	67 (8.4)	29 (16.4)	14 (10.8)	125.3 (3.3)
Age Groups					
0–20	11 (16.7)	24 (3.0)	11 (6.2)	8 (6.2)	897.5 (23.7)
21–40	23 (34.8)	225 (28.3)	76 (42.9)	41 (31.5)	1131.5 (29.9)
41–60	24 (36.4)	329 (41.4)	70 (39.5)	43 (33.1)	1199.4 (31.7)
>60	8 (12.1)	217 (27.3)	20 (11.3)	37 (28.5)	560.8 (14.8)

Tan Tock Seng Hospital (TTSH), Singapore. Diagnosis of IU was made at presentation, and classification of IU was done according to the International Uveitis Study Group (IUSG) [6] recommendations and affirmed by SUN Working Group [7] criteria described earlier. To obtain diagnoses for specific ocular entities or systemic disease associations, all IU patients underwent a standardized clinical history, systemic review, complete ophthalmological examination and standardized laboratory investigations. Laboratory tests, included a complete blood count (CBC), erythrocyte sedimentation rate (ESR), C-reactive protein (CRP), syphilis screen consisting of Venereal Disease Research Laboratory (VDRL), and treponemal serology (syphilis IgG) tests, immune markers consisting of rheumatoid factor (RF), anti-double-stranded deoxyribonucleic acid (DNA) (anti-dsDNA), anti-neutrophil cytoplasmic antibodies (ANCA), chest radiograph, *Mantoux* skin test and/or tuberculosis (TB) interferon gamma release assay (IGRA) (T-SPOT.*TB*, Oxford Immunotec Ltd, U.K.). Further ancillary investigations were performed based on clinical presentation and signs where necessary, including polymerase chain reaction (PCR) DNA analysis, serologic IgG analysis, and human leukocyte antigen (HLA) typing and vitreous biopsy. Magnetic resonance imaging was considered and performed if patients exhibited neurological symptoms or signs suggestive of MS.

The criteria for the most commonly diagnosed diseases in this cohort were as follows. Presumed TB-associated uveitis was diagnosed when there was exclusion of other known etiologies of uveitis, suggestive clinical history and signs, supportive investigations such as positive *Mantoux* reaction, TB IGRA and chest radiograph findings, and response to empirical anti-tuberculosis treatment, and in some, evidence of *Mycobacterium tuberculosis* or its DNA in ocular fluid/tissues [12–13]. Fuchs heterochromic iridocyclitis (FHI) was diagnosed when there are uveitis with

characteristic white stellate keratic precipitates, diffuse iris stromal atrophy with variable iris pigment epithelial atrophy and iris color changes [14]. All other systemic diseases were diagnosed according to current diagnostic criteria, with referral to the respective specialists. The term idiopathic was used for cases in which the intraocular inflammation was not characteristic of a recognized uveitic entity or could not be attributed to a specific underlying systemic disease. FHI was considered to be idiopathic. Severe vitritis was defined as IU with grade >2+ haze [5,15]. Masquerade syndrome was excluded if patients responded to standard immunosuppressive therapy.

Data collected included the demographics of the patients, including gender, race, age at presentation, year at presentation and eye(s) affected, as well as clinical and laboratory results. Other systemic co-morbidities and medical history were also noted. All descriptive data were entered into a computerized database system for descriptive analysis, and analyzed with IBM SPSS Statistics (version 19, IBM Corp, New York, USA) and R version 2.14.1. Fisher's Exact test was used to determine any association between etiologies with ethnicity, as well as etiologies with complications. Bonferroni correction was done for the comparison between the local ethnic distribution in Singapore and the ethnic distribution in our study, with statistical significance defined to be p<0.0167. Categorical-type data were analyzed with Pearson Chi-Square goodness-of-fit test, specifically the comparison of ethnic distribution between the data collected and the Singapore population. Spearman's rho was used to check for linear tendencies of etiologies and IU patients from 2004–2011. A p-value less than 0.05 was considered to indicate statistical significance.

The investigation adhered to the tenets of the Declaration of Helsinki. The study protocol obtained Institutional Review Board (IRB) approval from the National Healthcare Group Domain

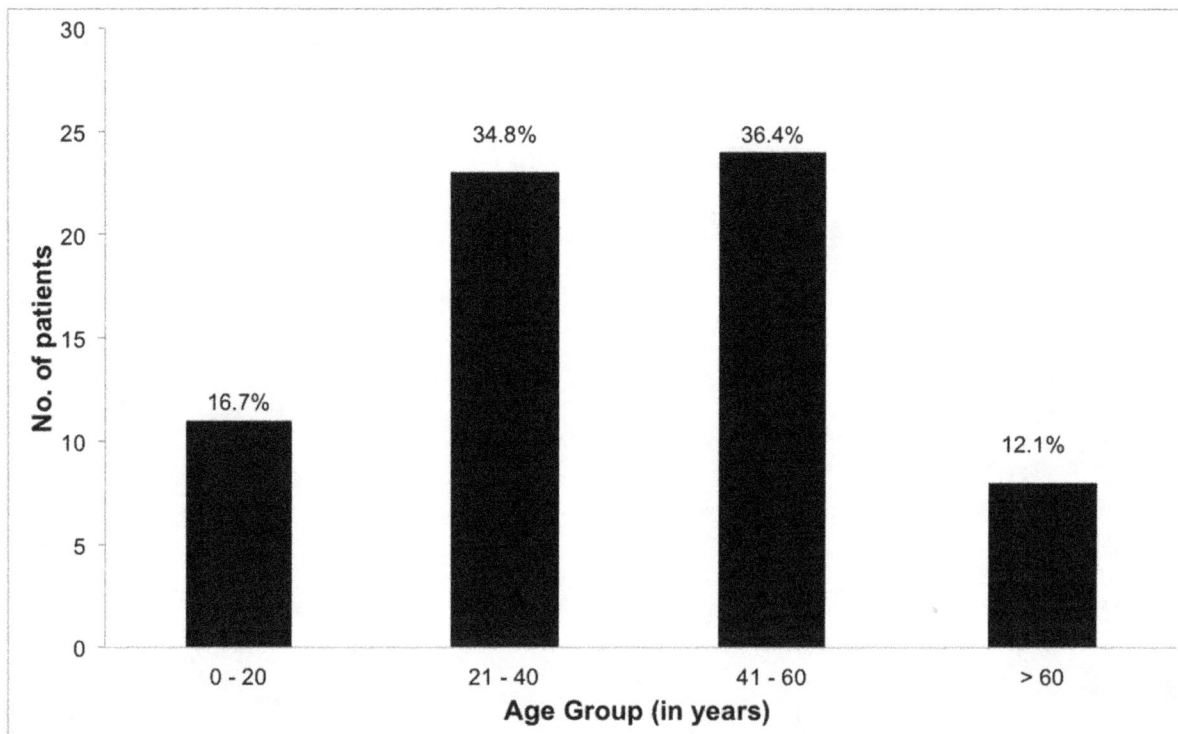

Figure 1. Age distribution of IU patients, showing that largest subgroup of the patients was in the age group of 41–60 years.

Table 2. Demographic profile of patients.

Etiology	Idiopathic		Infective		Immune-mediated		Masquerade	
Number of patients (n, %)	36		14		14		2	
Gender								
Male	15	(41.7)	6	(42.9)	9	(64.3)	0	(0.0)
Female	21	(58.3)	8	(57.1)	5	(35.7)	2	(100.0)
Race								
Chinese	23	(63.9)	6	(42.9)	8	(57.1)	1	(50.0)
Malay	3	(8.3)	4	(28.6)	3	(21.4)	1	(50.0)
Asian Indians	7	(19.4)	2	(14.3)	3	(21.4)	0	(0.0)
Others	3	(8.3)	2	(14.3)	0	(0.0)	0	(0.0)
Laterality								
Bilateral	21	(58.3)	6	(42.9)	10	(71.4)	0	(0.0)

Specific Review Board (NHG-DSRB), with waiver of informed consent.

Results

Demographics

Our study included 66 patients with newly diagnosed IU, comprising 5.7% of 1168 new patients diagnosed with uveitis between years of 2004 and 2011. In comparison with the other classifications of uveitis from 2004–2011, there were 795 AU patients (68.1%), 177 posterior uveitis patients (15.2%) and 130 panuveitis patients (11.1%). With the exception of IU, majority of all the other uveitis patients were males, and had unilateral disease. The profile of the Singapore population and detailed demographic profile of patients and laterality, stratified based on the various classification of uveitis, is listed in Table 1.

There were 30 males (45.5%) and 36 females (54.5%). The disease was bilateral in 37 patients (56.1%). The majority of patients were of Chinese ethnicity (n = 38, 57.6%), followed by Asian Indians (n = 12, 18.2%), and Malays (n = 11, 16.7%). The median age at diagnosis was 40.0 years (mean 39.4±15.9 years, range 6–71 years). The largest subgroup of the patients were in the age group of 41–60 years (36.4%), followed by 21–40 years (34.8%), then 0–20 years (16.7%), and finally >60 years (12.1%) (Figure 1). Three patients (4.5%) were in the pediatric age group, which is defined as younger than 16. Age distribution and demographic profile of the IU patients are shown in Figure 1 and Table 2. In total, there were 37 patients (56.1%) who had bilateral IU. The proportion of bilateral IU was 21 (58.3%), 6 (42.9%) and 10 (71.4%) for the idiopathic IU, infective IU and known immune-mediated IU patients respectively. The detailed demographic profile of patients and laterality, stratified based on etiology, is listed in Table 2.

There was a general statistically significant (p = 0.021) downward trend for the proportion of IU patients over the total uveitis patients (except 2006) in our tertiary referral eye center, with Spearman's rho (ρ) of −0.786 (Table 3 and Figure 2).

Etiology of Intermediate Uveitis

Majority of the cases were non-infectious (n = 52, 78.8%). Of the 66 patients over 8 years, 39 (59.1%) were idiopathic, 14 (21.2%) had an underlying infective cause, and another 11 (16.7%) had a known immune-mediated etiology. Masquerade syndromes (ocular lymphoma) were diagnosed in 2 patients (3.0%). Idiopathic IU was the commonest diagnosis across all age groups, but there were a high proportion of IU patients with known immune-mediated etiologies in the 21–40 age group (n = 7, 30.4%). Detailed trending of age groups by etiology is shown in Table 4 and Figure 3. Using the Fisher's Exact test, there was no statistically association between age groups and the etiology categories (p = 0.410).

There was an even spread of newly diagnosed IU patients over 2004–2007, with a subsequent general downward tendency noted from 2008–2011. Looking at the patterns of the various etiologies over 2004–2011, we noticed a general downward tendency for the infective etiology category (Spearman's rho (ρ) = −0.566, p = 0.143). The detailed pattern of etiologies over 2004–2011 is shown in Figure 4.

Of the 14 patients with infective etiology, the most common in our population was presumed TB (n = 10, 15.2%), followed by syphilis (n = 2, 3.0%). Eight of the 10 patients (80.0%) diagnosed with presumed TB were tested positive for TB IGRA, and 5 of these patients (50.0%) had positive Mantoux skin reactions of ≥ 8 mm. Three of these patients (30.0%) had both positive IGRA

Table 3. Incidence and proportion of IU and total uveitis patients.

Year	No. of IU patients	No. of uveitis patients	Percentage of IU/uveitis patients (%)
2004	10	103	9.7
2005	4	101	4.0
2006	10	73	13.7
2007	10	163	6.1
2008	11	203	5.4
2009	9	255	3.5
2010	7	177	4.0
2011	5	222	2.3

and *Mantoux* skin reaction. All of the patients diagnosed with presumed TB had suggestive clinical history and signs, while none of the 10 patients had positive chest radiograph findings or presence of TB DNA in ocular fluid/tissues. Among the patients with infective etiology, majority had unilateral IU (n = 8, 57.1%). Of the 11 patients with known immune-mediated etiologies, the most common etiology was sarcoidosis (n = 4, 6.1%), followed by Behcet's disease (n = 2, 3.0%) and MS (n = 2, 3.0%). Among the patients with known immune-mediated etiologies, majority had bilateral IU (n = 10, 71.4%).

The most common form of IU among Chinese (n = 25, 65.8%) and Asian Indians (n = 8, 66.7%) was idiopathic, while that in Malays (n = 4, 36.4%) was infective (Table 2). Using the Fisher's Exact test, there was no statistically significant association between ethnicity and etiology categories (p = 0.468). The most common form of IU among males (n = 15, 50.0%) and females (n = 21, 58.3%) was idiopathic. Males had a higher incidence of known immune-mediated IU (n = 9, 30.0%) compared to females (n = 5, 13.9%). Using the Pearson Chi-Square test, there was no statistically significant association between gender and etiology categories (p = 0.271).

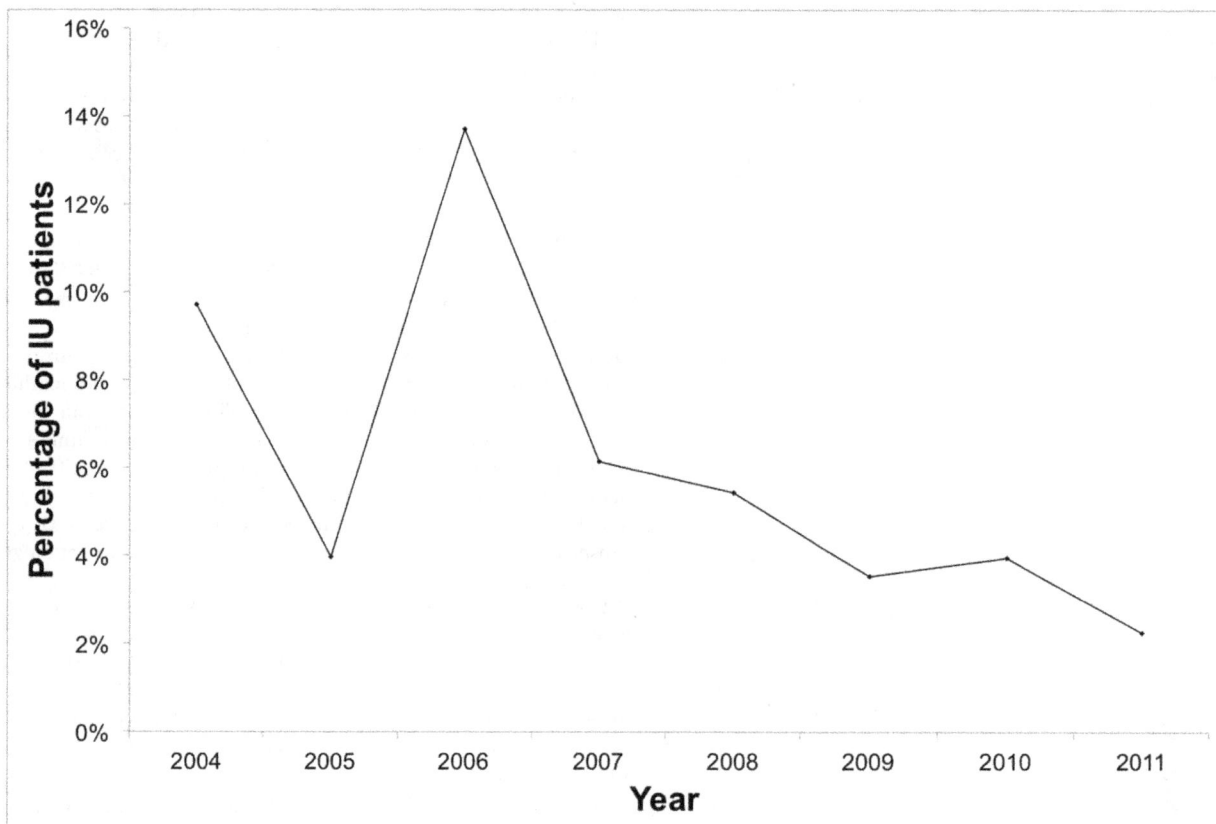

Figure 2. Proportion of IU patients over the total number of uveitis patients. This showed a statistically significant (p = 0.021) downward trend, with Spearman's rho of −0.786. This is possibly due to an increasing trend of the total number of uveitis patients, while the incidence of IU patients had been generally stable, in comparison.

Table 4. Classification of etiology by age groups.

	Age Groups (years)				Total
	0–20	21–40	41–60	>60	
No. of patients (n)	11	23	24	8	66
Idiopathic (n, %)*	7 (63.6)	11 (47.8)	15 (62.5)	6 (75.0)	39 (59.1)
Infective (n, %)*	2 (18.2)	5 (21.7)	6 (25.0)	1 (12.5)	14 (21.2)
TB	2 (18.2)	4 (17.4)	4 (16.7)	0 (0.0)	10 (15.2)
Syphilis	0 (0.0)	1 (4.3)	0 (0.0)	1 (12.5)	2 (3.0)
HSV†	0 (0.0)	0 (0.0)	1 (4.2)	0 (0.0)	1 (1.5)
HIV	0 (0.0)	0 (0.0)	1 (4.2)	0 (0.0)	1 (1.5)
Immune-mediated (n, %)*	2 (18.2)	7 (30.4)	2 (8.3)	0 (0.0)	11 (16.7)
Sarcoidosis	0 (0.0)	2 (8.7)	2 (8.3)	0 (0.0)	4 (6.1)
MS	0 (0.0)	2 (8.7)	0 (0.0)	0 (0.0)	2 (3.0)
Behcet	0 (0.0)	2 (8.7)	0 (0.0)	0 (0.0)	2 (3.0)
AS	1 (9.1)	0 (0.0)	0 (0.0)	0 (0.0)	1 (1.5)
Psoriasis‡	0 (0.0)	1 (4.3)	0 (0.0)	0 (0.0)	1 (1.5)
JIA	1 (9.1)	0 (0.0)	0 (0.0)	0 (0.0)	1 (1.5)
Masquerade (n, %)*	0 (0.0)	0 (0.0)	1 (4.2)	1 (12.5)	2 (3.0)

*expressed as percentage of patients within age group.
†HSV was diagnosed with a positive polymerase chain reaction test.
‡Psoriasis was diagnosed based on a clinical diagnosis of IU and dermatologic manifestations diagnosed as psoriasis by a dermatologist.
Abbreviations: TB, tuberculosis; HSV, Herpes simplex virus; HIV, human immunodeficiency virus; MS, multiple sclerosis; AS, ankylosing spondylitis; JIA, juvenile idiopathic arthritis.

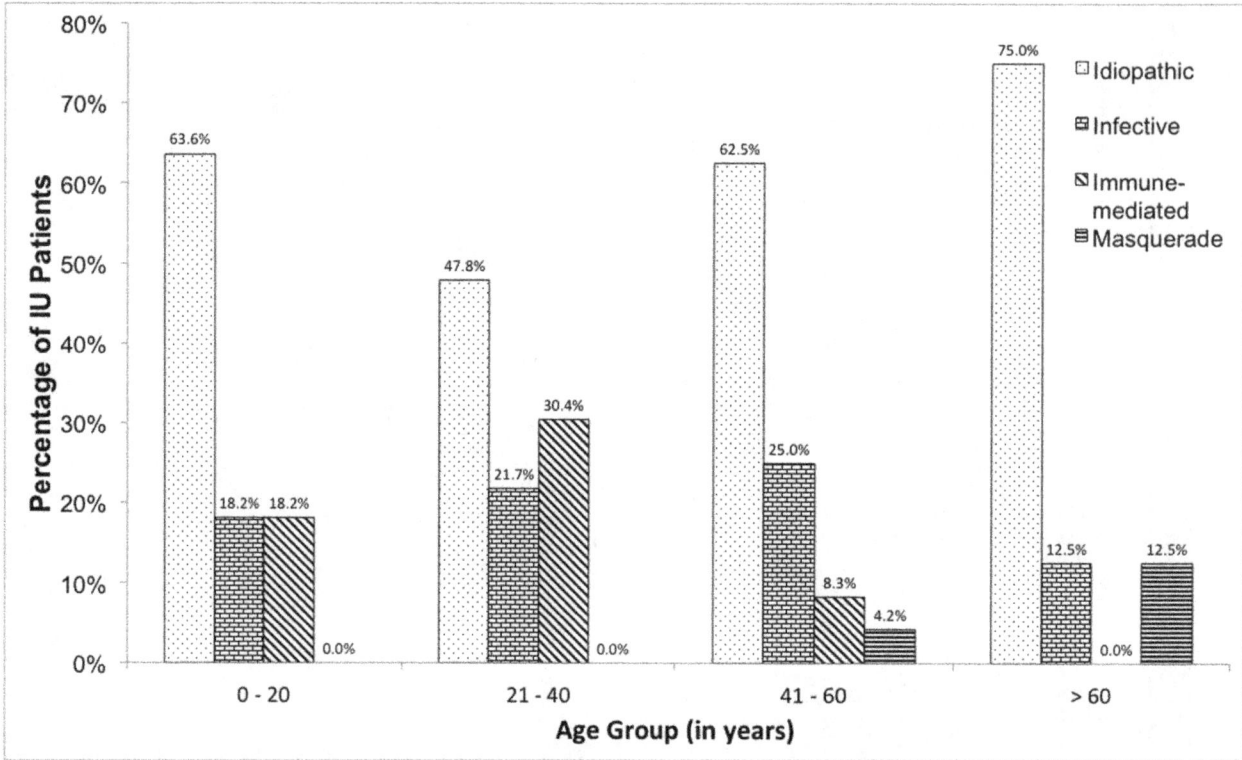

Figure 3. Etiology distribution of IU patients stratified by age groups. Idiopathic IU was the commonest diagnosis across all age groups, but there were a high proportion of IU patients with known immune-mediated etiology in the 21–40 age group (30.4%).

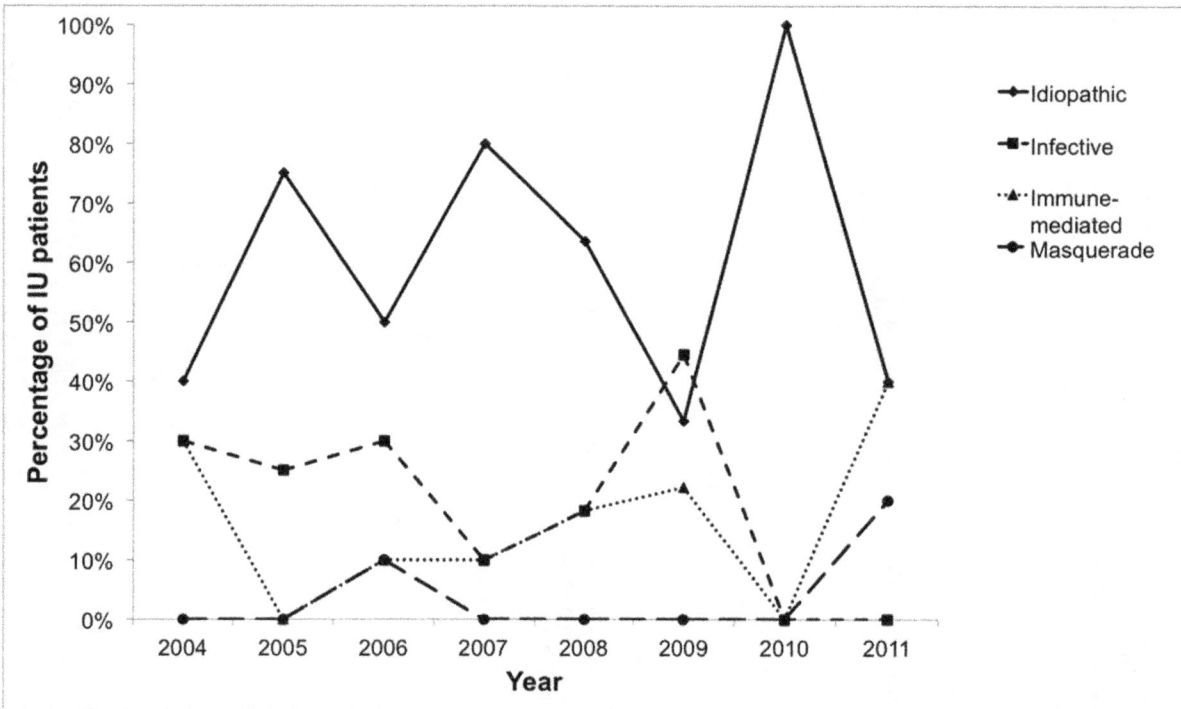

Figure 4. Stratification of etiologies of IU from 2004 to 2011. There was a general downward tendency for the infective etiologies, with Spearman's rho of −0.566.

In total, 21 IU patients (31.8%) developed complications, with cystoid macular edema (CME) being most common (n = 19, 28.8%). This was followed by chronic glaucoma (n = 4, 6.1%). Two (3.0%) patients with associated ocular hypertension were eventually diagnosed with masquerade syndrome secondary to intraocular lymphoma. There were 6 patients (9.1%) with severe vitritis associated with decreased visual acuity, of which 83.3% were diagnosed with TB uveitis. Using the Fisher's exact test, there is a statistically significant (p<0.001) association between severe vitritis and TB-associated IU.

Treatment

Fifty (75.8%) patients with IU required treatment. Corticosteroids were used in all treatments. Fifteen (22.7%) received topical therapy alone, 4 (6.1%) received systemic therapy alone, 11 (15.2%) received topical and systemic therapy, and 10 (15.2%) required adjuvant periocular steroids. Immunosuppressive treatment was used only in non-infective etiologies of IU, and 10 patients (15.2%) received concurrent immunosuppressive therapy. Seven patients (10.6%) received only 1 type of concurrent immunosuppressive therapy and 3 (4.5%) received 2 types of concurrent immunosuppressive therapy, on top of corticosteroid therapy. Immunosuppressive therapy used include that of methotrexate (n = 3, 4.5%), azathioprine (n = 6, 9.1%), cyclophosphamide (n = 1, 1.5%), tacrolimus (n = 2, 3.0%), and mycophenolate mofetil (n = 4, 6.1%). Presumed TB patients received full antibiotic treatment as per the WHO guidelines.

IU patients with CME, chronic glaucoma and severe vitritis were treated with systemic and/or periocular steroids. These patients made up 38.0%, 12.0% and 8.0% of treated patients respectively.

Discussion

The overall incidence of IU is the lowest anatomic type among uveitis occurrences in published Asian, European and Northern American studies, with incidence ranging from 5–20% [2,5,16–20]. We observed this similar trend in our center comprising only 5.7% of uveitis patients seen at our tertiary service. In our population, IU was most common in the Chinese population (57.6%), followed by Asian Indians (18.2%), and Malays (16.7%), which was statistically dissimilar (p<0.001) to our ethnic distribution in Singapore (Chinese 74.1%, Malays 13.4%, Asian Indians 9.2%) [21], suggesting a probable predisposition of the Singapore local Indian population for IU. This is contrasted with our previous findings in AU, which was commonest in the Chinese population (69.8%), followed by Malays (13.2%), and Asian Indians (11.4%) [11]. Our center had a slightly higher prevalence amongst females (54.5%), similar to other published studies (USA 64.0%, Japan 55.0%, India 54.9%) [6–7,22]. The age of presentation amongst our IU patients were in the fourth decade, which was similar to other Asian studies [5,15,23]. They were also older compared to patients with uveitis in general, which was reportedly common in the second-third decade [3,20,22,24–25]. We also had a low incidence of uveitis among our pediatric age group (4.5%), which is similar to other published studies (5–10%) [26]. We noticed a statistically significant (p = 0.021) downward trend for the proportion of IU patients over the total uveitis patients, with Spearman's rho (ρ) of −0.786. This is likely due to a decreasing trend of the IU patients while the incidence of the total number of uveitis patients had been generally stable in comparison in our tertiary eye center, especially between 2008 and 2011 (Table 3). The decreasing trend in our center could also be attributed to possible changes in referral patterns due to better management of the etiologies of IU in the primary care setting.

From our study, patients with IU had a relatively high incidence of an infective etiology, particularly TB (15.2%), especially in our age group of 30–40 years. This was consistent with our tuberculosis incidence rates among our population, with the highest incidence between the 4th to 7th decade [27]. This could be also due to a demographic difference or a later presentation of symptoms due to decreased awareness. Countries endemic with infective diseases such as TB have a much higher rate of presumed TB etiologies compared to our cohort, with our incidence of 15.2% compared to 46.7% (India) [4]. Of note, there was no significant (p>0.999) association between the Asian Indian IU patients in our study and TB, using the Fisher's Exact test. The likely cause could be that the Asian Indian patients in our study are mostly local patients who went through the legally mandatory Bacillus Calmette-Guérin (BCG) vaccination at birth. However, our incidence (15.2%) was higher than other less endemic areas, such as Japan and USA, with an incidence of 6.9% [5] and 7.0% [20] respectively. This correlates with World Health Organization (WHO) estimates of TB prevalence in Singapore to be of 35 per 100,000, compared to 185 per 100,000 in India, and only 4.1 per 100,000 in the USA. TB-associated uveitis is more commonly associated with posterior uveitis (choroiditis) or panuveitis than IU [10,13,28–30]. Severe vitritis is also reported to be significantly associated with latent TB uveitis in predominantly posterior segment inflammation [10]. Our study showed statistically significant association between severe vitritis and TB-associated IU (p<0.001). In our previously reported AU cases, there was a relatively low incidence of TB [11]. This may further indicate that TB uveitis possibly presents more commonly as IU or posterior uveitis than AU. This highlights the need for an increased index of suspicion of TB uveitis in IU patients with severe vitritis in TB endemic countries.

Most cases of IU were idiopathic. This was a similar finding in many other published studies in Asian and Caucasian nations, ranging from 70–90% in Africa, Europe and USA [2,9,16–17,20,24,31] and 42.3% in Japan [5]. Despite the increased use of investigational tools in determining the etiology of IU, this worldwide consistency suggests that typically, specific systemic etiologies of IU could not be determined. However, it could be possible that IU is commonly due to a local pathological process, rather than a systemic one. It is expected that with the advances in knowledge and diagnostic techniques, the proportion of idiopathic uveitis cases would decline over time [32]. Our incidence of 54.5% is more similar to that of Japan, compared to Africa, Europe and USA, consistent with genetic and geographical differences between Asians and Caucasians. These differences were also evidenced in other etiologies [5,9]. MS was strongly associated with IU in western population, ranging from 14.8%–16.2% [33–34], compared to 3.0% in our study. The prevalence of MS in South East Asia is low, with an incidence of only 2–3 per 100,000 [35], compared to 196 per 100,000 [36] amongst European and American Caucasians. MRI was thus not routinely performed as part of our workup for patients with intraocular inflammation in view of the low prevalence of MS in South East Asia. In Japan, there was a much higher prevalence of immune-mediated etiologies of IU, seen in Vogt-Koyanagi-Harada (VKH) disease (10.1% versus 0%), sarcoidosis (9.5% versus 6.1%), and Behcet's disease (5.8% versus 3.0%) [5].

The limitations of this study are the retrospective nature, and the relatively smaller number of patients. There is the problem of referral or selection bias, as our tertiary referral institution sees the more severe cases, resulting in the data reflecting a select subset of our population and not representative of the general population of Singapore. Nevertheless, IU is a relatively uncommon disease, and this data was obtained over a period of 8 years. Also, our tertiary institution has no bias in terms of referral patterns towards any particular age group or ethnicity. Moreover, the results of our study are consistent with other Asian studies and as such, this suggests that these results are representative.

In summary, our results suggest a statistically significant downward trend for the proportion of IU patients over the total uveitis patients in our tertiary referral eye center. In TB endemic countries, a high index of suspicion for TB-associated uveitis is required in patients with associated severe vitritis. Ocular complications developed in about one-third of cases with CME being the most common. Comparisons with other countries showed disparities indicating possible genetic and geographical differences in the etiology of IU.

Author Contributions

Conceived and designed the experiments: ST. Performed the experiments: SH WL. Analyzed the data: HM EW. Wrote the paper: HM ST.

References

1. Bloch-Michel E, Nussenblatt RB. (1987) International Uveitis Study Group Recommendations for the Evaluation of Intraocular Inflammatory Disease. Am J Ophthalmol 103: 234–235.
2. Jabs DA, Nussenblatt RB, Rosenbaum JT. (2005) Standardization of Uveitis (SUN) Working Group. Standardization of Uveitis Nomenclature for Reporting Clinical Data. Results of the First International Workshop. Am J Ophthalmol 140: 509–516.
3. Multicenter Uveitis Steroid Treatment Trial Research Group, Kempen JH, Altaweel MM, Holbrook JT, Jabs DA, et al. (2010) The multicenter uveitis steroid treatment trial: rational, design, and baseline characteristics. Am J Ophthalmol 149: 550–561.
4. Rothova A, Buitenhuis HJ, Meenken C, Brinkman CJ, Linssen A, et al. (1992) Uveitis and systemic disease. Br J Ophthalmol 76: 137–141.
5. Smit RL, Baarsma GS. (1995) Epidemiology of uveitis. Curr Opin Ophthal 6: 57–61.
6. Parchand S, Tandan M, Gupta V, Gupta A. (2011) Intermediate uveitis in Indian population. J Opthalmic Inflamm Infect 1: 65–70.
7. Wakabayashi T, Morimura Y, Miyamoto Y, Okada AA. (2003) Changing patterns of intraocular inflammatory diseases. Ocul Immunol Inflamm 11: 277–286.
8. Zierhut M, Foster CS. (1992) Multiple sclerosis, sarcoidosis and other diseases in patients with pars planitis. Dev Ophthalmol 23: 41–47.
9. Khairallah M, Yahia SB, Ladjimi A, Messaoud R, Zaouali S, et al. (2007) Pattern of uveitis in a referral centre in Tunisia, North Africa. Eye 21: 33–39.
10. Chang JH, Wakefield D. (2002) Uveitis: a global perspective. Ocul Immunol Inflamm 10: 263–279.
11. Tan WJ, Poh EW, Wong PY, Ho SL, Lim WK, et al. (2013) Trends in Patterns of Anterior Uveitis in a Tertiary Institution in Singapore. Ocul Immunol Inflamm 21: 270–275.
12. Gupta V, Gupta A, Rao NA. (2007) Intraocular tuberculosis-an update. Surv Ophthalmol 52: 561–587.
13. Cimino L, Herbort CP, Aldigeri R, Salvarani C, Bolardi L. (2009) Tuberculous uveitis, a resurgent and underdiagnosed disease. Int Ophthalmol 29: 67–74.
14. J Huang, Paul A Guadio. (2010) Ocular inflammatory disease and uveitis manual. Lippincott Williams & Wilkins: Philadelphia.
15. Ang M, Hedayatfar A, Zhang R, Chee SP. (2012) Clinical signs of uveitis associated with latent tuberculosis. Clin Experiment Ophthalmol 40: 689–696.
16. Al-Mezaine HS, Kangave D, Abu El-Asrar AM. (2010) Pattern of Uveitis in Patients Admitted to a university hospital in Riyadh, Saudi Arabia. Ocul Immunol Inflamm 18: 424–431.
17. Soheilian M, Heidari K, Yazdani S, Shahsavari M, Ahmadieh H, et al. (2004) Pattern of uveitis in a tertiary eye care center in Iran. Ocul Immunol Inflamm 12: 297–310.
18. Perkins ES, Folk J. (1984) Uveitis in London and Iowa. Ophthalmologica 189: 36–40.
19. Henderly DE, Genstler AJ, Smith RE, Rao NA. (1987) Changing patterns of uveitis. Am J Ophthalmol 103: 131–136.
20. Smit RL, Baarsma GS, de Vries J. (1993) Classification of 750 consecutive uveitis patients in the Rotterdam Eye Hospital. Int Ophthalmol 17: 71–75.
21. Department of Statistics, Singapore (2011). Singapore Residents by Age Group, Ethnic Group and Sex. Available at: http://www.singstat.gov.sg/pubn/reference/mdscontents.html#Demography [Accessed 12 May 2013].
22. Donaldson MJ, Pulido JS, Herman DC, Diehl N, Hodge D. (2007) Pars planitis: A 20-year study of incidence, clinical features, and outcomes. Am J Ophthalmol 144: 812–817.
23. Keino H, Nakashima C, Watanabe T, Taki W, Hayakawa R, et al. (2009) Frequency and clinical features of intraocular inflammation in Tokyo. Clin Experiment Ophthalmol 37: 595–601.
24. Sengun A, Karadag R, Karakurt A, Saricaoglu MS, Abdik O, et al. (2005) Causes of uveitis in a referral hospital in Ankara, Turkey. Ocul Immunol Inflamm 13: 45–50.
25. Hamade IH, Elkum N, Tabbara KF. (2009) Causes of uveitis at a referral center in Saudi Arabia. Ocul Immunol Inflamm 17: 11–16.
26. Cunningham ET Jr. (2000) Uveitis in children. Ocul Immunol Inflamm 8: 251–261.
27. Communicable Disease Center, Tan Tock Seng Hospital (2002). Trends in selected infectious diseases in Singapore. Available at: http://aidsdatahub.org/dmdocuments/Trends_in_Infectious_Disease_in_Singapore.pdf.pdf [Accessed 18 April 2013].
28. Bodaghi B, LeHoang P. (2000) Ocular tuberculosis. Curr Opin Ophthalmol 11: 443–448.
29. Hamade IH, Tabbara KF. (2010) Complications of presumed ocular tuberculosis. Acta Ophthalmol 88: 905–909.
30. Davis EJ, Rathinam SR, Okada AA, Tow SL, Petrushkin H, et al. (2012) Clinical spectrum of tuberculous optic neuropathy. J Ophthalmic Inflamm Infect 2: 183–189.
31. Cimino L, Aldigeri R, Salvarani C, Zotti CA, Boiardi L et al. (2010) The causes of uveitis in a referral centre of Northern Italy. Int Opthalmol 30: 521–529.
32. Wakefield D, Chang JH. (2005) Epidemiology of uveitis. Int Ophthalmol Clin 45: 1–13.
33. Raja SC, Jabs DA, Dunn JP, Fekrat S, Machan CH, et al. (1999) Pars planitis: clinical features and class II HLA associations. Ophthalmology 106: 594–599.
34. Malinowski SM, Pulido JS, Folk JC. (1993) Long-term visual outcome and complications associated with pars planitis. Opthalmology 100: 818–824.
35. Chong HT. (2008) Multiple sclerosis in South East Asia and diagnostic criteria for Asians. Neurology Asia 13: 145–146.
36. Aguirre-Cruz L, Flores-Rivera J, De La Cruz-Aguilera DL, Rangel-Lopez E, Corona T. (2011) Multiple sclerosis in Caucasians and Latino Americans. Autoimmunity 44; 571–575.

6

Green Tea Extract Treatment Alleviates Ocular Inflammation in a Rat Model of Endotoxin-Induced Uveitis

Yong Jie Qin[1], Kai On Chu[1], Yolanda Wong Ying Yip[1], Wai Ying Li[1], Ya Ping Yang[1], Kwok Ping Chan[1], Jia Lin Ren[2], Sun On Chan[2*◊], Chi Pui Pang[1*◊]

1 Department of Ophthalmology and Visual Sciences, The Chinese University of Hong Kong, Hong Kong, 2 School of Biomedical Sciences, The Chinese University of Hong Kong, Hong Kong, China

Abstract

Green tea extract (GTE) ingested by rats exerted anti-oxidative activities in various ocular tissues as shown in our previous studies. The present work investigated anti-inflammatory effects of GTE on endotoxin-induced uveitis (EIU). EIU was generated in adult rats by a footpad injection of 1 mg/kg lipopolysaccharide (LPS). Oral administration of GTE (550 mg/kg) was given one, two or four times after LPS injection. Twenty-four hours later, LPS produced severe hyperemia and edema in the iris. Immunocytochemical examinations showed an accumulation of infiltrating cells in the aqueous humor that were immunopositive for cluster of differentiation 43 (CD43) and CD68, markers for leucocytes and macrophages, respectively. Analyses of the aqueous humor showed an increase in pro-inflammatory mediators including tumor necrosis factor-alpha (TNF-α), interleukin-6 (IL-6) and monocyte chemoattractant protein-1 (MCP-1). GTE treatments improved the clinical manifestations and reduced infiltrating cells and protein exudation in the aqueous humor, which were not observed under half dose of GTE (275 mg/kg). The number of CD68 positive macrophages residing in the iris and ciliary was also reduced. GTE suppressed production of TNF-α, IL-6 and MCP-1 in the aqueous humor, which was associated with a down-regulation of LPS receptor complex subunits, Toll-like receptor 4 (TLR-4) and CD14, and suppression of nuclear factor-kappa Bp65 (NF-κBp65) in the iris and ciliary body. Our findings show that GTE is a potent anti-inflammatory agent against the inflammation of EIU, and suggest a potential use in treatment of acute uveitis.

Editor: Anand Swaroop, National Eye Institute, United States of America

Funding: This work was supported in part by a block grant of the University Grants Committee Hong Kong, a GRF Grant (Project No. CUHK461612), a seed grant from Lui Che Woo Institute of Innovative Medicine (Project No. 8303107) and the Endowment Fund for Lim Por-Yen Eye Genetics Research Centre, Hong Kong. The funders had no role in study design, data collection and analysis, decision to publish, or preparation of the manuscript.

Competing Interests: The authors have declared that no competing interests exist.

* Email: cppang@cuhk.edu.hk (CPP); sunonchan@cuhk.edu.hk (SOC)

◊ These authors contributed equally to this work.

Introduction

Uveitis, an ocular inflammatory condition, accounts for approximately 10–15% cases of total blindness and up to 20% of legal blindness in developed world [1,2]. The goal of uveitis treatment is to suppress inflammation and achieve regression when it occurs [3]. However inflammation can recur with various complications, such as cataract and permanent cumulative damages [4,5]. Administrations of corticosteroid are standard therapeutic strategy, but they have many potential side effects such as intraocular pressure increase, cataract formation and increase in infection susceptibility [6]. Therefore, alternative treatments which are safer and more long lasting are needed.

The rat model of endotoxin-induced uveitis (EIU) has been widely used for evaluating potential ocular anti-inflammatory compounds since it was reported in 1980 [7–12]. EIU can be induced by systemic injection of lipopolysaccharide (LPS), which generates inflammatory responses largely in the anterior uvea and mild responses in the posterior segments of the eye, mimicking the pathological conditions in human acute uveitis [12–14]. It has

been reported that LPS was recognized by membrane-bound cluster of differentiation 14 (mCD14) and Toll-like receptors (principally TLR-4) on the surface of macrophages. Receptors activation in these immune surveillance cells resulted in phosphorylation of nuclear factor-kappa B (NF-κB) and caused release of pro-inflammatory factors, such as tumor necrosis factor-α (TNF-α), interlukin-6 (IL-6) and monocyte chemoattractant protein-1 (MCP-1) [15–21]. As a crucial proximal mediator, TNF-α stimulates acute phase reaction of inflammation by influencing leukocyte activation and infiltration, and inducing production of other mediators such as IL-6, a major cytokine regulator of acute phase response [22,23]. MCP-1, a powerful chemotactic and activating factor [24], stimulates the activation of mitogen-activated protein kinases (MAPKs) to promote monocytes migration [25]. Another study shows that the blood-humor barrier is broken down two hours after LPS injection [26], which results in migration of polymorphonuclear and mononuclear cells into the aqueous humor. The inflammatory process reaches peak level at 18–24 hours after LPS injection [27].

Catechins, the major component in green tea extract (GTE), have been shown to exert anti-oxidative, anti-inflammatory, anti-angiogenic and anti-carcinogenic effects [28,29]. In a pharmacokinetic study, we have shown that catechins reach peak level in the ocular tissues of normal rats at 1 to 2 hours after ingestion, and produce significant reduction in oxidative stress within these tissues [30]. We have addressed in this study the hypothesis that orally administered GTE could serve as effective anti-inflammatory agents to alleviate inflammatory responses in anterior segments of the eye triggered by a systemic injection of LPS.

Materials and Methods

Endotoxin-induced uveitis and GTE treatment

All experiments were conducted according to the Association for Research in Vision and Ophthalmology (ARVO) statement on the use of animals. Ethics approval for this study was obtained from the Animal Ethics Committee of the Chinese University of Hong Kong. Sprague-Dawley rats (about 250 g, 6–8 weeks old) were obtained from the Laboratory Animal Service Center of the Chinese University of Hong Kong. Ethics approval for this study was obtained from the Animal Ethics Committee of the University. All animals were housed at 25°C with 12/12 hour light-dark cycles, and were allowed to access freely to food and water. Before the experiment, animals were fasted overnight and body weight was recorded.

EIU was induced by injection of 0.1 mL of pyrogen-free saline dissolved LPS (from Salmonella typhimurium; Sigma Chemical, St. Louis, MO, USA) at the dose of 1 mg/kg into one footpad. The dosage was selected according to results of a preliminary study, which showed that LPS at 1 mg/kg was the optimal dose in inducing moderate inflammation in both eyes without causing obvious lesion in the liver and kidney. The GTE Theaphenon E was kindly provided by Dr. Y. Hara, which contains EGCG (epigallocatechin gallate, >65%), EGC (epigallate catechins, <10%), EC (epicatechin, <10%) and ECG (epicatechin gallate, <10%) and other trace catechin derivatives. It was prepared as a 550 mg/kg GTE suspension in 0.5 mL distilled water and was fed intragastrically into the rat.

The rats were randomly divided into three treatment groups: i) GTE1, fed with GTE two hours after LPS injection (LPS+GTE1, n = 6); ii) GTE2, fed with GTE twice at two and eight hours after LPS injection (LPS+GTE2, n = 6); iii) GTE4, fed with GTE four times at two, five, eight and eleven hours after LPS injection (LPS+ GTE4, n = 6). Control groups consisted of: i) normal control, footpad injected with saline and fed with water two hours after injection (Saline+water, n = 3); (ii) LPS controls, footpad injected with LPS and fed with water (LPS+water, n = 6); (iii) Dxm controls, footpad injected with LPS and fed with Dexamethasone (Dxm) (1 mg/kg, distilled water suspension; Sigma Chemical, USA) two hours after LPS injection (LPS+Dxm, n = 6); and (iv) GTE controls, footpad injected with saline and fed with GTE four

times as in GTE4 group (Saline+GTE4, n = 3). Another eighteen rats were used for histological studies.

In another experiment, the dosage effect of GTE was tested in 23 rats: i) normal control (n = 5), footpad injected with saline followed by oral administration of water at the 2nd and 11th hours after footpad injection; ii) LPS group (n = 6), footpad injection of LPS followed by feeding of water at the 2nd and 11th hour after footpad injection; iii) 550 mg/kg GTE (n = 6), oral administration of the dose at the 2nd and 11th hour after footpad injection of LPS; iv) half dose GTE (n = 6), oral administration of 275 mg/kg GTE at the 2nd and 11th hour after the LPS injection.

Twenty four hours after LPS injection, the rats were anesthetized with intraperitoneal injection of 4.0 mL of ketamine-xylazine mixture (1.5:1, Alfasan International B.V., Holland) for collections of ocular tissues. They were terminated immediately by drawing the whole blood through heart puncture.

Clinical manifestations scoring

Clinical features of ocular inflammation in both eyes were evaluated using a slit lamp and graded from score 0 to score 4 by a masked observer 24 hours after LPS injection as described previously [31]. The grading is assigned as: 0 = no obvious inflammatory response; 1 = discrete dilation of iris and conjunctival vessels; 2 = moderate dilation and iris and conjunctival vessels with moderate flare in the anterior chamber; 3 = intense iridal hyperemia with intense flare in the anterior chamber; 4 = same clinical signs as 3 with presence of fibrinoid exudation and miosis.

Histological examination of infiltrating cells

Under deep anesthesia, the rats were perfused intracardially with 0.01 M sterile phosphate buffer saline (PBS) followed by 4% paraformaldehyde. Both eyes were removed and immersed in 10% formalin for 24 hours at room temperature. Some connective tissues were maintained on each eye to facilitate orientation. The eyes were embedded in paraffin and sectioned in 5 μm thickness along the vertical meridian and the optic nerve head. After deparaffinization and rehydration, the sections were stained with Hematoxylin and Eosin (H&E). The anterior and posterior segments of the eyeball were examined under a light microscope (DMRB, Leica Microsystems, Wetzlar, Germany). Total number of infiltrating cells located in anterior segments (anterior/posterior chamber) and posterior segments (vitreous body around optic nerve head) were counted in a masked fashion by an ocular pathologist as described previously [32].

Some sections were selected for immunostaining in order to determine the identity of infiltrating cells. The slides were heat to induce epitope retrieval using a pressure cooker (Biocare Medical, Walnut Creek, CA). After blocking with 0.1% bovine serum at room temperature, mouse anti-rat monoclonal antibody CD43 (1:80 dilution, AbD Serotec, Kidlington, UK) or CD68 (1:100 dilution, AbD Serotec, Kidlington, UK) was applied separately to the sections and incubated at 4°C overnight, which binds

Table 1. Primer sequences used for quantitative real-time PCR detection of rat-CD14, TLR-4 and GAPDH.

Gene	Identification	Forward, 5'-3'	Reverse, 5'-3'	Product size
CD14	NM_021744.1	TCACAATTCACTGCGGGATA	CGATGTCCTAGGAGCAAAGC	330 bp
TLR-4	NM_019178.1	TGATGCCTCTCTTGCATCTG	TCCAGCCACTGAAGTTGTGA	247 bp
GAPDH	NM_017008.4	GTGCCAGCCTCGTCTCATA	GTTGAACTTGCCGTGGGTAG	190 bp

CD14: cluster of differentiation 14; TLR-4: toll-like receptor 4; GAPDH: glyceraldehyde-3-phosphate dehydrogenase.

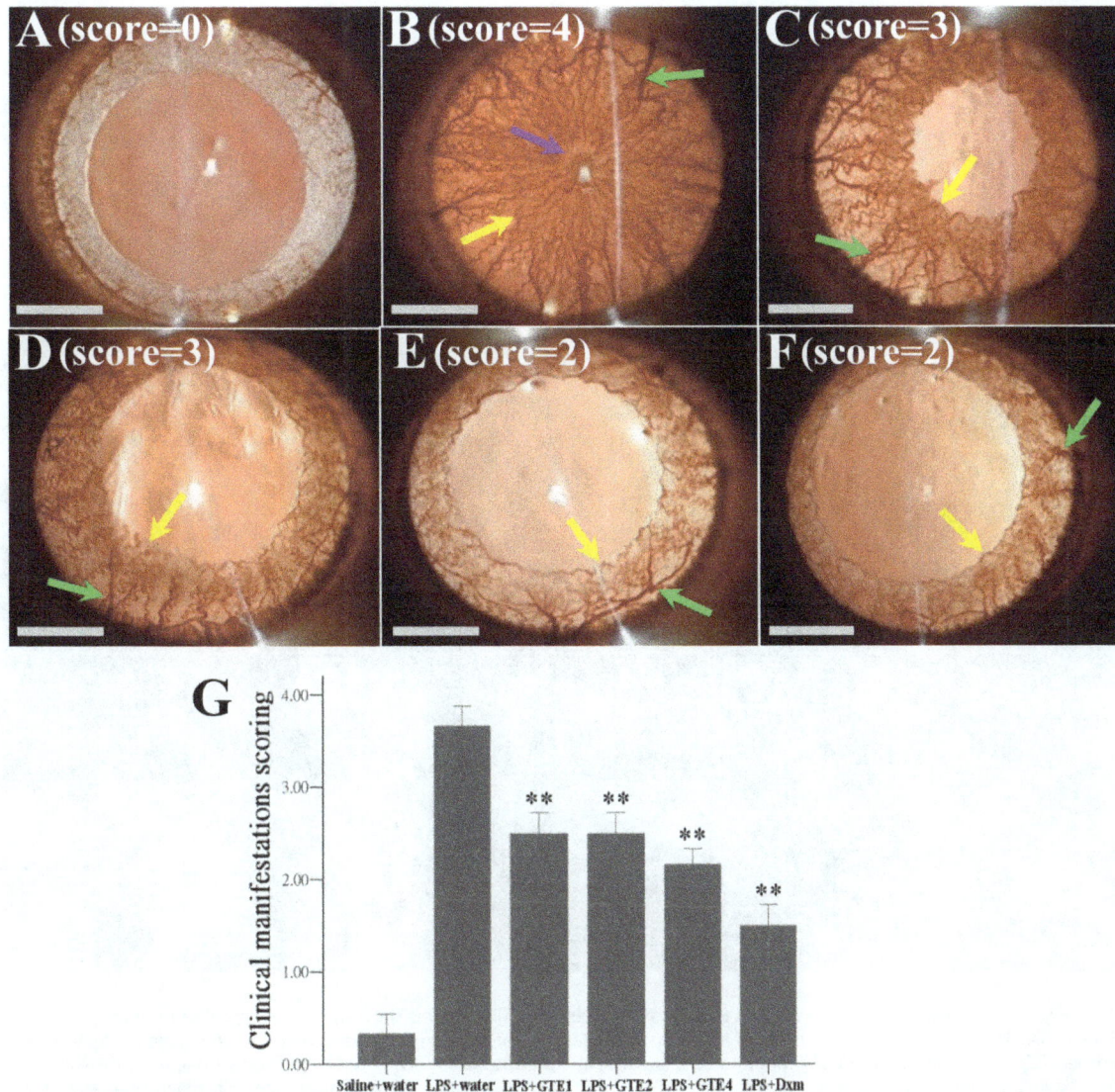

Figure 1. Clinical manifestations of ocular inflammation in rat eyes. Ocular inflammation was evaluated by slit lamp examination 24 hours after LPS injection. (A): No inflammatory feature was observed in normal control rats (saline+water). (B) and (C): Hyperemia (green arrow), edema (yellow arrow) and synachesia (purple arrow) occurred in the iris of LPS treated rats. (D) and (E): Inflammatory responses were subsided in rats treated with GTE1 (D) and GTE4 (E). (F): Inflammatory responses were also suppressed in rats treated with Dexamethasone (Dxm). (G): The scores of clinical features were reduced significantly after GTE and Dxm treatments (**$p < 0.05$, when compared with LPS+water). Saline+water, n = 3; LPS+water, n = 6; LPS+GTE1, n = 6; LPS+GTE2, n = 6; LPS+GTE4, n = 6; LPS+Dxm, n = 6. Data were shown as mean ± SE. Scar bar = 2 mm.

preferentially to leucocytes and macrophages, respectively. The sections were then washed and incubated in secondary antibody (1:1000 dilution; Alexa Fluor 488 for CD43, Alexa Fluor 594 for CD68; Invitrogen, Carlsbad, CA, USA) at room temperature for 1 hour. DAPI (4′,6-diamidino-2-phenylindole, 1:2000 dilution) was used for counter-stain of nuclei. The sections were mounted using aqueous mounting medium (GBI Labs, Manchester, UK) and examined under fluorescence microscope (Diagnostic Instruments, Sterling Heights, Michigan). Control sections were processed as above without primary antibody.

In another experiment, sections of the eye were processed for immunostaining of CD68 in order to determine whether GTE treatment reduced LPS-induced accumulation of macrophages in the stroma of iris and ciliary body. Four non-consecutive sections were collected from the eye of normal controls, and animals treated with LPS alone, LPS plus GTE or dexamethasone. The number of CD68 positive cells inside stroma of iris and ciliary body was counted in a masked fashion.

Cell count and protein assay in aqueous humor

Aqueous humor was collected by piercing the anterior chamber with a 30 gauge needle. One microliter aqueous humor was diluted with 9 μl 0.01 M PBS and suspended in an equal volume of Trypan-blue solution. The number of cells was counted by using a hemacytometer under a light microscope. Another portion of the aqueous humor was centrifuged at 2500 rpm for 15 minutes at 4°C. Cells-free supernatant was used for total protein assay in duplicate (Bio-Rad, Hercules, CA, USA).

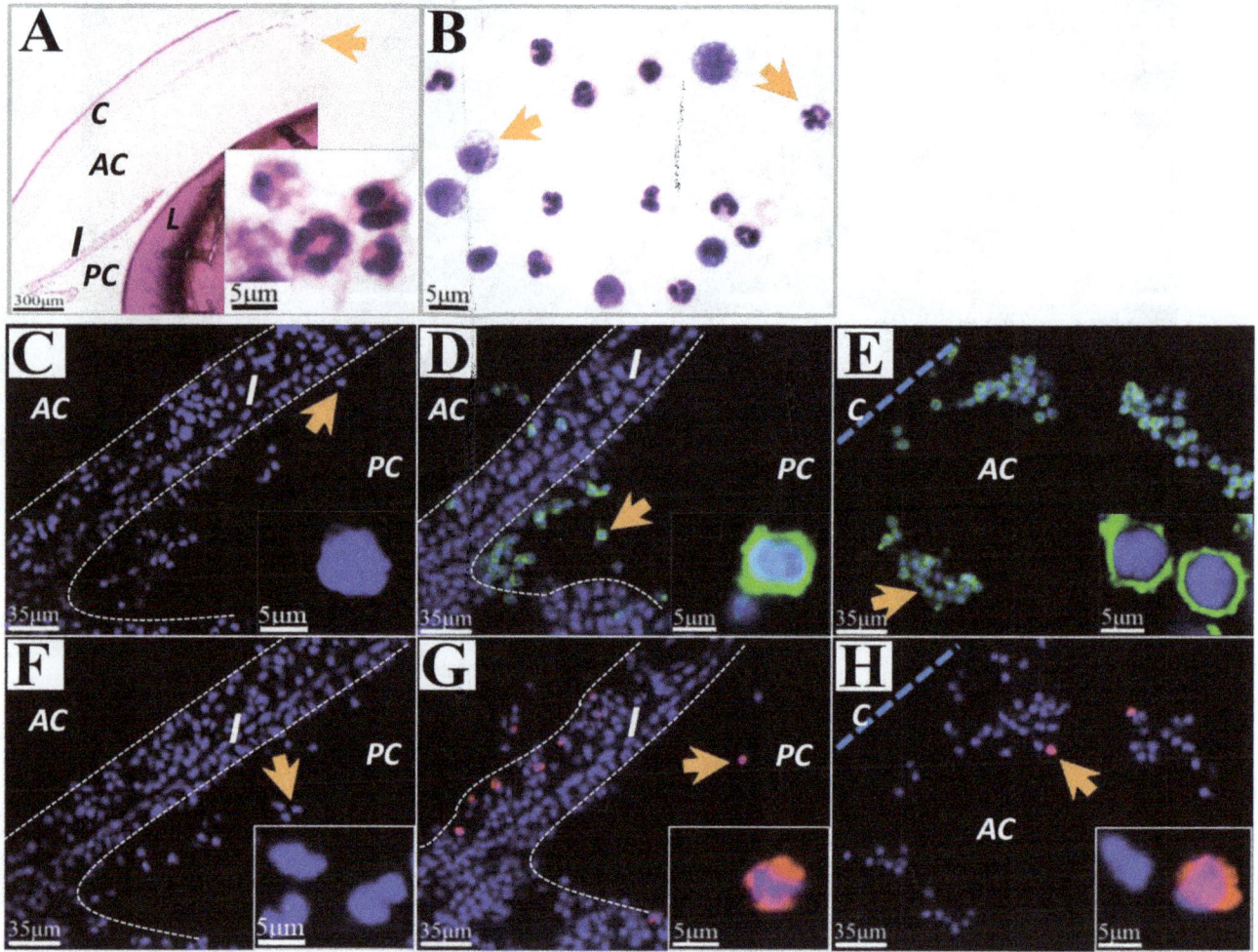

Figure 2. Histological features of infiltrating cells in ocular tissues. Paraffin sections showed infiltrating cells in the anterior segments of the eye after LPS insult. (A): H&E section showed clusters of infiltrating cells (arrow, magnified in the insert) with polymorphic nuclei in anterior (AC) and posterior chamber (PC). (B): Giemsa staining of infiltrating cells (arrows) in aqueous humor. (D) and (E): Fluorescent micrographs showing localization of CD43 on leukocytes (arrow, magnified in the insert) in iris (I), PC and AC. (G) and (H): CD68 was localized on macrophage/monocytes (arrows, magnified in the insert) in iris, PC and AC. No staining was observed in control sections treated without primary antibody against CD43 (C) or CD68 (F). C: cornea.

Determination of pro-inflammatory factors in the serum and aqueous humor

Blood samples were collected by heart puncture and clotted at room temperature for 2 hours in serum vial. They were centrifuged at 2500 rpm for 15 minutes at 4°C. The serum and cells-free aqueous humor were taken for determination of TNF-α and IL-6 (rat-ELISA kit, R&D Systems, Minneapolis, USA) and MCP-1 (rat-ELISA kit, Invitrogen, Camarillo, CA, USA), each in duplicate.

Quantification of CD14 and TLR-4 mRNA expression

Iris, ciliary body/process and retina were collected. After washing with 0.01 M cold sterile PBS, tissues were immersed in 300–500 μl Trizol reagent (Invitrogen, USA) and stored at −80°C until use. Total RNA were isolated and treated with RNase-free DNaseI according to the manufacturer's protocol (Qiagen, Hilden, Germany). RNA (0.5–1 μg) was reversely transcribed into cDNA using SuperScript III reverse transcriptase (Invitrogen, USA). PCR was performed using iCycler PCR instrument (Bio-Rad) and lightCycle 480 II real-time PCR system (Roche Applied Science,

Penzberg, Germany). Sequences of the gene-specific primers were designed using the online Primer 3 Input Program (version 0.4.0) (Table 1).

Quantitative real-time PCR (qPCR) was performed with SYRB green PCR mixture containing 10 μl of 2×480 SYRB green I Master (Roche, USA), 0.55 μl of 10 nM primers (Invitrogen), 1 μl cDNA and 8 μl double distilled water. The parameters were as follows: pre-incubation 95°C for 10 minutes, followed by 40 amplification cycles each with denaturation at 95°C for 15 seconds, annealing/extension at 60°C for 1 minute. The melt-curve analysis was performed using default settings of the instrument. Final qPCR products were electrophoresed in 2.0% agarose gel. Relative CD14 and TLR-4 mRNA expression of each sample was calculated as described [33]. In brief, after the threshold cycle value of the target gene (C_T *target*) was emendated with the value of internal control gene GAPDH (C_T *GAPDH*), the normalized expression value ($2^{-(CT\ target - CT\ GAPDH)}$) was calculated, then the expression fold change due to treatment were obtained according to the normalized expression value.

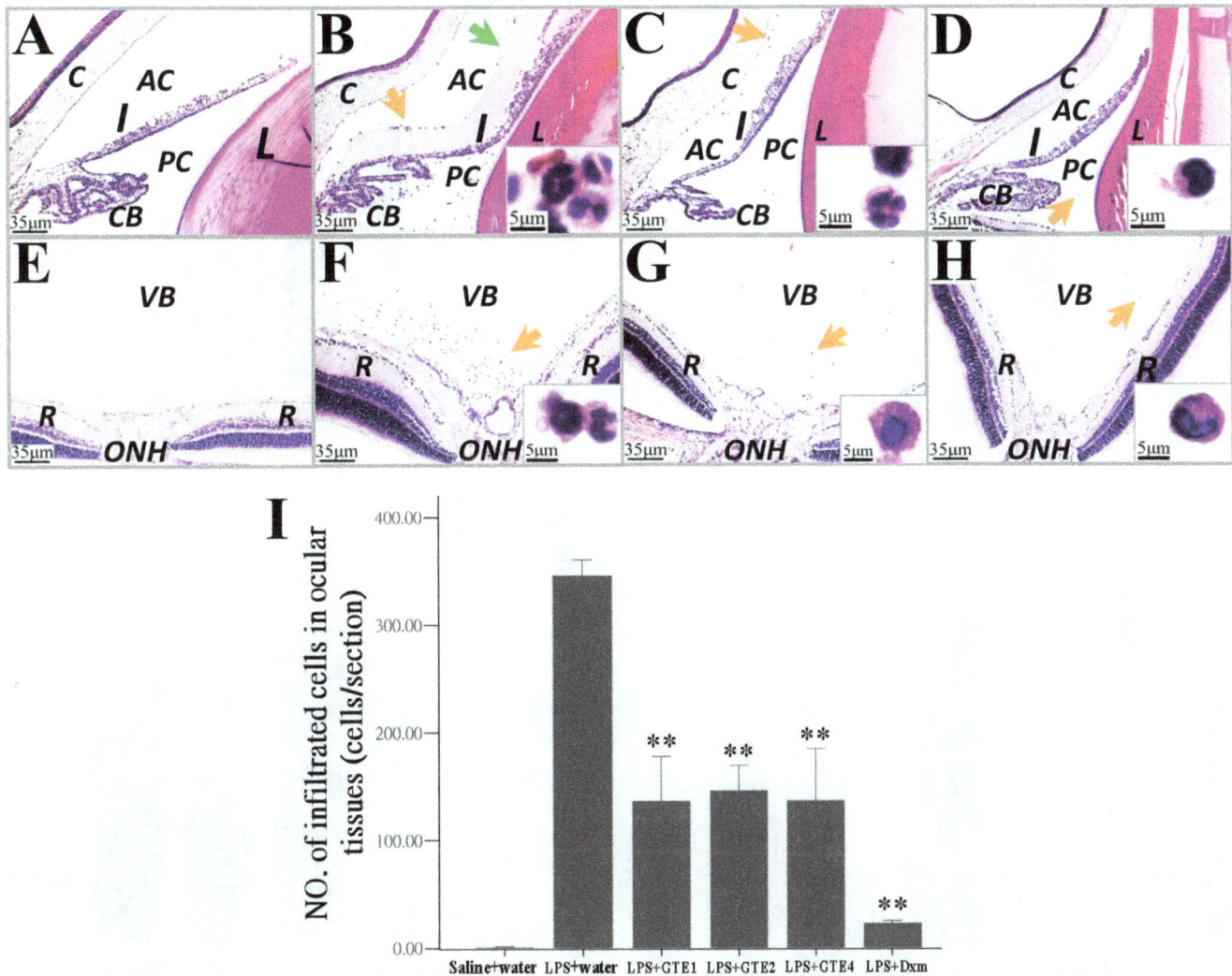

Figure 3. The number of infiltrating cells in ocular tissues after GTE treatments. (A), (B), (C) and (D): H&E sections showing accumulation of infiltrating cells (orange arrows, magnified in inserts) and protein exudation (green arrow) in anterior segments of the eye. (E), (F), (G) and (H): H&E sections showing infiltrating cells (arrows) in vitreous body (VB) around the optic nerve head (ONH). (A, E): Saline+water; (B, F): LPS+water; (C, G): LPS+GTE4; (D, H): LPS+Dxm. (I): The number of infiltrating cells in the anterior and posterior segments of the eye was reduced in rats treated with GTE (**$p < 0.05$) when compared with that with LPS and vehicle treatment. n = 3 in each group. Data were shown as mean ± *SE*. L: lens; CB: ciliary body; R: retina.

Western blot analysis

Nuclear proteins were isolated from iris and ciliary body by using ReadyPrepTM Protein Extraction Kit (Cytoplasmic/Nuclear, Bio-Rad, Hercules, CA, USA). Protein concentration was adjusted equally with protein assay kit (Bio-RAD, Hercules, CA, USA), then re-suspended in 5x sample loading buffer, heated for 5 min at 95°C and separated on 12.5% SDS-polyacrylamide gel electrophoresis (SDS-PAGE). The proteins were transferred onto a nitrocellulose membrane (AmershamTM HybondTM-ECL, GE Healthcare, UK), blocked with 5% Bovine albumin BSA (A9418, Sigma-Aldrich, USA), and incubated with NF-κBp65 antibody (1:300, sc-372, Santa Cruz Biotechnology, INC.) and Lamin B antibody (1:500, sc-6216, Santa Cruz Biotechnology, INC.) at 4°C overnight. After washing with TBS-0.05% tween-20 (TBST), HRP-coupled secondary antibodies (1:1000, Santa Cruz Biotechnology, INC.) were applied to the membrane for 1 hour at room temperature, followed by three washes with TBST. The immunoreactive bands were visualized with enhanced chemiluminescence reagents (GE Healthcare, UK) and images were captured by the Universal Hood II image system (Bio-Rad Laboratories, Segrate, Italy). Band intensities of NF-κBp65 were normalized with those of internal control (Lamin B) using NIH Image J software (version 1.47).

Statistical analysis

All data were analyzed by nonparametric Kruskal-Wallis Tests. Two group comparisons were done by Mann-Whitney Tests. The *p*-value less than 0.05 was considered statistically significant. All statistical analyses were performed using SPSS statistical software package (version 20.0).

Results

Clinical manifestations of inflammation in the eye

Slit lamp examination showed development of hyperemia and edema associated with miosis and fibril formation in the iris 24

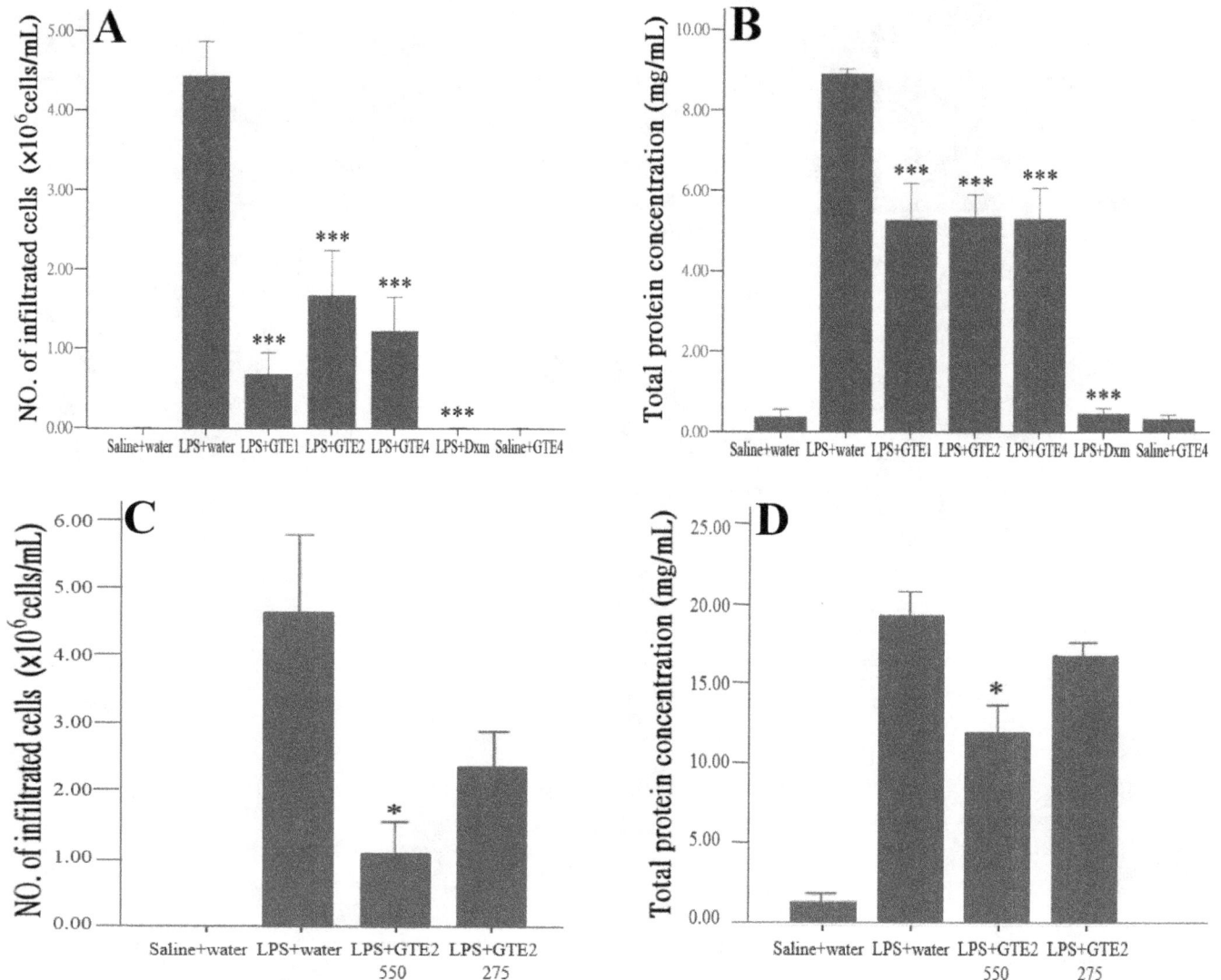

Figure 4. GTE treatment on cell infiltration and protein exudation in aqueous humor. (A) and (B): GTE caused a significant reduction in accumulation of cells (A) and protein exudation (B) in aqueous humor (***$p<0.01$) when compared with LPS+water. The differences among the GTE treatment groups were, however, not significant ($p>0.05$). Saline+water, n = 3; LPS+water, n = 6; LPS+GTE1, n = 6; LPS+GTE2, n = 6; LPS+GTE4, n = 6; LPS+Dxm, n = 6; Saline+water, n = 3. (C) and (D): In another experiment, significant reduction in infiltrating cells (C) and protein content (D) in aqueous humor was observed only in rats treated with 550 mg/kg GTE (*$p<0.05$), but not in those received half dose (275 mg/kg) of GTE. Saline+water, n = 5; n = 6 in LPS+water, LPS+GTE2 550 and LPS+GTE2 275. Data were shown as mean ± *SE.*

hours after LPS injection (Fig. 1B–C). These clinical features were not observed in the normal controls (Fig. 1A), and appeared less severe in the GTE treated rats (Fig. 1D–E) and rats treated with dexamethasone (Fig. 1F). Quantitative evaluation of these clinical scores showed a significant reduction in animals treated with 1 to 4 times oral administration of GTE ($p<0.05$) when compared with animals fed with water after LPS insult (Fig. 1G).

Infiltrating cells in anterior segments of the eye

Injection of LPS induced substantial accumulation of infiltrating cells in the anterior chamber and posterior chamber of the eye (Fig. 2A). Giemsa staining showed that these infiltrating cells in aqueous humor were variable in size and polymorphic in nuclear shape (Fig. 2B). Immunohistochemical studies on paraffin sections of LPS treated eye showed that most infiltrating cells in anterior and posterior chamber were CD43 positive leucocytes (Fig. 2D–E), whereas a few were CD68 positive macrophages (Fig. 2G–H).

A few CD43 and CD68 positive cells were found in the stroma of iris and ciliary body (Fig. 2D and G). No staining was detected in sections processed with the absence of primary antibody (Fig. 2C and F).

The effects of GTE treatment on ocular inflammation were investigated in paraffin sections of the eye. LPS induced an accumulation of infiltrating cells and proteineous substances in the anterior and posterior chamber (Fig. 3B), which was not observed in normal control animals (Fig. 3A). Treatment of GTE reduced substantially the infiltration of cells and accumulation of protein in the anterior and posterior chamber (Fig. 3C), which was further reduced in animals treated with Dxm (Fig. 3D). Similar observations were presented in their corresponding vitreous body around the optic nerve head (Fig. 3E–H), where the accumulation of infiltrating cells was highly reduced in both GTE (Fig. 3G) and Dxm (Fig. 3H) treated animals. Counting of infiltrating cells on these sections (in anterior and posterior chamber, and in vitreous

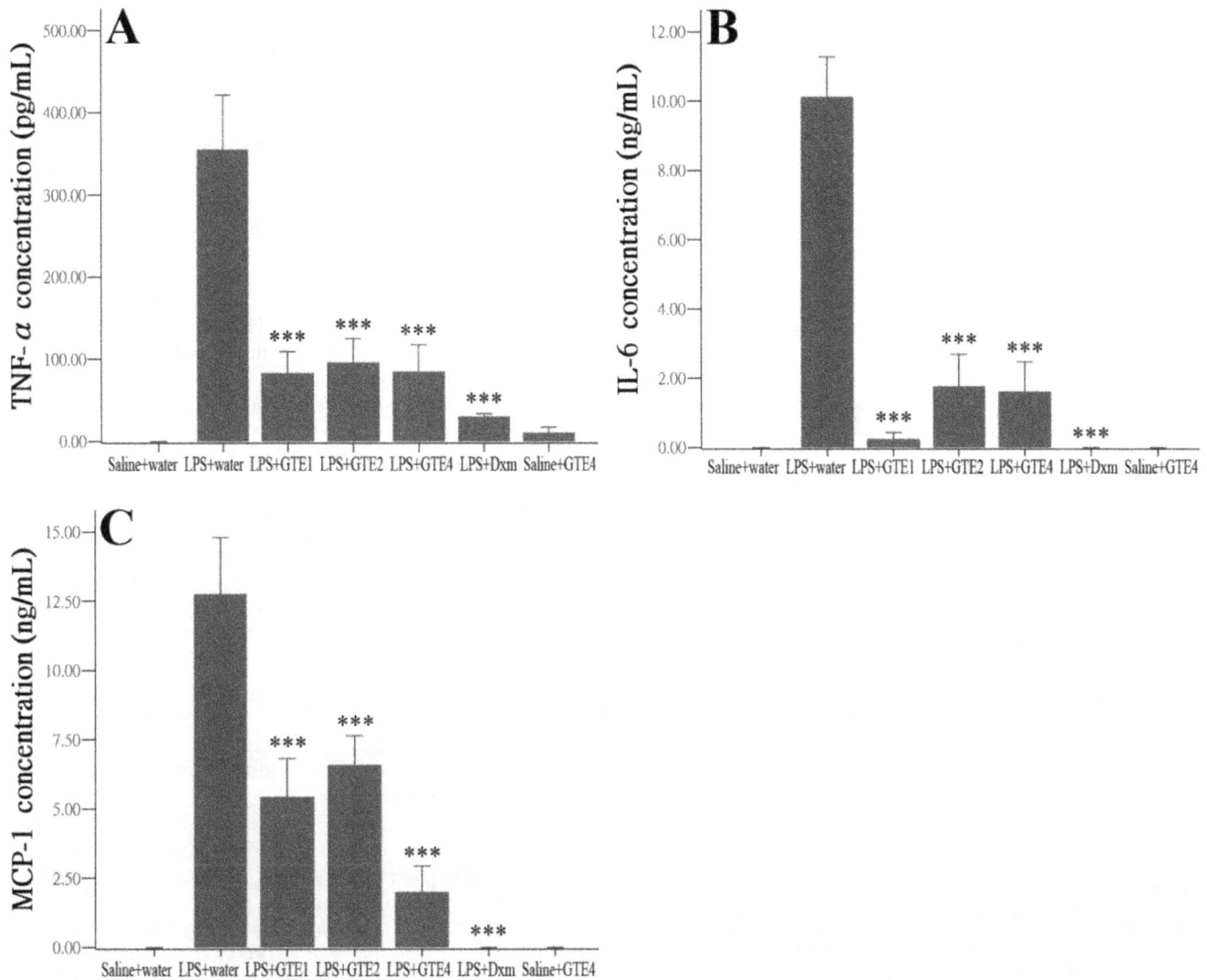

Figure 5. Effects of GTE on cytokine and chemokine production in aqueous humor. The pro-inflammatory factors TNF-α (A), IL-6 (B) and MCP-1 (C) were all reduced significantly after GTE treatments when compared with LPS+water (***$p<0.01$). Within group comparisons, however, did not show obvious differences among GTE treated groups ($p>0.05$). Sensitivity of the assays: 5 pg/mL for TNF-α, 21 pg/mL for IL-6, less than 8.0 pg/mL for MCP-1. Saline+water, n = 3; LPS+water, n = 6; LPS+GTE1, n = 6; LPS+GTE2, n = 6; LPS+GTE4, n = 6; LPS+Dxm, n = 6; Saline+water, n = 3. Data were shown as mean ± SE.

Table 2. TNF-α, IL-6 and MCP-1 concentration in the serum after different treatments.

Groups	Serum, mean ± SD				
	TNF-α (pg/mL)	IL-6 (ng/mL)	p value	MCP-1 (ng/mL)	p value
Saline+water (n = 3)	-	-	-	-	-
LPS+water (n = 6)	-	0.16±0.15	-	6.19±1.19	-
LPS+GTE1 (n = 6)	-	0.12±0.10	0.749	4.82±0.67	0.078
LPS+GTE2 (n = 6)	-	0.08±0.06	0.378	5.20±1.40	0.337
LPS+GTE4 (n = 6)	-	0.13±0.10	0.936	4.59±1.15	0.055
LPS+Dxm (n = 6)	-	0.05±0.08	0.121	1.74±2.07**	0.004
Saline+GTE4 (n = 3)	-	-	-	-	-

-: undetectable. Sensitivity of these assays is 5 pg/mL for TNF-α, 21 pg/mL for IL-6, less than 8.0 pg/mL for MCP-1.
Saline+water: saline injection and fed with water; LPS+water: LPS injection and fed with water; LPS+GTE1: GTE was fed once after LPS injection; LPS+GTE2: GTE was fed twice after LPS injection; LPS+GTE4: GTE was fed four times after LPS injection; LPS+Dxm: Dxm was fed once after LPS injection; Saline+GTE4: saline injection and fed as GTE4; **$p<0.05$, compared with LPS+water.

Table 3. CD14 and TLR-4 mRNA expression in the iris and ciliary body and the retina by quantitative real-time PCR analyses.

Groups	Iris-ciliary body C_T values, mean ± SD CD14	TLR-4	GAPDH	Fold change in expression due to treatment CD14	TLR-4	Retina C_T values, mean ± SD CD14	TLR-4	GAPDH	Fold change in expression due to treatment CD14	TLR-4
Saline+water (n = 3)	24.93±0.36	26.42±0.69	18.28±0.32	−11	−31	27.18±0.18	27.12±1.15	18.50±0.60	−37	−38
LPS+water (n = 6)	21.38±0.96	21.54±0.36	18.28±0.70	1	1	22.37±.74	20.84±0.29	18.51±0.42	1	1
LPS+GTE1 (n = 6)	22.65±0.51	24.32±0.44	19.09±0.30	−2	−3	22.25±1.12	23.10±0.90	17.84±1.12	−2	−4
LPS+GTE2 (n = 6)	22.23±1.31	23.57±0.51	18.39±0.97	−2	−4	25.00±1.44	25.81±0.76	18.97±0.81	−2	−11
LPS+GTE4 (n = 6)	22.92±0.83	24.05±0.29	18.71±0.48	−2	−4	25.49±1.90	27.06±1.43	17.80±0.42	−10	−30
LPS+Dxm (n = 6)	23.99±0.52	25.18±0.50	18.63±0.32	−5	−9	29.04±2.37	25.50±2.37	19.60±1.69	−10	−38
Saline+GTE4 (n = 3)	26.21±0.40	27.26±0.38	18.82±0.48	−19	−47	27.45±0.71	27.43±2.27	18.15±0.56	−37	−50

C_T: threshold cycle; Saline+water: saline injection and fed with water; LPS+water: LPS injection and fed with water; LPS+GTE1: GTE was fed once after LPS injection; LPS+GTE2: GTE was fed twice after LPS injection; LPS+GTE4: GTE was fed four times after LPS injection; LPS+Dxm: Dxm was fed once after LPS injection; Saline+GTE4: saline injection and fed as GTE4.

space) showed a significant reduction in GTE treated animals ($p<0.05$) when compared with the vehicle treated LPS group (LPS+water) (Fig. 3I).

Cell infiltration and protein exudation in aqueous humor

The changes in infiltrating cells and protein content in aqueous humor were also analyzed. Treatments of GTE produced significant decrease in infiltration cells ($p<0.05$) and accumulation of protein ($p<0.05$) when compared with vehicle treated LPS group (Fig. 4A–B), agreeing with the results in histological analyses, though these effects were not as potent as Dxm ($p<0.01$). No differences were observed among animals treated with one, two or four times of oral administrations of GTE, agreeing with the findings in the histological study. The reason of lack of effect for multiple dosage was unclear, but may be caused by the rapid decline of anti-oxidative property of GTE in the aqueous humor [30]. Treatment with GTE alone without injection of LPS produced neither an accumulation of cells nor an increase in protein exudation in the aqueous humor.

The dosage effect was tested in another experiment, in which the rats were fed with either 550 or 275 mg/kg GTE, 2 and 11 hours after LPS injection. The results showed that both infiltrating cell number and protein level in aqueous humor were significantly reduced at the dose of 550 mg/kg ($p<0.05$), but the effect became insignificant when the dose was reduced to half (Fig. 4C–D), indicating that 550 mg/kg is an effective dose in suppressing these inflammatory responses.

TNF-α, IL-6, and MCP-1 in aqueous humor

The pro-inflammatory factors TNF-α, IL-6 and MCP-1 were determined in the aqueous humor using ELISA. LPS caused a surge in TNF-α, IL-6 and MCP-1, which were barely detected in normal controls (Fig. 5A–C). All GTE treatments caused a significant reduction of these factors when compared with the LPS group (LPS+water) ($p<0.05$). However, no significant difference was detected within the GTE groups ($p>0.05$), suggesting that multiple treatments did not produce additional effect in reducing these pro-inflammatory factors. The effect of Dxm was more potent than both GTE1 and GTE2 only for MCP-1 (GTE1 vs Dxm, $p = 0.007$; GTE2 vs Dxm, $p = 0.002$) but not for TNF-α and IL-6. GTE alone did not produce any detectable change in these factors. Analyses of the serum showed no significant reduction of pro-inflammatory factors in animals treated with either GTE when compared with those treated with LPS and vehicle (Table 2). Dexamethasone treatment caused a significant reduction in MCP-1 ($p<0.01$) but not in IL-6. While TNF-α was beyond the detectable level in the serum, both GTE and Dxm treatments could not reduce the level of IL-6 and MCP-1 to that of normal control.

Expression of CD14 and TLR-4 mRNA, and NF-κBp65 activity in ocular tissues

Quantitative real-time PCR was used to determine the expression of TLR-4 and CD14, the respective receptor and co-receptor for LPS, after LPS injection and GTE treatment (Table 3). Expression of both TLR-4 and CD14 were up-regulated after LPS insult in the iris and ciliary body (Fig. 6A) and in the retina (Fig. 6B). These elevated expressions were suppressed significantly by GTE or Dxm treatment ($p<0.01$, Fig. 6A–B). GTE treatment alone without LPS injection did not caused obvious changes in TLR-4 and CD14 expression when compared with normal control.

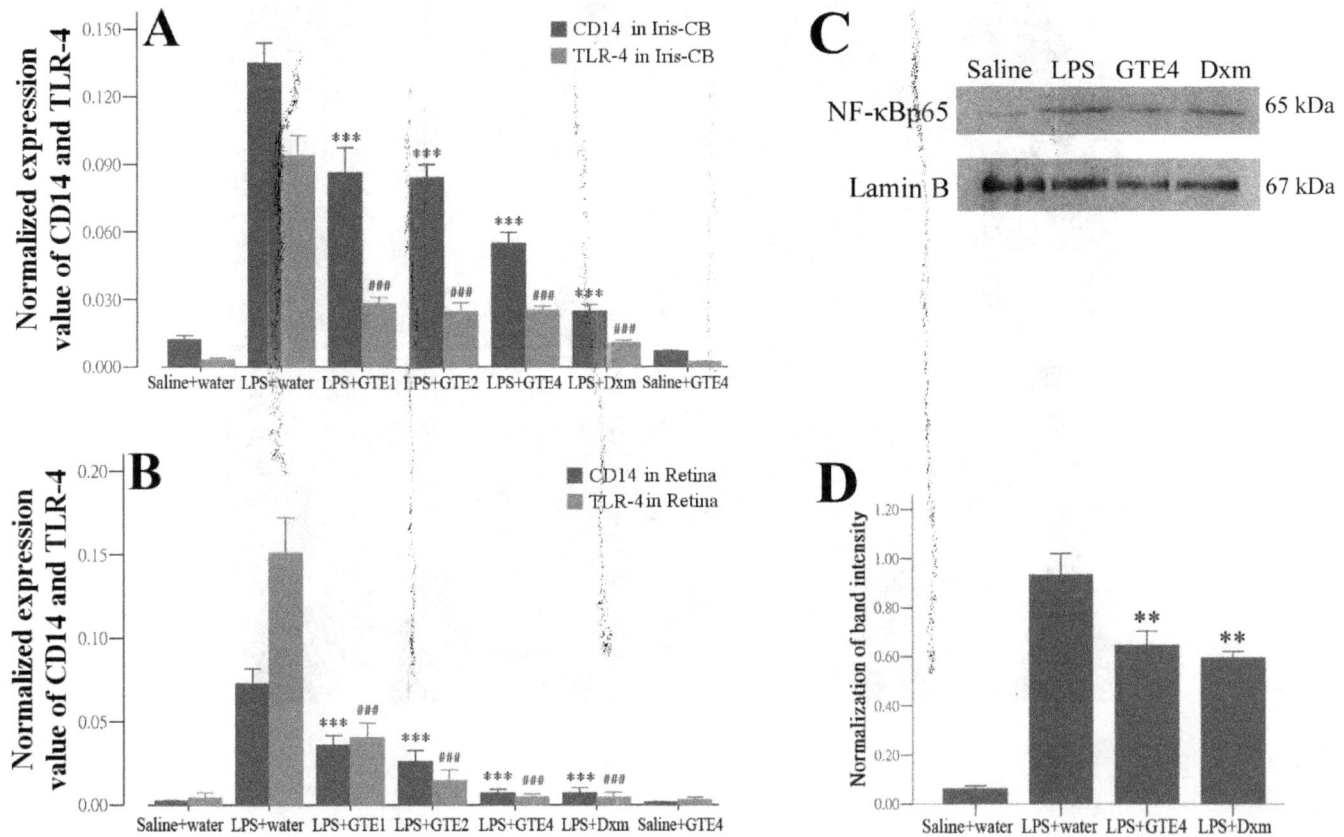

Figure 6. Effect of GTE on CD14 and TLR-4 mRNA expression and nuclear NF-κBp65 protein expression in ocular tissues. (A) and (B): Quantitative PCR analyses showing expression of CD14 and TLR-4 transcripts in the iris and ciliary body (A), and the retina (B). Both genes were reduced significantly after GTE or Dxm treatment, when compared with the values in LPS+water group. GTE treatments alone (saline+GTE4) did not generate obvious changes to these expression genes. Saline+water, n = 3; LPS+water, n = 6; LPS+GTE1, n = 6; LPS+GTE2, n = 6; LPS+GTE4, n = 6; LPS+Dxm, n = 6; Saline+GTE4, n = 3. (C): Nuclear proteins isolated from iris and ciliary body were analyzed using Western blot to detect the level of nuclear NF-κBp65. Lamin B was used as internal control. (D): Measurements of band intensity of NF-κBp65/Lamin B showed a significant reduction of nuclear NF-κBp65 after treatment with GTE or dexamethasone (Dxm). n = 3 in each plot. Data were shown as mean ± SE. **$p<0.05$, *** and ###: $p<0.01$, compared with LPS+water.

The level of nuclear NF-κBp65, a downstream molecule of TLR-4 signaling, was examined in the iris and ciliary body after LPS and GTE treatments. Western blot showed that this protein was upregulated in the tissues after LPS injection, and its expression was decreased substantially after treatment of GTE4 and Dxm (Fig. 6C). Measurements of band intensity with reference to that of Lamin B confirmed a significant reduction of nuclear NF-κBp65 after GTE4 or Dxm treatment ($p<0.05$) (Fig. 6D).

Effect of GTE on macrophages within iris and ciliary body

To investigate the effect of GTE treatment on the macrophages accumulating in the iris and ciliary body, sections of the eye were immunostained with antibody against CD68. In normal control only a few CD68 positive macrophages were observed in the stroma of iris and ciliary body (Fig. 7A). The number of macrophages was increased substantially after LPS treatment (Fig. 7B and E), and was reduced significantly after treatment of either GTE4 or Dxm ($p<0.05$) (Fig. 7C–E).

Discussion

Results of this study show that oral administration of GTE, at the dose of 550 mg/kg, produces anti-inflammatory effects against LPS-induced ocular inflammation. The major findings include: i) GTE alleviates clinical manifestations of ocular inflammation; ii) it reduces infiltration of leukocytes and macrophages, and leakage of protein into aqueous humor and vitreous body; iii) it also suppresses production of pro-inflammatory biomarkers TNF-α, IL-6 and MCP-1 in aqueous humor; iv) these anti-inflammatory effects are associated with down-regulation of LPS receptors, TLR-4 and CD14, and reduction of nuclear NF-κBp65, v) GTE also reduces accumulation of macrophages in the stroma of iris and ciliary body. These results provide evidence for the first time that GTE is a potent anti-inflammatory agent for acute ocular inflammation.

We have shown in this study that the levels of pro-inflammatory mediators, TNF-α, IL-6 and MCP-1, were elevated significantly in the aqueous humor twenty-four hours after LPS injection. TNF-α has been shown in rats to be the major player in LPS-induced leukocyte adhesion, vascular leakage and cell death in the rats' eyes [34]. In mice deficient of MCP-1, inflammatory responses are reduced in a model of EIU [32]. The surge of infiltrating leukocytes and macrophages in the aqueous humor is thus likely caused by an increased production of pro-inflammatory factors as a response to the LPS insult. LPS also induces an accumulation of macrophages in the stroma of iris and ciliary body, either by recruitment of circulating macrophages or activation of resident

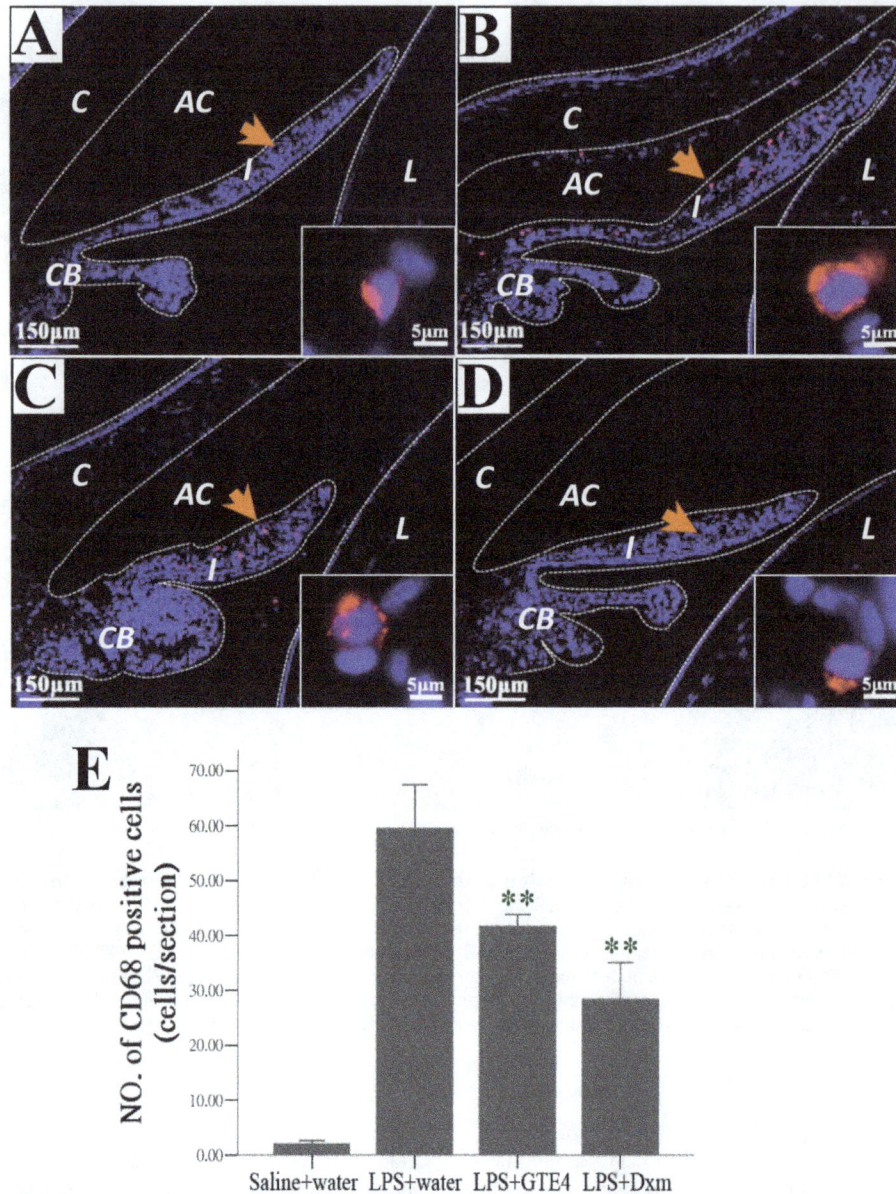

Figure 7. Effect of GTE on macrophages within iris and ciliary body. (A)–(D): Fluorescent micrographs showing some cells were immunopositive to CD68, a marker for macrophages (arrows, magnified in inserts) 24 hours after treatment with (A): saline+water, (B): LPS+water, (C): LPS+GTE4, (D): LPS+Dxm. (E): A significant reduction in number of macrophages presented in the stroma of iris and ciliary body was observed after treatment with GTE and dexamethasone (Dxm). n = 3 in each group. Data were shown as mean ± SE. **p<0.05 compared with LPS+water. C: cornea; AC: anterior chamber; I: iris; PC: posterior chamber; L: lens; CB: ciliary body.

cells in these tissues. GTE exerts its anti-inflammatory actions through a suppression of production of these pro-inflammatory factors, and thereby reducing the infiltration of leucocytes and macrophages and exudation of protein into the aqueous humor, and recruitment or activation of macrophages residing in the iris and ciliary body. These anti-inflammatory effects seem to be specific to ocular tissues as shown by the results that significant reduction of IL-6 and MCP-1 after GTE treatment is observed only in the aqueous humor but not in the serum. The specific changes agree with previous findings that TNF-α, IL-6 and MCP-1 are elevated in aqueous humor of patients with infectious or noninfectious uveitis but not in the serum [35,36]. Reduction of TNF-α was detected only in the aqueous humor but not in the

serum, possibly because its properties of brief production [37] and high hepatic clearance [38] in the circulatory system.

Juxtaposition of CD14 and TLR-4 in the anterior uvea contributes to the sensitivity of iris and ciliary body to LPS [39]. CD14 does not have a trans-membrane segment and so needs TLR-4, a trans-membrane protein, to transduce the LPS stimulation. LPS binds primarily to resident macrophages or epithelial cells lining the iris and ciliary processes [39,40]. When LPS-CD14-TLR4 cluster activation is inhibited by lipid raft-disrupting drug or lipid A mimetic antagonists, LPS-induced cellular cascading reaction is interrupted [41,42]. We have shown in this study that GTE suppresses LPS induced elevation of CD14 and TLR-4 mRNA in the anterior uvea and the retina, suggesting that GTE treatment may alleviate ocular inflammation by suppressing formation of the LPS receptor complex. These findings are consistent with previous reports showing that EGCG is able to block the interaction between LPS and TLR-4 and downregulate TLR-4 mRNA expression *in vitro* [43,44]. However, other receptor components, such as HSP 70/90 (heat-shock proteins 70 and 90), CXCR4 (chemokine receptor 4), and DAF (decay-accelerating factor) also participate in the LPS-CD14-TLR4 cluster activation, probably acting as additional LPS-transfer molecules [45]. Moreover, EGCG has also been shown to suppress inflammatory responses by binding to the surface molecule 67-kDa laminin receptor (76LR), which results in reduction of expression of pro-inflammatory mediators, such as TNF-α, IL-6 and cyclooxygenase-2 [43]. Whether GTE may modulate function of these molecules remains to be investigated.

Anti-inflammatory properties of GTE have been reported in other experimental disease models. Epigallocatechin-3-gallate (EGCG), the major constituent of GTE, has shown to reduce expression of inflammatory biomarkers in human cell lines such as chondrocytes and corneal epithelium, and experimental models of dry eye [46–48]. These effects are related to a suppression of IκB kinase-β (IKKβ) and TANK-binding kinase-1 (TBK1) [49], or inhibition of the proteasome-mediated degradation pathway that induces accumulation of NF-κB inhibitors, p27^{Kip1} and IκB-α

[50]. We have shown in the current study that LPS induced nuclear NF-κBp65 is significantly reduced after GTE treatment, probably caused by a reduced level of TLR-4-CD14 receptor complex, and leads eventually to a reduced expression of genes coding for cytokines and chemokines.

To our knowledge, this is the first report to demonstrate anti-inflammatory effects of GTE on acute ocular inflammation. The findings in this study support strongly that GTE is a potent therapeutic agent for treatment of acute anterior uveitis.

Acknowledgments

We are indebted to Prof. Yukihiko Hara for his generous donation of green tea extract (Theaphenon E, Tea Solutions, Hara Office Inc., Japan). We thank Ms Pancy O. S. TAM and Dr. Ka Sin LAW for their expert technical advice.

Author Contributions

Conceived and designed the experiments: CPP SOC KOC. Performed the experiments: YJQ YWWY WYL YPY KPC JLR. Analyzed the data: YJQ YWWY WYL. Contributed reagents/materials/analysis tools: WYL YPY KPC. Wrote the paper: YJQ CPP SOC KOC.

References

1. Durrani OM, Tehrani NN, Marr JE, Moradi P, Stavrou P, et al. (2004) Degree, duration, and causes of visual loss in uveitis. Br J Ophthalmol 88: 1159–1162.
2. Gritz DC, Wong IG (2004) Incidence and prevalence of uveitis in Northern California; the Northern California Epidemiology of Uveitis Study. Ophthalmology 111: 491–500.
3. Siddique SS, Shah R, Suelves AM, Foster CS (2011) Road to remission: a comprehensive review of therapy in uveitis. Expert Opin Investig Drugs 20: 1497–1515.
4. Nguyen QD, Callanan D, Dugel P, Godfrey DG, Goldstein DA, et al. (2006) Treating chronic noninfectious posterior segment uveitis: the impact of cumulative damage. Proceedings of an expert panel roundtable discussion. Retina Suppl: 1–16.
5. Nguyen QD, Hatef E, Kayen B, Macahilig CP, Ibrahim M, et al. (2011) A cross-sectional study of the current treatment patterns in noninfectious uveitis among specialists in the United States. Ophthalmology 118: 184–190.
6. Lee FF, Foster CS (2010) Pharmacotherapy of uveitis. Expert Opin Pharmacother 11: 1135–1146.
7. Poulaki V, Iliaki E, Mitsiades N, Mitsiades CS, Paulus YN, et al. (2007) Inhibition of Hsp90 attenuates inflammation in endotoxin-induced uveitis. Faseb J 21: 2113–2123.
8. Ohgami K, Ilieva I, Shiratori K, Koyama Y, Jin XH, et al. (2005) Anti-inflammatory effects of aronia extract on rat endotoxin-induced uveitis. Invest Ophthalmol Vis Sci 46: 275–281.
9. Yang X, Jin H, Liu K, Gu Q, Xu X (2011) A novel peptide derived from human pancreatitis-associated protein inhibits inflammation in vivo and in vitro and blocks NF-kappa B signaling pathway. PLoS One 6: e29155.
10. Kalariya NM, Reddy AB, Ansari NH, VanKuijk FJ, Ramana KV (2011) Preventive effects of ethyl pyruvate on endotoxin-induced uveitis in rats. Invest Ophthalmol Vis Sci 52: 5144–5152.
11. Suzuki J, Manola A, Murakami Y, Morizane Y, Takeuchi K, et al. (2011) Inhibitory effect of aminoimidazole carboxamide ribonucleotide (AICAR) on endotoxin-induced uveitis in rats. Invest Ophthalmol Vis Sci 52: 6565–6571.
12. Rosenbaum JT, McDevitt HO, Guss RB, Egbert PR (1980) Endotoxin-induced uveitis in rats as a model for human disease. Nature 286: 611–613.
13. Okumura A, Mochizuki M, Nishi M, Herbort CP (1990) Endotoxin-induced uveitis (EIU) in the rat: a study of inflammatory and immunological mechanisms. Int Ophthalmol 14: 31–36.
14. Da SP, Girol AP, Oliani SM (2011) Mast cells modulate the inflammatory process in endotoxin-induced uveitis. Mol Vis 17: 1310–1319.
15. Smith JR, Hart PH, Williams KA (1998) Basic pathogenic mechanisms operating in experimental models of acute anterior uveitis. Immunol Cell Biol 76: 497–512.
16. Wakefield D, Gray P, Chang J, Di Girolamo N, McCluskey P (2010) The role of PAMPs and DAMPs in the pathogenesis of acute and recurrent anterior uveitis. Br J Ophthalmol 94: 271–274.
17. Poltorak A, He X, Smirnova I, Liu MY, Van Huffel C, et al. (1998) Defective LPS signaling in C3H/HeJ and C57BL/10ScCr mice: mutations in Tlr4 gene. Science 282: 2085–2088.
18. de Vos AF, Klaren VN, Kijlstra A (1994) Expression of multiple cytokines and IL-1RA in the uvea and retina during endotoxin-induced uveitis in the rat. Invest Ophthalmol Vis Sci 35: 3873–3883.
19. Heiligenhaus A, Thurau S, Hennig M, Grajewski RS, Wildner G (2010) Anti-inflammatory treatment of uveitis with biologicals: new treatment options that reflect pathogenetic knowledge of the disease. Graefes Arch Clin Exp Ophthalmol 248: 1531–1551.
20. Kawai T, Akira S (2010) The role of pattern-recognition receptors in innate immunity: update on Toll-like receptors. Nat Immunol 11: 373–384.
21. Lin S, Yin Q, Zhong Q, Lv FL, Zhou Y, et al. (2012) Heme activates TLR4-mediated inflammatory injury via MyD88/TRIF signaling pathway in intracerebral hemorrhage. J Neuroinflammation 9: 46.
22. Pooran N, Indaram A, Singh P, Bank S (2003) Cytokines (IL-6, IL-8, TNF): early and reliable predictors of severe acute pancreatitis. J Clin Gastroenterol 37: 263–266.
23. Serhan CN (2010) Novel lipid mediators and resolution mechanisms in acute inflammation: to resolve or not? Am J Pathol 177: 1576–1591.
24. Chertin B, Farkas A, Puri P (2003) Epidermal growth factor and monocyte chemotactic peptide-1 expression in reflux nephropathy. Eur Urol 44: 144–149.
25. Jimenez-Sainz MC, Fast B, Mayor FJ, Aragay AM (2003) Signaling pathways for monocyte chemoattractant protein 1-mediated extracellular signal-regulated kinase activation. Mol Pharmacol 64: 773–782.
26. Bhattacherjee P, Williams RN, Eakins KE (1983) An evaluation of ocular inflammation following the injection of bacterial endotoxin into the rat foot pad. Invest Ophthalmol Vis Sci 24: 196–202.
27. Okumura A, Mochizuki M (1988) Endotoxin-induced uveitis in rats: morphological and biochemical study. Jpn J Ophthalmol 32: 457–465.
28. Masukawa Y, Matsui Y, Shimizu N, Kondou N, Endou H, et al. (2006) Determination of green tea catechins in human plasma using liquid chromatography-electrospray ionization mass spectrometry. J Chromatogr B Analyt Technol Biomed Life Sci 834: 26–34.
29. Stangl V, Dreger H, Stangl K, Lorenz M (2007) Molecular targets of tea polyphenols in the cardiovascular system. Cardiovasc Res 73: 348–358.
30. Chu KO, Chan KP, Wang CC, Chu CY, Li WY, et al. (2010) Green tea catechins and their oxidative protection in the rat eye. J Agric Food Chem 58: 1523–1534.
31. Pouvreau I, Zech JC, Thillaye-Goldenberg B, Naud MC, Van Rooijen N, et al. (1998) Effect of macrophage depletion by liposomes containing dichloromethylene-diphosphonate on endotoxin-induced uveitis. J Neuroimmunol 86: 171–181.
32. Tuaillon N, Shen DF, Berger RB, Lu B, Rollins BJ, et al. (2002) MCP-1 expression in endotoxin-induced uveitis. Invest Ophthalmol Vis Sci 43: 1493–1498.
33. Schmittgen TD, Livak KJ (2008) Analyzing real-time PCR data by the comparative C(T) method. Nat Protoc 3: 1101–1108.
34. Koizumi K, Poulaki V, Doehmen S, Welsandt G, Radetzky S, et al. (2003) Contribution of TNF-alpha to leukocyte adhesion, vascular leakage, and apoptotic cell death in endotoxin-induced uveitis in vivo. Invest Ophthalmol Vis Sci 44: 2184–2191.
35. de Visser L, Rijkers GT, Wiertz K, Rothova A, de Groot-Mijnes DF (2009) Cytokine and chemokine profiling in ocular fluids of patients with infectious

uveitis. In: de Visser L, editor. Infectious uveitis. New developments in etiology and pathogenesis. Gildeprint Drukkerijen: Enschede, NL, 148–173.

36. Ooi KG, Galatowicz G, Calder VL, Lightman SL (2006) Cytokines and chemokines in uveitis: is there a correlation with clinical phenotype? Clin Med Res 4: 294–309.

37. van Kessel KP, van Strijp JA, Verhoef J (1991) Inactivation of recombinant human tumor necrosis factor-alpha by proteolytic enzymes released from stimulated human neutrophils. J Immunol 147: 3862–3868.

38. Grewal HP, Mohey EDA, Gaber L, Kotb M, Gaber AO (1994) Amelioration of the physiologic and biochemical changes of acute pancreatitis using an anti-TNF-alpha polyclonal antibody. Am J Surg 167: 214–218, 218–219.

39. Brito BE, Zamora DO, Bonnah RA, Pan Y, Planck SR, et al. (2004) Toll-like receptor 4 and CD14 expression in human ciliary body and TLR-4 in human iris endothelial cells. Exp Eye Res 79: 203–208.

40. Su GL (2002) Lipopolysaccharides in liver injury: molecular mechanisms of Kupffer cell activation. Am J Physiol Gastrointest Liver Physiol 283: G256–G265.

41. Piazza M, Rossini C, Della FS, Pozzi C, Comelli F, et al. (2009) Glycolipids and benzylammonium lipids as novel antisepsis agents: synthesis and biological characterization. J Med Chem 52: 1209–1213.

42. Triantafilou M, Miyake K, Golenbock DT, Triantafilou K (2002) Mediators of innate immune recognition of bacteria concentrate in lipid rafts and facilitate lipopolysaccharide-induced cell activation. J Cell Sci 115: 2603–2611.

43. Hong BE, Fujimura Y, Yamada K, Tachibana H (2010) TLR4 signaling inhibitory pathway induced by green tea polyphenol epigallocatechin-3-gallate through 67-kDa laminin receptor. J Immunol 185: 33–45.

44. Lin YL, Lin JK (1997) (-)-Epigallocatechin-3-gallate blocks the induction of nitric oxide synthase by down-regulating lipopolysaccharide-induced activity of transcription factor nuclear factor-kappaB. Mol Pharmacol 52: 465–472.

45. Triantafilou M, Triantafilou K (2002) Lipopolysaccharide recognition: CD14, TLRs and the LPS-activation cluster. Trends Immunol 23: 301–304.

46. Akhtar N, Haqqi TM (2011) Epigallocatechin-3-gallate suppresses the global interleukin-1beta-induced inflammatory response in human chondrocytes. Arthritis Res Ther 13: R93.

47. Cavet ME, Harrington KL, Vollmer TR, Ward KW, Zhang JZ (2011) Anti-inflammatory and anti-oxidative effects of the green tea polyphenol epigallocatechin gallate in human corneal epithelial cells. Mol Vis 17: 533–542.

48. Lee HS, Chauhan SK, Okanobo A, Nallasamy N, Dana R (2011) Therapeutic efficacy of topical epigallocatechin gallate in murine dry eye. Cornea 30: 1465–1472.

49. Youn HS, Lee JY, Saitoh SI, Miyake K, Kang KW, et al. (2006) Suppression of MyD88- and TRIF-dependent signaling pathways of Toll-like receptor by (-)-epigallocatechin-3-gallate, a polyphenol component of green tea. Biochem Pharmacol 72: 850–859.

50. Nam S, Smith DM, Dou QP (2001) Ester bond-containing tea polyphenols potently inhibit proteasome activity in vitro and in vivo. J Biol Chem 276: 13322–13330.

7

Acute Increase of Children's Conjunctivitis Clinic Visits by Asian Dust Storms Exposure - A Spatiotemporal Study

Lung-Chang Chien[1], Yi-Jen Lien[2], Chiang-Hsin Yang[3], Hwa-Lung Yu[2]*

1 Division of Biostatistics, University of Texas School of Public Health at San Antonio Regional Campus, San Antonio, Texas, United States of America, 2 Department of Bioenvironmental Systems Engineering, National Taiwan University, Taipei, Taiwan, 3 Department of Health Care Management, National Taipei University of Nursing and Health Sciences, Taipei, Taiwan

Abstract

Adverse health impacts of Asian dust storms (ADS) have been widely investigated and discussed in respiratory disease, but no study has examined the association between ADS events and their impact on eye diseases, especially in children. The impact of ADS events on the incidence of children's conjunctivitis is examined by analyzing the data from children's clinic visits registered in the 41 districts of Taipei area in Taiwan during the period 2002–2007. The structural additive regression modeling approach was used to assess the association between ADS events and clinic visits for conjunctivitis in children with consideration of day-of-the-week effects, temperature, and air quality levels. This study identifies an acute increase in the relative rate for children's conjunctivitis clinic visits during ADS periods with 1.48% (95% CI = 0.79, 2.17) for preschool children (aged <6 years old) and 9.48% (95% CI = 9.03, 9.93) for schoolchildren (aged ≥6 years old), respectively. The relative rates during post-ADS periods were still statistically significant, but much lower than those during ADS periods. The spatial analysis presents geographic heterogeneity of children's conjunctivitis clinic visits where higher relative rates were more likely observed in the most populated districts Compared to previous ADS studies related to respiratory diseases, our results reveals significantly acute impacts on children's conjunctivitis during ADS periods, and much influence on schoolchildren. Vulnerable areas were also identified in high density population.

Editor: Chen-Wei Pan, Medical College of Soochow University, China

Funding: This research and data collection was supported by funds from the National Science Council of Taiwan (NSC101-2628-E-002-017-MY3 and NSC101-2628-E-002-003) and the Environmental Protection Department of the New Taipei City Government (Taiwan). The funders had no role in study design, data collection and analysis, decision to publish, or preparation of the manuscript.

Competing Interests: The authors have declared that no competing interests exist.

* Email: hlyu@ntu.edu.tw

Introduction

Asian dust storm (ADS) events, severe wide-spread disasters that spawn from Mongolia and North China, cause many diseases including respiratory diseases, cardiovascular diseases, asthma, chronic obstructive pulmonary disease, pneumonia, and stroke. The health outcomes of these diseases range from death to various stages of illness that may require hospital admissions, emergency room visits, and clinic visits [1–7]. ADS events diversely impact human health primarily due to a rapid elevation of concentrated levels of air pollutants over a large scale area in a short period of time [8]. Inhalation of air pollutants during these storms has been implicated as the leading cause of adverse health effects. However, eye exposure to direct contact with air pollutants during these storms and the subsequent development of conjunctivitis has rarely been discussed.

The eyes are particularly vulnerable and highly sensitive to direct contact with air pollutants due to the dense neuronal innervations on the ocular surface [9]. For eye-related diseases which are highly correlated with exposure to air pollutants, conjunctivitis is the most significant Conjunctivitis, defined as an irritation or an inflammation of the conjunctiva, usually elicits symptoms of eye irritation and itching. Previous research has established an association between the development of conjunctivitis and the ambient levels of outdoor air pollution or airborne allergens, such as fungal spores and pollen grains [10–12]. Indoor air pollution, such as the cooking smoke from the combustion of biomass (e.g., charcoal, wood, and dung), has also been investigated as a causal agent in the development of conjunctivitis and other eye diseases [13]. ADS events are characterized by extremely high concentrations of air pollutants and allergens compared to the concentrations of these same pollutants and allergens during general periods. Thus, the development of conjunctivitis as a result of exposure during ADS events would be highly likely [14]. However, epidemiological research on the ADS effects to eye health is still rare,, and has not yielded any significant findings [15].

Children, in particular, are very susceptible to the adverse effects of airborne exposures because their immune systems are not as fully developed as those of adults [16]. Previous studies focused on the adverse effects of air pollution on children's health in terms of both short-term [17–21] and long-term exposure [22–24], These pediatrics researches have been centered on investigating pulmonary and lung dysfunction, asthma and respiratory symptoms, and pneumonias, especially for the case of the studies regarding to the influence of ADS events In addition, findings regarding the health impact of ADS events are commonly uncertain because of limited health observations [25]. In the other words, previous ADS and children's health studies have seldom focused on conjunctivitis and analyzed large scale populations of children observed over long periods of time and at varied locations [26]. Due to the availability of nationwide health insurance data in Taiwan, it allows the population-based analysis to reveal the epidemiological linkages between ADS events and the diseases of concern, e.g. conjunctivitis [27,28].

The main purpose of this study was to investigate the spatiotemporal influence of ADS events on the development of conjunctivitis in children by using a large, population-based database taken from daily clinic visits registered in hospitals and clinics in Northern Taiwan from 2002–2007. Specifically, three main questions were addressed: (1) whether there is an increase in children's clinic visits for conjunctivitis during ADS events and for one week after the storm; (2) whether preschool children are more vulnerable than school children to the impact of ADS events as they relate to the development of conjunctivitis; and (3) whether geographic location plays a role in the impact of ADS events on children's conjunctivitis clinic visits.

Materials and Methods

Ethic statement: The data were obtained from National Health Research Institute of Taiwan (NHRI). All of the data request should be approved by IRB of NHRI. The approval number of this study is NHIRD-102-097. Due to concerns regarding personal confidentiality, all individually identifiable health information (e.g., personal identification or hospital identification number) is encrypted prior to release.

Children's clinic visit data

This study retrieve the children's clinic visit data from Taiwan's National Health Insurance (NHI) database which covers the claim data of over 99.6% of the inhabitants of the entire Taiwan, including both emergency and ambulatory visits for various diseases and diagnosis. The database uses International Classification of Diseases, Ninth Revision, Clinical Modification (ICD-9-CM) classification codes to record cause-specific data. Due to concerns regarding personal confidentiality, all individually identifiable health information (e.g., personal identification or hospital identification number) is encrypted prior to release from Bureau of NHI. This study retrieved patients aged ≤14 years with recorded conjunctival disorders (ICD-9: 372). Because children older than 6 years old in Taiwan receive compulsory education, this population was categorized into a preschool group for <6 years-old and a schoolchildren group aged ≥6 years old. This population-based data also contained space-time information for any clinic and hospital visits of children with the diagnosis of conjunctivitis in Taipei City and New Taipei City from 2002–2007. These visits included both ambulatory and emergency room encounters.

Study Area

Taipei has more than six million citizens within an area of approximately 2324.37 km^2. Taipei is best described as a geographic location in Northern Taiwan that contains two administrative regions, Taipei City and New Taipei City. Among them, New Taipei City surrounds Taipei City. The northern boundary is the coastline for to the Taiwan Straits and the Pacific Ocean. This northern coastline border offers no geographic barrier to ADS events that sweep in from the north. In addition, Taipei City has a characteristic basin type of topography that is geographically bounded by three different Mountains to the north, the west, and the southeast. The basin topography reduces air diffusion and increases air pollutant concentrations. According to insurance administrative divisions, a total of 41 districts are contained in the study area with 12 districts for Taipei City and 29 districts for New Taipei City, as shown in Figure 1.

Asian dust storm and air pollution data

A total of 30 ADS events occurring from 2002–2007 were identified by the Taiwan Environmental Protection Agency (TWEPA), during a total of 90 days (Table 1). The TWEPA defines the criteria to determine the incidence of a ADS event, including performing a dust storm track nowcasting along with Taiwan Central Weather Bureau, interpreting remote sensing data, and observing the PM$_{10}$ level at the four ADS indicator stations, i.e., Matsu, Wanli, Guanyin, and Yilan. If forecasting results reveal a high probability that ADS events are headed toward Taiwan, the TWEPA will issue warnings when at least one of the four indicator stations measure PM$_{10}$ concentrations > 100 μg/m^3 [29]. For the analyses purposes the study period from 2002 to 2007 was divided into three sub-periods. First, the time period of the actual ADS event (Table 1) is defined as the ADS period. Second, the time period up to and including 7 days after an ADS event has ended is defined as the post-ADS period. Third, all the other days in the study period are defined as the other period. In addition to the ADS data, PM$_{10}$ concentrations have been regularly monitored at TWEPA stations across Taiwan since 1994. Both the PM$_{10}$ concentrations and temperature measurements used in our analysis were based on the daily observations at the Jhongshan monitoring station located in the most populated area of Taipei City (see Figure 1).

Statistical Modeling Analysis

We analyzed the spatiotemporal pattern of children's conjunctivitis clinic visits in the 41 study districts from 2002 to 2007 using a structured additive regression (STAR) model. The count data for clinic visits followed a Poisson distribution, and can be modeled via a Poisson model framework taking into account both linear and nonlinear explanatory variables, i.e.,

$$Y_{dt}|\mu_{dt} \sim \text{Poisson}(\mu_{dt})$$

Y_{ct} is the number of children's conjunctivitis clinic visits in district d (d = 1, 2,..., 41) at day t (t = 1, 2,..., 2191).

$$\log(\mu_{dt}) = \text{intercept} + X'\beta + Z'\gamma + f(TP) + f(T) + f_{spat}(d) + \log(POP),$$

where μ_{dt} is the expected value of Y_{dt}. The β is a vector of categorical fixed effects $X = [I_{MON}, I_{TUE}, I_{WED}, I_{THUR}, I_{FRI}, I_{SAT}, I_{ADS}, I_{POST-ADS}]'$ corresponding to six dummy variables for day-of-the-week (DOW) from Monday to Saturday plus two dummy

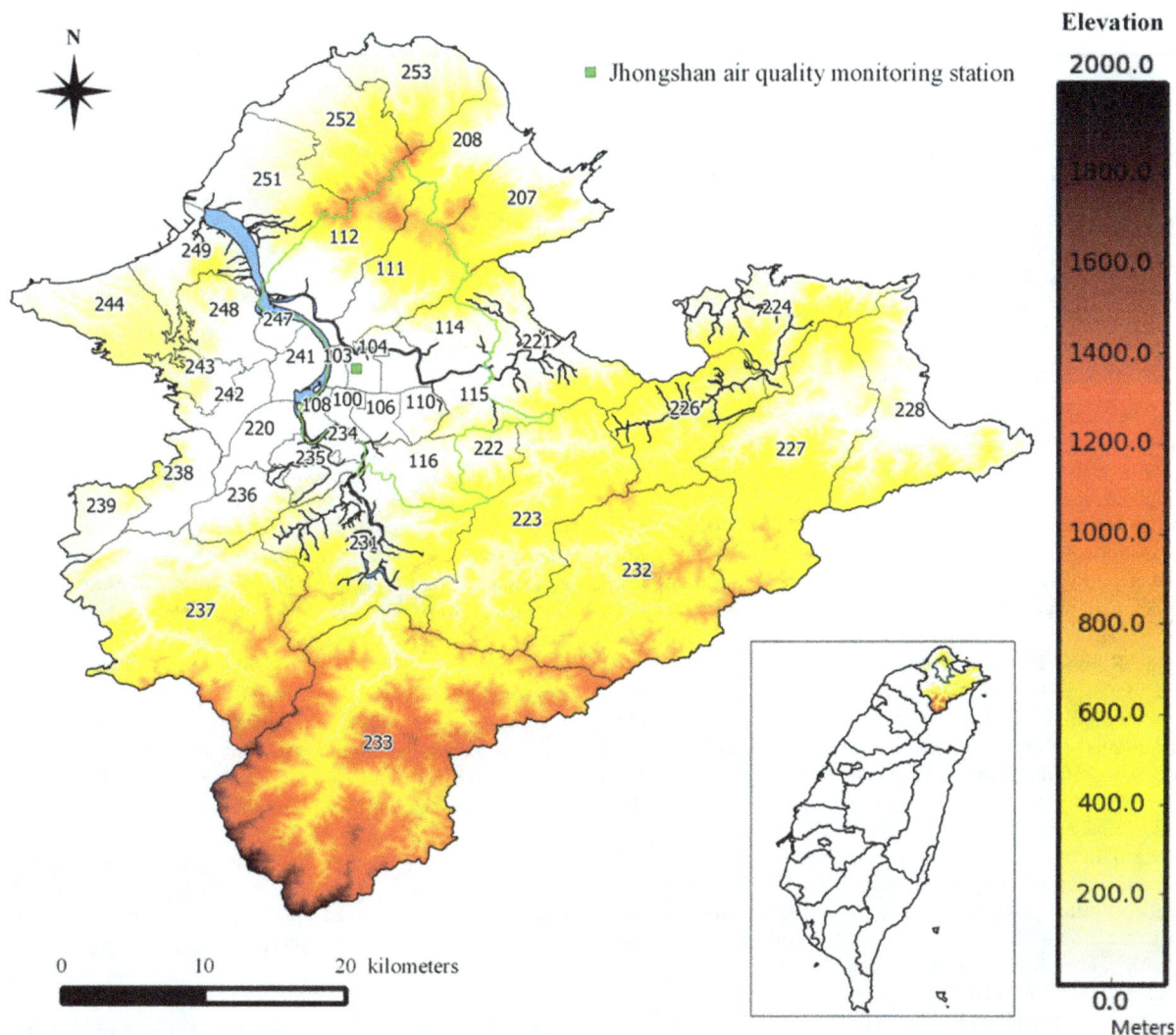

Figure 1. Map of Taipei City (surrounded by green boundaries) and New Taipei City, along with the map of their geographical locations in the Taiwan Island. The district names are denoted by their zip codes with the names shown at the table below. The Jhongshan air quality monitoring station is highlighted by a green square.

Zip code	District name	Zip code	District name	Zip code	District name	Zip code	District name	Zip code	District name
100	Jhongjheng	112	Beitou	222	Shenkeng	233	Wulai	242	Sinjhuang
103	Datong	114	Neihu	223	Shihding	234	Yonghe	243	Taishan
104	Jhongshan	115	Nangang	224	Rueifang	235	Jhonghe	244	Linkou
105	Songshan	116	Wunshan	226	Pingsi	236	Tucheng	247	Lujhou
106	Daan	207	Wanli	227	Shuangsi	237	Sansia	248	Wugu
108	Wanhua	208	Jinshan	228	Gongliao	238	Shulin	249	Bali
110	Sinyi	220	Banciao	231	Sindian	239	Yingge	251	Danshui
111	Shilin	221	Sijhih	232	Pinglin	241	Sanchong	252	Sanjhih
								253	Shihmen

variables for the ADS period and post-ADS period. Theoretically, DOW variables are mainly used to adjust for short-term temporal autoregressive correlations. From a practical standpoint, we are able to investigate the peak number of children's conjunctivitis clinic visits within one week of an ADS event which reflects a special attribute of medical service in Taiwan. Two ADS variables can be used to evaluate the impact of ADS on children's conjunctivitis clinic visit during the ADS period and the post-ADS period compared to other period. The γ is the vector of continuous confounders Z, which contains at least one of five air

pollutants (CO, NO_x, O_3, PM_{10}, and SO_2). Two nonlinear smoothing functions for calendar time T and for daily mean temperature TP applied a B-spline with a second order random walk penalty [30,31] to adjust for long-term temporal trends and the effects of weather. The spatial function $f_{spat}(d)$ is defined by a structured spatial effect using the Markov random fields [32] with a normally distributed conditional autoregressive prior:

$$f_{spat}(d')|d \neq d' \sim N(\Sigma_{d' \in \Theta d} f_{spat}(d')/N_d, \sigma_d^2/N_d),$$

Table 1. Dust storm events in Taiwan, 2002–2007.

Year	Date	# of events	# of days
2002	2/11-2/12, 3/6-3/9, 3/23-3/24, 3/31-4/1, 4/8-4/15, 4/17-4/19	6	21
2003	2/18-2/19, 2/23-2/25, 3/6-3/9, 3/25-3/30, 4/25-4/28	5	19
2004	1/1-1/4, 1/13-1/14, 1/21-1/22, 1/24-1/25, 2/6-2/12, 2/14-2/16, 2/26-2/27, 3/3-3/7, 4/2-4/4	9	30
2005	3/18-3/19, 11/29-11/30, 12/21-12/22	3	6
2006	3/19-3/20, 3/29-3/30, 4/20-4/21	3	6
2007	1/28-1/29, 4/2-4/3, 4/17-4/18, 12/30-12/31	4	8

where the denominator N_d in both the mean and the variance is the number of neighboring districts adjacent to district d, and θ_d is a subset of neighbors of district d. The variance σ^2_d and unknown smoothing parameters are estimated simultaneously with hyperpriors following an inverse Gamma distribution IG(0.001, 0.001). Last, the term log(POP) is the offset defined by the logarithm of the district-level population of children approximated by multiplying the proportion of children in Taipei by the total population of each district.

The STAR model's estimates are calculated according to an empirical Bayes influence that utilizes a restricted maximum likelihood method. This is a surrogate of the maximum likelihood method designed to avoid the loss of degrees of freedom and to prevent biasing estimated coefficients toward zero [33,34]. Model selection for choosing the best combinations of air pollutants utilized the Akaike Information Criterion (AIC) [35]. Specifically, seven one-pollutant models were fitted for selecting significant positive estimated coefficients of air pollutants. Then, several two-pollutant and three-pollutant models were fitted retaining the significant air pollutants from one-pollutant models. Only the models with positively significant air pollutants were included in the selection to determine the final model according to the smallest AIC separately for preschool children and schoolchildren. In these models, the estimated coefficient of this fixed effect can be explained by the percentage change in the relative rate (RR) of children's conjunctivitis clinic visits compared to the reference level. The spatial function can be interpreted by the RR in district 'd' compared with the mean value for the population as a whole and accounting for spatial autocorrelations by taking a logarithm of it [36]. The spatial effect in each district has a posterior distribution which can be used to generate a 95% credible interval (CI) in order to determine the significance of each spatial estimate according to the 95% posterior probability. For a more meaningful presentation, the spatial effect can be categorized into: (1) a strictly positive effect if 95% of the posterior distribution is above one; (2) a strictly negative effect if 95% of the posterior distribution is below one; (3) a non-significant effect if 95% of the posterior distribution contains one. Maps for the estimated spatial effects with corresponding 95% posterior probability were constructed to highlight the spatial pattern of children's conjunctivitis clinic visits. Data were cleaned and managed by using SAS v9.3 software (SAS Institute Inc., Cary, NC), and the spatiotemporal data analyses were accomplished by the BayesX v2.01 software package [37].

Results

Figure 2 depicts the crude rate of daily children's conjunctivitis clinic visits among the 41 districts in Taipei, clearly demonstrating that the crude clinic visit rate was not uniformly distributed across the study area. By city, the crude rate per 100,000 children in Taipei City ranged from 47.98 to 266.28, but there was a wider range from 0.72 to 400.89 in New Taipei City, which means that the geographic disparity of children's conjunctivitis morbidity there may be larger than that in Taipei City. Table 2 documents that the daily average measurements of O_3 and PM_{10} were elevated during the ADS period. Their averages decreased during the post-ADS period, but were still higher than levels during other period. The other air pollutants had decreased average measurements from the other period through the ADS period, but these were increased during the post-ADS period.

Figure 3 gives ranked values of AIC for the fit and complexity of the selected models. It suggests that among those 31 models, the AIC was when more air pollutants were included, and the smallest AIC appeared in the five-pollutant models. Models shown in red dots in Figure 3 were not considered because they had non-significant or significantly negative estimates even if they had a smaller AIC. Therefore, the four-pollutant model $NO_x+O_3+PM_{10}+SO_2$ for preschool children and the two-pollutant model NOx+O3 for schoolchildren were finally determined as the best final models.

Table 3 displays the percentage change of RR for children's conjunctivitis clinic visits, suggesting: (1) Compared to Sunday, a relatively higher percentage of RR increase for preschool children's and schoolchildren's conjunctivitis clinic visits was more likely happened on a Monday, a Wednesday, and a Saturday; (2) schoolchildren had a higher increased percentage change in RR than preschool children for conjunctivitis clinic visits during ADS periods; (3) a lasting positive impact (i.e., an increased percentage change of RR) during post-ADS periods was noted in schoolchildren; and (4) both NO_2 and O_3 were significantly and positively associated with children's conjunctivitis clinic visits. Specifically, the strongest DOW effect appeared on Monday for preschool children with a 47.90% (95% CI = 47.33, 48.47) elevated RR and on Saturday for schoolchildren with a 29.20% (95% CI = 28.67, 29.72) elevated RR, compared to Sunday, a day on which the clinics are closed. During the ADS period, the RR significantly increased 1.48% (95% CI = 0.79, 2.17) for preschool children's conjunctivitis clinic visits, while the percentage increased over 6-fold to 9.48% (95% CI = 9.03, 9.93) for schoolchildren. This impact did not extend through the post-ADS period for preschool children and the effect showed a negative decline with a −2.16% (95% CI = −2.68, −1.63) RR. However, schoolchildren were still significantly affected during the post-ADS period with a 2.32% (95% CI = 1.98, 2.66) elevation in the RR for conjunctivitis clinic visits. Moreover, air pollutants, NO_x and O_3, also had a stronger influence on conjunctivitis clinic visits for schoolchildren than for preschool children. Interestingly, O_3 had a stronger impact than NO_x for both groups.

(a)

■	91012.2 - 101021.0
■	81003.5 - 91012.2
■	70994.7 - 81003.5
■	60985.9 - 70994.7
■	50977.2 - 60985.9
■	40968.4 - 50977.2
■	30959.6 - 40968.4
■	20950.8 - 30959.6
■	10942.1 - 20950.8
■	933.3 - 10942.1

(b)

■	360.8 - 400.9
■	320.8 - 360.8
■	280.8 - 320.8
■	240.8 - 280.8
■	200.8 - 240.8
■	160.7 - 200.8
■	120.7 - 160.7
■	80.7 - 120.7
■	40.7 - 80.7
■	0.7 - 40.7

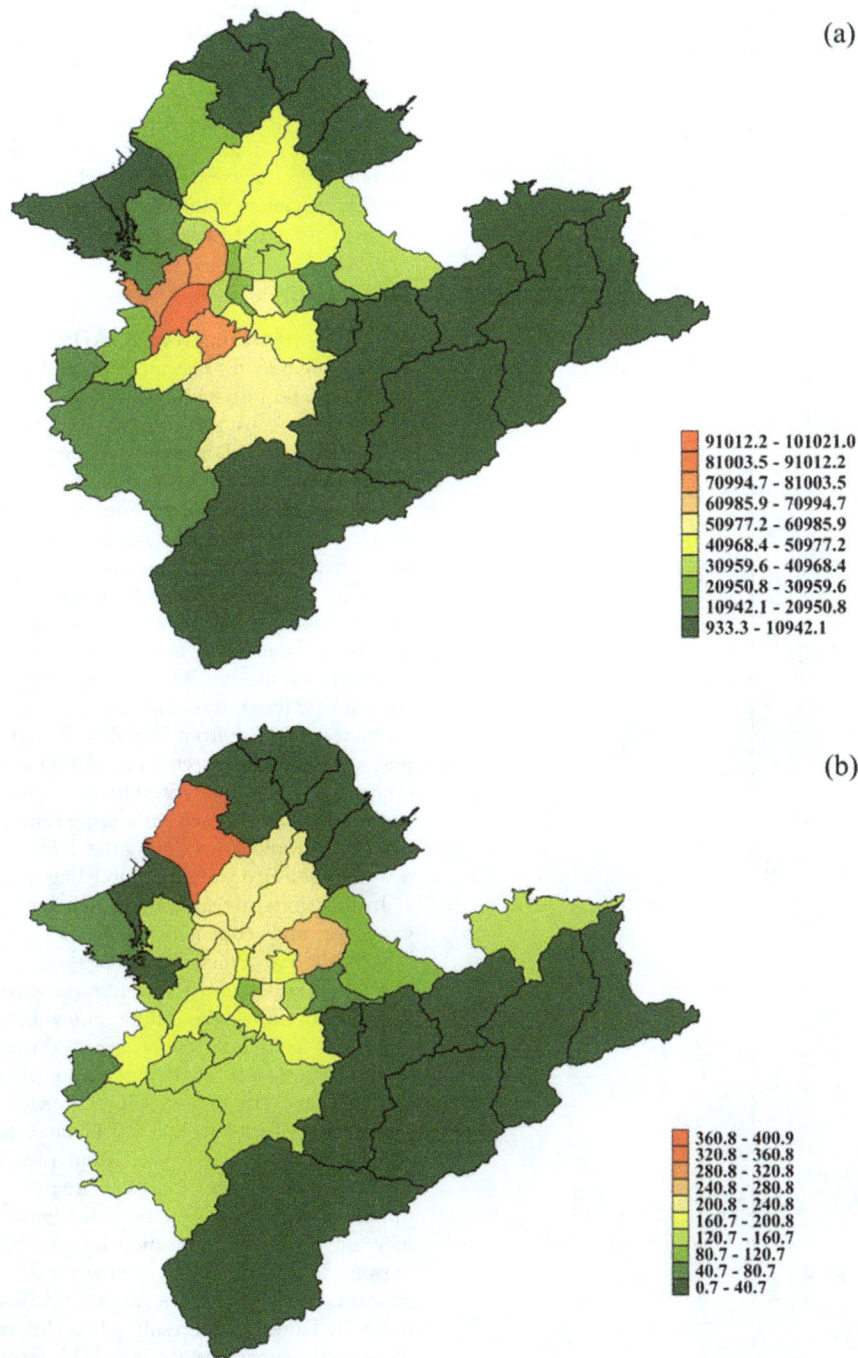

Figure 2. Maps of (a) spatial distribution of the average children population and (b) crude daily children's conjunctivitis clinic visit rate per 100,000 children population in Taipei, 2002–2007.

The influences of time and temperature on children's conjunctivitis clinic visits demonstrated a greater RR during summers when the temperature was hotter (see Figure 4). In particular, in preschool children there was a consistent significantly positive association between conjunctivitis clinic visits and temperature, especially when the temperature increased from 23.92°C to 26.19°C. The greatest RR = 1.18 (95% CI = 1.12, 1.25) appeared at an extremely hot temperature (33.76°C). For schoolchildren, a significant RR >1 for conjunctivitis clinic visits happened between

temperatures of 21.80°C to 26.61°C, and the greatest RR of 1.11 (95% CI = 1.07, 1.16) occurred at a temperature of 24.84°C.

Figure 5 depicts the distribution of spatial effects attributed to children's conjunctivitis clinic visits across 41 districts. It suggests that the significant RR >1, appeared in the more populated areas which included 11 of the 12 districts in Taipei City and 16 of the 29 districts in New Taipei City. Districts near the mountains in the southwest and the coastlines in the north exhibited a significant RR<1. The two maps of 95% posterior probability in the two children's groups were almost identical, except for the Nangang

Table 2. Average measurement of air pollutants during ADS periods, post-ADS periods and Other periods in Taipei, Taiwan, 2002–2007.

Air pollutant	ADS period		Post-ADS period		Other period		P-value[††]
	Mean	Std[†]	Mean	Std[†]	Mean	Std	
CO (ppm)	0.82	0.30	1.01	0.33	0.88	0.32	<.0001
NO$_x$ (ppb)	45.50	17.43	60.10	23.38	49.77	19.51	<.0001
O$_3$ (ppb)	25.13	7.40	20.60	8.00	18.99	8.29	<.0001
PM$_{10}$ (μg/m^3)	81.11	35.41	63.04	25.44	53.32	22.51	<.0001
SO$_2$ (ppb)	3.91	2.03	4.17	2.28	4.35	2.08	<.0001

[†]Std = standard deviation.
[††]P-value was determined by the ANOVA test with null hypothesis H$_0$: $\mu_{ADS} = \mu_{post\text{-}ADS} = \mu_{other}$.

District. Moreover, out of all the 27 districts with a significantly elevated RR, the average RR was 2.70 for preschool children and 3.80 for schoolchildren. The Danshui District displayed the strongest spatial effect contributing to conjunctivitis clinic visits for both children's groups. Comparisons between the two children's groups reveal that 25 of the 41 districts had larger RRs for schoolchildren's conjunctivitis clinic visits than for preschool children's conjunctivitis clinic visits. Of these districts, 11 were in Taipei City and 14 were in New Taipei City.

Discussion

As extreme weather events, ADS bring a higher concentration of air pollutants to Taiwan, and lead to increased risk of disease incidence and hospitalizations. This risk has been documented to be heterogeneous across space and time [38]. Previous studies emphasized the ADS impact on upper respiratory tract diseases, pneumonia and cardiovascular diseases [4,5,39]. Thus far, no significant finding related to the impact of ADS on the development of conjunctivitis had been documented [15]. This may have been due to inadequate sample sizes and the lack of inclusion of spatiotemporal associations leading to insufficient power and possible biases [15]. This research reveals the statistically significant associations between ADS exposure and children's eye health. Based on the large Taiwan National Health Insurance dataset, this study has a lower risk of containing biased estimates resulting from sampling limitations. In addition, spatial and temporal autocorrelations relating to health outcomes are also controlled in this analysis. Therefore, this study reliably provides objective findings based on a large sample size that also covers a broad geographic area during the defined study period and utilizes a well-established statistical modeling approach.

In this study, we found a significant association between ADS exposure and conjunctivitis in both preschool children and schoolchildren. Previous findings showed a similar association between ADS exposure and respiratory diseases in children [26–28]. Importantly, this study notes that increased impacts of children's conjunctivitis occurred during ADS periods; while increased impacts of children's respiratory illnesses occurred during post-ADS periods [26–28]. Moreover, during the ADS period, schoolchildren had a 6.41 times higher percentage of RR for conjunctivitis clinic visits than preschool children. Previous research has shown that the increase of PM concentration outdoors during ADS events is significantly higher than the increase of PM concentration indoors [40]. While the prevalent seasons for ADS events, winter and spring, overlap the two academic semesters, there is not an ADS-related class suspension policy in Taiwan. As a result, schoolchildren have a higher chance of outdoor exposures during ADS events, going to and from school, than preschool children. Schoolchildren may also have more outdoor activities than preschool children. This exposure most likely explains a greater increase in the conjunctivitis clinic visit rates for schoolchildren. The influence of schoolchildren and preschool children had opposite directions during post-ADS period where schoolchildren still positively affected by ADS with an increased RR% (2.32%) while preschool children's RR% became negative (−2.16%). This situation may be explained by the distinct behavior patterns between the two groups of children. Schoolchildren, as compared to preschool children, have a greater opportunity for ADS exposures during and after the ADS events because they experience more outdoor activities. The negative RR% in preschool children could be interpreted by a protective mentality of parents who feel uncertainty about when the ADS finishes, and may bring children outside to look for eye doctors

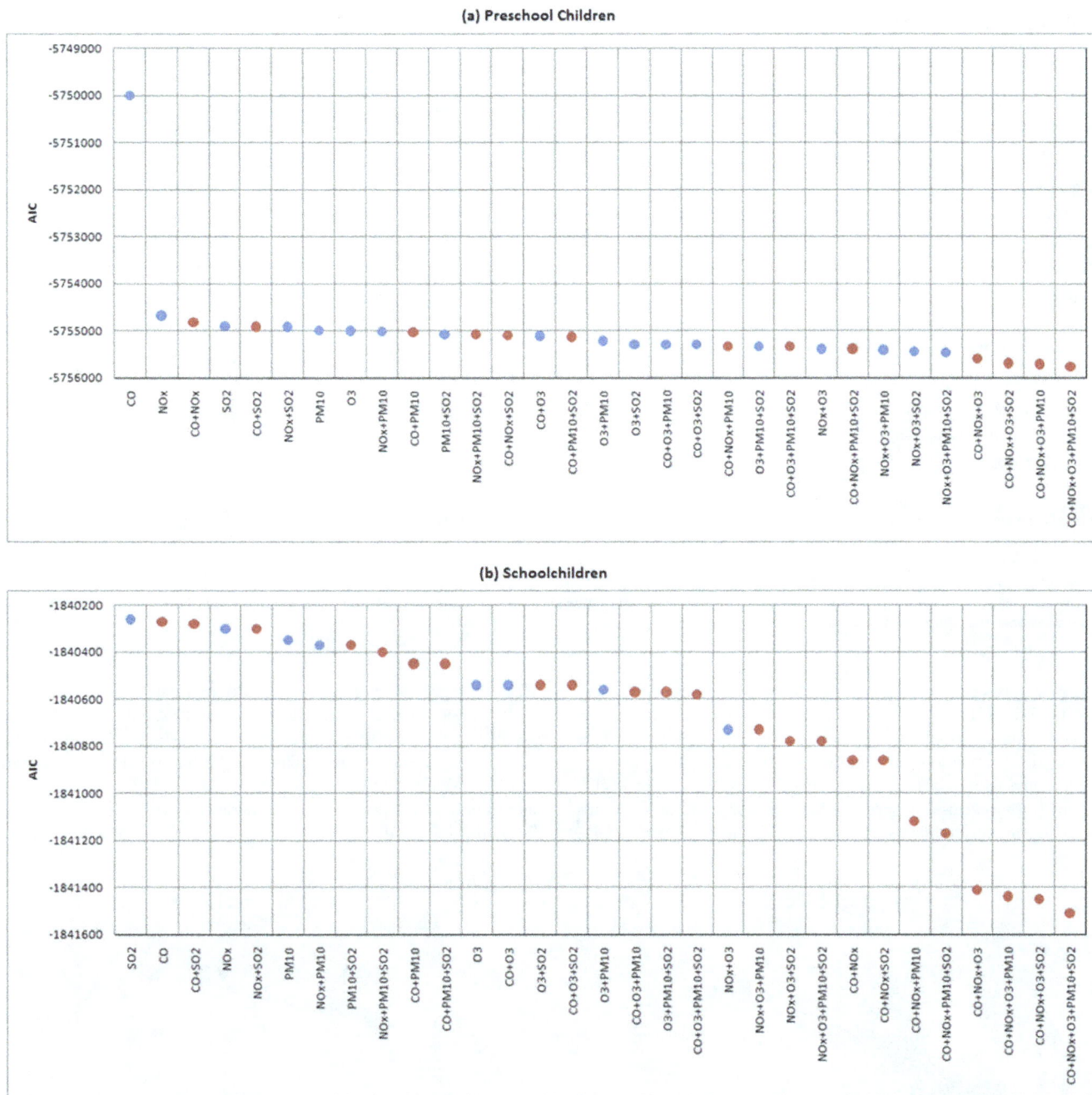

Figure 3. The model selection for (a) preschool children and (b) schoolchildren, where blue dots represent models with all significantly positive estimates for air pollutants, and red dots represent models with at least one non-significant or significantly negative estimate for air pollutants. Our final models were only considered among blue dots.

instead of directly using medicines which can be bought from pharmacy stores without prescriptions.

In order to delineate the health impact of ADS events in regards to conjunctivitis, the short-term and long-term temporal patterns of conjunctivitis clinic visit rates were also analyzed. Among them, the day-of-week pattern is an important confounding factor for clinic visits, and this is true for other diseases as shown in previous studies [26,27]. In Taiwan, major medical services in both hospitals and clinics are closed from Saturday afternoon until Monday morning. Therefore, there is a strong incentive to visit clinics on Saturday (before the weekend effect) and Monday (after

the weekend effect). The day-of-the-week clinic visit pattern observed in this study is quite consistent with the medical care-seeking pattern that has resulted under the current national health care delivery system in Taiwan. Moreover, the highly elevated relative rates on Monday essentially accounts for those patients unable to seek medical treatments from Saturday through Sunday. In the case of children, who are incapable of accessing clinic care independently and are dependent on a parent's working schedule which allows for only nighttime availability, this may be especially true. In addition, while the implementation of NHI in Taiwan increases the accessibility of medical services with relatively low co-

Table 3. Percentage change of relative rate in children's conjunctivitis clinic visits.

Variable	Preschool children		Schoolchildren	
	%	95% CI	%	95% CI
Day-of-week[†]				
Monday	47.90	(47.33, 48.47)	26.75	(26.41, 27.10)
Tuesday	6.91	(6.44, 7.38)	−7.13	(−7.41, −6.84)
Wednesday	14.43	(13.95, 14.92)	26.82	(26.48, 27.17)
Thursday	3.18	(2.72, 3.63)	−13.23	(−13.50, −12.96)
Friday	6.42	(5.96, 6.89)	4.17	(3.87, 4.47)
Saturday	29.20	(28.67, 29.72)	74.70	(74.29, 75.12)
ADS episode[†]				
ADS period	1.48	(0.79, 2.17)	9.48	(9.03, 9.93)
Post-ADS period	−2.16	(−2.68, −1.63)	2.32	(1.98, 2.66)
Air pollutant (interquartile range)[††]				
NO_x (22.16 ppb)	1.63	(1.34, 1.92)	3.49	(3.34, 3.66)
O_3 (11.22 ppb)	3.26	(2.93, 3.59)	6.21	(6.02, 6.40)
PM_{10} (29.88 µg/m³)	0.42	(0.10, 0.74)	–	–
SO_2 (2.63 ppb)	1.19	(0.87, 1.51)	–	–

[†]The reference level of day-of-week and ADS episode are Sunday and the other days, respectively.
[††]The estimate was presented by the increase percentage of relative rate for an interquartile range change in air pollutants, calculated from [exp(interquartile range×estimated coefficient)−1]×100%.

payments, prescription medications can only be issued for a three day period [41]. After three days, the patient must see the physician again to obtain more medication if necessary. This prescription regulation may induce higher clinic visit rates on Wednesdays as noted in this study and in previous studies [27].

This study reveals a geographic heterogeneity for conjunctivitis incidence as verified by studying the documented clinic visits.

Notably, there is a decreasing trend in relative rates from the northwestern coastal districts to the urban areas. In particular, the Danshui District has a greater RR than its surrounding coastal districts, i.e., the Sanjhih District, Shihmen District, Jinshan District, Wanli District, and Bali District. This result can be attributed to the imbalance of medical resources in the area. Though the northwestern coastal districts are noted for their

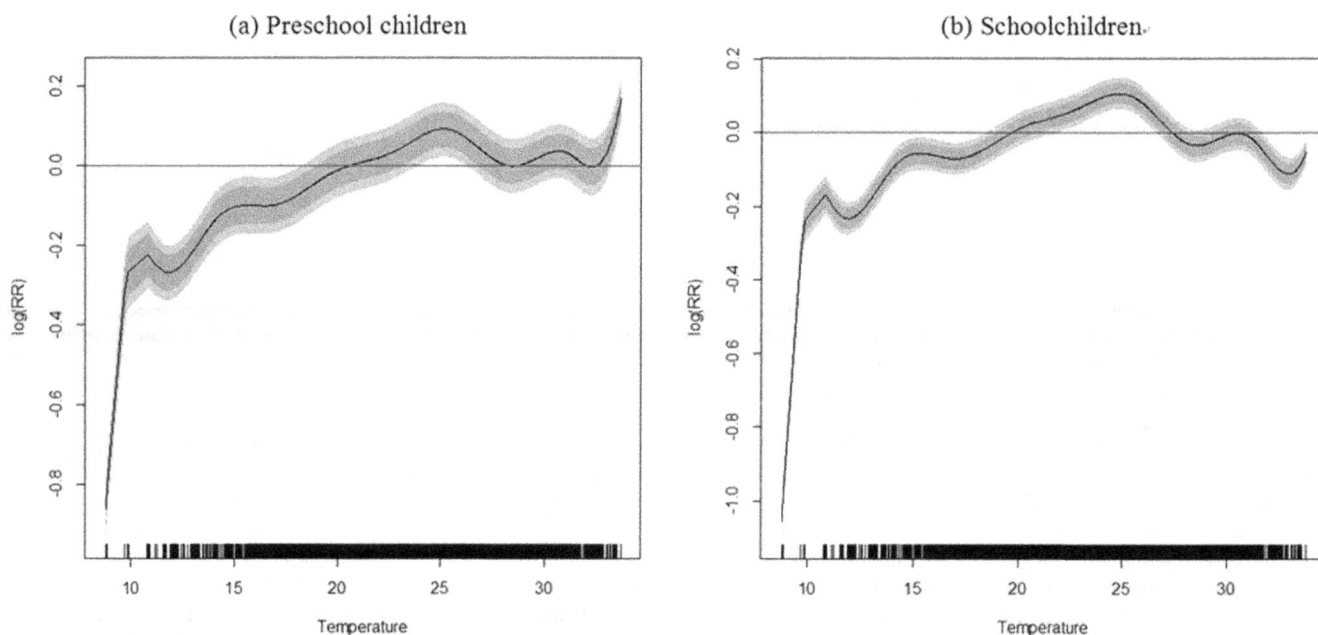

Figure 4. Temperature smoother for (a) preschool children's and (b) schoolchildren's conjunctivitis clinic visits. Dark grey and light grey colors represent 80% and 95% credible intervals, respectively.

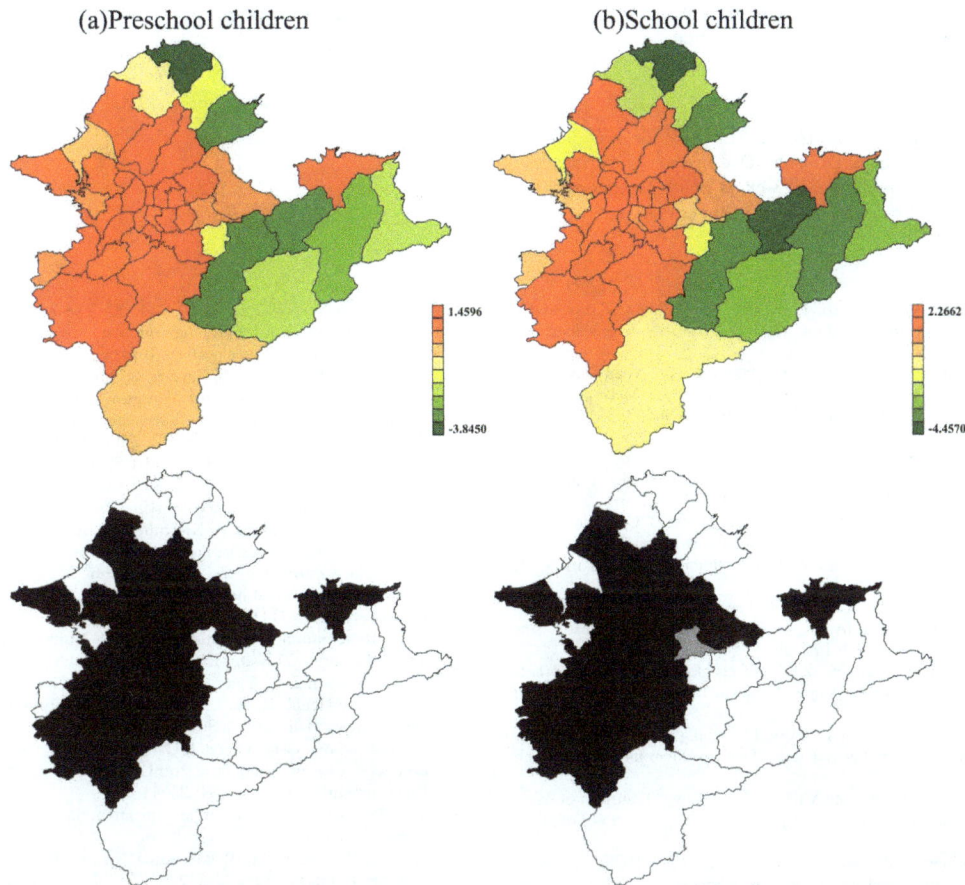

Figure 5. Maps of spatial effects (upper) with corresponding significance (lower) for (a) preschool children's and (b) schoolchildren's conjunctivitis clinic visits in Taipei, Taiwan, 2002–2007, presented by RR. In upper plots, the red color signifies higher RR, and the green color signifies lower RR. In lower plots, black and white areas demonstrate districts where the RR is statistically greater than 1 and smaller than 1, respectively. Grey areas demonstrate no significant difference.

popular oceanic recreational areas for swimmers and tourists, the numbers of well-equipped hospitals and clinics are much less numerous than in the Danshui District. In addition, the lack of eye departments in coastal area might propel residents to consult the medical center in Danshui district. Convenient transportation is another advantage in that eye clinics in the Danshui District are more accessible than nearby areas. As a result, medical services located in the Danshui District are most often the first choice for the tourists and local residents. Another important factor contributing to the increase in conjunctivitis clinic visits in this district relates to its geographical location. The Danshui District is located near an outlet where the Danshui River flows into the Taiwan Strait and therefore, sits at the opening of the Taipei Basin. Because of this location, wind speeds are generally higher in the Danshui District [42]. Studies have shown that dust and wind are the major irritating factors that often trigger eye diseases, such as conjunctivitis [12,43,44]. The distinct features of the spatial function in the STAR model not only control for spatial autocorrelation, but also facilitate the analysis of the geographical heterogeneity in conjunctivitis clinic visit. In addition, short-term and long-term temporal pattern modeling could be performed as in other diseases and health outcomes [26–28]. After consideration of the general spatial and temporal patterns of conjunctivitis clinic visit rates and their associations with covariates, ambient pollutants may better differentiate the health impact from ADS exposure on the subsequent development of conjunctivitis.

This study has three main limitations: First, the study period of this research is restricted to only 6 years because of inconsistent disease coding without the use of ICD-9 before 2002 plus a funding shortage after 2007. Second, some potential allergies to conjunctivitis, such as pollen grain and fungal spores, do not have district-level measurements, so this study is unable to include them as confounding predictors. Third, the STAR model has a complicated estimating algorithm in that, sometimes, unknown parameters cannot converge. This is especially when considering pre-ADS periods for 7 days prior to ADS periods or longer post-ADS periods up to 14 days.

Conclusions

This study demonstrates significantly elevated risks in children's clinic visits due to conjunctivitis in both preschool children and schoolchildren during ADS periods in Taipei, Taiwan. This acute impact produced an increased percentage of RR for clinic visits due to conjunctivitis in schoolchildren during the ADS period, and lasted during the 1 week post-ADS period. In addition, new evidence about the spatial disparities for the adverse effects of ADS events on children's eye health in northern Taiwan was also discovered. Children in all ages are suggested to reduce their overall outdoor exposure time during the ADS period and the post-ADS period, especially for schoolchildren who live in high risk districts. The results and findings of this study should be of particular concern to policy makers or media outlets that are responsible for issuing ADS warnings in advance.

Acknowledgments

We appreciate the Bureau of National Health Insurance for providing the clinic visit database. We also thank Dr. Shyh-Dye Lee for his constructive comments for the result interpretation, as well as Mary Trottier and Dr. Robert Woods for editing the English writing of the article.

References

1. Tam WWS, Wong TW, Wong AHS, Hui DSC (2011) Effect of dust storm events on daily emergency admissions for respiratory diseases. Respirology: no-no.
2. Lee EC, Leem J, Hong YC, Kim H, Kim HC (2008) Effects of Asian Dust Storm Events on Daily Admissions for Asthma and Stroke in Seven Metropolitans of Korea. Epidemiology 19: S145 110.1097/1001.ede.0000339954.000035923.cc.
3. Chiu HF, Tiao MM, Ho SC, Kuo HW, Wu TN, et al. (2008) Effects of Asian dust storm events on hospital admissions for chronic obstructive pulmonary disease in Taipei, Taiwan. Inhalation toxicology 20: 777–781.
4. Cheng MF, Ho SC, Chiu HF, Wu TN, Chen PS, et al. (2008) Consequences of exposure to Asian dust storm events on daily pneumonia hospital admissions in Taipei, Taiwan. Journal of toxicology and environmental health Part A 71: 1295–1299.
5. Chan CC, Chuang KJ, Chen WJ, Chang WT, Lee CT, et al. (2008) Increasing cardiopulmonary emergency visits by long-range transported Asian dust storms in Taiwan. Environmental Research 106: 393–400.
6. Yang CY, Tsai SS, Chang CC, Ho SC (2005) Effects of Asian dust storm events on daily admissions for asthma in Taipei, Taiwan. Inhalation toxicology 17: 817–821.
7. Chen YS, Sheen PC, Chen ER, Liu YK, Wu TN, et al. (2004) Effects of Asian dust storm events on daily mortality in Taipei, Taiwan. Environmental research 95: 151–155.
8. Lee HN, Tanaka T, Chiba M, Igarashi Y (2003) Long Range Transport of Asian Dust from Dust Storms and its Impact on Japan. Water, Air, & Soil Pollution: Focus 3: 231–243.
9. Tuominen IS, Konttinen YT, Vesaluoma MH, Moilanen JA, Helinto M, et al. (2003) Corneal innervation and morphology in primary Sjogren's syndrome. Investigative ophthalmology & visual science 44: 2545–2549.
10. Novaes P, do Nascimento Saldiva PH, Kara-Jose N, Macchione M, Matsuda M, et al. (2007) Ambient levels of air pollution induce goblet-cell hyperplasia in human conjunctival epithelium. Environmental health perspectives 115: 1753–1756.
11. Cakmak S, Dales RE, Burnett RT, Judek S, Coates F, et al. (2002) Effect of airborne allergens on emergency visits by children for conjunctivitis and rhinitis. The Lancet 359: 947–948.
12. Bourcier T, Viboud C, Cohen J-C, Thomas F, Bury T, et al. (2003) Effects of air pollution and climatic conditions on the frequency of ophthalmological emergency examinations. British Journal of Ophthalmology 87: 809–811.
13. Ezzati M, Saleh H, Kammen DM (2000) The Contributions of Emissions and Spatial Microenvironments to Exposure to Indoor Air Pollution from Biomass Combustion in Kenya. Environmental health perspectives 108: 833–839.
14. Ma C-J, Kasahara M, Höller R, Kamiya T (2001) Characteristics of single particles sampled in Japan during the Asian dust-storm period. Atmospheric Environment 35: 2707–2714.
15. Yang C-Y (2006) Effects of Asian Dust Storm Events on Daily Clinical Visits for Conjunctivitis in Taipei, Taiwan. Journal of Toxicology and Environmental Health, Part A 69: 1673–1680.
16. Schwartz J (2004) Air pollution and children's health. Pediatrics 113: 1037–1043.
17. Dockery DW, Ware JH, Ferris BG Jr, Speizer FE, Cook NR, et al. (1982) Change in pulmonary function in children associated with air pollution episodes. Journal of the Air Pollution Control Association 32: 937–942.
18. Dassen W, Brunekreef B, Hoek G, Hofschreuder P, Staatsen B, et al. (1986) Decline in children's pulmonary function during an air pollution episode. Journal of the Air Pollution Control Association 36: 1223–1227.
19. van der Zee S, Hoek G, Boezen HM, Schouten JP, van Wijnen JH, et al. (1999) Acute effects of urban air pollution on respiratory health of children with and without chronic respiratory symptoms. Occupational and environmental medicine 56: 802–812.
20. Boezen HM, van der Zee SC, Postma DS, Vonk JM, Gerritsen J, et al. (1999) Effects of ambient air pollution on upper and lower respiratory symptoms and peak expiratory flow in children. Lancet 353: 874–878.
21. Pope CA 3rd (1989) Respiratory disease associated with community air pollution and a steel mill, Utah Valley. American Journal of Public Health 79: 623–628.

22. Jedrychowski W, Flak E, Mroz E (1999) The adverse effect of low levels of ambient air pollutants on lung function growth in preadolescent children. Environmental health perspectives 107: 669–674.
23. Horak F Jr, Studnicka M, Gartner C, Spengler JD, Tauber E, et al. (2002) Particulate matter and lung function growth in children: a 3-yr follow-up study in Austrian schoolchildren. The European respiratory journal: official journal of the European Society for Clinical Respiratory Physiology 19: 838–845.
24. McConnell R, Berhane K, Gilliland F, London SJ, Vora H, et al. (1999) Air pollution and bronchitic symptoms in Southern California children with asthma. Environmental health perspectives 107: 757–760.
25. Middleton N, Yiallouros P, Kleanthous S, Kolokotroni O, Schwartz J, et al. (2008) A 10-year time-series analysis of respiratory and cardiovascular morbidity in Nicosia, Cyprus: the effect of short-term changes in air pollution and dust storms. Environmental health: a global access science source 7: 39.
26. Chien L-C, Yang C-H, Yu H-L (2012) Estimated Effects of Asian Dust Storms on Spatiotemporal Distributions of Clinic Visits for Respiratory Diseases in Taipei Children (Taiwan). Environmental health perspectives 7: e41317.
27. Yu H-L, Chien L-C, Yang C-H (2012) Asian Dust Storm Elevates Children's Respiratory Health Risks: A Spatiotemporal Analysis of Children's Clinic Visits across Taipei (Taiwan). PloS one 7: e41317.
28. Yu H-L, Yang C-H, Chien L-C (2013) Spatial vulnerability under extreme events: A case of Asian dust storm's effects on children's respiratory health. Environment international 54: 35–44.
29. TWEPA (2011) Dust storm identification. in Asian dust storm monitoring network. Taipei.
30. Lang S, Brezger A (2004) Bayesian P-Splines. Journal of Computational and Graphical Statistics 13: 183–212.
31. Brezger A, Lang S (2008) Simultaneous probability statements for Bayesian P-splines. Statistical Modelling 8: 141–168.
32. Kindermann R, Snell JL, American Mathematical Society (1980) Markov random fields and their applications. Providence, R.I.: American Mathematical Society. ix, 142 p. p.
33. Belitz C, Lang S (2008) Simultaneous selection of variables and smoothing parameters in structured additive regression models. Computational Statistics & Data Analysis 53: 61–81.
34. Fahrmeir L, Lang S (2001) Bayesian Inference for Generalized Additive Mixed Models Based on Markov Random Field Priors. Journal of the Royal Statistical Society Series C (Applied Statistics) 50: 201–220.
35. Akaike H (1974) A new look at the statistical model identification. Automatic Control, IEEE Transactions on 19: 716–723.
36. Fromont A, Binquet C, Sauleau EA, Fournel I, Bellisario A, et al. (2010) Geographic variations of multiple sclerosis in France. Brain: a journal of neurology 133: 1889–1899.
37. Belitz C, Brezger A, Kneib T, Lang S (2012) BayesX - Software for Bayesian inference in structured additive regression models. Version 2.1.
38. Chen PS, Tsai FT, Lin CK, Yang CY, Chan CC, et al. (2010) Ambient Influenza and Avian Influenza Virus during Dust Storm Days and Background Days. Environmental Health Perspectives 118: 1211–1216.
39. Yang CY, Cheng MH, Chen CC (2009) Effects of Asian dust storm events on hospital admissions for congestive heart failure in Taipei, Taiwan. Journal of toxicology and environmental health Part A 72: 324–328.
40. Kuo H-W, Shen H-Y (2010) Indoor and outdoor PM2.5 and PM10 concentrations in the air during a dust storm. Building and Environment 45: 610–614.
41. TWDOH (2012) Regulations Governing the Medical Services Covered under National Health Insurance. In: Department of Health EY, editor. Taipei, Taiwan.
42. NCU (2005) Taiwan Wind Query System. Chungli, Taiwan: National Central University.
43. Liu Z (2009) Acute Conjunctivitis. Essentials of Chinese Medicine: 443–445.
44. Stoss M, Michels C, Peter E, Beutke R, Gorter RW (2000) Prospective cohort trial of Euphrasia single-dose eye drops in conjunctivitis. The Journal of Alternative and Complementary Medicine 6: 499–508.

Author Contributions

Conceived and designed the experiments: HLY LCC. Performed the experiments: LCC YJL CHY. Analyzed the data: LCC YJL. Contributed reagents/materials/analysis tools: LCC CHY HLY. Wrote the paper: HLY LCC.

8

A Forward Phenotypically Driven Unbiased Genetic Analysis of Host Genes That Moderate Herpes Simplex Virus Virulence and Stromal Keratitis in Mice

Richard L. Thompson[1]*, **Robert W. Williams**[2], **Malak Kotb**[1], **Nancy M. Sawtell**[3]*

1 Department of Molecular Genetics, Microbiology, and Biochemistry, University of Cincinnati College of Medicine, Cincinnati, Ohio, United States of America, 2 Center of Genomics and Bioinformatics and Department of Anatomy and Neurobiology, University of Tennessee Health Science Center, Memphis, Tennessee, United States of America, 3 Division of Infectious Diseases, Cincinnati Children's Hospital Medical Center, Cincinnati, Ohio, United States of America

Abstract

Both viral and host genetics affect the outcome of herpes simplex virus type 1 (HSV-1) infection in humans and experimental models. Little is known about specific host gene variants and molecular networks that influence herpetic disease progression, severity, and episodic reactivation. To identify such host gene variants we have initiated a forward genetic analysis using the expanded family of BXD strains, all derived from crosses between C57BL/6J and DBA/2J strains of mice. One parent is highly resistant and one highly susceptible to HSV-1. Both strains have also been fully sequenced, greatly facilitating the search for genetic modifiers that contribute to differences in HSV-1 infection. We monitored diverse disease phenotypes following infection with HSV-1 strain 17syn+ including percent mortality (herpes simplex encephalitis, HSE), body weight loss, severity of herpetic stromal keratitis (HSK), spleen weight, serum neutralizing antibody titers, and viral titers in tear films in BXD strains. A significant quantitative trait locus (QTL) on chromosome (Chr) 16 was found to associate with both percent mortality and HSK severity. Importantly, this QTL maps close to a human QTL and the gene proposed to be associated with the frequency of recurrent herpetic labialis (cold sores). This suggests that a single host locus may influence these seemingly diverse HSV-1 pathogenic phenotypes by as yet unknown mechanisms. Additional suggestive QTLs for percent mortality were identified—one on Chr X that is epistatically associated with that on Chr 16. As would be anticipated the Chr 16 QTL also modulated weight loss, reaching significance in females. A second significant QTL for maximum weight loss in male and female mice was mapped to Chr 12. To our knowledge this is the first report of a host genetic locus that modulates the severity of both herpetic disease in the nervous system and herpetic stromal keratitis.

Editor: Stacey Efstathiou, University of Cambridge, United Kingdom

Funding: The work was supported by NIH RC1 AI087336, www.nih.gov/. The funders had no role in study design, data collection and analysis, decision to publish, or preparation of the manuscript.

Competing Interests: The authors have the following interests.

* E-mail: richard.thompson@uc.edu (RLT); nancy.sawtell@cchmc.org (NMS)

Introduction

Over 5 billion people are infected worldwide with herpes simplex virus type 1 (HSV-1) and will remain so for life constituting a reservoir of virus with the potential to infect new hosts. While many infections are asymptomatic, serious disease occurs in some individuals and HSV is the leading cause of both sporadic necrotizing encephalitis and infectious blindness in the United States [1–4]. Significantly, genital infection with HSV-2 is associated with a two-fold increased risk of transmission in sexually transmitted cases of HIV [5–7]. The ubiquity of HSV in the human population is the result of its ability to establish latent infections in sensory neurons and subsequently reactivate to cause recurrent disease and transmission to new hosts. No effective vaccine is yet available. Effective anti-HSV drugs exist, but resistant strains can develop [8–10], and antivirals cannot eliminate the latent viral reservoir. Advances in genomics present the opportunity to gain insight into host genetic variation that predispose to serious disease outcomes. This knowledge in turn can lead to enhanced treatment protocols, the design of new strategies to reduce latent reservoirs, and the potential to discover biomarkers to identify individuals at greater risk of severe herpetic disease.

About 40 years ago it was shown that both viral and host genetics contribute greatly to the outcome of experimental infection in mice [11,12]. Other factors that impact HSV disease outcome in mice include the age of the host at the time of infection, the route of infection and the inoculation titer. Traditional reverse genetic approaches (e.g. gene knock out, knock down, or over expression strategies) have provided insight into the viral genes that regulate pathogenic processes and the role that the components of the host immune system plays in the formation of herpetic stromal keratitis [13–17]. However, little is known about naturally occurring host gene variants and molecular networks that modulate the infectious process or predispose the host to severe outcomes. A very early study suggested that a gene or genes residing close to the immunoglobulin heavy chain locus were involved in keratitis in mice [18]. Cantin and colleagues describe three loci on mouse chromosome (Chr) 6 involved in neutrophil function and resistance to fatal disease in mice [19].

Recently a human genetic locus associated with frequency of recurrent HSV-1 *labialis* (cold sores) has been mapped to Chr 21 [20,21]. Despite these successes, there is much left to learn about the naturally occurring gene variants and molecular networks that contribute to protection against severe disease caused by herpes simplex virus.

We employed the BXD advanced recombinant inbred (ARI, [22]) lines of mice to identify novel gene variants that impact the severity of several important HSV-1 disease phenotypes including percent mortality (viral invasion of the central nervous system resulting in death) and herpetic stromal keratitis, in a well-characterized mouse model of HSV-1 corneal infection. The BXD gene reference population (GRP) is particularly well-suited for these studies for several reasons. First, the lines result from a cross of C57BL/6J (B6 or B) and DBA/2J (D2 or D) inbred strains of mice that are highly resistant and highly susceptible to HSV infection respectively [12]. In addition both parental strains have been deeply and completely sequenced and the BXD lines have been densely genotyped. Thus interval mapping for the identification of quantitative trait loci (QTL) is greatly expedited. The BXD lines have been used by researchers throughout the world in many diverse studies including those centered on the eye and nervous system (for example see [23–27]), as well as several infectious agents (for example [28–31]). The BXD family is one of the largest GRP, presently containing ~160 lines of mice, each line of which is isogenic except for sex chromosomes. This large family permits the efficient identification of naturally occurring gene variants and molecular networks that regulate biologic properties. In addition a large number of previously published and as yet unpublished phenotypes and omics data sets on these strains can be accessed directly using the GeneNetwork.org site that also incorporates software for mapping and statistical analysis of the BXD and many other populations.

Here we infected the BXD lines and the parental strains with HSV-1 strain 17syn+ via the cornea and systematically phenotyped mice for >30 days post-infection. We report a novel QTL on Chr 16 that controls both virulence and HSK severity. This Chr 16 locus is also linked to maximum weight loss in females. A second QTL for maximum weight loss maps to Chr 12. The Chr 16 interval is homologous to human Chr 21, and the region identified here maps close to, but appears to be distinct from, the region on human Chr 21 that influences cold sore frequency in humans [20]. Our findings suggest that a single host locus may regulate both percent mortality and HSK severity in mice (and perhaps recurrent disease frequency in humans [20]) by some common as yet unidentified mechanism, which is discussed further below.

Methods

Ethics Statement

This study was carried out in complete accordance with the recommendations in the Guide for the Care and Use of Laboratory Animals of the National Institutes of Health. Animals were housed in American Association for Laboratory Animal Care-approved quarters. The protocol (internal protocol number 2E06052) was approved by the Animal Care and Use Committee of the Cincinnati Children's Hospital Medical Center (PHS assurance# - A3108-01). No surgical procedures were performed.

Infection and phenotyping

Herpes simplex virus type 1 (HSV-1) infection: HSV-1 strain 17syn+ was propagated on cultured rabbit skin cells (RSC, originally obtained from Bernard Roizman at the University of

Chicago) and viral titers were determined by serial-dilution plaque assay as previously detailed [32–34]. The wild type HSV-1 laboratory strain 17syn+ was originally obtained from John H. Subak-Sharpe at the MRC Virology Unit in Glasgow, Scotland. Animals were housed in American Association for Laboratory Animal Care approved quarters. Male and female C57BL/6J and DBA/2J mice (4 to 6 weeks old) were obtained from Jackson Laboratories. At least four male and four female mice (4 to 6 weeks old) of the various BXD strains were employed and most strains were analyzed more than once throughout the multi-year study. BXD mice were obtained from the colony at the University of Tennessee Health Science Center or a colony maintained at the University of Cincinnati.

Prior to inoculation, mice were anesthetized by intraperitoneal injection of sodium pentobarbital (50 mg/kg of body weight). A 10 µl drop containing 1×10^6 pfu of HSV strain 17syn+ was placed onto each scarified corneal surface as previously detailed [32–34]. Virus titers in tear films were assayed on day 4 p.i. Mice were observed daily and weighed every other day until weight returned to that recorded prior to infection. Mice were euthanized if 30% of starting body weight was lost. Percent mortality was scored from 48 hours through 21 days p.i. Any deaths occurring outside of this range were not attributed to acute viral infection. Eyes were examined by two independent observers and scored on a 0 to 5 point scale: 0 = no visible corneal opacity; 1 = up to 25% cornea involvement; 2 = 25–50% cornea involvement; 3 = 50–75% cornea involvement; 4 = 75–100% cornea involvement; and 5 = penetrating keratitis, essentially as previously detailed [35–37]. At 30 to 35 days p.i., mice were necropsied, major organs and draining lymph nodes were examined grossly, spleen weights recorded, and blood samples taken for serum virus neutralizing antibody titer analysis. Eyes were routinely processed for histological examination. Following overnight fixation in 4% paraformaldehyde, eyes were embedded in paraffin, sectioned and stained with cresyl violet for histological examination of the cornea.

Genome wide data analysis

QTL mapping. Quantitative trait locus (QTL) mapping was performed with the GeneNetwork analysis tools (www. genenetwork.org). Single marker regression was performed across the entire mouse complement of chromosomes at markers typed across BXD strains. A likelihood ratio statistic (LRS) was calculated at each marker comparing the hypothesis that the marker is associated with the phenotype with the null hypothesis that there is no association between marker and phenotype. Genome-wide significance was determined by performing 2000 permutations. Significant QTLs were found on Chr 12 and 16 (weight loss), Chr X and 16 (percent mortality) and Chr 16 (herpetic stromal keratitis severity). Other tools available at www. genenetwork.org were employed for pair-wise scans and Spearman rank correlation statistical analyses.

Results

Thirty-two fully inbred BXD strains were phenotyped. Groups of each line, including males and females in approximately equal numbers, were infected with wild type HSV-1 strain 17syn+ on the cornea as detailed in Methods. A single investigator infected all of the mice to ensure high technical consistency. Infected mice were observed daily, weighed every other day, and tear films were collected on day 4 post-infection (p.i.) to evaluate viral titers. Eyes were independently scored by two investigators for the severity of herpetic stromal keratitis essentially as previously described

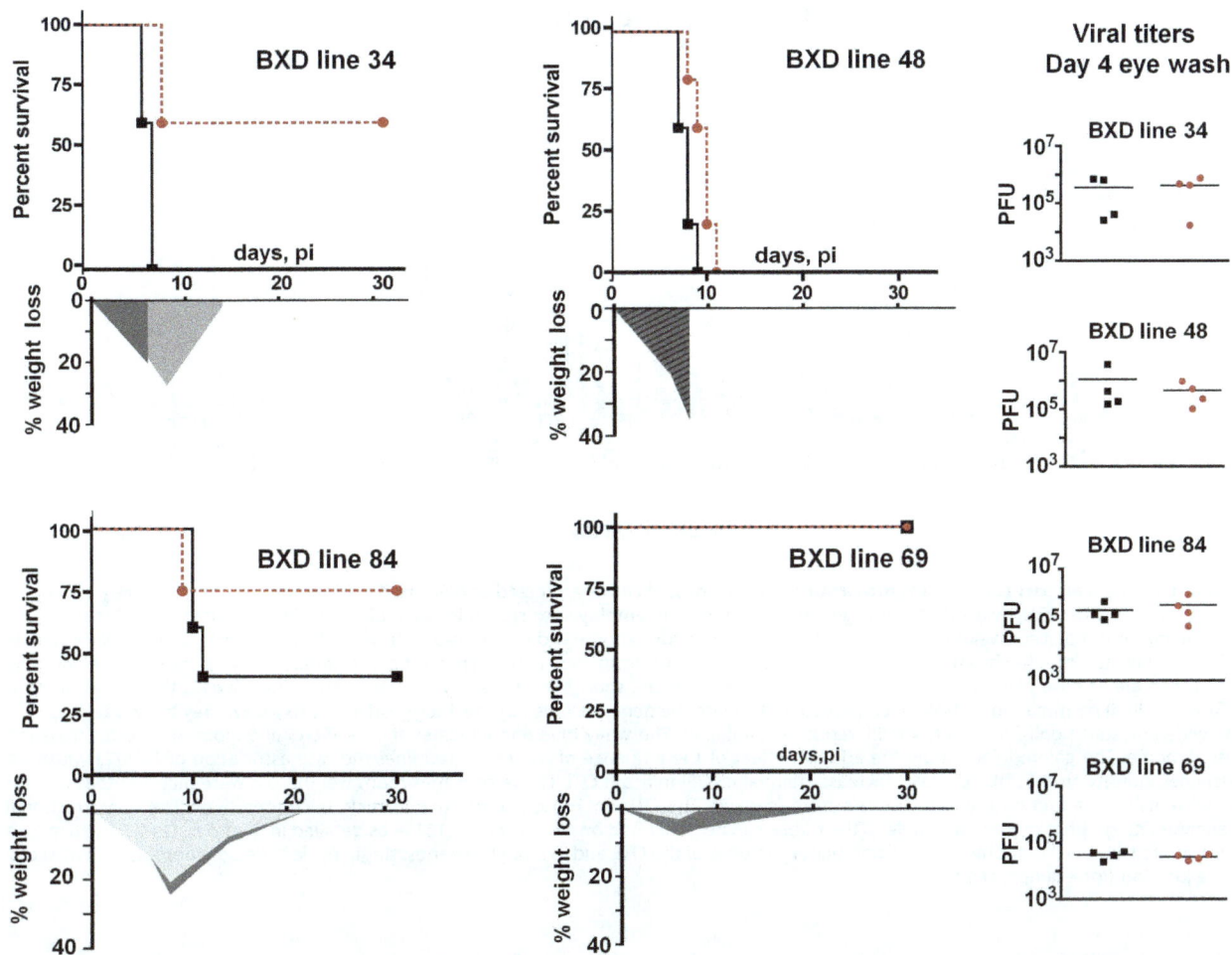

Figure 1. Representitive results with several BXD strains. Shown are representitive data from four different BXD lines. The top Y axis in each panel is the percent survival and the bottom Y axis is the percent weight loss. The X axis is the time in Days post infection (p.i.). The scattergrams on the right show the tear film titers of individual mouse eyes at 4 days p.i. Red circles and dashed lines = female; Black squares and solid lines = male. In the experiment shown, which is a small subset of the data generated, four male and four female mice of each BXD strain were employed.

[35,36], and as detailed further below and in methods. The parental strains and most BXD lines were analyzed more than once throughout the multi-year study in groups ranging from 3–10. In all cases the reproducibility of the disease phenotypes displayed within individual lines was consistent. In contrast, extensive variability in the phenotypes was displayed between lines.

General patterns of disease

Clinical and postmortem findings in humans combined with animal model studies provide a temporal and spatial understanding of primary HSV infection. In the mouse corneal infection model with viral strains of moderate virulence, viral replication occurs in an overlapping wave in three distinct tissue compartments including corneal epithelium, innervating trigeminal ganglion (TG), and connecting central nervous system (CNS). This acute phase of primary infection resolves in 8–12 days. Viral replication on the cornea peaks at day 4 p.i. By 2 days p.i. virus that has transported through sensory neuron axons to the TG begins to replicate and viral titers reach their peak on day 4 p.i. in TG, and infectious virus is cleared within 8 to 9 days p.i. During this time virus enters the CNS, and it is the timing and extent of

viral replication here that determines whether or not lethal encephalitis ensues [33,38–42].

With respect to susceptibility to fatal encephalitis, four general patterns were observed (fig. 1). Some of the BXD lines were highly resistant as is the B6 parent strain. This outcome is typified by BXD69. In this line, 100% of both males and females survived infection with minimal weight loss. At its maximum, less than 10% of original body weight was lost which had returned to preinfection values within 12 days p.i. In contrast, other lines were highly susceptible with no survivors, similar to the D2 parent at the inoculation titer employed. The BXD48 line typifies the response of these susceptible lines. Both males and females of this line continuously lost weight and succumbed to infection by day 12 p.i.

In some lines, males and females exhibited susceptibility differences as typified in BXD34 strain (fig.1). This sex bias in mouse susceptibility to HSV infection is a recognized phenomenon and there is some suggestion that the same bias exists in humans [43,44]. In general, mice in these groups lost about 25% of their body weight within days 8 p.i. In those lines surviving, body weight was recovered over the next 10 days. We noted that males in these groups lost less weight at the time of death than surviving females in the same group. Viral replication on the eye

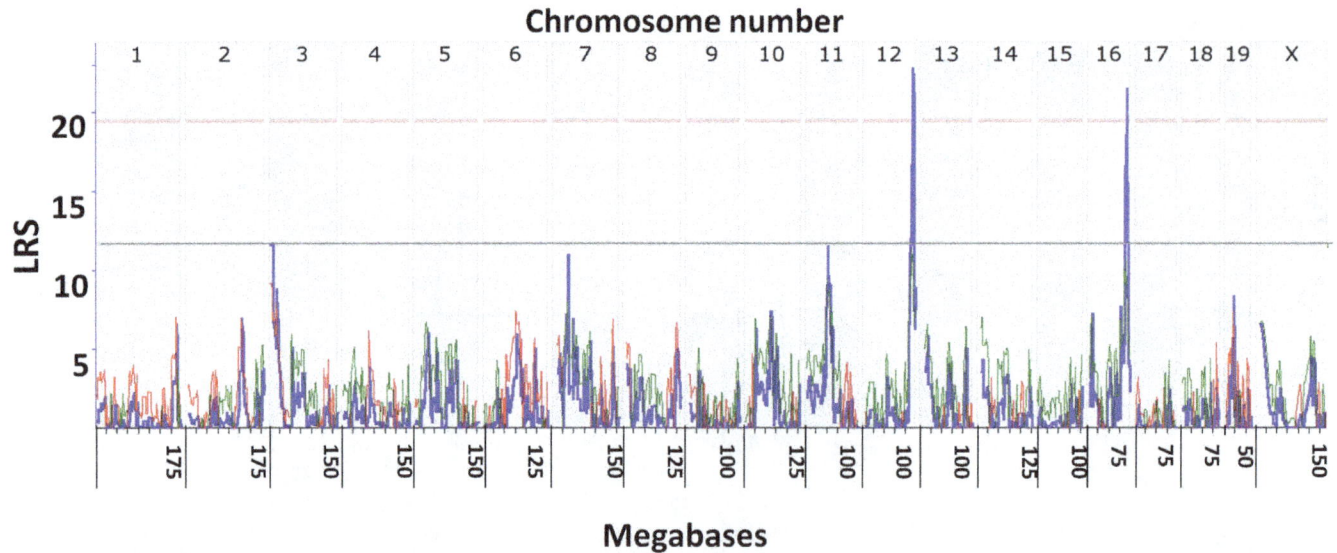

Figure 2. Quantitative trait loci for percent maximum weight loss. Mice were infected as described in methods and weighed every other day. Analysis tools in genenetwork (GN) available at www.genenetwork.org were employed to search for possible quantitative trait loci (QTL) in male and female mice. The maximum percent weight loss was employed to search for genome wide association. Shown is a screen capture from GN for female mice. The X axis shows the mouse chromosomes from chromosome 1 to X from the centromere to the end (mouse chromosomes have only one arm). The long ticks are at base pair number 1 of each chromosome and the short ticks are every 25 megabases. The Y axis is the likelihood ratio statistic (LRS) score. 2000 permutation tests were employed to estimate the genome wide adjusted suggestive LRS (p = 0.37, grey horizontal line) and the genome wide adjusted significant LRS (p = 0.05, red horizontal line). The wavy blue line indicates the local LRS at various SNPs etc. across the entire mouse genome. The colored lines show the additive effect of the influence of the locus (red lines indicate association of DBA/2J with trait values, green lines indicate that C57BL/6J alleles increase trait values). Significant QTL for percent maximum weight loss were mapped to Chr12 for both male and female mice and on Chr16 for female mice (shown). The QTL on 16 was suggestive in male mice (not shown). A fully functional interactive analysis and graphic interface available to the public can be generated on GN for trait ID:16194 as detailed in methods. On GN the user can restrict the output to the specific chromosomal region under the peak of the QTL and explore the genes, single nucleotide polymorphisms (SNPs) etc. present in the location (for example see fig. 7).

was similar for both males and females in these groups (fig. 1 and data not shown). A sex difference in susceptibility was not universal, however, as many lines exhibited a similar percent mortality in males and females (fig. 1, e.g. BXD69, BXD48), indicating that host genetic loci can moderate the effect of sex.

Interval mapping and identification of significant QTL. Gene mapping methods systematically evaluate the statistical significance of linkage between genetic markers (e.g. SNPs or microsatellites) across the whole genome and differences in phenotypes. We performed mapping using the GeneNetwork. Interval maps are computed using the Haley-Knott regression method (for review see [45]). Permutation analysis was used to estimate the empirical genome-wide p values associated with a given likelihood ratio statistic (LRS) score. The LRS is mathematically related to the log of odds (LOD) ratio that is often employed in genetic analyses and LRS can be converted to LOD by dividing the LRS score by 4.61.

Genome wide linkage scan interval mapping for maximum weight loss. Weight loss is an effective measure of infectious disease severity. We detected significant QTL for percent maximum weight loss on Chr 12 and 16 in female mice (see fig. 2) and on Chr 12 in male mice, which also had a suggestive QTL on Chr 16 (not shown). Figure 2 is a screen shot of an interactive graphic interface in GN and shows the result of a genome wide analysis of percent weight loss in female mice. The peak LRS was 22 on Chr 12 at ~114.5 Mb. We detected a second significant QTL on Chr 16 in female mice with an LRS of 21 at ~89.4 Mb. This region of Chr 12 was previously associated with keratitis by analysis of congenic mouse strains [18]. In contrast, the Chr 16 interval has not been identified previously for HSV disease

resistance. The results of a pair scan analysis that tests for all possible two-locus epistatic interactions did not suggest any interaction between the loci on Chr 12 and 16. Note that the original data consisting of 11 herpes-associated phenotypes generated as part of this study, along with high resolution, dynamic, and interactive plots and maps can be easily regenerated by searching GeneNetwork for *Species* = Mouse, *Group* = BXD, *Type* = Phenotypes, and then entering the search string "herpes".

Genome wide linkage scan interval mapping for percent mortality. We also detected a significant QTL associated with percent mortality on the distal portion of chromosome 16 (maximum LRS = 29 at 86.2 Mb, fig. 3). Infected mice of susceptible strains showed signs of central nervous system disease including hunched posture, roughened fur, convulsions and/or ataxia, indicating that death was the result of herpetic encephalitis. Several suggestive QTL were found on Chrs 4, 11, 12, and X. The strongest of these suggestive QTL with an LRS of 17.5 was on Chr 4. Of interest, the susceptibility allele at the Chr 4 locus is inherited from the resistant B6 parent (red line in fig. 3). A pair scan analysis suggested a possible interaction between Chr 16 and the suggestive QTL on Chr X (not shown). We performed composite mapping to control for possible masking effects of the QTL on Chr 16. Epistasis, the moderation of the phenotypic effect of alleles at one gene by alleles of another gene, can sometimes be revealed by this approach and secondary, but still significant loci can be identified. We detected a significant locus on the proximal part of Chr X with a peak LRS of 24 when we controlled for SNP rs4213268 on Chr 16 (fig. 3B bottom panel, green arrow and line).

Genome wide linkage scan interval mapping for herpetic stromal keratitis. Two independent investigators scored the

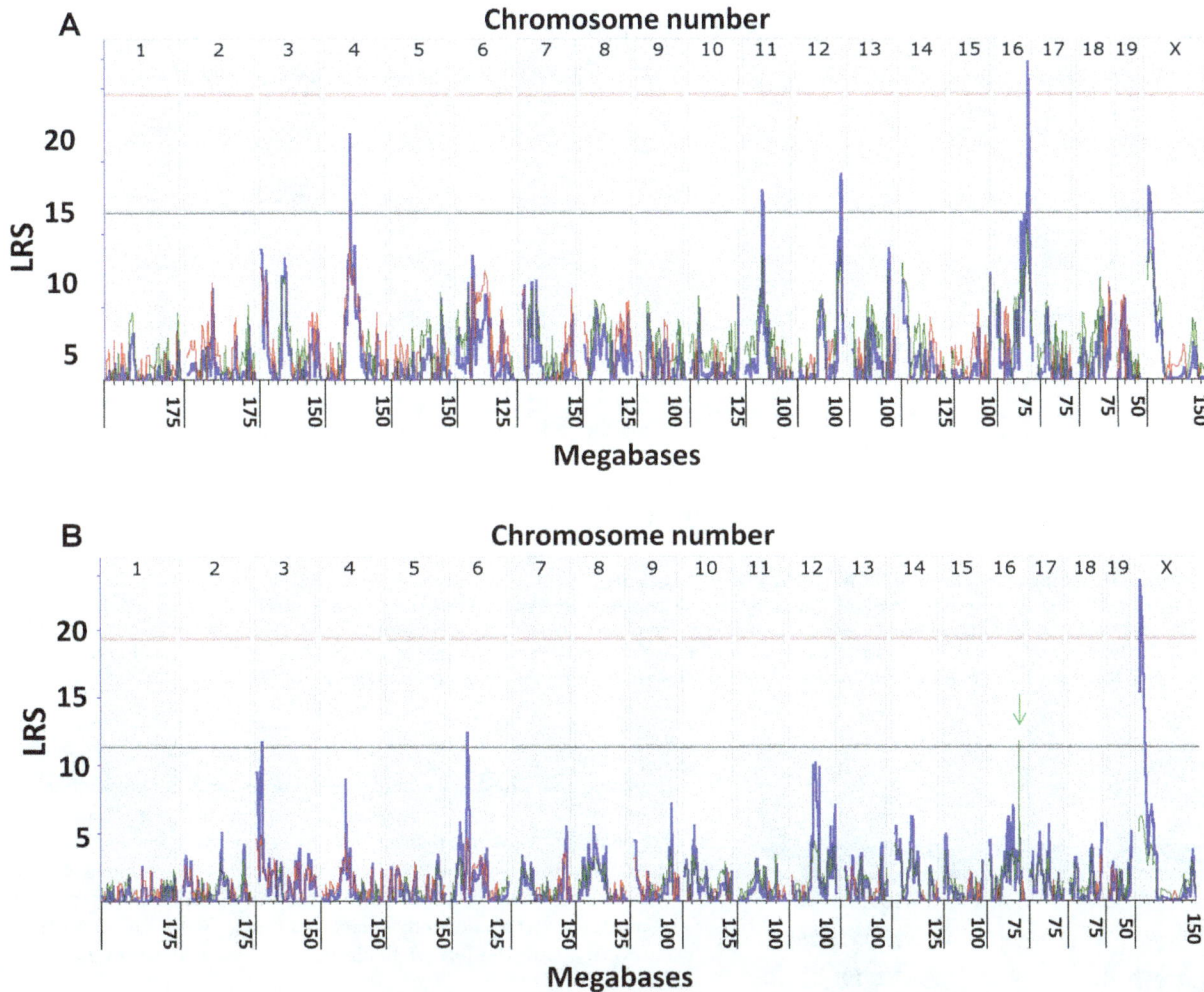

Figure 3. Quantitative trait loci for percent survival. Percent survival of male and female mice combined was employed to search for QTL associated with mortality. See the legend for fig. 2 for an explanation of the lines in the figure. A significant QTL was mapped to the distal end of Chr 16 and suggestive QTL were localized to Chr 4, 11, 12 and X (panel A). A pair scan analysis revealed a possible interaction between the locus on 16 and the suggestive locus on X (not shown). The marker regression function was used to identify SNPs with high LRS scores on Chr 16 and X, and the composite scan analysis was then employed to control for the Chr 16 or the Chr X locus. Controlling for the QTL on 16 (green arrow and line) revealed that the suggestive QTL on X was significant (panel B).

severity of herpetic stromal keratitis throughout the acute stage of infection, and final scores were obtained on day 30 p.i. A scale 0 to 5 was based on previously published criteria [35–37,46] as detailed in methods and also by histochemical analysis of corneal tissues. The average score of all the eyes in a group ± standard error was employed for interval mapping. A statistically significant QTL for HSK severity was localized to the same region of the distal arm of Chr 16 as was significant for percent mortality. The peak LRS for virulence mapped to 86.45 Mb (fig. 3A) and the peak LRS for HSK mapped to 86.16 Mb (fig. 4). Suggestive QTL were also observed on Chrs 3, 8, 11, 12, and 18. Controlling for the QTL on Chr 16 did not reveal any additional significant QTL. Likewise pair scans did not detect interactions.

Representative photographs of whole eyes and photomicrographs of sectioned corneas are shown in fig. 5. As seen in the photographs of live animals at 30 days p.i., eyes of BXD70 appear normal, whereas those of BXD102 have significant opacity covering most of the cornea. Microscopic examination of the corneas extended these findings. Corneas from BXD70 appear normal, whereas thickening and derangement of the epithelial and

stromal layers, and neovascularization of the stromal layer is pervasive in BXD102 corneas (fig. 5.).

The BXD70 and BXD102 differ at the HSK locus on 16 QTL, with line BXD70 having the C57BL/6J haplotype and BXD102 having the DBA/2J haplotype across the entire region. This region co-maps with percent mortality, although these particular lines had 100 percent survival of both males and females. Weight loss, a general measure of disease severity, was significantly greater in BXD102 mice (p ≤ 0.05, Student t test). BXD70 mice had very little eye disease with an average score of 0.2 compared to an average score of 4.5 for BXD102.

In general, those BXD strains that exhibited more severe disease signs or greater mortality had higher serum antibody neutralization titers. A QTL for serum neutralization titer was not obtained, and this may be due at least in part to the fact that many and in some cases all of the animals of a susceptible BXD strain succumbed to infection before serums were obtained at 30 days p.i. Strains in which sera from at least three survivors was obtained were included in the analysis. Since the phenotypes of percent mortality, percent maximum weight loss and HSK had QTL that

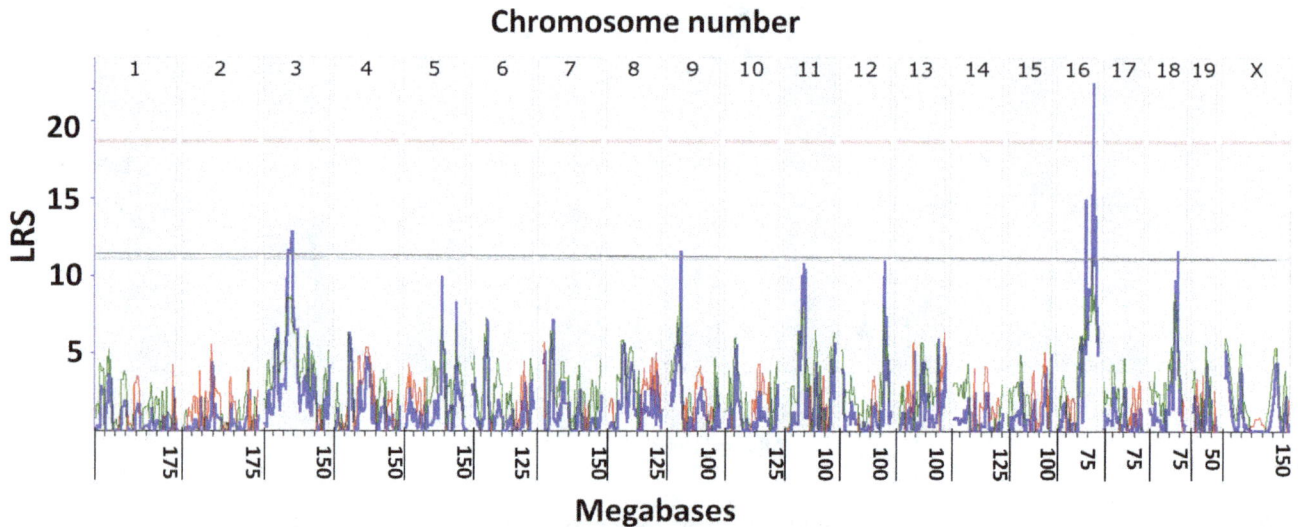

Figure 4. Quantitative trait loci associated with herpetic stromal keratitis. BXD strains of mice were infected via the cornea and the severity of stromal keratitis in male and female mice combined determined by two independent observers using a 5 point scale (0 = no disease, 5 = penetrating stromal keratitis). Analysis tools in genenetwork available at www.genenetwork.org were employed to search for possible quantitative trait loci (QTL). See the legend for fig. 2 for an explanation of the lines in the figure. A significant quantitative trait locus (QTL) for severity of herpetic stromal keratitis was identified on Ch 16. A fully functional interactive analysis and graphic interface is available on GN for trait ID:16186.

BxD strain	70	102
Survival (%)	100	100
max weight loss (%)	5.7 (2.7-7.9)	21.4 (15-25)
Viral titers (eye, d4)	$1.1 \times 10^5 \pm 4 \times 10^4$	$1.1 \times 10^5 \pm 1 \times 10^5$
Neut. Antibody	1/500	1/2000
Spleen weight (gm)	0.15±0.05	0.13±0.03
Eye Score	0.2 (0-0.5)	4.5 (3.0-5.0)

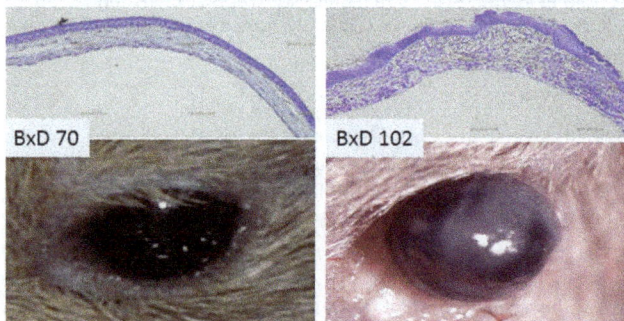

Figure 5. Representitive data in BXD lines that differ at the HSK QTL on Chr 16. Groups of male and female mice were infected as described in methods with 1×10^6 pfu of HSV-1 strain 17syn+. The indicated parameters were assayed as described in the text and eyes were scored at 30 days p.i. by two independent investigators. The top micrographs are of cresyl violet stained corneal sections processed at 30 days p.i. Deranged and thickened corneal epithelium, neovascularization, derangned stromal keratocytes and greatly thickened stromal layer with immune cellular infiltrate is seen in the BXD102 strain. The BXD70 cornea appears normal. The bottom photos are of representitive live mouse eyes 30 days p.i. The BXD70 mouse eye appears normal. Neovascularization and stromal opacity covering more than 75% of the cornea is seen in the BXD102 eye.

mapped to Chr 16, we performed Spearman rank correlations to determine if the co-mapping was statistically significant. The Spearman rank correlation is a non-parametric measure that assesses how well the relationship between two variables can be described using a monotonic function. We found that percent mortality was significantly correlated to both weight loss and HSK severity, with the former being the stronger association (fig. 6).

Discussion

Translating the advances in genomic technology into progress toward realizing the broad benefits promised by individualized medicine will require protocols to determine each individual's susceptibility to disease states and sensitivity to treatment and prevention regimens. Analysis of genetic reference populations (GRP) coupled with genome wide association studies (GWAS) can lead to the identification of naturally occurring gene variants associated with severe disease outcomes and deduction of the gene networks to which they contribute. This information in turn can identify biomarkers of susceptibility and also suggest potential new treatment strategies. Herpes simplex virus type 1 (HSV-1) infection is an example of an infectious disease which is normally relatively benign in most individuals but can cause severe disease sequelae in otherwise healthy people. There is at present no way to predict who might be susceptible to these rare severe manifestations of herpetic disease.

Our current understanding of HSV-1 disease mechanisms comes largely from reverse genetics approaches such as gene deletions in mice and the virus or RNAi knock downs of viral or host genes. A large body of literature defines the importance of many viral genes and host immune modulating factors, cellular infiltrates, cytokines and angiogenic factors, and potential autoimmunity in viral virulence and/or the formation of the corneal scaring and loss of visual acuity (reviewed in [13,16,36,47–50]. However, these studies do not identify those individuals potentially at high risk. We employed an unbiased forward phenotypically driven systems genetics approach to begin to identify unknown

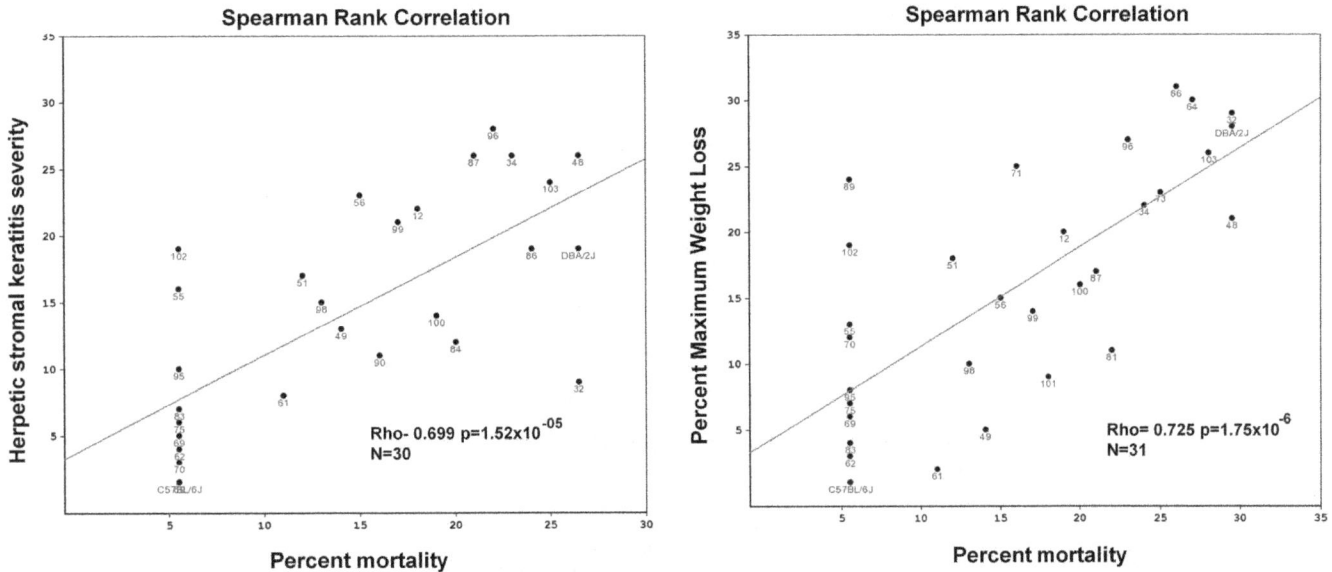

Figure 6. Correlations between phenotypes that map to the distal end of Chr 16. Spearman Rank correlations were performed bewteen percent mortality and herpetic stromal keratitis datasets (left panel, $p = 1.52 \times 10^{-05}$) or percent maximum weight loss of both male and female mice combined and percent mortality of male and female mice combined (right panel, $p = 1.75 \times 10^{-06}$).

gene variants and potential molecular networks of the host that contribute to these severe herpetic disease states, with the ultimate goals of disease risk prediction and improved treatment outcomes. It is of interest that none of the aforementioned host genes or molecular mechanisms was directly implicated in the QTLs we identified.

In this study a single well-characterized HSV-1 laboratory isolate (17syn+) and a single inoculation titer were employed in the BXD family using a generally well characterized model of ocular HSV infection. The BXDs are particularly well suited for these studies because the parental strains are either very resistant to HSV-1 (C57BL/6J) or very sensitive (DBA/2J). The BXD lines have the advantage of being widely available and they have a 40-year history of use [51]. The BXDs have also been thoroughly genotyped and phenotyped and many large omics data sets generated in prior studies can be mined to, for example, identify relevant pleiotropic interactions and expression QTL (eQTL) in many tissues and cell types.

Our analysis revealed and mapped significant QTLs on Chr12 and 16 (weight loss), Chr X and 16 (percent mortality) and Chr 16 (herpetic stromal keratitis severity). Somewhat surprisingly a common QTL for all three of these phenotypes overlaps on the distal end of Chr 16. Virulence of a given virus strain and its ability to cause HSK are not linked [35,36]. Note however, that in one study, passage of viral isolates in vivo co-selected for increased neuroinvasiveness and increased HSK severity [35,36]. A major common host QTL for both percent mortality (neuroinvasion) and HSK, while not predictable, may have important implications for how the process leading to HSK is initiated. This is currently under investigation.

There is a paucity of forward genetic analyses of HSV disease. Prior studies in mice implicated a region on Chr 6 that confers resistance to HSV infection that appears to be an autosomal dominant but is nevertheless strongly sex-biased [19]. Our studies did not detect this locus, presumably because the underlying variants are not segregating in the BXDs. Analysis of the eight parent Collaborative Cross mouse lines, when they become widely available, would cover more than 90% of mouse genetic diversity.

An early study employed congenic lines of mice that varied at the immunoglobin heavy chain (IgH) locus and found an association with the locus on Chr 12 and keratitis [18]. A study performed on 129/SVEV x C57BL/6)F(2) mice at the ten centimorgan (cM) level revealed loci on Chr 3, 5, 12, 13 and 14 with impacts on general disease, and 10 and 17 associated with keratitis in complex with other loci [52]. Our study uncovered a highly significant QTL on Chr 12 locus for percent maximum weight loss. The QTL on the distal end of Chr 12 (106–119 Mb) contains the Igh locus, and this same region reached the suggestive linkage criterion for percent mortality and HSK severity. This region contains over 200 genes and further studies will be required to reduce this number of positional candidates to a manageable number.

While it is possible that IgH family members are involved in resistance to HSV, there was no direct correlation between serum neutralizing antibody titers in BXDs and percent mortality. A mechanism of molecular mimicry of an IgH locus and viral antigen leading to HSK has been described [47], but is limited to specific viral and mouse strains and dominant only under conditions of low viral load [53], which were not duplicated in our studies. Other potentially interesting genes within this region include YinYang1 (YY1), a transcription factor that can both up or down regulate genes through its cognate binding sites and is known to regulate HSV-1 genes [54,55]. The YY1 gene contains a non-synonymous SNP between B6 and D2 and also has a cis expression QTL (cis-eQTL) at 110.06 Mb (determined with the Hippocampus Consortium data set in GN [56]), which regulates levels of expression in the nervous system. Such cis-eQTL are often implicated in disease phenotypes. This region of Chr 12 also contains the *Rest* gene. REST and co-REST proteins are thought to help silence the viral genome in cultured cells, and there is evidence this occurs in sensory neurons in vivo [57,58]. The *Rest* gene has a cis-eQTL at ~112.35 Mb.

A few forward genetic analyses of HSV disease severity in humans have been reported. In a series of phenotypically driven GWAS studies in highly inbred human populations, Cassanova and colleagues have demonstrated the importance of the innate immune response in protection. In particular, they found TOLL

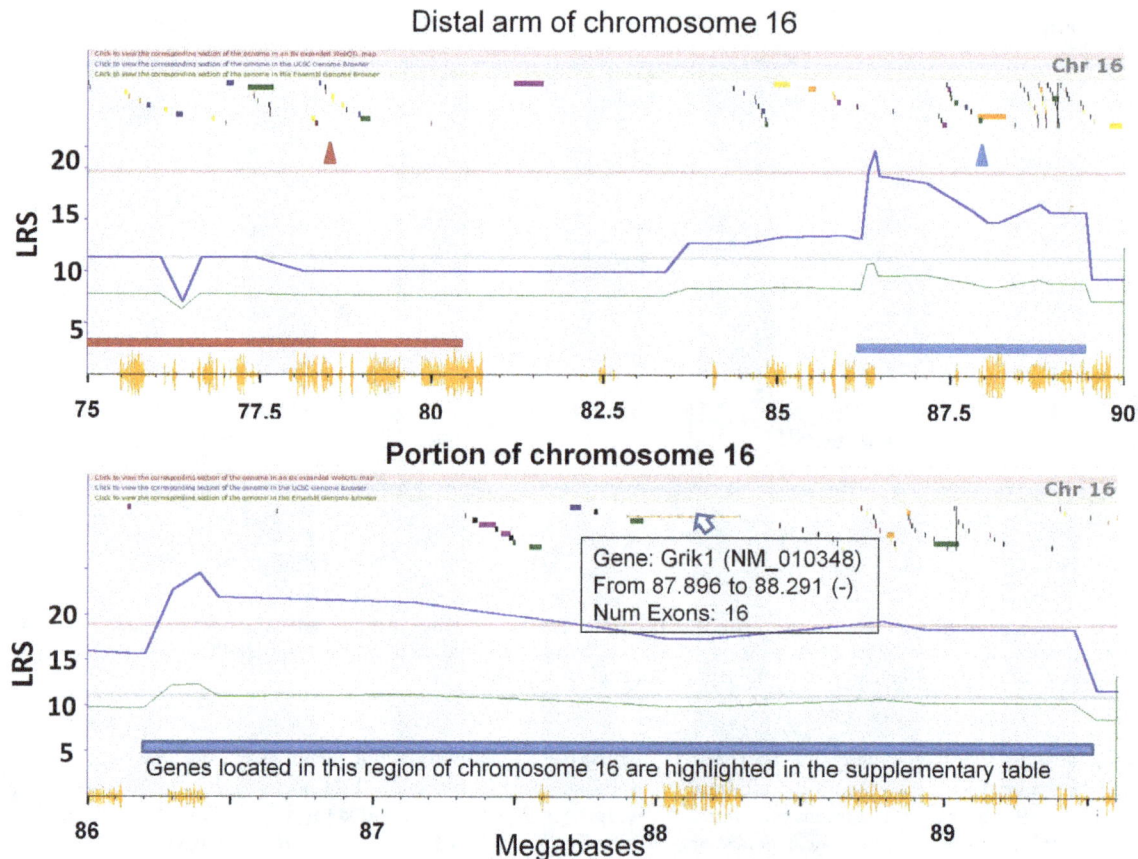

Figure 7. Schematic representation of the region of mouse Chr 16 from 75 to 90 mb. Suggestive (grey horizontal line) and significant (red horizontal line) LRS for HSV virulence (HSE) in male and female mice combined are indicated. The wavy blue line is the local LRS. The gold seismic graph along the X axis indicates local SNP density. The mouse susceptibility QTL region is deliniated by a solid blue rectangle just above the SNP seismic graph. The region equivalent to the human cold sore frequency QTL is designated by a solid red rectangle just above the seismic graph at 75–82 mb. The location of the mouse equivalent (D16Ertd472e) to the human "cold sore" gene (C21orf91) is indicated by a red triangle. A blue triangle indicates the 3′ end of the Grik1 gene that is an expression QTL for Grik1 in the nervous system. C21orf91 is a short gene shown as a gold box, which is not clearly discernable at this magnification (Top panel). Bottom panel. A three megabase region comprising the peak of the QTL is shown. Grik1, which is 395 kb in length is also shown as a gold rectangle and the other variously colored shapes indicate known or predicted genes and transcripts in the region. In GN, hovering the mouse cursor over the colored shapes (indicated by the open arrow in fig. 7, bottom) gives brief information about each gene. Clicking on the shapes calls up all related entries in the NCBI Gene database. The bands along the top are clickable and either increase the magnification, go to the respective region of the UCSC genome browser, or go to the respective region of the Ensemble genome browser. A fully functional and interactive figure can be generated and further explored on genenetwork.org for trait 16185 by performing the interval mapping function for Chr16.

receptor signaling/interferon gamma pathways important for protection of the central nervous system from HSV-1 encephalitis. Rare individuals with defects in these pathways can suffer repeated bouts of HSE [59–61]. However the vast majority of people who experience HSE do not have frank defects in these pathways and there is as yet no evidence that certain alleles predispose to greater risk. These studies are akin to and confirm prior reverse genetic studies performed in mouse models in that the defects ablated gene function and emphasize the importance of the innate interferon response pathways in preventing serious CNS infection [62–66].

A forward approach in a genetically more diverse human GRP examined frequency of herpes labialis (cold sores) and mapped frequent recurrent disease to a locus on human Chr 21, which is homologous to part of mouse Chr 16. The putative "cold sore" gene (*C21orf91*) which encodes a protein of unknown function, maps near to but is distinct from the QTL we have identified for percent mortality (HSE) and stromal keratitis severity (HSK, see fig. 7). A putative mouse gene highly homologous to *C21orf91* (also designated *D16Ertd472e*, *EURL*, *YG91*, and *CSSG1*) resides at the

expected location of 78.54 Mb on mouse Chr 16 and there is one nonsynonymous SNP between the parental mouse strains. However, this gene does not overlap the murine QTL (fig. 7 top panel). There are at least two possible explanations for this result. The same gene may be involved in neuroinvasiveness/ HSK in mice and cold sore frequency in humans, and the studies map it to different locations due to mapping resolution. Alternately, distinct HSV resistance loci and genes may exist in this region of human Chr 21 and mouse Chr 16.

We examined the regions under and near the Chr 16 locus to identify candidate genes that might affect these phenotypic properties. The list was filtered down to a list of 63 candidates using factors such as the LRS value (fig. 7 bottom panel), known gene functions, known transcription levels in neural tissues and eyes (from Affymetrix and Illumina array and RNAseq databases in Genenetwork.org) as well as the density of SNPs (see Table S1). The 45 genes distal to 88.6 Mb are part of a keratin protein cluster [67] and are not likely to be involved. Of the remaining 18 genes under the locus only one—*Grik1*— is known to be expressed in sensory neurons [68]. *Grik1* encodes the GluR5 subunit of the kainate 1 ionotropic glutamate receptor that is detected in more than half of the neurons in dorsal root ganglia [68]. In addition *Grik1* mRNA levels in the nervous system are controlled by an expression QTL (eQTL) at 87.9 Mb and there is a very high SNP density within and around *Grik1* (fig 7). For these reasons *Grik1* is a top candidate gene for regulation of percent mortality (neuroinvasion) and severity of stromal keratitis. GluR5 is a ligand (glutamate) binding component of a kainate receptor that is involved in a large array of nervous system phenotypes such as complex behaviors and cocaine addiction (reviewed in [69]) including some previously associated with HSV infection such as schizophrenia [70,71]. Other possible candidates include *Bach1*, a transcription factor thought to be ubiquitously expressed and implicated in spinal injury repair [72]. Listerin E3 ubiquitin ligase 1 (*Ltn1*, aka *Zfp294*) is expressed developmentally in neurons of the PNS and CNS [73]. These latter genes are somewhat less promising candidates than *Grik1* because they are associated with few if any C57BL/6J versus DBA/2J non-synonymous SNPs, indels, or cis-eQTLs.

Although the precise sequence variants involved in disease susceptibility to HSV-1 remain to be identified, the fact that host functions that regulate disease severity in mice (HSE and HSK, this study) and frequency of recurrent disease in humans [20,74] map closely together implies there may be a previously unknown association between viral interaction with the nervous system and the severity of HSK. One potential mechanism is a host function that regulates the efficiency of the virus to transport in axons in the anterograde direction from neuron cell bodies in the trigeminal ganglia to the brain (i.e. percent mortality) or cornea (HSK severity) and possibly to the mucocutaneous region around the mouth in humans (cold sore frequency, [20]). Further studies may clarify whether the locus identified on mouse Chr 16 and/or the human Chr 21 is associated with an increased risk of HSK in humans. Finally, our studies have revealed BXD lines relatively resistant to HSE that are either highly susceptible, or highly resistant to the development of HSK. By analyzing the infectious disease dynamics in these selected strains using powerful omics approaches, it should be practical now to identify molecular networks and biomarkers associated with high risk for the formation of severe HSK.

Supporting Information

Table S1 Shown are the known and predicted genes under and near the Chr 16 QTL for percent mortality detailed in figure 7. Genes within the QTL are highlited in light blue (entries 7 to 70). An interactive table containing more information can be generated at www.genenetwork.org by using the GeneNetwork Interval Analyst for Chr 16 gated between 85 and 90 Mb.

Acknowledgments

We thank Katie Burke for expert technical assistance

Author Contributions

Conceived and designed the experiments: RLT RWW NMS MK. Performed the experiments: RLT NMS. Analyzed the data: RLT NMS RWW. Contributed reagents/materials/analysis tools: RLT RWW MK NMS. Wrote the paper: RLT RWW NMS.

References

1. Levitz RE (1998) Herpes simplex encephalitis: a review. Heart Lung 27: 209–212.
2. Whitley RJ (1990) Viral encephalitis. N Engl J Med 323: 242–250.
3. Whitley RJ (2002) Herpes simplex virus infection. Semin Pediatr Infect Dis 13: 6–11.
4. Smith G (2012) Herpesvirus transport to the nervous system and back again. Annu Rev Microbiol 66: 153–176.
5. Corey L (2007) Synergistic copathogens—HIV-1 and HSV-2. N Engl J Med 356: 854–856.
6. Corey L, Wald A, Celum CL, Quinn TC (2004) The effects of herpes simplex virus-2 on HIV-1 acquisition and transmission: a review of two overlapping epidemics. J Acquir Immune Defic Syndr 35: 435–445.
7. Glynn JR, Biraro S, Weiss HA (2009) Herpes simplex virus type 2: a key role in HIV incidence. Aids 23: 1595–1598.
8. Horsburgh BC, Chen SH, Hu A, Mulamba GB, Burns WH, et al. (1998) Recurrent acyclovir-resistant herpes simplex in an immunocompromised patient: can strain differences compensate for loss of thymidine kinase in pathogenesis? J Infect Dis 178: 618–625.
9. Griffiths A, Chen SH, Horsburgh BC, Coen DM (2003) Translational compensation of a frameshift mutation affecting herpes simplex virus thymidine kinase is sufficient to permit reactivation from latency. J Virol 77: 4703–4709.
10. Griffiths A, Coen DM (2003) High-frequency phenotypic reversion and pathogenicity of an acyclovir-resistant herpes simplex virus mutant. J Virol 77: 2282–2286.
11. Plummer G, Goodheart CR, Miyagi M, Skinner GR, Thouless ME, et al. (1974) Herpes simplex viruses: discrimination of types and correlation between different characteristics. Virology 60: 206–216.
12. Lopez C (1975) Genetics of natural resistance to herpesvirus infections in mice. Nature 258: 152–153.
13. Steiner I, Benninger F (2013) Update on herpes virus infections of the nervous system. Current neurology and neuroscience reports 13: 414.
14. Metcalf JF, Michaelis BA (1984) Herpetic keratitis in inbred mice. Invest Ophthalmol Vis Sci 25: 1222–1225.
15. Hazlett LD, Hendricks RL (2010) Reviews for immune privilege in the year 2010: immune privilege and infection. Ocular immunology and inflammation 18: 237–243.
16. Gimenez F, Suryawanshi A, Rouse BT (2013) Pathogenesis of herpes stromal keratitis—a focus on corneal neovascularization. Prog Retin Eye Res 33: 1–9.
17. Veiga-Parga T, Suryawanshi A, Mulik S, Gimenez F, Sharma S, et al. (2012) On the role of regulatory T cells during viral-induced inflammatory lesions. J Immunol 189: 5924–5933.
18. Foster CS, Tsai Y, Monroe JG, Campbell R, Cestari M, et al. (1986) Genetic studies on murine susceptibility to herpes simplex keratitis. Clin Immunol Immunopathol 40: 313–325.
19. Lundberg P, Welander P, Openshaw H, Nalbandian C, Edwards C, et al. (2003) A locus on mouse chromosome 6 that determines resistance to herpes simplex virus also influences reactivation, while an unlinked locus augments resistance of female mice. J Virol 77: 11661–11673.
20. Kriesel JD, Jones BB, Matsunami N, Patel MK, St Pierre CA, et al. (2011) C21orf91 genotypes correlate with herpes simplex labialis (cold sore) frequency: description of a cold sore susceptibility gene. J Infect Dis 204: 1654–1662.
21. Hobbs MR, Jones BB, Otterud BE, Leppert M, Kriesel JD (2008) Identification of a herpes simplex labialis susceptibility region on human chromosome 21. J Infect Dis 197: 340–346.
22. Peirce JL, Lu L, Gu J, Silver LM, Williams RW (2004) A new set of BXD recombinant inbred lines from advanced intercross populations in mice. BMC Genet 5: 7.
23. Lu H, Li L, Watson ER, Williams RW, Geisert EE, et al. (2011) Complex interactions of Tyrp1 in the eye. Mol Vis 17: 2455–2468.
24. Geisert EE, Lu L, Freeman-Anderson NE, Templeton JP, Nassr M, et al. (2009) Gene expression in the mouse eye: an online resource for genetics using 103 strains of mice. Mol Vis 15: 1730–1763.
25. Carneiro AM, Airey DC, Thompson B, Zhu CB, Lu L, et al. (2009) Functional coding variation in recombinant inbred mouse lines reveals multiple serotonin transporter-associated phenotypes. Proc Natl Acad Sci U S A 106: 2047–2052.
26. Rulten SL, Ripley TL, Hunt CL, Stephens DN, Mayne LV (2006) Sp1 and NFkappaB pathways are regulated in brain in response to acute and chronic ethanol. Genes Brain Behav 5: 257–273.
27. Alexander RC, Wright R, Freed W (1996) Quantitative trait loci contributing to phencyclidine-induced and amphetamine-induced locomotor behavior in inbred mice. Neuropsychopharmacology 15: 484–490.
28. Aziz RK, Kansal R, Abdeltawab NF, Rowe SL, Su Y, et al. (2007) Susceptibility to severe Streptococcal sepsis: use of a large set of isogenic mouse lines to study genetic and environmental factors. Genes Immun 8: 404–415.
29. Zumbrun EE, Abdeltawab NF, Bloomfield HA, Chance TB, Nichols DK, et al. (2011) Development of a murine model for aerosolized ebolavirus infection using a panel of recombinant inbred mice. Viruses 4: 3468–3493.

30. Nedelko T, Kollmus H, Klawonn F, Spijker S, Lu L, et al. (2012) Distinct gene loci control the host response to influenza H1N1 virus infection in a time-dependent manner. BMC Genomics 13: 411.

31. Yadav JS, Pradhan S, Kapoor R, Bangar H, Burzynski BB, et al. (2011) Multigenic control and sex bias in host susceptibility to spore-induced pulmonary anthrax in mice. Infect Immun 79: 3204–3215.

32. Sawtell NM, Thompson RL (2004) Comparison of herpes simplex virus reactivation in ganglia in vivo and in explants demonstrates quantitative and qualitative differences. J Virol 78: 7784–7794.

33. Thompson RL, Preston CM, Sawtell NM (2009) De novo synthesis of VP16 coordinates the exit from HSV latency in vivo. PLoS Pathog 5: e1000352.

34. Thompson RL, Sawtell NM (2011) The herpes simplex virus type 1 latency associated transcript locus is required for the maintenance of reactivation competent latent infections. J Neurovirol 17: 552–558.

35. Brandt CR (2004) Virulence genes in herpes simplex virus type 1 corneal infection. Curr Eye Res 29: 103–117.

36. Brandt CR (2005) The role of viral and host genes in corneal infection with herpes simplex virus type 1. Exp Eye Res 80: 607–621.

37. Brandt CR, Coakley LM, Grau DR (1992) A murine model of herpes simplex virus-induced ocular disease for antiviral drug testing. J Virol Methods 36: 209–222.

38. Shimeld C, Tullo AB, Hill TJ, Blyth WA, Easty DL (1985) Spread of herpes simplex virus and distribution of latent infection after intraocular infection of the mouse. Archives of virology 85: 175–187.

39. Whitley RJ (2001) Chapter 73: Herpes Simplex Viruses. In: P. M. H. David M Knipe, editor editors. Field's Virology. Lippincott Williams & Wilkins. pp. 2461–2510.

40. Thompson RL, Stevens JG (1983) Biological characterization of a herpes simplex virus intertypic recombinant which is completely and specifically non-neurovirulent. Virology 131: 171–179.

41. Thompson RL, Cook ML, Devi-Rao GB, Wagner EK, Stevens JG (1986) Functional and molecular analyses of the avirulent wild-type herpes simplex virus type 1 strain KOS. J Virol 58: 203–211.

42. Thompson RL, Rogers SK, Zerhusen MA (1989) Herpes simplex virus neurovirulence and productive infection of neural cells is associated with a function which maps between 0.82 and 0.832 map units on the HSV genome. Virology 172: 435–450.

43. Hill TJ, Yirrell DL, Blyth WA (1986) Infection of the adrenal gland as a route to the central nervous system after viraemia with herpes simplex virus in the mouse. J Gen Virol 67 (Pt 2): 309–320.

44. Han X, Lundberg P, Tanamachi B, Openshaw H, Longmate J, et al. (2001) Gender influences herpes simplex virus type 1 infection in normal and gamma interferon-mutant mice. J Virol 75: 3048–3052.

45. Broman KW (2001) Review of statistical methods for QTL mapping in experimental crosses. Lab Anim (NY) 30: 44–52.

46. Brandt CR, Akkarawongsa R, Altmann S, Jose G, Kolb AW, et al. (2007) Evaluation of a theta-defensin in a Murine model of herpes simplex virus type 1 keratitis. Invest Ophthalmol Vis Sci 48: 5118–5124.

47. Zhao ZS, Granucci F, Yeh L, Schaffer PA, Cantor H (1998) Molecular mimicry by herpes simplex virus-type 1: autoimmune disease after viral infection. Science 279: 1344–1347.

48. Suryawanshi A, Veiga-Parga T, Rajasagi NK, Reddy PB, Sehrawat S, et al. (2011) Role of IL-17 and Th17 cells in herpes simplex virus-induced corneal immunopathology. J Immunol 187: 1919–1930.

49. Veiga-Parga T, Gimenez F, Mulik S, Chiang EY, Grogan JL, et al. (2012) Controlling herpetic stromal keratitis by modulating lymphotoxin-alpha-mediated inflammatory pathways. Microbes and infection / Institut Pasteur 15: 677–687.

50. Inoue Y (2008) Immunological aspects of herpetic stromal keratitis. Semin Ophthalmol 23: 221–227.

51. Taylor BA, Heiniger HJ, Meier H (1973) Genetic analysis of resistance to cadmium-induced testicular damage in mice. Proc Soc Exp Biol Med 143: 629–633.

52. Norose K, Yano A, Zhang XM, Blankenhorn E, Heber-Katz E (2002) Mapping of genes involved in murine herpes simplex virus keratitis: identification of genes and their modifiers. J Virol 76: 3502–3510.

53. Huster KM, Panoutsakopoulou V, Prince K, Sanchirico ME, Cantor H (2002) T cell-dependent and -independent pathways to tissue destruction following herpes simplex virus-1 infection. Eur J Immunol 32: 1414–1419.

54. Gu W, Huang Q, Hayward GS (1995) Multiple Tandemly Repeated Binding Sites for the YY1 Repressor and Transcription Factors AP-1 and SP-1 Are Clustered within Intron-1 of the Gene Encoding the IE110 Transactivator of Herpes simplex Virus Type 1. J Biomed Sci 2: 203–226.

55. Lieu PT, Wagner EK (2000) Two leaky-late HSV-1 promoters differ significantly in structural architecture. Virology 272: 191–203.

56. Overall RW, Kempermann G, Peirce J, Lu L, Goldowitz D, et al. (2009) Genetics of the hippocampal transcriptome in mouse: a systematic survey and online neurogenomics resource. Front Neurosci 3: 55.

57. Roizman B, Gu H, Mandel G (2005) The first 30 minutes in the life of a virus: unREST in the nucleus. Cell Cycle 4: 1019–1021.

58. Du T, Zhou G, Khan S, Gu H, Roizman B (2010) Disruption of HDAC/CoREST/REST repressor by dnREST reduces genome silencing and increases virulence of herpes simplex virus. Proc Natl Acad Sci U S A 107: 15904–15909.

59. Guo Y, Audry M, Ciancanelli M, Alsina L, Azevedo J, et al. (2011) Herpes simplex virus encephalitis in a patient with complete TLR3 deficiency: TLR3 is otherwise redundant in protective immunity. J Exp Med 208: 2083–2098.

60. Sancho-Shimizu V, Perez de Diego R, Lorenzo L, Halwani R, Alangari A, et al. (2011) Herpes simplex encephalitis in children with autosomal recessive and dominant TRIF deficiency. J Clin Invest 121: 4889–4902.

61. Zhang SY, Abel L, Casanova JL (2013) Mendelian predisposition to herpes simplex encephalitis. Handb Clin Neurol 112: 1091–1097.

62. Cantin E, Tanamachi B, Openshaw H (1999) Role for gamma interferon in control of herpes simplex virus type 1 reactivation. J Virol 73: 3418–3423.

63. Cantin E, Tanamachi B, Openshaw H, Mann J, Clarke K (1999) Gamma interferon (IFN-gamma) receptor null-mutant mice are more susceptible to herpes simplex virus type 1 infection than IFN-gamma ligand null-mutant mice. J Virol 73: 5196–5200.

64. Leib DA, Harrison TE, Laslo KM, Machalek MA, Moorman NJ, et al. (1999) Interferons regulate the phenotype of wild-type and mutant herpes simplex viruses in vivo. J Exp Med 189: 663–672.

65. Everett RD, Boutell C, McNair C, Grant L, Orr A (2010) Comparison of the biological and biochemical activities of several members of the alphaherpesvirus ICP0 family of proteins. J Virol 84: 3476–3487.

66. Halford WP, Weisend C, Grace J, Soboleski M, Carr DJ, et al. (2006) ICP0 antagonizes Stat 1-dependent repression of herpes simplex virus: implications for the regulation of viral latency. Virol J 3: 44.

67. Pruett ND, Tkatchenko TV, Jave-Suarez L, Jacobs DF, Potter CS, et al. (2004) Krtap16, characterization of a new hair keratin-associated protein (KAP) gene complex on mouse chromosome 16 and evidence for regulation by Hoxc13. J Biol Chem 279: 51524–51533.

68. Bourane S, Mechaly I, Venteo S, Garces A, Fichard A, et al. (2007) A SAGE-based screen for genes expressed in sub-populations of neurons in the mouse dorsal root ganglion. BMC Neurosci 8: 97.

69. Piers TM, Kim DH, Kim BC, Regan P, Whitcomb DJ, et al. (2012) Translational Concepts of mGluR5 in Synaptic Diseases of the Brain. Front Pharmacol 3: 199.

70. Conejero-Goldberg C, Torrey EF, Yolken RH (2003) Herpesviruses and Toxoplasma gondii in orbital frontal cortex of psychiatric patients. Schizophr Res 60: 65–69.

71. Rantakallio P, Jones P, Moring J, Von Wendt L (1997) Association between central nervous system infections during childhood and adult onset schizophrenia and other psychoses: a 28-year follow-up. Int J Epidemiol 26: 837–843.

72. Kanno H, Ozawa H, Dohi Y, Sekiguchi A, Igarashi K, et al. (2009) Genetic ablation of transcription repressor Bach1 reduces neural tissue damage and improves locomotor function after spinal cord injury in mice. J Neurotrauma 26: 31–39.

73. Chu J, Hong NA, Masuda CA, Jenkins BV, Nelms KA, et al. (2009) A mouse forward genetics screen identifies LISTERIN as an E3 ubiquitin ligase involved in neurodegeneration. Proc Natl Acad Sci U S A 106: 2097–2103.

74. Kriesel JD, Gebhardt BM, Hill JM, Maulden SA, Hwang IP, et al. (1997) Anti-interleukin-6 antibodies inhibit herpes simplex virus reactivation. J Infect Dis 175: 821–827.

9

Staphylococcus aureus Ocular Infection: Methicillin-Resistance, Clinical Features, and Antibiotic Susceptibilities

Chih-Chun Chuang[1,2,3◊], Ching-Hsi Hsiao[1,4◊], Hsin-Yuan Tan[1,4], David Hui-Kang Ma[1,4], Ken-Kuo Lin[1,4], Chee-Jen Chang[5,6], Yhu-Chering Huang[4,7]*

1 Department of Ophthalmology, Chang Gung Memorial Hospital, Linkou, Taiwan, 2 Department of Ophthalmology, Changhua Christian Hospital, Changhua, Taiwan, 3 Department of Ophthalmology, Yuan-Sheng Hospital, Changhua, Taiwan, 4 College of Medicine, Chang Gung University, Taoyuan, Taiwan, 5 Graduate Institute of Clinical Medical Science, Chang Gung University, Taoyuan, Taiwan, 6 Clinical Informatics and Medical Statistics Research Center, Chang Gung University, Taoyuan, Taiwan, 7 Division of Pediatric Infectious Diseases, Department of Pediatrics, Chang Gung Memorial Hospital, Linkou, Taiwan

Abstract

Background: Methicillin-resistant *Staphylococcus aureus* (MRSA) infection is an important public health issue. The study aimed to determine the prevalence of ocular infections caused by MRSA and to identify the clinical characteristics and antibiotic susceptibility of ocular MRSA infections by comparing those of ocular methicillin-sensitive *S. aureus* (MSSA) infections.

Methodology/Principal Findings: The medical records of the patients (n = 519) with culture-proven *S. aureus* ocular infections seen between January 1, 1999 and December 31, 2008 in Chang Gung Memorial Hospital were retrospectively reviewed. Two hundred and seventy-four patients with MRSA and 245 with MSSA ocular infections were identified. The average rate of MRSA in *S. aureus* infections was 52.8% and the trend was stable over the ten years (*P* value for trend = 0.228). MRSA ocular infections were significantly more common among the patients with healthcare exposure (*P* = 0.024), but 66.1% (181/274) patients with MRSA ocular infections had no healthcare exposure. The most common clinical presentation for both MRSA and MSSA ocular infections was keratitis; MRSA and MSSA caused a similar disease spectrum except for lid infections. MRSA was significantly more resistant than MSSA to clindamycin, erythromycin and sulfamethoxazole/trimethoprim (all *P*<0.001).

Conclusions/significance: We demonstrated a paralleled trend of ocular MRSA infection in a highly prevalent MRSA country by hospital-based survey. Except for lid disorder, MRSA shared similar spectrum of ocular pathology with MSSA. Since *S. aureus* is a common ocular pathogen, our results raise clinician's attention to the existence of highly prevalent MRSA.

Editor: Mark Alexander Webber, University of Birmingham, United Kingdom

Funding: This work was supported in part by Chang Gung Memorial Hospital, Linkou, Taiwan, grant number CMRPG381511. No additional external funding received for this study. The funders had no role in study design, data collection and analysis, decision to publish, or preparation of the manuscript.

Competing Interests: The authors have declared that no competing interests exist.

* E-mail: ychuang@adm.cgmh.org.tw

◊ Chih-Chun Chuang and Ching-Hsi Hsiao contributed equally to this manuscript.

Introduction

Staphylococcus aureus is among the most important and commonly isolated human bacterial pathogens. *S. aureus* isolates resistant to methicillin, usually also resistant to other β-lactam antimicrobial drugs, are termed methicillin-resistant *S. aureus* (MRSA). MRSA, first identified in the 1960s, was traditionally associated with healthcare facilities, but is now a dominant pathogen in community-associated infections. [1] MRSA is of particular concern as a serious cause of morbidity and mortality worldwide, because of its multiple drug resistance, leaving limited treatment options and its believed increasing prevalence.

Previous data on ocular MRSA infections were generally limited to case reports and small case series, [2–7] but a variety of more recent publications have presented substantially larger analyses of ocular MRSA in the United States. [8–18] Case series of catastrophic eye infections caused by MRSA has been reported recently in patients after refractive and cataract surgery. [11,15,16] According to the report from American Society of Cataract and Refractive Surgery, MRSA has replaced nontuberculous mycobacteria to be the most common pathogen causing infections after laser-assisted in situ keratomileusis. [19] MRSA has been reported to account for 18.2% (6/33) culture-proven endophthalmitis in a referral vitreoretinal practice. [15] The proportion of MRSA in ocular *S. aureus* infections from a single institution varies from 3% to 30%, with some reports showing increasing incidence of MRSA. [8–10] The Surveillance Network, which monitors antimicrobial susceptibility patterns of bacterial pathogens in the United States, reported an increase in the proportion of MRSA among *S. aureus* ocular infections, from

29.5% in 2000 to 41.6% in 2005, which showed MRSA is a rising menace in ocular field. [12] In Taiwan, the rate of MRSA among *S. aureus* clinical isolates, was about 60% during 1997–2000, [20,21] a rate higher than that reported in other regions of the world, [20] but the rate of ocular infections caused by MRSA remains unknown.

Here, we conducted a 10-year retrospective study to determine the rate of ocular MRSA infections and to identify the clinical characteristics and antibiotic susceptibility of ocular MRSA infection by comparing those of ocular methicillin sensitive *S. aureus* (MSSA) infections seen in Chang Gung Memorial Hospital, a 3000-bed tertiary referral hospital in Taiwan.

Methods

Ethics

The study was approved by the institute review boards from Chang Gung Memorial Hospital, which allowed retrieve of the patients list from the electronic microbiology database, review of the medical information. A waiver of consent was granted given the retrospective nature of the project and anonymous analysis of the data.

Participants and Procedures

From the microbiologic laboratory database, we identified all the patients with an ocular specimen, collected by ophthalmologists, sent for bacterial culture and positive for *S. aureus* between January 1, 1999 and December 31, 2008. We included no more than one isolate per patient. We determined susceptibility of the isolates to seven antibiotics (oxacillin, penicillin, erythromycin, clindamycin, trimethoprim/sulfamethoxazole, vancomycin and teicoplanin) using the disc diffusion method according to the Clinical and Laboratory Standard Institute (CLSI) standards for antimicrobial susceptibility testing. We used oxacillin, which was replaced by cefoxitin since March 2006, to test for β-lactam antibiotic resistance. We reviewed patient charts to collect demographic and clinical information. Based on the structures involved, we classed ocular infections into one of seven diagnoses: conjunctivitis, keratitis, lid disorder, lacrimal system disorder, wound infection, endophthalmitis and other (e.g., blebitis, buckle or implant infection and sclera ulcer). If the chart showed more than one diagnosis, we chose the primary pathology or the more severe diagnosis. If the patients had either: 1) a MRSA infection identified after 48 hours of admission to a hospital; 2) a history of hospitalization, surgery, dialysis, or residence in a long-term care facility within one year of the MRSA culture date; 3) a permanent indwelling catheter or percutaneous medical device present at the time of culture; or 4) a known positive culture for MRSA prior to the study period, they were thought to have healthcare exposure [22].

Statistical Analysis

Patients with MSSA ocular infections constituted the control group and patients with MRSA ocular infections were the study group. Nominal variables were analyzed with the chi square test. Continuous variables were analyzed with Student's *t* test. Trend analysis was performed by the chi square test for trends. For comparison, we grouped the data into two five-year study periods, from January 1999 to December 2003 and from January 2004 to December 2008. All analyses were two-tailed, and *P*<0.05 was considered statistically significant. We performed all statistical analyses using R (The R Foundation for Statistical Computing, Vienna, Austria; available at: http://www.R-project.org).

Results

During the 10-year study period, *S. aureus* was isolated from 519 patients. Of these, 274 were MRSA and 245 were MSSA.

The Rate of MRSA in *S. aureus* Ocular Infections

As illustrated in Figure 1, the average annual rate of MRSA among ocular *S. aureus* infections was 52.8%, ranging from 41.9% in 2000 to 76.5% in 2006, and the trend was stable for the 10-year interval (*P* value for trend = 0.228).

Characteristics of Ocular MRSA and MSSA Infections (Table 1)

The groups had similar median ages, 41.3 years (range, 1 month to 89 years) for patients with ocular MRSA infections and 37.3 years (range, 2 months to 84 years) for those with ocular MSSA infections. Of the 281 males and 238 females infected, significantly more males than females had MSSA (*P*=0.036). The groups did not differ in eye involvement (laterality). Ninety three patients (93/274, 33.9%) with MRSA ocular infections and 60 patients (60/245, 24.5%) with MSSA ocular infections had healthcare exposure; MRSA infections were significant more common among the patients with healthcare exposure (*P*=0.024). Patients with MRSA did not differ significantly from MSSA patients in the presence of underlying comorbidities or use of immunosuppressants. In MRSA group, the rate of the patients with healthcare exposure significantly decreased from 44.8% to 25.9% (*P*=0.002) in the most recent five years. There was no change in other demographics of both MRSA and MSSA groups between the two study periods.

Clinical Diagnoses Associated with Ocular MRSA and MSSA Infections (Table 2)

Keratitis was the most common ocular diagnosis in all patients and accounted for 36.1% and 40.0% of cases of MRSA and MSSA, respectively. About 20% of patients in both groups had conjunctivitis. In MRSA group, the rate of lid disorder significantly increased from 23.9% to 76.1% (*P*<0.001), while the rate of keratitis significantly decreased from 55.6% to 44.4% during the last five years (*P*=0.001). The rate of various diagnoses caused by MSSA did not change between the two study periods. By comparison, patients with MRSA infections presented with lid disorder significantly more often than patients with MSSA infections (24.5% vs. 16.7%, *P*=0.040), but the rate of patients presenting with other diagnoses did not differ significantly between both groups. MRSA and MSSA did not differ in their association with a diagnosis of vision-threatening disorders (i.e., keratitis, orbital cellulitis or endophthalmitis).

Antibiotics Susceptibility of MRSA and MSSA for Ocular Infections (Table 3)

As expected, MRSA was significantly more resistant than MSSA to several antibiotics including clindamycin, erythromycin and sulfamethoxazole/trimethoprim. Seventy-eight percent of MRSA isolates were susceptible to sulfamethoxazole/trimethoprim. All MRSA and MSSA isolates were susceptible to vancomycin and teicoplanin. Susceptibility of both MRSA and MSSA groups to all seven antibiotics did not change significantly in the most recent five years.

Discussion

To our knowledge, the current study represents the largest reported case series of ocular *S. aureus* infections. Our findings

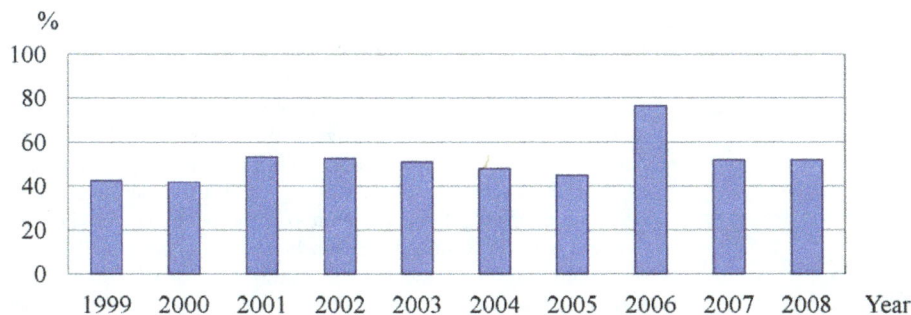

Figure 1. Percentage of patients with ocular methicillin-resistant *Staphylococcus aureus* **(MRSA) by year.**

show that 52.8% of ocular *S. aureus* infections were MRSA and the trend was stable over a 10-year interval at our hospital. MRSA ocular infections were significant more common among the patients with healthcare exposure. Except for lid disorder, MRSA and MSSA caused a similar disease spectrum and severity of ocular disorders. MRSA was significantly more resistant than MSSA to clindamycin, erythromycin and sulfamethoxazole/trimethoprim.

Our data showed a relatively high and stable rate of ocular isolates of MRSA in our hospital, although most other studies reported increasing MRSA prevalence. Blomquist showed an increase in the incidence of ophthalmic MRSA from 12% to 33% over a 5-year period (2000 to 2004) in an urban health care system in the United States. [9] Freidlin et al. reported a similar increase in the proportion of ocular MRSA infections from 4.1% in 1998 to 1999 to 16.7% in 2005–2006. [10] The Surveillance Network demonstrated an increase in the proportion of culture-positive ocular MRSA from 29.5% in 2000 to 41.6% in 2005 in serious *S. aureus* ocular infections, predicting that MRSA could be more common than MSSA within two to three years, based on the rate of increase. [13] Instead, our results were in line with the prevalence reported for our hospital and Taiwan. MRSA was first documented in the early 1980s in Taiwan and its prevalence has increased remarkably since. [23] Based on data from 12 major hospitals in Taiwan, MRSA accounted for 53% to 83% of all *S. aureus* clinical isolates in 2000. [24] In our hospital, an average of 63.9% of all *S. aureus* infections were MRSA (range, 59.0% to 70.0%), with no trend change over a 10-year interval, similar to ocular infections due to *S. aureus*. These data indicate that MRSA is prevalent and with a stable rate of *S. aureus* infections in our hospital, perhaps in the plateau stage, in the past decade.

As expected, a statistically significantly greater number of the patients with MRSA ocular infections had healthcare exposure than those with MSSA ocular infections in this study. However, it is noteworthy that two thirds of the patients (181/274, 66.1%) with MRSA ocular infections had no healthcare exposure, which meant the isolates were potentially community associated. MRSA was once associated with healthcare facilities, but more recent reports showed an increasing frequency of isolates from community-associated MRSA infections in Taiwan as elsewhere. [25–30] Since most ophthalmologic patients are seen and treated as outpatients instead of inpatients, community-associated MRSA may play an important role in MRSA ocular infections. Further analysis of community associated ocular MRSA infection has been conducted and published separately [31].

In our study, the most common presentation of ocular MRSA infections was keratitis (36.1%), followed by lid disorder (24.5%) and conjunctivitis (20.1%); nearly half (47.8%) of ocular MRSA infections were vision-threatening. However, previous large case series studies showed that the most common manifestation of ophthalmic MRSA infection was conjunctivitis [8,10] or lid disorder [9]; vision-threatening infections were relatively uncommon. [8–10] Our results may have differed due to selection bias, because there were more severe cases in our hospital, a tertiary referred center. Also, physicians may differ in which cases they sent for diagnostic testing; some may tend to culture only the most serious cases. Third, we may exclude some patients with ocular infections, while the cultures were not done by ophthalmologists.

MRSA is believed to cause a more severe disease than MSSA, but this observation has not reached consensus. [32,33] Our results did not show that MRSA caused more severe ocular diseases than MSSA; this agrees with Freidlin's study, which

Table 1. Comparison of demographics and characteristics of ocular 274 methicillin-resistant *Staphylococcus aureus* and 245 methicillin-sensitive *Staphylococcus aureus* infections.

Characteristics	MRSA (n = 274)	MSSA (n = 245)	p value*
Age (Mean ±SD years)	41.3±26.6	37.3±27.3	0.096
Gender (F/M)	138/136	100/145	0.036
Eye (R/L/B)	123/115/36	106/110/29	0.776
Healthcare exposure	93	60	0.024
Comorbidities	82	57	0.218
Immunosuppressive treatment (Local/Systemic/Nil)	17/20/237	11/8/226	0.079

*Two-sample *t* test for age comparison, Chi-square test for others.
MRSA: methicillin-resistant *Staphylococcus aureus*, MSSA: methicillin-sensitive *Staphylococcus aureus*, F: female, M: male, R: right eye, L: left eye, B: both eyes.

Table 2. Comparison of clinical diagnoses associated with ocular 274 methicillin-resistant *Staphylococcus aureus* and 245 methicillin-sensitive *Staphylococcus aureus* infections.

Diagnosis	MRSA (n = 274) No. (%)	MSSA (n = 245) No. (%)	p-value
Keratitis	99 (36.1)	98 (40.0)	0.414
Lid disorder*	67 (24.5)	41 (16.7)	0.040
Conjunctivitis	55 (20.1)	49 (20.0)	1
Lacrimal system disorder[†]	29 (10.6)	37 (15.1)	0.158
Wound infection	10 (3.6)	7 (2.9)	0.795
Endophthalmitis	9 (3.3)	4 (1.6)	0.357
Others[‡]	5 (1.8)	9 (3.7)	0.305
Vision-threatening disorder[§]	131 (47.8)	121 (49.4)	0.786

*Lid disorders including cellulitis, lid abscess and hordeolum.
[†]Lacrimal system disoder including dacrocystitis and canaliculitis.
[‡]Others including blebitis, sclera ulcer, buckle infection and hydroxyapatite implant infection.
[§]Vision-threatening disorder including keratitis, cellulitis and endophthalmitis.
MRSA: methicillin-resistant *Staphylococcus aureus*, MSSA: methicillin-sensitive *Staphylococcus aureus*.

reported MRSA and MSSA caused similar eye disease. [10] We did find that patients with MRSA were more likely to have lid infections. In addition, the rate of lid disorder caused by MRSA significantly increased, but the rate of keratitis caused by MRSA significantly decreased during the last five years. Community-associated MRSA has a reported predilection for causing skin and soft tissue infections, [22,34] and we also found that lid and lacrimal system disorders were more common, but keratitis, endophthalmitis and wound infection were less common among community associated MRSA cases than healthcare associated MRSA cases. [31] Thus, 66.1% of patients with MRSA ocular infections were community-associated and the paralleled significant increase in the rate of the MRSA patients without healthcare exposure (i.e. community-associated MRSA) in the most recent five years may explain these results.

According to antibiotic susceptibility profiles, vancomycin was the most active agent against ocular MRSA isolates, whereas sulfamethoxazole-trimethoprim retained some degree of activity

against MRSA, but was less effective than in previous studies. [9,10,13] Although vancomycin retains extremely high efficacy against MRSA, *S. aureus* with reduced susceptibility to vancomycin was identified. [35] Since prior vancomycin use is a risk factor for MRSA with reduced vancomycin susceptibility, [36] and no convincing evidence shows that routine vancomycin prophylaxis is effective in elective cataract surgery, [37] we recommend that ophthalmologists follow guideline of the Centers for Disease Control and Prevention [38] and the American Academy of Ophthalmology [39] against the routine use of vancomycin for prophylaxis to halt the spread of resistance. Several recent studies have reported that MRSA has a high rate of *in vitro* resistance to fluoroquinolones, including new generation ones, the most popular empiric therapy in ocular infections. [9,10,12,13,15,16,40] We did not test fluoroquinolones in our study because they were not included in the recommended list of antibiotics published by the CLSI. In Taiwan, National data from 2000 (TSAR program) has demonstrated 40% *S. aureus* (including MSSA and MRSA) in vitro resistance to ciprofloxacin. [21] We may extend the antibiotic susceptibility profiles to include commonly used topical antibiotics in future studies.

Eight ocular MRSA isolates from pediatric patients were stored and available for genotyping analysis, including pulsed-filed gel electrophoresis (PFGE) typing, SCC*mec* elements and the detection of PVL genes in this study. The only one healthcare associated MRSA isolate was characterized as PFGE type A/SCC*mec* IIIA/PVL-negative, which was compatible with those of healthcare associated MRSA isolates (sequence type (ST) 239, Hungary clone) in our previous studies. [29,41] Four of seven isolates classified as community-associated MRSA were characterized by PFGE type D/SCC*mec* VT/PVL positive, and the other three were characterized by PFGE type C/SCCmec IV/PVL-negative. Both clones shared the common genetic characteristics of community-associated MRSA strains in Taiwan (ST 59, Taiwan clone). [29,41] These molecular results, though limited, further confirmed the classification of community-associated and health-care-associated MRSA based on epidemiologic data in the present study was confident.

The currently recommended disc diffusion method to determine resistance against methicillin for *S. aureus* uses cefoxitin rather than oxacillin, because cefoxitin results are easier to interpret and are more sensitive for the detection of *mecA*-mediated resistance than oxacillin results, especially for identifying community associated MRSA, which may have low MIC to oxacillin. [42,43] Our Clinical Microbiology Laboratories started using cefoxitin instead

Table 3. Antibiotic susceptibility of 274 methicillin-resistant *Staphylococcus aureus* and 245 methicillin-sensitive *Staphylococcus aureus* isolates for ocular infections.

Antibiotics	MRSA (n = 274) No. (%)	MSSA (n = 245) No. (%)	p value[†]
Clindamycin	24 (8.8)	179 (73.1)	<0.001
Erythromycin	14 (5.1)	153 (62.5)	<0.001
Penicillin	0 (0)	20 (8.2)	<0.001
Sulfamethoxazole/Trimethoprim	214 (78.1)	241 (99.2)	<0.001
Vancomycin	274 (100)	245 (100)	
Teicoplanin*	260 (100)	226 (100)	

*No sensitivity test for teicoplanin in 1999.
[†]Two-proportional *t* test.
MRSA: methicillin-resistant *Staphylococcus aureus*, MSSA: methicillin-sensitive *Staphylococcus aureus*.

of oxacillin to test for β-lactam antibiotic resistance since March 2006 as the performance standard from the CLSI was revised. When we made a comparison between MRSA and MSSA ocular infections from March 2006 to the end of 2008, the results were the same as those in the 10-year study interval except there was no significant difference in the proportion of the patients with healthcare exposure in MRSA and MSSA. It was probably due to the increase in community-associated MRSA over time in our hospital [31].

Our study has the inherent flaws of a retrospective design. The patient selection criteria may influence data interpretation. Since our study population attended a referral-based, tertiary-care hospital, results may not be applicable to other populations. In addition, we used oxacillin/cefoxitin testing as a surrogate for detecting the *mec*A gene in the identification of resistant species of *Staphylococcus*; and we distinguished community-associated MRSA from healthcare-associated MRSA based on epidemiological differences, not genetic characterization. Our Clinical Microbiology Laboratories retain only isolates from blood for long-term storage, so we did not have the ocular isolates for further analysis. Thus, misclassification bias may limit applicability of the results. Furthermore, resistance found *in vitro* based on serum systemic standards does not always correlate with clinical resistance, because there are no susceptibility standards for topical therapy. Finally, the scope of our study primarily focused on the epidemiology and included a broad spectrum of diseases, so the treatment and visual outcomes were not intended to be discussed.

Infectious diseases may differ by regions in epidemiologic patterns, spectrum and severity of disease, and profiles of antibiotic susceptibility. In this 10-year retrospective study, we found that MRSA was common in ocular *S. aureus* infections in our hospital, which paralleled trends of systemic MRSA infections, in this highly prevalent MRSA country. While we failed to demonstrate a difference in virulence between MRSA and MSSA, vision-threatening disorders were common in both. All MRSA isolates were susceptible to vancomycin. Establishing the baseline characteristics of MRSA ocular infections helps us track future progress and choose the most appropriate treatment.

Acknowledgments

The authors thank Mr. Lin Yu-Jr in the Biostatistical Center for Clinical Research, Chang Gung Memorial Hospital, Taiwan for the assistance in statistical analyses.

Author Contributions

Conceived and designed the experiments: CCC CHH HYT. Performed the experiments: CCC CHH. Analyzed the data: CCC CHH YCH. Contributed reagents/materials/analysis tools: DHKM KKL CJC YCH. Wrote the paper: CHH YCH.

References

1. Deresinski S (2005) Methicillin-resistant Staphylococcus aureus: an evolutionary, epidemiologic, and therapeutic odyssey. Clin Infect Dis 40: 562–573.
2. Fukuda M, Ohashi H, Matsumoto C, Mishima S, Shimomura Y (2002) Methicillin-resistant Staphylococcus aureus and methicillin-resistant coagulase-negative Staphylococcus ocular surface infection efficacy of chloramphenicol eye drops. Cornea 21: S86–89.
3. Sotozono C, Inagaki K, Fujita A, Koizumi N, Sano Y, et al. (2002) Methicillin-resistant Staphylococcus aureus and methicillin-resistant Staphylococcus epidermidis infections in the cornea. Cornea 21: S94–101.
4. Donnenfeld ED, O'Brien TP, Solomon R, Perry HD, Speaker MG, et al. (2003) Infectious keratitis after photorefractive keratectomy. Ophthalmology 110: 743–747.
5. Kotlus BS, Rodgers IR, Udell IJ (2005) Dacryocystitis caused by community-onset methicillin-resistant Staphylococcus aureus. Ophthalmic Plastic & Reconstructive Surgery 21: 371–375.
6. Kotlus BS, Wymbs RA, Vellozzi EM, Udell IJ (2006) In vitro activity of fluoroquinolones, vancomycin, and gentamicin against methicillin-resistant Staphylococcus aureus ocular isolates. American Journal of Ophthalmology 142: 726–729.
7. Rutar T, Chambers HF, Crawford JB, Perdreau-Remington F, Zwick OM, et al. (2006) Ophthalmic manifestations of infections caused by the USA300 clone of community-associated methicillin-resistant Staphylococcus aureus. Ophthalmology 113: 1455–1462.
8. Shanmuganathan VA, Armstrong M, Buller A, Tullo AB (2005) External ocular infections due to methicillin-resistant Staphylococcus aureus (MRSA). Eye 19: 284–291.
9. Blomquist PH (2006) Methicillin-resistant Staphylococcus aureus infections of the eye and orbit (an American Ophthalmological Society thesis). Transactions of the American Ophthalmological Society 104: 322–345.
10. Freidlin J, Acharya N, Lietman TM, Cevallos V, Whitcher JP, et al. (2007) Spectrum of eye disease caused by methicillin-resistant Staphylococcus aureus. American Journal of Ophthalmology 144: 313–315.
11. Solomon R, Donnenfeld ED, Perry HD, Rubinfeld RS, Ehrenhaus M, et al. (2007) Methicillin-resistant Staphylococcus aureus infectious keratitis following refractive surgery. American Journal of Ophthalmology 143: 629–634.
12. Asbell PA, Colby KA, Deng S, McDonnell P, Meisler DM, et al. (2008) Ocular TRUST: nationwide antimicrobial susceptibility patterns in ocular isolates. Am J Ophthalmol 145: 951–958.
13. Asbell PA, Sahm DF, Shaw M, Draghi DC, Brown NP (2008) Increasing prevalence of methicillin resistance in serious ocular infections caused by Staphylococcus aureus in the United States: 2000 to 2005. J Cataract Refract Surg 34: 814–818.
14. Cavuoto K, Zutshi D, Karp CL, Miller D, Feuer W (2008) Update on bacterial conjunctivitis in South Florida. Ophthalmology 115: 51–56.
15. Deramo VA, Lai JC, Winokur J, Luchs J, Udell IJ (2008) Visual outcome and bacterial sensitivity after methicillin-resistant Staphylococcus aureus-associated acute endophthalmitis. Am J Ophthalmol 145: 413–417.
16. Major JC Jr, Engelbert M, Flynn HW Jr, Miller D, Smiddy WE, et al. (2010) Staphylococcus aureus endophthalmitis: antibiotic susceptibilities, methicillin resistance, and clinical outcomes. Am J Ophthalmol 149: 278–283 e271.
17. Adebayo A, Parikh JG, McCormick SA, Shah MK, Huerto RS, et al. (2011) Shifting trends in in vitro antibiotic susceptibilities for common bacterial conjunctival isolates in the last decade at the New York Eye and Ear Infirmary. Graefes Archive for Clinical and Experimental Ophthalmology 249: 111–119.
18. Haas W, Pillar CM, Torres M, Morris TW, Sahm DF (2011) Monitoring Antibiotic Resistance in Ocular Microorganisms: Results From the Antibiotic Resistance Monitoring in Ocular MicRorganisms (ARMOR) 2009 Surveillance Study. Am J Ophthalmol 152: 567–574 e563.
19. Solomon R, Donnenfeld ED, Holland EJ, Yoo SH, Daya S, et al. (2011) Microbial keratitis trends following refractive surgery: results of the ASCRS infectious keratitis survey and comparisons with prior ASCRS surveys of infectious keratitis following keratorefractive procedures. J Cataract Refract Surg 37: 1343–1350.
20. Diekema DJ, Pfaller MA, Schmitz FJ, Smayevsky J, Bell J, et al. (2001) Survey of infections due to Staphylococcus species: frequency of occurrence and antimicrobial susceptibility of isolates collected in the United States, Canada, Latin America, Europe, and the Western Pacific region for the SENTRY Antimicrobial Surveillance Program, 1997–1999. Clin Infect Dis 32 Suppl 2: S114–132.
21. McDonald LC, Lauderdale TL, Shiau YR, Chen PC, Lai JF, et al. (2004) The status of antimicrobial resistance in Taiwan among Gram-positive pathogens: the Taiwan Surveillance of Antimicrobial Resistance (TSAR) programme, 2000. Int J Antimicrob Agents 23: 362–370.
22. Naimi TS, LeDell KH, Como-Sabetti K, Borchardt SM, Boxrud DJ, et al. (2003) Comparison of community- and health care-associated methicillin-resistant Staphylococcus aureus infection.[see comment]. JAMA 290: 2976–2984.
23. Chen ML, Chang SC, Pan HJ, Hsueh PR, Yang LS, et al. (1999) Longitudinal analysis of methicillin-resistant Staphylococcus aureus isolates at a teaching hospital in Taiwan. J Formos Med Assoc 98: 426–432.
24. Hsueh PR, Liu CY, Luh KT (2002) Current status of antimicrobial resistance in Taiwan. Emerg Infect Dis 8: 132–137.
25. Chambers HF (2001) The changing epidemiology of Staphylococcus aureus? Emerg Infect Dis 7: 178–182.
26. Chen CJ, Huang YC, Chen C-J, Huang Y-C (2005) Community-acquired methicillin-resistant Staphylococcus aureus in Taiwan. Journal of Microbiology, Immunology & Infection 38: 376–382.
27. Zetola N, Francis JS, Nuermberger EL, Bishai WR (2005) Community-acquired meticillin-resistant Staphylococcus aureus: an emerging threat. Lancet Infect Dis 5: 275–286.
28. Huang YC, Su LH, Wu TL, Lin TY, Huang Y-C, et al. (2006) Changing molecular epidemiology of methicillin-resistant Staphylococcus aureus bloodstream isolates from a teaching hospital in Northern Taiwan. Journal of Clinical Microbiology 44: 2268–2270.

29. Huang YC, Ho CF, Chen CJ, Su LH, Lin TY (2008) Comparative molecular analysis of community-associated and healthcare-associated methicillin-resistant Staphylococcus aureus isolates from children in northern Taiwan. Clinical Microbiology & Infection 14: 1167–1172.

30. Wang JL, Chen SY, Wang JT, Wu GH, Chiang WC, et al. (2008) Comparison of both clinical features and mortality risk associated with bacteremia due to community-acquired methicillin-resistant Staphylococcus aureus and methicillin-susceptible S. aureus. Clin Infect Dis 46: 799–806.

31. Hsiao CH, Chuang CC, Tan HY, Ma DH, Lin KK, et al. (2012) Methicillin-Resistant Staphylococcus aureus Ocular Infection: A 10-Year Hospital-Based Study. Ophthalmology 119: 522–527.

32. Cosgrove SE, Sakoulas G, Perencevich EN, Schwaber MJ, Karchmer AW, et al. (2003) Comparison of mortality associated with methicillin-resistant and methicillin-susceptible Staphylococcus aureus bacteremia: a meta-analysis. Clin Infect Dis 36: 53–59.

33. Melzer M, Eykyn SJ, Gransden WR, Chinn S (2003) Is methicillin-resistant Staphylococcus aureus more virulent than methicillin-susceptible S. aureus? A comparative cohort study of British patients with nosocomial infection and bacteremia. Clin Infect Dis 37: 1453–1460.

34. Skiest DJ, Brown K, Cooper TW, Hoffman-Roberts H, Mussa HR, et al. (2007) Prospective comparison of methicillin-susceptible and methicillin-resistant community-associated Staphylococcus aureus infections in hospitalized patients. J Infect 54: 427–434.

35. Hawser SP, Bouchillon SK, Hoban DJ, Dowzicky M, Babinchak T (2011) Rising incidence of Staphylococcus aureus with reduced susceptibility to vancomycin and susceptibility to antibiotics: a global analysis 2004–2009. Int J Antimicrob Agents 37: 219–224.

36. Fridkin SK, Hageman J, McDougal LK, Mohammed J, Jarvis WR, et al. (2003) Epidemiological and microbiological characterization of infections caused by Staphylococcus aureus with reduced susceptibility to vancomycin, United States, 1997–2001. Clin Infect Dis 36: 429–439.

37. Gordon YJ (2001) Vancomycin prophylaxis and emerging resistance: are ophthalmologists the villains? The heroes? Am J Ophthalmol 131: 371–376.

38. (1995) CDC issues recommendations for preventing spread of vancomycin resistance. Am J Health Syst Pharm 52: 1272–1274.

39. Force A-CT (1999) The prophylactic use of vancomycin for intraocular surgery. Quality of Care Publications, Number 515, American Academy of Ophthalmology, San Francisco, CA, October.

40. Marangon FB, Miller D, Muallem MS, Romano AC, Alfonso EC (2004) Ciprofloxacin and levofloxacin resistance among methicillin-sensitive Staphylococcus aureus isolates from keratitis and conjunctivitis. American Journal of Ophthalmology 137: 453–458.

41. Huang YC, Chen CJ (2011) Community-associated meticillin-resistant Staphylococcus aureus in children in Taiwan, 2000s. Int J Antimicrob Agents 38: 2–8.

42. Broekema NM, Van TT, Monson TA, Marshall SA, Warshauer DM (2009) Comparison of cefoxitin and oxacillin disk diffusion methods for detection of mecA-mediated resistance in Staphylococcus aureus in a large-scale study. J Clin Microbiol 47: 217–219.

43. Chen FJ, Hiramatsu K, Huang IW, Wang CH, Lauderdale TL (2009) Panton-Valentine leukocidin (PVL)-positive methicillin-susceptible and resistant Staphylococcus aureus in Taiwan: identification of oxacillin-susceptible mecA-positive methicillin-resistant S. aureus. Diagnostic Microbiology and Infectious Disease 65: 351–357.

10

Genetic Characteristics of the Coxsackievirus A24 Variant Causing Outbreaks of Acute Hemorrhagic Conjunctivitis

Bin Wu, Xian Qi, Ke Xu, Hong Ji, Yefei Zhu*, Fenyang Tang, Minghao Zhou

Department of Acute Infectious Disease Control and Prevention, Jiangsu Province Center for Disease Control and Prevention, Nanjing, Jiangsu, China

Abstract

During September 2010, an outbreak of acute hemorrhagic conjunctivitis reemerged in Jiangsu, three years after the nationwide epidemic in China in 2007. In total, 2409 cases were reported, 2118 of which were reported in September; 79.8% of those affected were students or teachers, with a median age of 16 years. To identify and demonstrate the genetic characteristics of the etiological agent, 52 conjunctival swabs were randomly collected from four different cities. After detection and isolation, 43 patients were positive for coxsackievirus A24 variant according to PCR and 20 according to culture isolation. Neither adenovirus nor EV70 was detected. A phylogenetic study of the complete 3Cpro and VP1 regions showed that the Jiangsu isolates clustered into a new lineage, GIV-C5, with two uniform amino-acid mutations that distinguished them from all previous strains. Another new cluster, GIV-C4, formed by Indian isolates from 2007 and Brazilian isolates from 2009, was also identified in this study. Interestingly, our isolates shared greatest homology with the GIV-C4 strains, not with the isolates that were responsible for the nationwide acute hemorrhagic conjunctivitis epidemic in China in 2007. Although all our isolates were closely related, they could be differentiated into two subclusters within GIV-C5. In conclusion, our study suggests that a new cluster of coxsackievirus A24 variant that had already evolved into diverse strains was associated with the acute hemorrhagic conjunctivitis outbreaks in Jiangsu in September 2010. These viruses might have originated from the virus isolated in India in 2007, rather than from the epidemic strains isolated in China in 2007.

Editor: Xue-Jie Yu, University of Texas Medical Branch, United States of America

Funding: The study was supported by Jiangsu Province Health Development Project with Science and Education (ZX201109, RC2011084 and RC2011085). The funders had no role in study design, data collection and analysis, decision to publish, or preparation of the manuscript.

Competing Interests: The authors have declared that no competing interests exist.

* E-mail: jszyf@jscdc.cn

Introduction

Acute hemorrhagic conjunctivitis (AHC), characterized by the sudden onset of ocular pain, swelling of the eyelids, a "foreign body" sensation or irritation, epiphora (excessive tearing), eye discharge, and photophobia, is mainly caused by enterovirus 70 (EV70), coxsackievirus A24 variant (CA24v), or adenoviruses [1–3]. In China, the first AHC outbreak was reported in 1971 [4]. Because AHC is a notifiable infectious disease in China, all cases diagnosed by physicians have been registered in the National Disease Supervision Information Management System (NDSIMS). In 2007, a nationwide AHC epidemic caused by CA24v was reported in China, with a total of 74,263 AHC cases [5,6], after which the number of AHC cases returned to baseline in 2008 and 2009. In 2010, outbreaks of AHC reemerged around the world [7–11]. In China, outbreaks were reported in Zhejiang, Guangdong, Guangxi, Shandong, Henan, Fujian, Beijing, and Chongqing [7,12]. Several studies demonstrated that the outbreaks were caused by CA24v. However, to the best of our knowledge, in China in2010, the complete sequences of the VP1 and 3Cpro regions of CA24v, which are usually used for phylogenetic analyses, were only determined in Zhejiang and Guangdong Provinces and submitted to GenBank. These sequences indicated that the CA24v strains causing these outbreaks belonged to Group IV [7,8]. The objectives of the present study were to investigate the AHC outbreak in Jiangsu Province, China, in September 2010 and to identify the etiological agent causing this outbreak and determine its genetic characteristics.

Results

The Outbreak

Of the 4276 cases of AHC in Jiangsu Province reported to the NDSIMS between January 1 2007 and December 31 2010, 2409 were officially reported in 2010, which was approximately 25-fold higher than in 2009 and 20-fold higher than in 2008, and even 0.5-fold higher than in 2007 (**Table 1**). Unlike previous years, approximately 88% of the patients in 2010 were reported during September in 13 cities of Jiangsu Province. Of all the patients, 79.8% were students, kindergarten children, or teachers (**Table 1**). Reports began to increase from September 5, reached a peak on September 13, and returned to baseline on October 1 (**Fig. 1**). All the patients had conjunctival congestion and a clear history of contact with people presenting similar symptoms. No death from AHC was reported.

Virus Detection and Isolation

Neither adenovirus nor EV70 was detected in 52 patients with acute conjunctivitis.

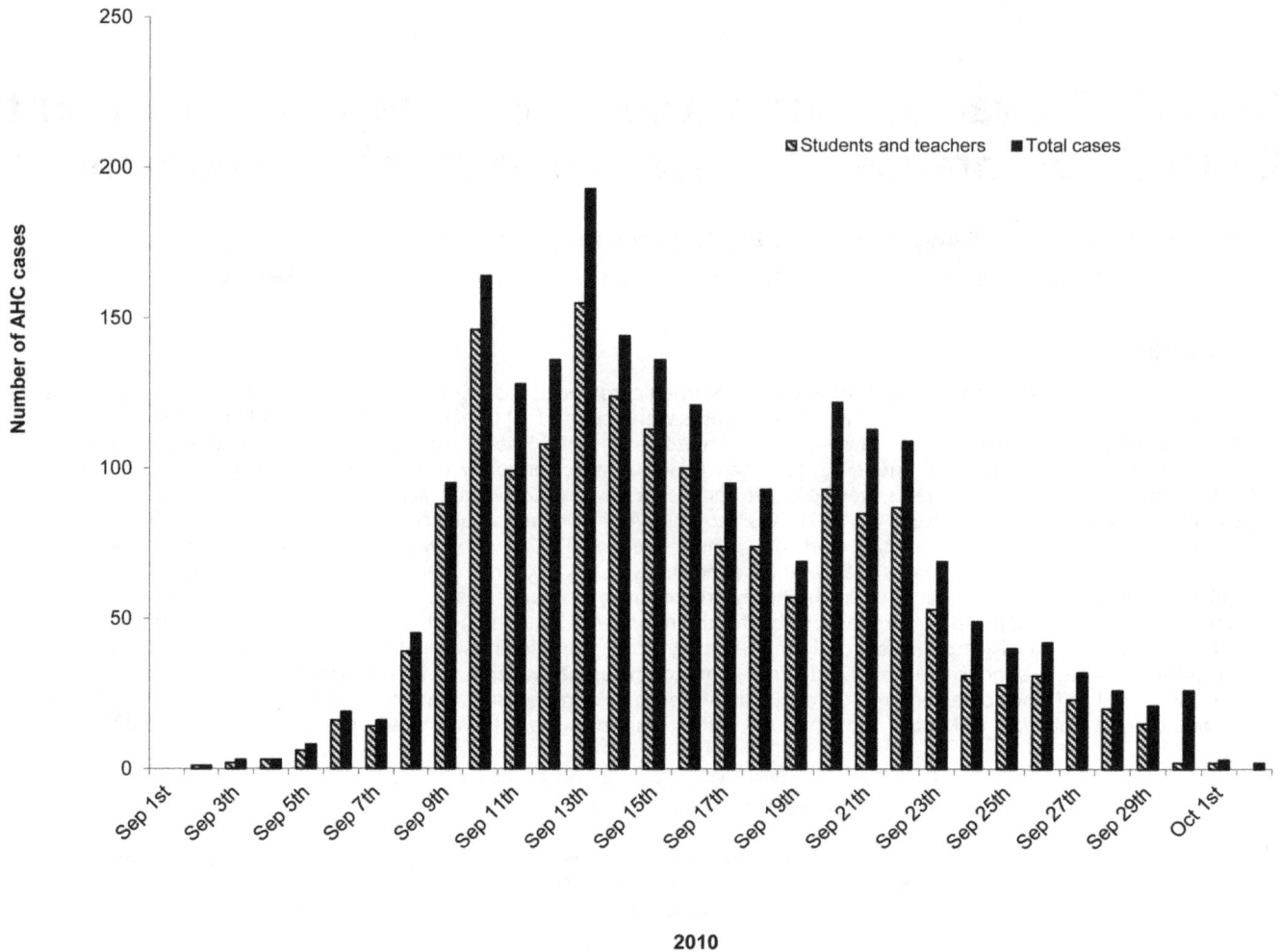

Figure 1. Distribution of the reported AHC cases in Jiangsu Province during the outbreak of September 2010.

However, 82.7% (43 of 52) of the patients were positive for CA24v according to PCR and 38.5% (20 of 52) according to culture isolation, suggesting that CA24v was the causative agent of the outbreak.

Phylogenetic Analysis of the 3Cpro Region

As in previous studies [8,13], phylogenetic analysis of the 3Cpro region showed that all the CA24v strains could be divided into four major groups. Our strains belonged to Group IV and formed a new cluster, C5, with strains isolated throughout the world after 2010. Another new cluster (C4) formed by strains from India (2007) and Brazil (2009) was also identified in this study (**Fig. 2**).

Analysis of the sequence identities of all five clusters of Group IV (**Table 2**) showed that our isolates shared the greatest homology with the C4 strains, rather than with the C3 strains, which were responsible for the nationwide AHC epidemic in China in 2007.

Further analyses showed that our strains clustered in two subclusters: C5A and C5B (**Fig. 2**). C5A, consisting of isolates P19, P29, and P41, with sequence identities of 99.6%–100%, shared greatest homology with strain GD03/2010 (99.6%). C5B, formed by other strains sharing 99.3%–100% homology, clustered with strain 378/India/2010 (99.3%–99.5%). The homology between our strains and Zhejiang strains isolated in 2010 ranks

Table 1. AHC cases reported to NDSIMS in Jiangsu from 2007 to 2010.

Year	Total cases	Cases in September	Student cases	Median age	Male:Female
2007	1649	984	702	25 years	1.99:1
2008	122	31	38	30 years	1.44:1
2009	96	8	20	27 years	2.10:1
2010	2409	2118	1690	16 years	1.69:1

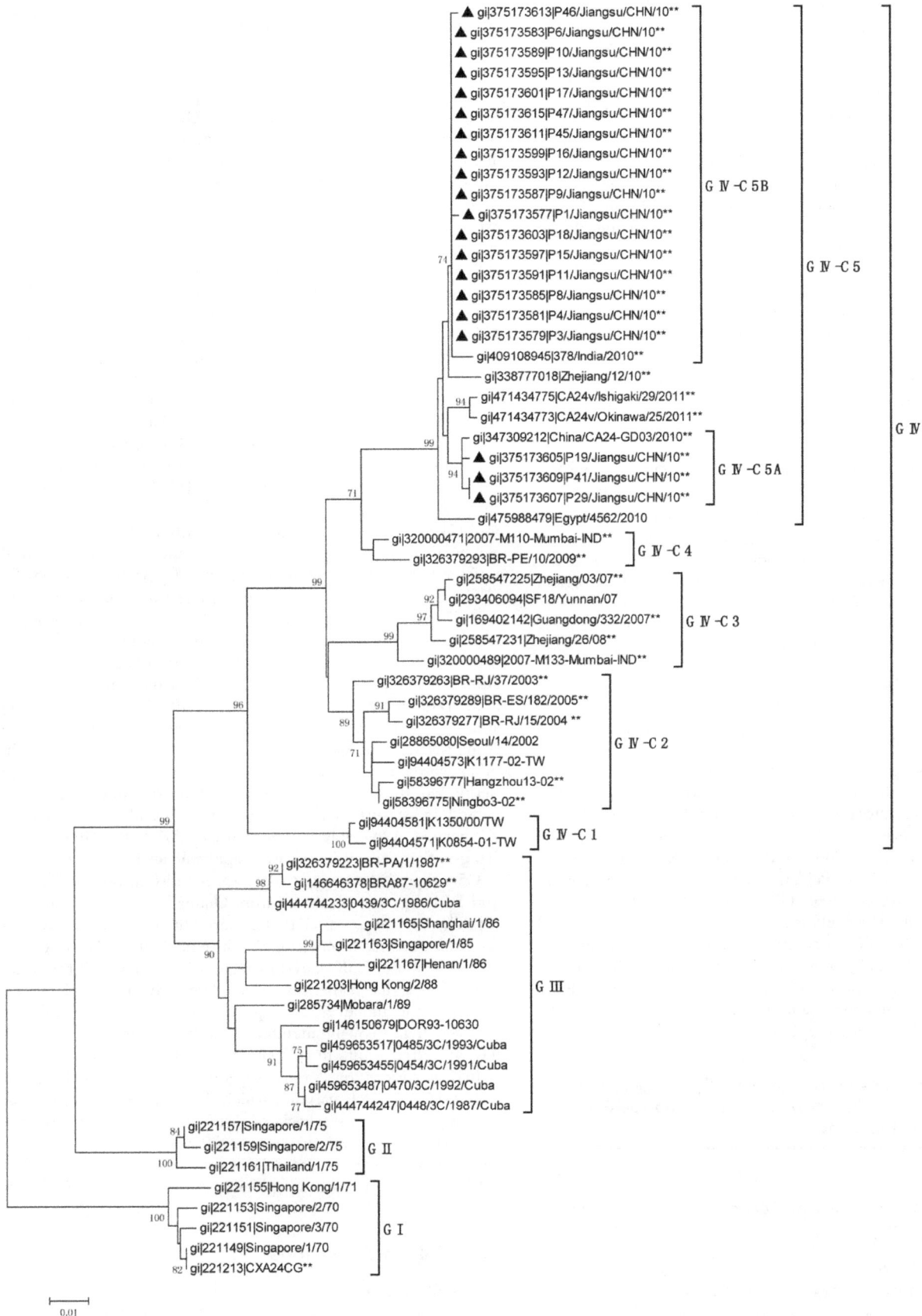

Figure 2. Phylogenetic analysis based on the 549-nucleotide 3Cpro gene of CA24v. All Jiangsu CA24v isolates identified in this study, marked with black triangles, were compared with strains available in GenBank. Strains for which the complete sequences of both the 3Cpro and VP1

regions were available are indicated with **. The MEGA 4.0 software was used for the phylogenetic analysis. The stability of the nodes was assessed using neighbor-joining cluster analysis with 1000 bootstrap replications, and only bootstrap values >70% are shown at the nodes.

second to the Indian strain (98.9%–99.1%), which is identical to the homology between C5A and C5B (98.9%–99.1%).

Phylogenetic Analyses of the VP1 Region

The sequence homology of the VP1 region confirmed the findings of the 3Cpro region analysis (**Fig. 3** and **Table 3**). The C5 lineage, which included our strains, also shared the highest sequence identities with the C4 lineage, which contained the same strains as in the 3C region analysis. The subclusters C5A and C5B were similarly identified with the VP1 region. The sequence identity between C5A and C5B ranged from 97.4% to 98.3%. As before, C5A shared greatest homology with strain GD03/2010 (99.2%–99.7%). However, because there were no complete VP1 sequences for the Indian strains isolated in 2010, we demonstrated that C5B clustered and shared its greatest homology with strain Zhejiang/12/10 (99.0–99.6%).

Amino Acid Sequence Analyses of the 3Cpro and VP1 Regions

An amino acid sequence analysis revealed two uniform mutations in all the strains that formed the C5 lineage after 2010. One was the *isoleucine* at position 54 of the 3Cpro region, and the other was the *aspartic acid* at position 301 of the VP1 region, whereas these two positions contained *valine* and *asparagine*, respectively, in all the other strains available in the GenBank before 2010 (**Table 4** and **Table 5**).

Discussion

Our study demonstrates that CA24v was the causative agent of the AHC outbreak in Jiangsu Province in September 2010. CA24v is a major etiological agent of AHC. After its first description in Singapore in 1970, AHC outbreaks caused by CA24v have occurred periodically throughout the world [2,4,8–11,13–17]. According to previous studies, four genotypes of CA24v can be distinguished and identified by phylogenetic analysis of the 3Cpro and VP1 regions [18,19]. Pei-Yu Chua reported that the CA24v strains of the fourth genotype, GIV, isolated from 2000 to 2007, can be divided into three different clusters: GIV-C1, GIV-C2, and GIV-C3 [13]. The Chinese isolates isolated in Guangdong, Yunnan, and Zhejiang provinces in 2007 and 2008 were all clustered within GIV-C3 [5–6,8]. In this study, two new clusters were identified containing strains isolated after 2007. Our strains belonged to GIV-C5, and the strains from India (2007) and Brazil

(2009) formed GIV-C4 (**Fig. 2** and **Fig. 3**). Contrary to previous studies [7,8], the differentiation of GIV-C5 and GIV-C4 is supported by phylogenetic analyses. First, our strains shared the highest sequence identities with the other strains within their clusters, whereas the identities were much lower with isolates that were categorized outside their clusters. The sequence identities were similar to the scores for the strains of other clusters (C1, C2, and C3) when compared with intra- and extra-clusters (**Table 2** and **Table 3**). Second, amino acid analyses revealed two uniform mutations that were only present in all the strains that formed the C5 lineage (**Table 4** and **Table 5**). These results suggest that the CA24v strain that caused the AHC outbreak in Jiangsu in September 2010 belonged to the new C5 cluster.

Interestingly, the new C5 cluster shared greatest homology and clustered with the C4 strains, which were represented by Indian strain M110 isolated in 2007 and Brazilian strain BR-PE/10 isolated in 2009 [10,15], and not with C3, which was responsible for the nationwide AHC epidemic in China in 2007. However, other Indian strains, such as M133 of GIV-C3, were also isolated in 2007. These results suggest that clues to the differentiation of C3 and C4 can be found retroactively as early as 2007 in India. C5 might then have evolved from C4, and has since evolved differently from the Chinese isolates of 2007 (**Fig. 2** and **Fig. 3**).

Our isolates were also differentiated as two subclusters within C5. The C5A cluster, formed by P19, P29, and P41, grouped together with the strains isolated in Guangdong Province in China in 2010 [8], whereas the others that formed C5B clustered with the strains isolated in Zhejiang Province in China in 2010. In an analysis of all the strains available in GenBank, we found that no strain isolated in 2010 in Guangdong clustered with C5B and no strain isolated in the same year in Zhejiang clustered with C5A. In other words, in 2010, at least when and where the studies were performed, the CA24v outbreaks in Guangdong might have been caused by strains that clustered with C5A alone, whereas in Zhejiang, CA24v only clustered with C5B [7,8]. However, in Jiangsu, the two subclusters were epidemic at the same time.

C5A shared the greatest sequence identity in both the 3Cpro and VP1 regions with strains from Guangdong Province in 2010 [8]. The VP1 region of C5B also shared the greatest identity with the strains isolated in Zhejiang Province in 2010 [7]. However, the 3Cpro region of C5B shared its highest homology with the strain isolated in India in the same year. Although the complete VP1 region of the Indian isolate was not available in GenBank, we deduced that frequent mutations and/or recombination events have occurred within the C5 cluster, generating its diversity.

In conclusion, our study suggests that a new cluster of coxsackievirus A24 variant, which had already evolved into diverse strains, was associated with the acute hemorrhagic conjunctivitis outbreak in Jiangsu in September 2010. These viruses might have originated from the Indian strains isolated in 2007, rather than from the epidemic strains present in China in 2007.

Materials and Methods

Ethics Statement

This study was approved by the Ethics Committee of the Jiangsu Provincial Center for Disease Control and Prevention. Written informed consent for the use of the 52 clinical specimens for virus isolation and detection was obtained from all the patients

Table 2. Homology of the complete 3Cpro regions of the strains in different clusters within CA24v genotype GIV investigated in this study.

Homology (%)	GIV-C5	GIV-C4	GIV-C3	GIV-C2	GIV-C1
GIV-C5	98.0–100.0	–	–	–	–
GIV-C4	95.8–97.0	98.7	–	–	–
GIV-C3	92.8–94.2	95.8–96.8	98.0–99.8	–	–
GIV-C2	93.8–96.8	95.4–97.0	94.6–96.4	98.0–99.6	–
GIV-C1	91.0–91.9	92.5–93.4	91.9–93.6	93.0–94.2	99.5

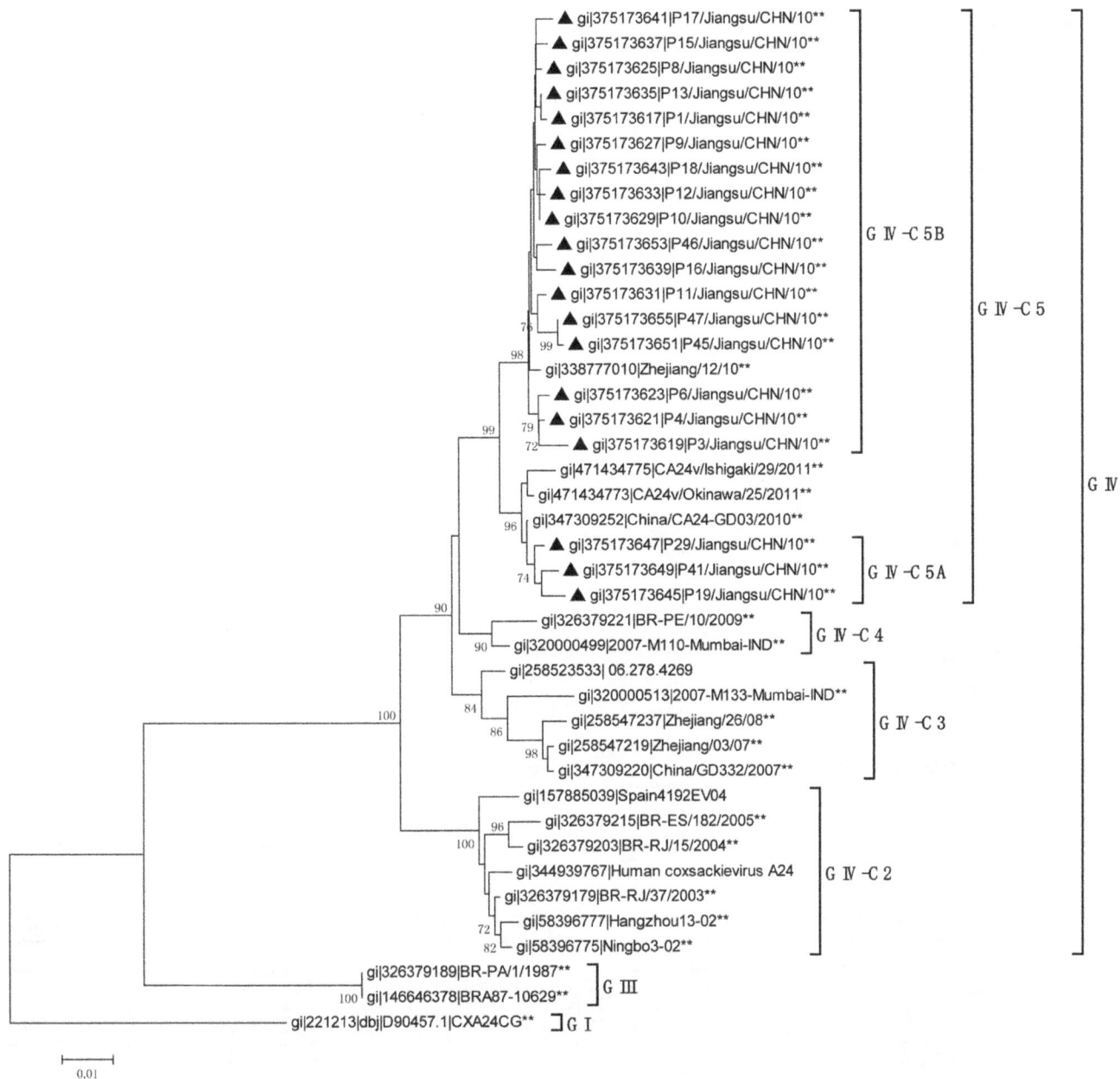

Figure 3. Phylogenetic analysis based on the 915-nucleotide VP1 gene of CA24v. All Jiangsu CA24v isolates identified in this study, marked with black triangles, were compared with strains available in GenBank. Strains for which the complete sequences of both the 3Cpro and VP1 regions were available are indicated **. The MEGA 4.0 software was used for the phylogenetic analysis. The stability of the nodes was assessed using neighbor-joining cluster analysis with 1000 bootstrap replications, and only bootstrap values >70% are shown at the nodes.

Table 3. Homology of the complete VP1 regions of the strains in different clusters within CA24v genotype GIV in this study.

Homology (%)	GIV-C5	GIV-C4	GIV-C3	GIV-C2
GIV-C5	97.3–99.9	–	–	–
GIV-C4	96.5–97.7	98.9	–	–
GIV-C3	94.1–97.3	96.1–97.5	97.4–99.8	–
GIV-C2	94.1–95.4	94.5–95.8	94.5–96.3	98.0–99.6

or the legal guardians of child patients. The Ethics Committee waived the requirement for the consent of the patients or guardians to use the basic information about the 4276 cases of AHC obtained from NDSIMS, because no samples were acquired from those patients. Patient identifiers, including names, addresses, and case numbers, were removed from any parts of the documents used in this study to ensure patient confidentiality.

Clinical Information and Specimen Collection

The 4276 cases of AHC in Jiangsu Province that were reported to NDSIMS between January 1 2007 and December 31 2010 were investigated in this study. In total, 52 conjunctival swabs from AHC patients aged 7–56 years (28 males and 24 females in the

Table 4. Amino acid mutations in the 3Cpro region in different genotypes of CA24v.

Genotype	Strains	Amino acid site in the 3Cpro region																	
		8	15	31	47	49	54	68	76	78	92	114	118	139	151	154	158	160	182
GI	gi|221213|CXA24CG	V	I	H	I	I	V	T	K	K	T	V	A	N	I	T	I	M	S
	gi|221149|Singapore/1/70	.	.	.	.	.	.	.	.	.	.	.	.	.	.	.	.	.	.
GII	gi|221161|Thailand/1/75	.	.	.	V	.	.	.	.	.	.	.	.	H	.	V	.	.	N
	gi|221159|Singapore/2/75	.	.	.	.	.	.	.	.	.	.	.	.	H	.	V	M	.	N
GIII	gi|221167|Henan/1/86	.	V	Y	.	.	.	.	.	.	A	.	T	H	.	.	.	.	.
	gi|146646378|BRA87-10629	I	V	.	.	.	.	.	R	.	A	.	A	.	H	.	.	.	.
GIV-C1	gi|94404581|K1350/00/TW	.	V	.	.	.	.	I	.	.	.	.	.	H	.	.	.	.	.
	gi|94404571|K0854-01-TW	.	V	.	.	.	.	I	.	.	.	.	.	H	.	.	.	.	.
GIV-C2	gi|58396777|Hangzhou13-02	.	V	.	.	.	.	I	.	.	.	.	.	H	V	.	.	I	.
	gi|58396775|Ningbo3-02	.	V	.	.	.	.	I	.	.	.	I	.	H	V	.	.	I	.
	gi|326379277|BR-RJ/15/2004	.	V	.	.	.	.	I	.	.	.	I	.	H	V	.	.	I	.
GIV-C3	gi|320000489|2007-M133-IND	.	V	.	V	.	V	.	.	.	.	I	.	H	.	.	.	I	.
	gi|169402142|Guangdong/332/2007	.	V	Y	.	.	V	.	.	.	.	I	.	H	.	.	.	I	.
	gi|258547231|Zhejiang/26/08	.	V	Y	.	.	V	.	.	.	.	I	.	H	.	.	.	I	.
GIV-C4	gi|320000471|2007-M110-IND	.	V	.	.	.	.	.	.	.	.	I	.	H	V	.	.	I	.
	gi|326379293|BR-PE/10/2009	.	V	.	.	.	.	.	.	.	.	I	.	H	V	.	.	I	.
GIV-C5	gi|475988479|Egypt/4562/2010	.	V	.	.	I*	.	.	.	.	.	I	.	H	V	.	.	I	.
	gi|409108945|378/India/2010	.	.	.	.	I*	.	.	.	.	.	I	.	H	V	.	.	I	.
	gi|375173607|P29/Jiangsu/CHN/10	.	V	.	.	I*	.	.	.	.	.	I	.	H	V	.	.	I	.
	gi|347309212|GD03/2010	.	V	.	.	I*	.	.	.	.	.	I	.	H	V	.	.	I	.
	gi|338777018|Zhejiang/12/10	.	V	.	.	I*	.	.	.	R	.	I	.	H	V	.	.	I	.
	gi|471434775|Ishigaki/29/2011	.	V	.	.	I*	.	.	.	.	.	I	.	H	V	.	.	I	.

*Amino acid mutation only present in all GIV-C5 strains.

Table 5. Amino acid mutations in the VP1 region in different genotypes of CA24v.

Genotype	Strains	Amino acid site in the VP1 region																
		11	25	32	51	56	89	100	103	146	151	168	196	250	255	256	297	301
GI	gi|221213|CXA24CG	S	L	S	V	I	M	E	K	T	Y	R	I	F	I	I	I	N
GII	gi|146646378|BRA87-10629	T	S	P	A	V	I	.	.	A	H	.	M	Y	.	T	T	.
GIV-C2	gi|58396775|Ningbo3-02	T	P	L	A	V	I	D	R	A	H	.	M	Y	.	T	T	.
	gi|58396777|Hangzhou13-02	T	P	L	A	V	I	D	R	A	H	.	M	Y	V	T	T	.
	gi|326379179|BR-RJ/37/2003	T	P	L	A	V	I	D	R	A	H	.	M	Y	.	T	T	.
	gi|157885039|Spain4192EV04	T	P	L	A	V	I	D	R	A	H	.	M	Y	.	T	T	.
	gi|326379209|BR-ES/93/2005	T	P	L	A	V	I	D	R	A	H	.	M	Y	.	T	T	.
GIV-C3	gi|347309220|GD332/2007	T	H	L	A	V	I	D	R	A	H	.	M	Y	.	T	T	.
	gi|320000513|2007-M133-IND	T	H	L	A	V	I	D	R	A	H	.	M	Y	.	T	T	.
	gi|258547237|Zhejiang/26/08	T	H	L	A	V	I	D	R	A	H	Q	M	Y	.	T	T	.
GIV-C4	gi|320000499|2007-M110-IND	T	H	L	A	V	I	D	R	A	H	.	M	Y	.	T	T	.
	gi|326379219|BR-PE/9/2009	T	H	L	A	V	I	D	R	A	H	.	M	Y	.	T	T	.
GIV-C5	gi|338777010|Zhejiang/12/10	T	H	L	A	V	I	D	R	A	H	.	M	Y	.	T	T	D*
	gi|347309252|CA24-GD03/2010	T	H	L	A	V	I	D	R	A	H	.	M	Y	.	T	T	D*
	gi|375173647|P29/Jiangsu/10	T	H	L	A	V	I	D	R	A	H	.	M	Y	.	T	T	D*
	gi|471434775|Ishigaki/29/2011	T	H	.	A	V	I	D	R	A	H	.	M	Y	.	T	T	D*

*Amino acid mutation only present in all GIV-C5 strains.

acute phase), were randomly collected from four hospitals in different cities (13 from Nanjing, eight from Taizhou, 15 from Yancheng, and 16 from Lianyungang) during September 2010 (1–5 days after the onset of symptoms).

Virus Detection and Isolation

Viral nucleic acid was extracted from the swabs with the QIAamp Mini Viral RNA Extraction Kit and the DNeasy Blood & Tissue Kit (Qiagen, Hilden, Germany). RT–PCR was performed with primers specific for CA24v and EV70 (CA24v-S: 5′-GTGAGTGCTTGCCCAGATTT-3′/CA24v-A: 5′-CTCCACTAGTGAGCGGTGTG-3′; and EV70-S: 5′-AGG-GATTCACCAGACATTGG-3′/EV70-A: 5′-ATTTTCCAC-CAGGCACTCTG-3′) and nested PCR was used for the generic detection of adenoviruses [20]. The PCR products were analyzed with 1% agarose electrophoresis. All 52 swabs were cultured in fresh monolayers of HEP-2 cells. The cultures were incubated at 36°C and observed daily for a cytopathic effect. Two blind passages were performed when no cytopathic effect was observed.

Nucleotide Sequencing and Phylogenetic Analyses

The 3Cpro and VP1 genes of the isolates were amplified from the RNAs extracted from the culture supernatants and cycle sequenced with primers 3C1/3C2 and CA24v-2407S/CA24v-3438A, respectively [6]. The products were analyzed with an ABI PRISM 3100 Genetic Analyzer (Applied Biosystems, Hitachi, Japan). The MEGA 4.0 software [21] was used for the phylogenetic analysis. The homologies among the genotypes were calculated using the Kimura two-parameter model. The phylogenetic trees were assessed using neighbor-joining cluster analysis with 1000 bootstrap replications, and only bootstrap values >70% are shown at the nodes.

Nucleotide Sequence Accession Numbers

All sequences reported in this study were deposited in GenBank under accession number JN788169–JN788308. In total, 276 strains with complete 3Cpro sequences and 139 strains with complete VP1 sequences that were available in GenBank (isolated between 1970 and 2011) were investigated. Sixty-three 3Cpro sequences and 41 VP1 sequences, selected for their representativeness, were used to construct the phylogenetic trees. Of these strains, 38 had complete sequences for both the 3Cpro and Vp1 regions. The GenBank accession numbers of the downloaded strains are shown on the trees (**Fig. 2** and **Fig. 3**).

Acknowledgments

The authors thank Drs Changjun Bao and Ling Gu for their excellent technical assistance.

Author Contributions

Conceived and designed the experiments: BW YZ MZ. Performed the experiments: BW XQ KX HJ. Analyzed the data: BW FT MZ. Contributed reagents/materials/analysis tools: XQ KX HJ FT MZ. Wrote the paper: BW YZ.

References

1. Babalola OE, Amoni SS, Samaila E, Thaker U, Darougar S (1990) An outbreak of acute haemorrhagic conjunctivitis in Kaduna, Nigeria. Br J Ophthalmol 74: 89–92.
2. Mirkovic RR, Schmidt NJ, Yin-Murphy M, Melnick JL (1974) Enterovirus etiology of the 1970 Singapore epidemic of acute conjunctivitis. Intervirology 4: 119–127.
3. Chang CH, Sheu MM, Lin KH, Chen CW (2001) Hemorrhagic viral keratoconjunctivitis in Taiwan caused by adenovirus types 19 and 37: applicability of polymerase chain reaction-restriction fragment length polymorphism in detecting adenovirus genotypes. Cornea 20: 295–300.
4. Mu GF (1989) [An etiological study of acute hemorrhagic conjunctivitis in Beijing area in 1984]. Zhonghua Yan Ke Za Zhi 25: 20–22.
5. Wu D, Ke CW, Mo YL, Sun LM, Li H, et al. (2008) Multiple outbreaks of acute hemorrhagic conjunctivitis due to a variant of coxsackievirus A24: Guangdong, China, 2007. J Med Virol 80: 1762–1768.
6. Yan D, Zhu S, Zhang Y, Zhang J, Zhou Y, et al. (2010) Outbreak of acute hemorrhagic conjunctivitis in Yunnan, People's Republic of China, 2007. Virol J 7: 138.
7. Yan JY, Chen Y, Li Z, Gong LM, Lu YY, et al. (2011) [Study on the pathological and molecular characteristics of AHC epidemic in Zhejiang Province in 2010]. Bing Du Xue Bao 27: 421–426.
8. De W, Huanying Z, Hui L, Corina M, Xue G, et al. (2012) Phylogenetic and molecular characterization of coxsackievirus A24 variant isolates from a 2010 acute hemorrhagic conjunctivitis outbreak in Guangdong, China. Virol J 9: 41.
9. Ayoub EA, Shafik CF, Gaynor AM, Mohareb EW, Amin MA, et al. (2013) A molecular investigative approach to an outbreak of acute hemorrhagic conjunctivitis in Egypt, October 2010. Virol J 10: 96.
10. Shukla D, Kumar A, Srivastava S, Dhole TN (2013) Molecular identification and phylogenetic study of coxsackievirus A24 variant isolated from an outbreak of acute hemorrhagic conjunctivitis in India in 2010. Arch Virol 158: 679–684.
11. (2010) Notes from the field: acute hemorrhagic conjunctivitis outbreaks caused by coxsackievirus A24v – Uganda and southern Sudan, 2010. MMWR Morb Mortal Wkly Rep 59: 1024.
12. Yang J, Lin Y, Wang HY, Tao ZX, Li Y, et al. (2012) [Identification and genetic characterization of coxsackievirus A24 isolated from patients with acute hemorrhagic conjunctivitis in Shandong Province]. Bing Du Xue Bao 28: 663–669.
13. Chu PY, Ke GM, Chang CH, Lin JC, Sun CY, et al. (2009) Molecular epidemiology of coxsackie A type 24 variant in Taiwan, 2000–2007. J Clin Virol 45: 285–291.
14. Ishiko H, Takeda N, Miyamura K, Kato N, Tanimura M, et al. (1992) Phylogenetic analysis of a coxsackievirus A24 variant: the most recent worldwide pandemic was caused by progenies of a virus prevalent around 1981. Virology 187: 748–759.
15. Triki H, Rezig D, Bahri O, Ben Ayed N, Ben Yahia A, et al. (2007) Molecular characterisation of a coxsackievirus A24 that caused an outbreak of acute haemorrhagic conjunctivitis, Tunisia 2003. Clin Microbiol Infect 13: 176–182.
16. Tavares FN, Campos Rde M, Burlandy FM, Fontella R, de Melo MM, et al. (2011) Molecular characterization and phylogenetic study of coxsackievirus A24v causing outbreaks of acute hemorrhagic conjunctivitis (AHC) in Brazil. PLoS One 6: e23206.
17. Fonseca MC, Sarmiento L, Resik S, Pereda N, Rodriguez H, et al. (2012) Isolation of Coxsackievirus A24 variant from patients with hemorrhagic conjunctivitis in Cuba, 2008–2009. J Clin Virol 53: 77–81.
18. Tavares FN, Costa EV, Oliveira SS, Nicolai CC, Baran M, et al. (2006) Acute hemorrhagic conjunctivitis and coxsackievirus A24v, Rio de Janeiro, Brazil, 2004. Emerg Infect Dis 12: 495–497.
19. Oh MD, Park S, Choi Y, Kim H, Lee K, et al. (2003) Acute hemorrhagic conjunctivitis caused by coxsackievirus A24 variant, South Korea, 2002. Emerg Infect Dis 9: 1010–1012.
20. Mitchell S, O'Neill HJ, Ong GM, Christie S, Duprex P, et al. (2003) Clinical assessment of a generic DNA amplification assay for the identification of respiratory adenovirus infections. J Clin Virol 26: 331–338.
21. Tamura K, Dudley J, Nei M, Kumar S (2007) MEGA4: Molecular Evolutionary Genetics Analysis (MEGA) software version 4.0. Mol Biol Evol 24: 1596–1599.

11

Pathogen Induced Changes in the Protein Profile of Human Tears from *Fusarium* Keratitis Patients

Sivagnanam Ananthi[1], Namperumalsamy Venkatesh Prajna[2], Prajna Lalitha[3], Murugesan Valarnila[1], Kuppamuthu Dharmalingam[4]*

1 Dr. G. Venkataswamy Eye Research Institute, Aravind Medical Research Foundation, Aravind Eye Care System, Madurai, India, 2 Cornea Clinic, Aravind Eye Hospital, Aravind Eye Care System, Madurai, India, 3 Department of Microbiology, Aravind Eye Hospital, Aravind Eye Care System, Madurai, India, 4 School of Biotechnology, Madurai Kamaraj University, Madurai, India

Abstract

Fusarium is the major causative agent of fungal infections leading to corneal ulcer (keratitis) in Southern India and other tropical countries. Keratitis caused by *Fusarium* is a difficult disease to treat unless antifungal therapy is initiated during the early stages of infection. In this study tear proteins were prepared from keratitis patients classified based on the duration of infection. Among the patients recruited, early infection (n = 35), intermediate (n = 20), late (n = 11), samples from five patients in each group were pooled for analysis. Control samples were a pool of samples from 20 patients. Proteins were separated on difference gel electrophoresis (DIGE) and the differentially expressed proteins were quantified using DeCyder software analysis. The following differentially expressed proteins namely alpha-1-antitrypsin, haptoglobin α2 chain, zinc-alpha-2-glycoprotein, apolipoprotein, albumin, haptoglobin precursor - β chain, lactoferrin, lacrimal lipocalin precursor, cystatin SA III precursor, lacritin precursor were identified using mass spectrometry. Variation in the expression level of some of the proteins was confirmed using western blot analysis. This is the first report to show stage specific tear protein profile in fungal keratitis patients. Validation of this data using a much larger sample set could lead to clinical application of these findings.

Editor: Vishnu Chaturvedi, New York State Health Department and University at Albany, United States of America

Funding: KD thanks the Department of Biotechnology, Government of India, New Delhi, India for grants no. BT/INF/22/2/2007, BT/PR13879/MED/12/458/2010 and BT/PR7592/MED/12/290/2006 for DBT Distinguished Biotechnology Research Professorship BT/HRD/35/03/2010. The funders had no role in study design, data collection and analysis, decision to publish, or preparation of the manuscript.

Competing Interests: The authors have declared that no competing interests exist.

* E-mail: dharmalingam.k@gmail.com

Introduction

Corneal ulceration is the most common cause of corneal blindness in developing countries [1]. A retrospective population based study in the Madurai district of southern Tamil Nadu, India, estimated an annual incidence of corneal ulceration of 11.3 per 10,000 in the populations [2], which is ten times higher than the reported incidence from a study from the United States [3]. *Fusarium* and *Aspergillus*, are the predominant etiological agents responsible for 44% of all corneal ulcers [4]. Reports from Ghana [5] and northern Tanzania [6] also showed fungi as the etiological agent in over 50% of culture positive cases of keratitis. *Fusarium* species is more commonly associated with fungal keratitis in southern India, while *Aspergillus* species is more often implicated in northern India and Nepal [7]. The visual outcome following mycotic keratitis is generally poorer when compared to bacterial keratitis [8] and Natamycin, which is still the drug of choice for antifungal treatment is ineffective during late stages of the disease [9]. Therapeutic keratoplasty performed for mycotic keratitis is known to have a poorer prognosis [6,10–11]. *Fusarium* sp., sometimes invade the anterior chamber and form a lens-iris-fungus mass at the pupillary area, thereby interfering with the normal drainage of the aqueous humor and leading to a rise in intraocular pressure [12,13]. Predictive or diagnostic markers are not available to detect the preclinical infections, a stage that is suitable for effective treatment. Neither the molecular mechanism underlying the susceptibility of the host and virulence of the pathogen examined.

In this study we have examined the tear profile of patients with keratitis caused by *Fusarium*. The tear proteins play an important role in maintaining healthy ocular surface, and changes in tear protein components have been shown to reflect the changes in the health of the ocular surface [14–20]. Proteomics is a valuable approach to find patterns of protein markers for a given disease [21]. Gel based proteomic approach has been used to show the alterations induced at the post translational level in an infectious disease [22,23]. Proteomic analysis can provide insights about protein expression patterns, which are associated with various pathological conditions and the identification of those tear proteins and their posttranslational modifications have the potential to reveal the mechanism of the disease [19,24–28]. The best method available at present to examine lower-abundance proteins and to quantify expression changes with high confidence is fluorescence two-dimensional difference gel electrophoresis (2D-DIGE) [29]. This multiplex technology allows the detection and quantitation of differences between samples resolved on the same gel, or across multiple gels, when linked by an internal standard [30]. 2D-DIGE circumvents the main drawbacks associated with conventional bidimensional polyacrylamide gel electrophoresis (2D-PAGE),

Table 1. The DIGE Experimental Design for Minimal Labeling with Cy Dyes used in this study.

Gel No	Cy 3	Cy 5	Cy 2
1	*Fusarium* early (30 µg)	Control(30 µg)	Pooled Internal standard
2	Control(30 µg)	*Fusarium* early(30 µg)	Pooled Internal standard
3	*Fusarium* intermediate(30 µg)	Control(30 µg)	Pooled Internal standard
4	Control(30 µg)	*Fusarium* intermediate(30 µg)	Pooled Internal standard
5	*Fusarium* late(30 µg)	Control(30 µg)	Pooled Internal standard
6	Control(30 µg)	*Fusarium* late(30 µg)	Pooled Internal standard

A total of 90 µg of labeled proteins were loaded on each gel for 2D electrophoresis; Tear sample from early, intermediate and late stage keratitis patients were used. Labeling, construction of pooled standards are described under materials and methods. 250 pmoles of dye per 30 µg protein was used.

such as low sensitivity, reduced dynamic range, and gel-to-gel variability, enabling more accurate and sensitive quantitation of proteins [31]. We have shown earlier variation in the expression level of tear proteins (prolactin inducible protein, serum albumin precursor, cystatin S precursor, cystatin SN precursor, cystatin, and human tear lipocalin) in fungal keratitis patients [15].

The present study aims to identify quantitative changes in the keratitis tear protein obtained from *Fusarium* keratitis patients using 2D DIGE. We have used tear fluid from different stages of *Fusarium* infection. As far as we know, this is the first report showing quantitative proteome level analysis of tear fluid from mycotic keratitis patients. Further these changes are fungal infection specific.

Results

2D DIGE analysis of Tear Proteins

The experimental design of 2D DIGE is described in Table 1, and eighteen images from six gels of a typical experiment are shown in Figure 1. The spot position in the fluorescent images generated by the Typhoon trio system was comparable to the silver or coomassie stained gels (data not shown).

The protein co-detection of the three different CyDye labeled images in each gel was first performed by the DIA module of the software. To perform reliable quantification, there is a built-in normalization function (using the internal standard) to compensate for experimental variations, such as differences in laser power, fluorescence labeling, and sample loading. DIA module used in addition for quantitation of protein volume ratios between the co detected Cy3, Cy5 & Cy2 signals from a single gel. Cy2 forming the internal standard and the ratio of Cy3/Cy2 and Cy5/Cy2 were calculated in the DIA module. In this module variable of one (N = 1) is considered. In Figure 2 protein spots were plotted with the log volume ratio on the x-axis and the left y-axis shows the number of spots and the right y-axis shows the spot volume. Table 2 shows the DIA data of the spot pairs detected, and the total number of spots used in the calculation is also given. In Figure 2, the spots that show less than two fold variation are within the two vertical lines. Spots outside the vertical lines represent the spots that show more than two fold variation. The normalized spot volume data against internal standard allowed a rapid overview of the differential protein expressions.

Comparison of quantitative changes in protein expression across gels

Differential protein expression of those co-detected pairs between the keratitis and control tear across all six gels representing different stages of infection were quantified using the BVA module. In order to avoid gel to gel variability, Isoelectric focusing and second dimension analysis were done using IPGphor III and Ettan Dalt six equipments, which allow simultaneous analysis of six samples. To detect variation in expression levels, relatively conservative selection criteria were used in image analysis. Differentially expressed proteins that fulfilled the following criteria alone were used for further analysis, 1) Minimum mean difference between the infected and control protein samples should be 1.5 fold or more, in terms of spot volume. 2) In all experiments an internal standard as described under materials and methods was included. 3) Built in t-test or one way ANOVA statistics software was used to detect significance of fold change (p≤0.05). 4) These spots were checked manually to confirm that they were true protein spots and not artifacts. More than 281 protein pairs (showed 1.5 fold variation or more in expression) were statistically significant (ANOVA p<0.05). However, upon application of the above stringent criteria only 140 protein pairs could be selected for further analysis. Among these 140 protein pairs, 116 spots showed higher expression level and 24 spots were down-regulated. Therefore, up-regulation of proteins seems to be the dominant features in the expression profiles after fungal infection. Similar analysis procedure was followed for all the gel comparisons and Table 3 shows the data. The data for ten differentially expressed proteins are shown in Figure 3, 4 and 5. Protein expression changes of a particular spot in each of the six gels in terms of the spot volume between the keratitis and control tears are shown. In addition, the 3-D representations of the spot volume are also shown. The BVA data was analyzed individually for Cy3 & Cy5 labeled gels (Table S1) to confirm the EDA data.

Image Analysis by DeCyder Extended Data Analysis (EDA)

Extended Data Analysis (EDA) module was used for principal component analysis and clustering studies. Matched spots that showed significant (ANOVA p≤0.01) variation in their expression were transferred to the EDA module of the software. Default settings were used for intra and intergel statistical analyses allowing the characterization and classification of biological samples based on protein expression data. Principle component analysis (PCA), which is a statistical method to eliminate redundant variables and reduce data complexity, was also performed and the results are shown in Figure 6. An unsupervised clustering analysis was performed by selecting the hierarchical clustering algorithm available within the EDA software and Figure 7 shows the result. In all these analysis default settings of the software were used and hence the confidence of the data is assured.

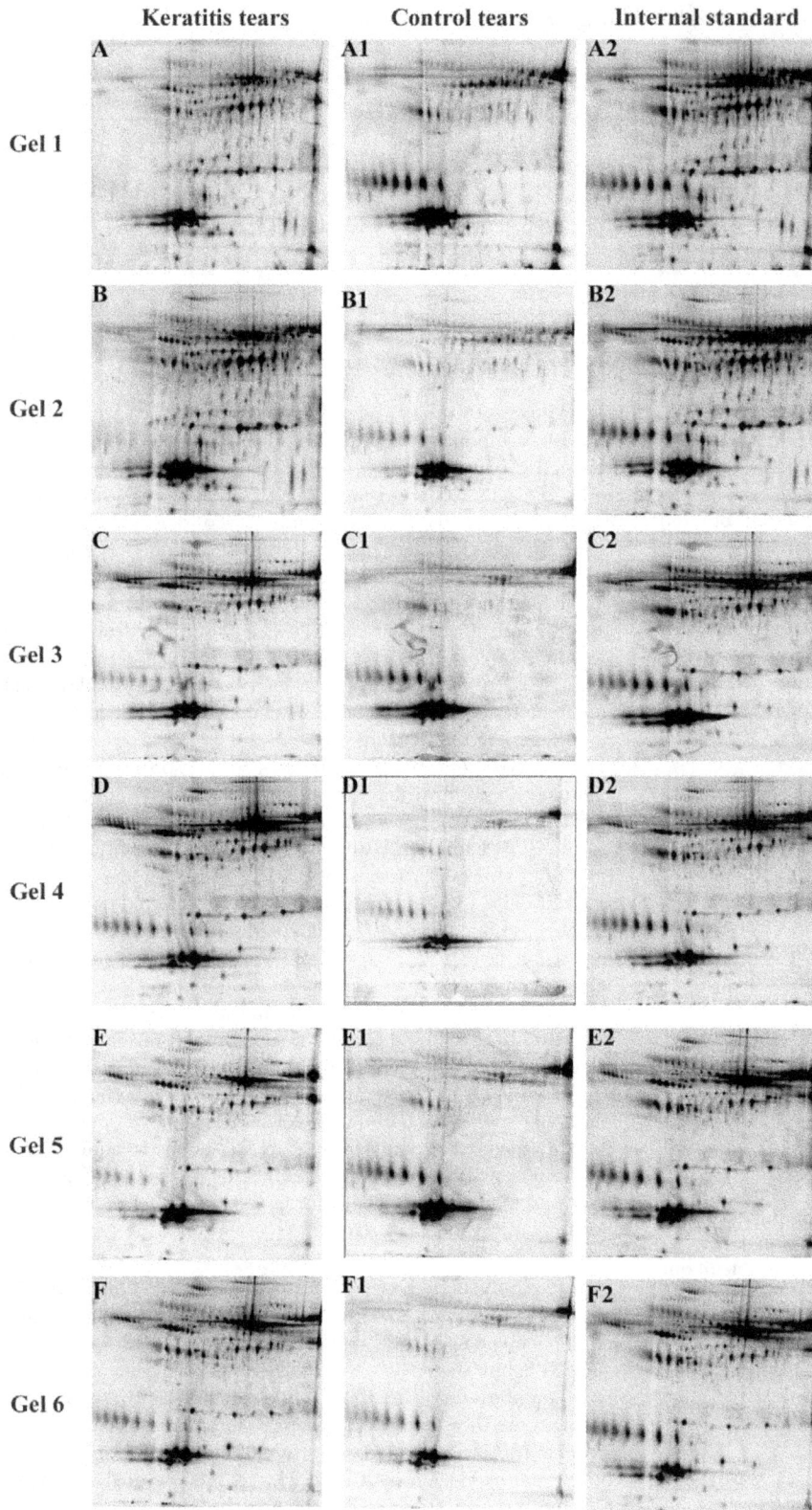

Figure 1. Fluorescent protein profiles of a set of six gels. Experimental design is described in Table 1. A&B represents *Fusarium* early keratitis; C&D represents *Fusarium* intermediate keratitis; E&F represents *Fusarium* late keratitis; A1–F1 represents control tears; A2–F2 represents the pooled internal standard. Each gel contained 90 µg of total protein separated by a pH 4–7 IPG strip in the first dimension and 12.5% polyacrylamide gel in the second dimension electrophoresis. Images were captured using a Typhoon Trio Variable Mode Imager.

Gel 1

Gel 3

Gel 5

Gel 2

Gel 4

Gel 6

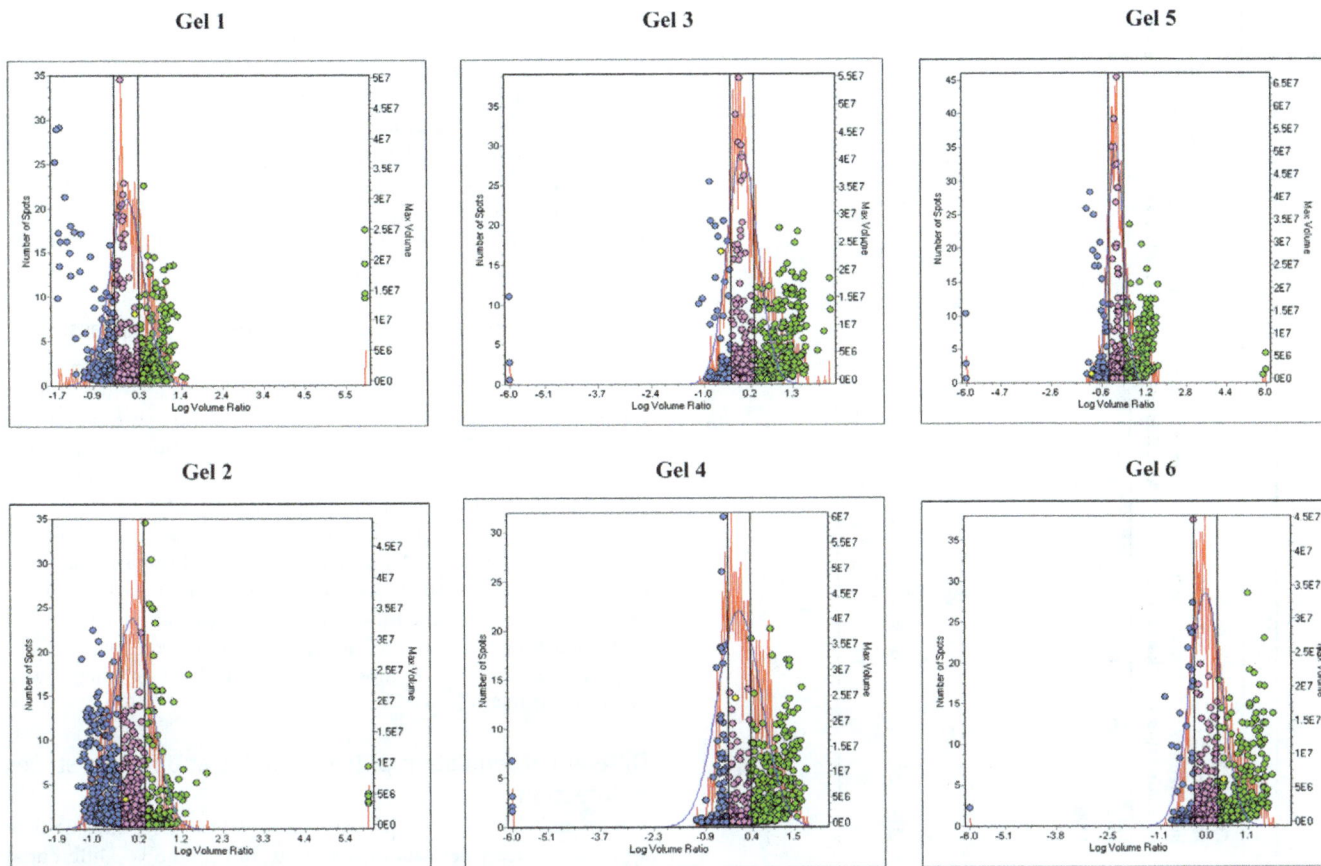

Figure 2. Discrimination of differentially expressed proteins in six gels. The histograms were generated by DeCyder DIA software, plotting spot frequency (left y-axis) against log volume ratio (x-axis), and a normal distribution model (red line) was fitted to the main peak of the frequency histogram. A 2 fold variation in expression level was set as threshold. The threshold values are represented by vertical black lines in the histogram, and the differentially expressed spot features are shown as blue spots (volume decreased) and green spots(volume increased). Table 2 describes the details of spots which show variable expression.

Dye swapping to minimize dye specific labeling efficiency

It has been reported that there was preferential lysine labeling of Cy2 to particular protein spot which has not been identified [32]. Since DIGE technology has not been applied extensively to tear sample, we have examined preferential labeling using a reciprocal labeling of the same protein. Therefore, with the reciprocal

staining approach, any possible false positive results caused by the preferential labeling of dyes could be identified and corrected.

Protein Identification by LC–MS/MS

Sixty four tear proteins were identified (Figure 8) using mass spectrometry as described under materials and methods. Some of the protein spots were isoforms and hence a total of 23 different

Table 2. Details of spot detection and spot quantitation using DIA software.

GelNo	Cy3	Cy5	Spots detected	Max Volume Threshold	Decreased	Similar	Increased
1	*Fusarium* early	Control	1149	2	225(19.6%)	592(51.5%)	332(28.9%)
2	Control	*Fusarium* early	1455	2	316(21.7%)	682(46.9%)	457(31.4%)
3	*Fusarium* intermediate	Control	1578	2	253(16%)	824(52.2%)	501(31.7%)
4	Control	*Fusarium* intermediate	1533	2	350(22.8%)	641(41.8%)	542(35.4%)
5	*Fusarium* late	Control	1567	2	229(14.6%)	915(58.4%)	423(27%)
6	Control	*Fusarium* late	1525	2	242(51.9%)	792(51.9%)	491(32.2%)

DIA analysis was done as described in DeCyder software manual using default settings. Data for the threshold value of two alone is given. Dye swapping was performed to normalize variations in labeling.

Table 3. BVA analysis of the data.

S.No	Description	Control Vs Fusarium (early, intermediate & late) keratitis tears	Control Vs Fusarium early keratitis tears	Control Vs Fusarium intermediate keratitis tears	Control Vs Fusarium late keratitis tears	Fusarium early Vs intermediate keratitis tears	Fusarium early Vs late keratitis tears	Fusarium intermediate Vs late keratitis tears
(A)	Total no. of paired spots detected	1578	1578	1578	1578	1578	1578	1578
(B)	Among (A) differentially expressed spots >1.5 fold difference in spot volume average ratio	1009	858	1129	854	750	551	496
(C)	Among (B) spots with ANOVA ≤0.05	281	243	279	261	163	124	90
(D)	Among (C) manually confirmed true spots	140	132	140	133	68	60	30
(E)	Among (D) Total number up regulated spots	116	109	116	110	54	49	12
(F)	Among (E) total number of spots identified	11	18	23	22	20	25	4
(G)	Among (D) Total number down regulated spots	24	23	24	23	14	11	18
(H)	Among (G) total number of spots identified	14	14	14	14	1	0	2

proteins from 64 spots were identified. The details of the identified proteins are shown in Table S2. Among them ten proteins were found to have statistically significant variation in expression level. Cystatin SA III precursor (spot ID 10), lacrimal lipocalin precursor (spot ID 24) and lacritin precursor (spot ID 30) were down regulated, while alpha 1 antitrypsin (spot ID 63), apolipoprotein (spot ID 32), haptoglobin (spot ID 18 & 19), albumin (spot ID 58), zinc α 2 glycoprotein (ZAG) (spot ID 38), lactoferrin (spot ID 52), were up regulated in the keratitis tear compared to control tear (Table 4 & Figure 8).

Gene ontology annotation of differentially expressed proteins

In order to better understand the biological function of differentially expressed proteins, gene annotation was performed using DAVID [33] 6.7 (a database for annotation, visualization and integrated discovery). Selected proteins were classified into three categories of cellular component, molecular function, and biological process (Table S3). All the proteins that showed altered expression levels were extracellular proteins. Proteins that have enzyme inhibitor activity (two were upregulated and two were downregulated) were the most common proteins in the category of molecular function. In the biological process category defense response proteins were most common and all of them were upregulated (n = 4).

Differential regulation of tear proteins at different stages of infection

The patients with keratitis were classified as early, intermediate and late as described under materials and methods. Differential expression of the proteins were observed in all the three infective stages (Table 5) and progressive up regulation of the seven proteins was observed as the disease progressed towards late stages of infection. Expression of cystatin SA III precursor and lacrimal lipocalin precursor declined during the late stage of infection. Lacritin precursor level was reduced to negligible amounts in the early infective stage itself compared to control (Figure 5). DIGE analysis shows that haptoglobin β chain (spots 40 & 43; Figure 8) and α2 chains (spots 18, 19, & 20; Figure 8) were upregulated in infected tear samples. Further two isoforms of beta chain and all three isoforms of α2 chains could also be detected. However, based on database entry all these are classified as haptoglobin precursors by MS/MS search as was shown earlier [22].

Immunodetection of Lacritin, Lipocalin and Haptoglobin in Tear Fluid

Among the differentially regulated proteins, expression level of three proteins was confirmed using western blot analysis. 1D western blot analysis confirmed the reduction of lacritin and lipocalin levels and the increase of haptoglobin in tears from patients with *Fusarium* keratitis compared with control tears. The band volumes as determined using ImageQuantTL (GE Healthcare, Uppsala, Sweden) are shown in (Figure 9). 2D western analysis was performed to examine expression of isoforms. Western blot analysis confirmed that lacritin protein was totally absent in early stage of infection. Interestingly expression variation of lacritin and lipocalin isoforms in keratitis tears was also confirmed by western analysis (Figure 10). Upregulation of haptoglobin α and β chains in fungal keratitis tears was also confirmed using western blot analysis.

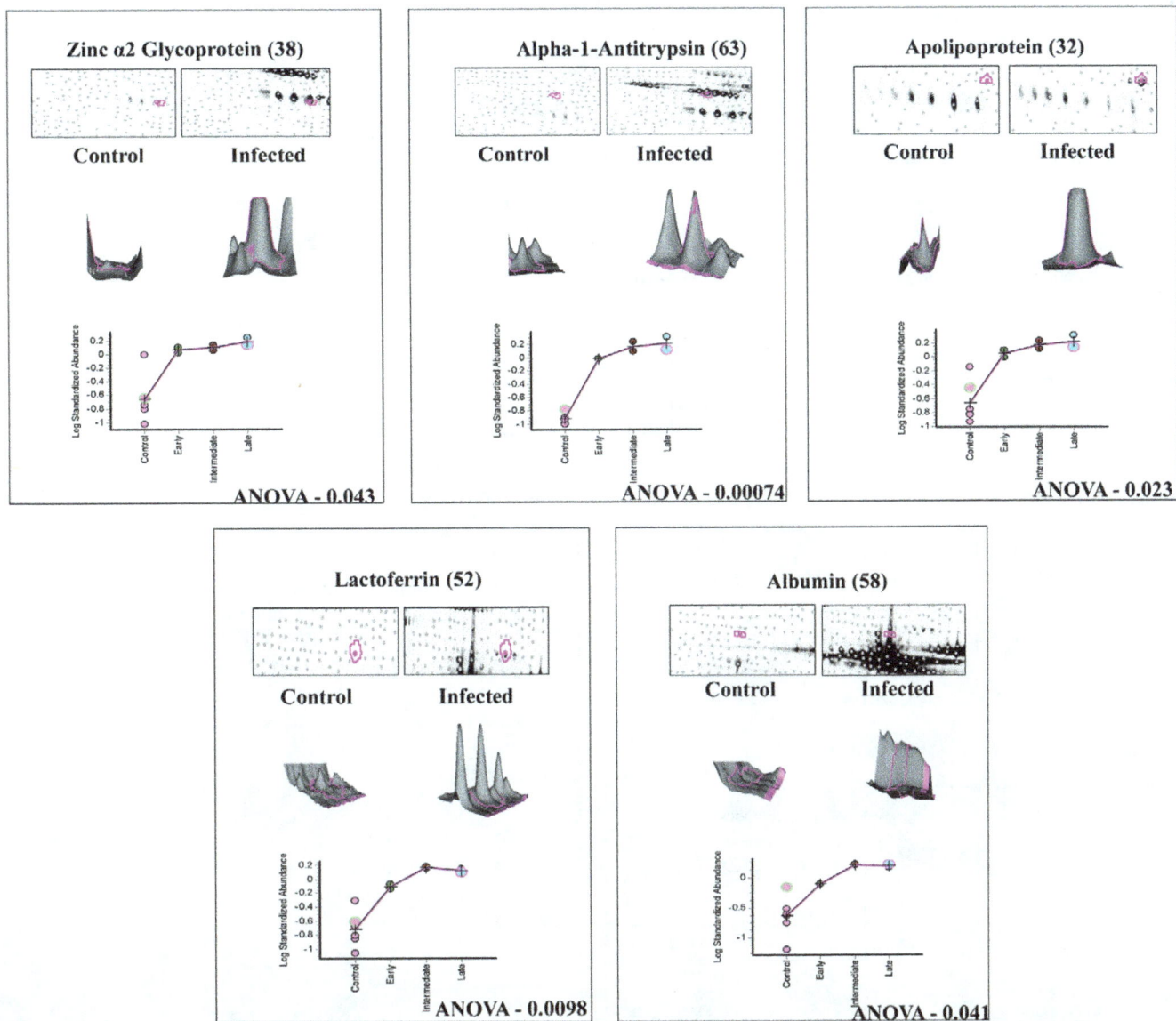

Figure 3. 3D and graphical representation of expression of up regulated proteins. Graphic views show the standardized log abundance of spot volume (y-axis) against the changes of proteins between the control and infected groups (x-axis) in all six gels. 3-D view of control and late stage infection sample spots is also shown.

Discussion

Tear proteins are derived from main and accessory lacrimal glands as well as proteins locally produced by corneal and conjunctival epithelial cells. Therefore tear is a useful sample to examine the expression of proteins in corneal infection.

One of the key steps that need careful attention in the tear proteomics is the method of collecting the tear. A recent study finds that there is no significant difference in the protein concentration in tears collected by capillary and schirmer collections, which are representatives of the reflex tear [34]. On loading the same amount of tear protein from normal and healthy control subjects, SDS PAGE reflected no significant change in the proteins as seen by the densitometry analysis. Most of the studies have used the capillary tear sample for the 2-D and MS analysis [35,15–16,28]. Capillary tear collection has been used for the 2-DE in disease conditions such as diabetic [20] and blepharitis

patients [19]. Since the tear secretion is profusing, the capillary collection has been used in pathological conditions like infectious keratitis.

Another study [36] aimed to compare methods of tear film collection (i.e., capillary collection versus Schirmer collection). There were 84 proteins identified from protein associated with the Schirmer method and 43 identified from the capillary method. Only 30 total proteins identified overlapped between the two collection methods. The study proposes that this difference arises through the Schirmer strip's interaction with the epithelium of the ocular surface (whereas the capillary method does not). To help examine this hypothesis, analysis of the various classifications/ functions of the proteins identified were grouped based on their general function as follows transport, metabolism, immune response, structure, antioxidation, protease inhibitors, unclassified, cell signaling, and protein folding. There are several cellular proteins (i.e., not secreted) observed from the Schirmer method

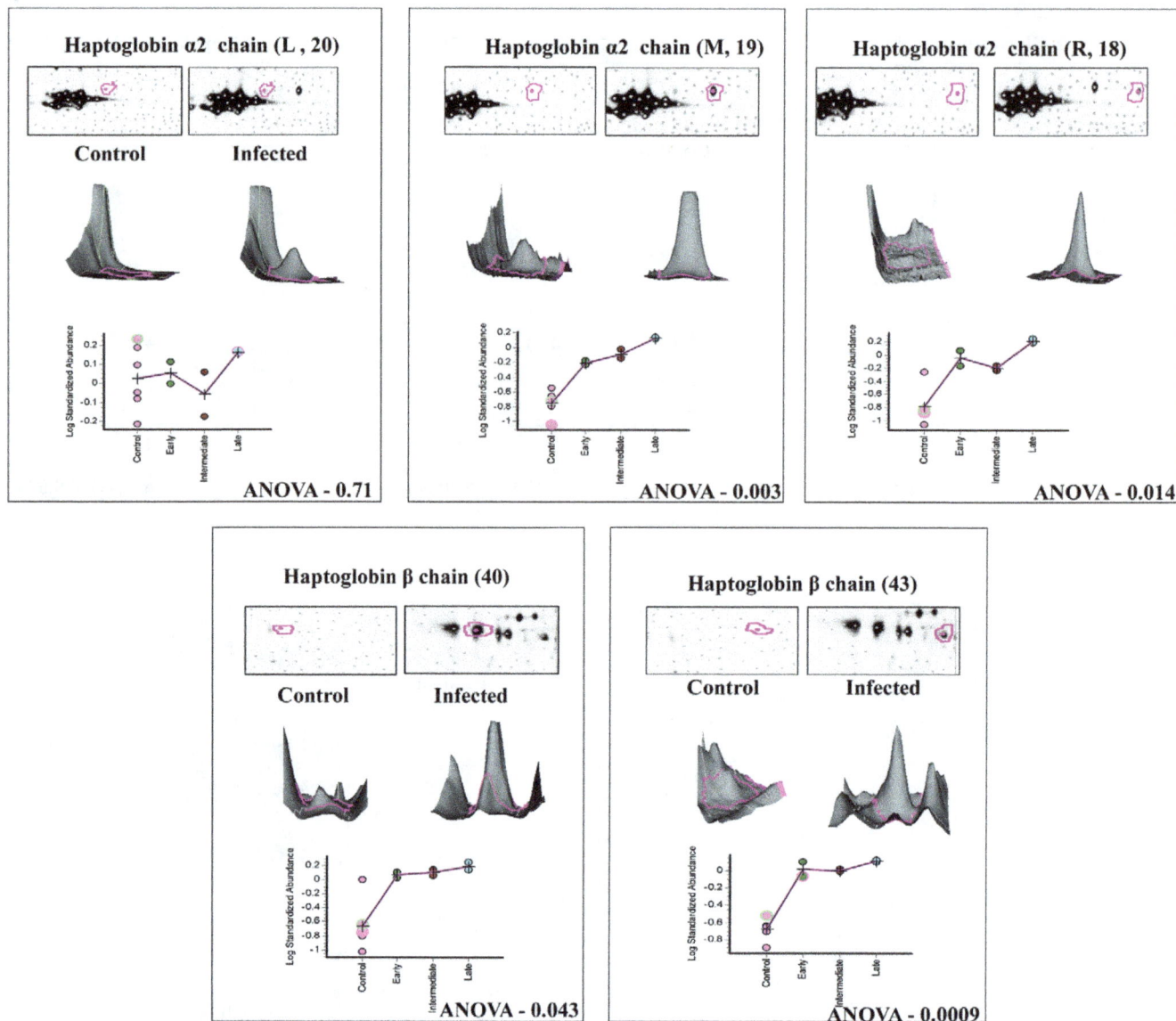

Figure 4. 3D and graphical representation of expression of Haptoglobin α2 & β chain. Graphic views show the standardized log abundance of spot volume (y-axis) against the changes of proteins between the control and infected groups (x-axis) in all six gels. 3-D view of control and late stage infection sample spots is also shown.

that were not found in tear film collected by capillary such as the S100 calcium binding series of proteins. Interestingly, serum albumin was detected at much higher levels in the tears collected using the Schirmer collection method.

Four fold decrease of lacrimal lipocalin precursor was observed in the tears of patients with fungal keratitis. Lipocalin-1, is a major tear protein secreted by lacrimal glands and acts as the principal lipid binding protein and is involved in the general protection of epithelial cell surfaces. Tear lipocalin protein level in human tears ranges between 0.5 and 1.5 g/l, making up 10%–20% of the total tear protein content in tears and is considered tear-specific [37,38]. Tissue specificity and concentration reflects the importance of lipocalin in the protection of the ocular surface [39]. Based on their possible role in lipid transport [40] lipocalin were called as tear-specific prealbumin [41].

Cystatins are cysteine proteinase inhibitors belonging to the cystatin superfamily. The role of cystatins as proteinase inhibitors

is well established. The balance between proteases secreted by the pathogen and protease inhibitor is believed to play a significant role in maintaining the normal ocular surface condition [42]. Human salivary cystatins are represented as Cystatin S. It contains three molecular species (cystatin S, cystatin SN and cystatin SA), which have distinct amino-acid sequences. Cystatin S binds cysteine proteases and inhibit their activity, thereby preventing uncontrolled proteolysis and tissue damages [43–46]. Cystatin S precursor was shown to be upregulated in healthy female tears compared to healthy male tears [47]. In tears of patients with blepharitis, significantly lower levels of cystatins SA have been reported [19]. The three fold reduction of cystatins in the tears of patients with fungal keratitis correlates well with their functional role. Cysteine protease inhibitors are reduced in several pathological conditions [48].

Ten fold reduction in the level of lacritin in the infected group compared to control may have relevance to resistance to fungal

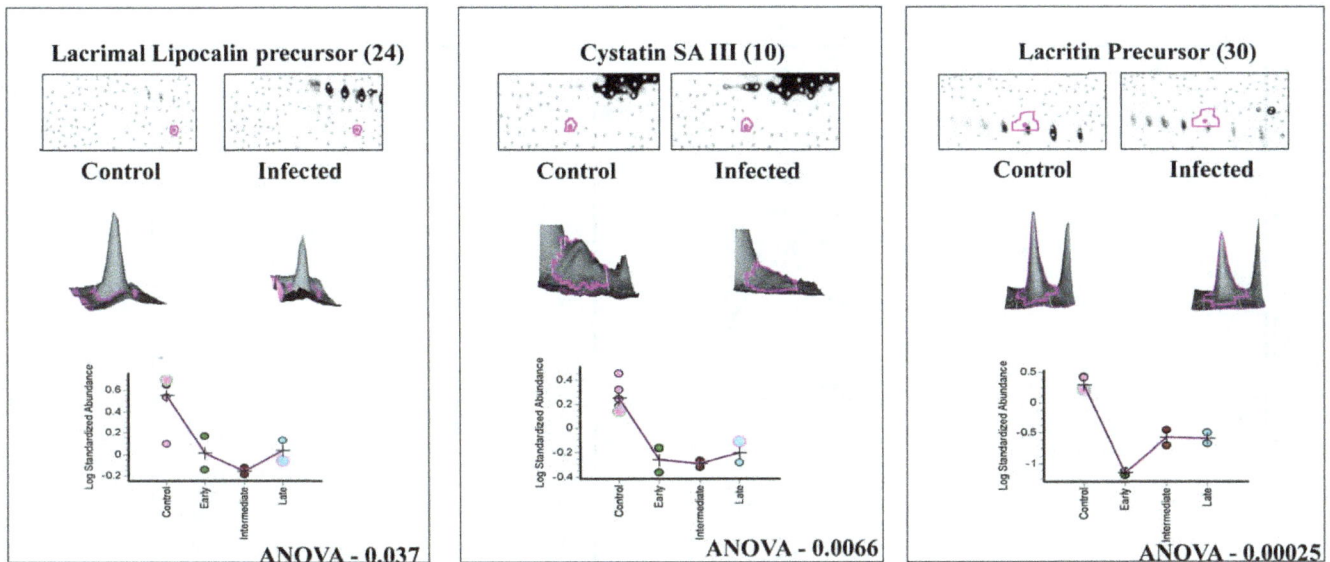

Figure 5. 3D and graphical representation of expression of down regulated proteins. Graphic views show the standardized log abundance of spot volume (y-axis) against the changes of proteins between the control and infected groups (x-axis) in all six gels. 3-D view of control and late stage infection sample spots is also shown.

infection. Lacritin is a glycoprotein found in the tears that is primarily produced by the lacrimal gland, but has also been shown to be produced by the meibomian glands, corneal and conjunctival epithelia. The protein is an extracellular growth factor thought to be associated with cell proliferation as a secretory mitogen [49,50]. It is a new lacrimal functional unit specific growth factor in human tears and flows through the ducts to target corneal epithelial cells on the ocular surface. This protein enhances unstimulated secretion and rapid tyrosine phosphorylation in lacrimal acinar cells, and it also stimulates corneal epithelial cell calcium signaling. Therefore, lacritin may play a key role in the function of the lacrimal gland-corneal axis and its deficiency could lead to cause some alterations in the defense mechanism. Lacritin might be important for tear secretion and maintaining normal tear conditions. Lacritin has been shown to be decreased in conditions altering tear film such as blepharitis [19] and dry eye, indicating the crucial role of this protein in infection and other conditions [34,51–52]. Reductions in the level of lipocalin precursor and lacritin have direct effect in the pathogenesis and susceptibility of host corneal tissue. Inhibition of the protease inhibitor cystatins may lead to better survival of the pathogen.

Alpha-1 antitrypsin is an enzyme that controls the activity of diverse proteolytic enzymes such as trypsin, chymotrypsin, collagenase, thrombin, fibrinolysin, granulocytic proteases and caseins by cleaving their catalytic sites [53]. This protein is found in a number of body fluids such as tears, perilymph, lymph, saliva, colostrum, breast milk, duodenal fluid, gallbladder bile, synovial fluid, cervical mucus, semen and amniotic fluid [54–57] and plays an important role in both physiological and pathological condition by inactivating enzymes activated by bacteria or other agents. This protein also regulates [58] the immune response by inhibiting the transformation and migration of lymphocytes. The increased level of tear alpha-1 antitrypsin in corneal ulcer and other diseases have been reported [59,60]. It has been shown that tear alpha-1 antitrypsin levels may increase in inflamed eyes in the absence of corneal involvement, for example, in cases of rosacea keratitis and allergic conjunctivitis [61,62]. All these studies imply that alpha-1-antitrypsin might be an acute-phase reactant [63]. In fungal

keratitis, the increase in alpha-1-antitrypsin could be due to the inflammation induced by the pathogen or a specific pathogen component may be involved.

Haptoglobin (Hp) is a plasma glycoprotein, the main biological function of which is to bind free hemoglobin (Hb). It is also a positive acute-phase protein with immunomodulatory properties [64–66]. Increase in tear haptoglobin alpha levels has been shown in conjunctivitis [65]. In our study haptoglobin β chain isoforms and α2 chain isoforms were upregulated in infected tear samples but not in control tear. The fungal infection presumably leads to the increased synthesis and export into tear samples. Since both α & β forms are found, it is interesting to examine whether functional α2β complexes are formed in the tear.

Zinc α2-glycoprotein (ZAG) is a 40-kDa single-chain polypeptide, which is secreted in various body fluids such as plasma, saliva, and tears [67]. It stimulates lipid breakdown in adipocytes [68] and is associated with the extreme weight loss that occurs in some cancers [69]. ZAG is shown to be increased in patients with Graves's ophthalmopathy [70]. The exact function of ZAG in tears and its possible role in lipid degradation are not demonstrated [70]. In our study, we detected significant upregulation of ZAG in keratitis patients, implying the alteration in the lipidome profile of tear in infection.

Apolipoproteins are proteins that bind to lipids (oil-soluble substances such as fat and cholesterol) to form lipoproteins, which transport the lipids through the lymphatic and circulatory systems. Apolipoproteins also serve as enzyme cofactors, receptor ligands and lipid transfer carriers that regulate the metabolism of lipoproteins and their uptake in tissues. Increased secretion of native apo A-I from the main lacrimal gland in patients with advanced diabetic retinopathy has been reported [71]. Apolipoprotein level was increased fivefold in all the three stages of fungal keratitis tears compared to control tears.

The mean albumin level in serum was reported as 44.7 mg/ml in the healthy individuals from India [72]. Albumin levels in tear fluids were reported to be 11.5 mg/l in healthy males and 12.7 mg/l in healthy females from Indian population [60]. In cases of allergic conjunctivitis tear levels of serum albumin reach

Proteins (Score Plot)   Spot Maps (Loading Plot)

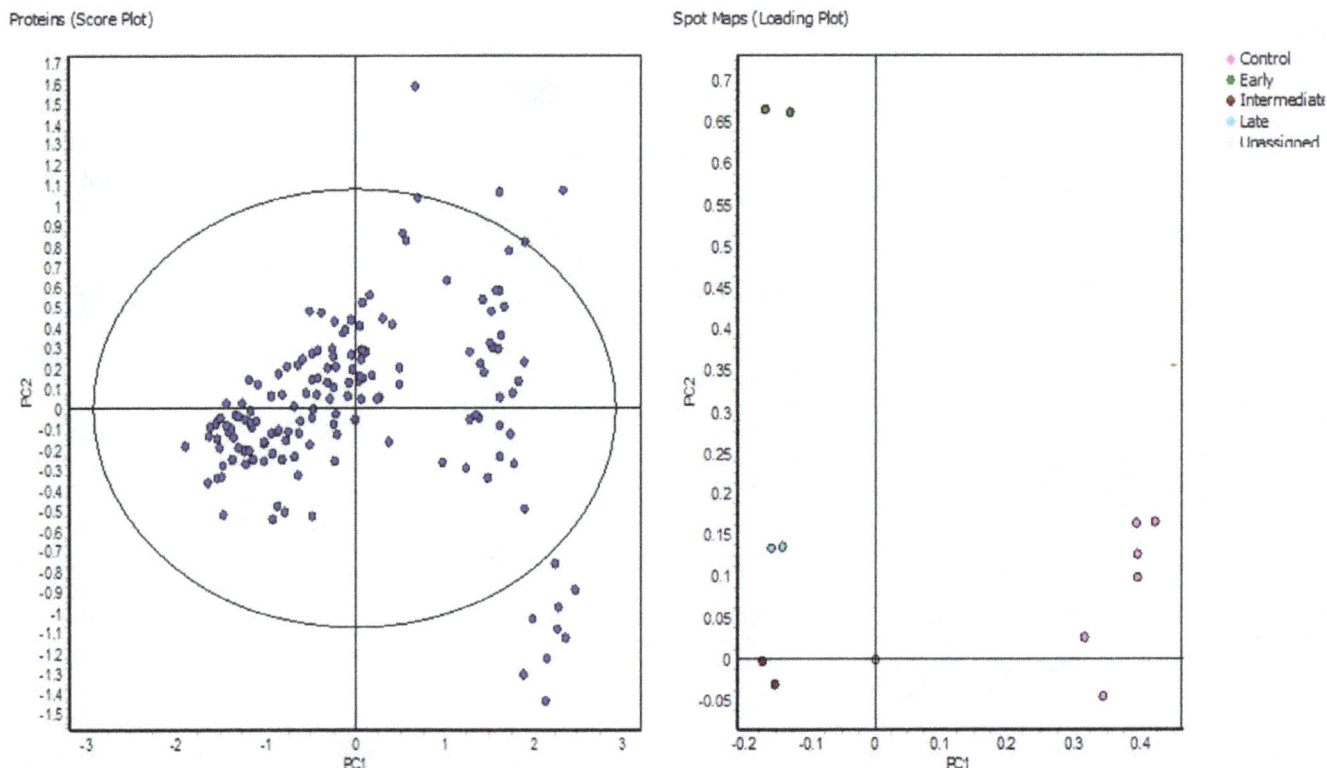

Figure 6. Clustering analysis of fusarium infected tear samples. Principal component analysis (PCA) has been performed across different experimental groups. A subset of those proteins whose expression varied within the 95th confidence level (ANOVA; $p < 0.01$) was created. In this analysis the default settings of the software were used.

serum levels rapidly, indicating a direct leak from inflamed vessels. The albumin content of tears also increases in cases of corneal ulceration [59]. Our earlier report [15] and our present results show albumin upregulation in keratitis tear sample indicating that during fungal infection there might be a leakage of this protein from inflamed vessels.

Tear lactoferrin (formerly known as lactotransferrin) is an 82 kDa protein produced by the acinar cells of the lacrimal gland. Lactoferrin is present in normal tears of humans and its level was found to be invariant through age. Lactoferrin is a glycoprotein, and a member of the transferrin family, belong to those proteins capable of binding and transferring Fe_{3+} ions [73]. Due to the increase in its concentration during most inflammatory reactions and some viral infections, several reports classify lactoferrin as an acute-phase protein [74]. Its concentration increases in all biological fluids, but the highest levels have been detected in the nidus of inflammation [75]. Lactoferrin has a wide variety of biological functions, many of which do not appear to be connected with its iron binding ability [76]. Its role in fungal infection is not clear as of now.

Functional Implication of Differentially Expressed Tear Proteins at different infective stages

As the infective stage progressed seven acute phase proteins were upregulated. Interestingly 2D western analysis reveals lipocalin and lacritin isoforms are at a negligible level in the early stage of fungal infection, but their level increase marginally during intermediate stage. This increase could be due to the fungal elaboration and the induction of inflammatory response. Taken

together these observations imply that the treatment options needs to be tailored based on the stage of infection.

2D-DIGE analysis of tears from fungal keratitis patients allowed the confident quantification of several differentially expressed proteins in comparison to normal tears. Fungal infection of cornea clearly induce increased expression of alpha 1 antitrypsin, apolipoprotein, haptoglobin, albumin, zinc α 2 glycoprotein (ZAG), lactoferrin, haptoglobin precursor, proteins related to inflammatory events. Expression of proteins related to host immune response such as cystatin SA III potential precursor, lacrimal lipocalin precursor, lacritin precursor is reduced in infection. Quantitation of lacritin levels showed that this protein is down regulated significantly in fungal keratitis when compared to bacterial keratitis tears (data not shown). This information and other results (unpublished) show that the changes reported in this paper are specific to fungal keratitis.

Additional studies focusing on the functional properties of these proteins in the pathogenesis of fungal keratitis may contribute to a better understanding of the disease. In addition these proteins form putative candidate biomarkers that could aid in the diagnosis, prognosis and treatment of fungal keratitis.

Materials and Methods

Tear Samples

Written Informed consents were obtained from study subjects and the study was approved by the Institutional Review Board of Aravind Medical Research Foundation (Madurai, India). The Declaration of Helsinki was adhered to when enrolling subjects. Reflex tear samples (100–150 µl) were collected from the keratitis eye of culture positive (*Fusarium*) patients who were categorized

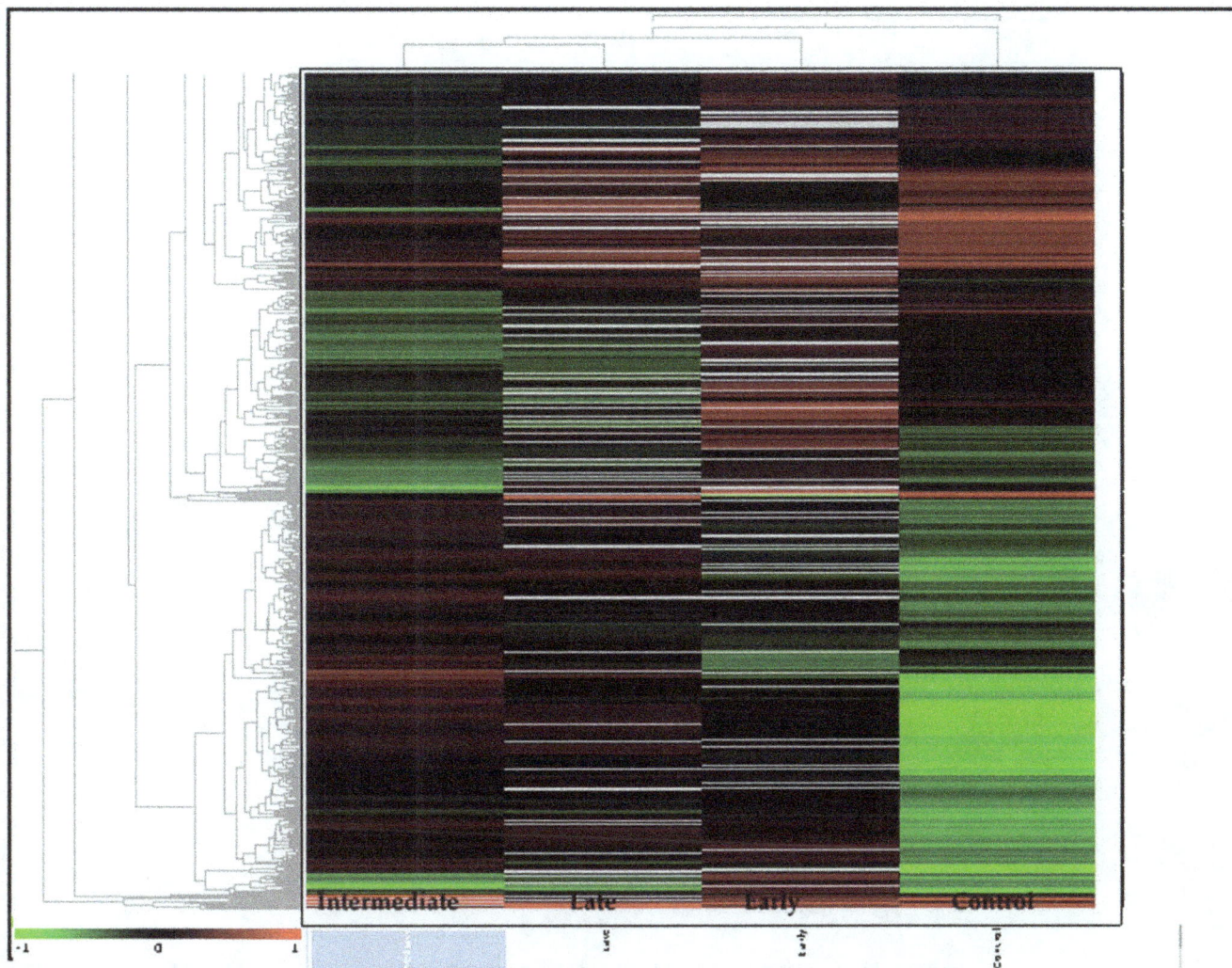

Figure 7. Unsupervised hierarchical of the expressed proteins. Log-transformed normalized protein spot volumes were used to perform unsupervised hierarchical cluster analysis. Green indicates decreased expression; red indicates increased expression. Patient groups; control and fusarium infected (Early, Intermediate and Late).

based on the duration of the infection as early (within 7 days), intermediate (7–14 days) and late (after 14 days) stage of infection. Tears from healthy individuals (whose corneas were clear and devoid of any infection & inflammation) served as controls (60–80 µl). All the tear samples were obtained from male individuals with the age range from 20–60 yrs. The total number of tear samples collected for each category of presentation is as follows, early −35 ; intermediate − 20 ; late − 11. Among them five samples from each category were included for this study. Tear samples were collected using 10 µl-capillary tubes without touching the eye globe or the lid. The samples were centrifuged at 7800× g for 10 min at 4°C to remove cellular debris and stored in liquid nitrogen until analysis. Samples were collected from patients before treatment. Protein concentration was estimated using Bradford's method [77]. Samples used in this study were described in table S4.

Two-dimensional difference gel electrophoresis

Sample preparation. Tears samples from *Fusarium* keratitis patients were pooled (250 µg of protein per patient). Three pools each were made from early, intermediate and late stage infection samples. Each pool was made from tear from five patients. Tear

samples from 20 healthy individuals were pooled and used as control samples (100 µg of protein per healthy individual). Pooled tear samples were concentrated using 3 kDa Amicon Ultra centrifugal device (MILLIPORE, County Cork, Ireland) as per manufactures instructions with minor modifications. Briefly, tear sample (2000–2500 µg) was diluted to 600 µl with MilliQ water and placed into a 3 kDa Amicon Ultra centrifugal device and centrifuged at 13,000× g for 10 min; under these conditions the volume of the concentrate was reduced to 100 µl. An additional 500 µl of MilliQ water was added and the mixture was centrifuged as above.

Proteins Labeling with CyDyes

Lysine labeling protocol, (minimal labeling) was used in this study. Each dye (2 nmol) was reconstituted with 5 µL anhydrous *N,N*-dimethylformamide (Sigma Aldrich chemical co.) and 400 pmol/µl stock dye was stored at −20°C. The stock dye was further diluted to 100 pmol/µl and this working dye solution was used immediately. The processed tear proteins were then labeled individually with dyes Cy3 and Cy5 while the pooled tear proteins prepared by mixing equal aliquot of protein from all samples in an experimental set up were labeled with Cy2 and was used as

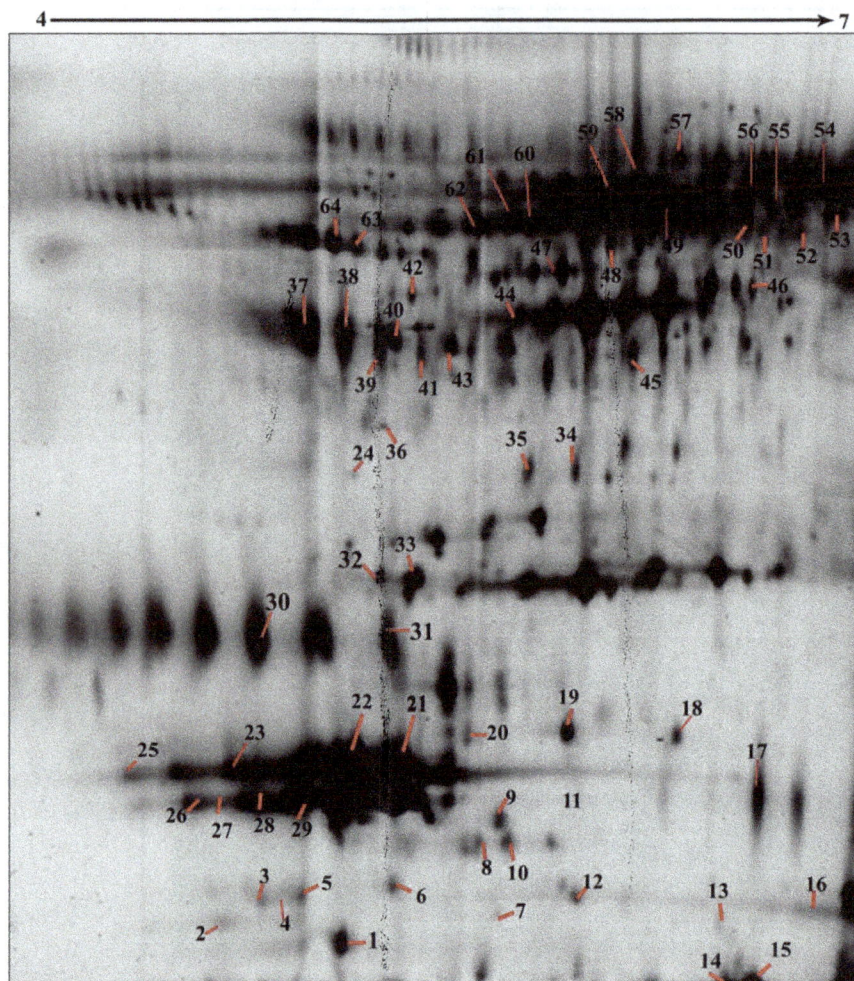

Figure 8. Tear protein profile showing the annotations of the identified tear proteins. 2D DIGE gel contained 30 μg of Cy2 labeled internal standard as described in Table 1 was separated by a pH 4–7 IPG strip in the first dimension and 12.5% polyacrylamide gel in the second dimension electrophoresis. Image was captured using a Typhoon Trio Variable Mode Imager.

internal standard. A 30 μg portion of each group was mixed with 2.5 μL of dye and incubated on ice for 30 min in the dark. In the case of Cy2 labeling, total mix was labeled and 30 μg aliquot was used in each gel. The labeling reactions were quenched with 2 μL of 10 mM lysine and incubation was continued on ice for 10 min. Cy3 & Cy5 labeled samples were mixed with the Cy2-labeled samples, and an equal volume of lysis buffer containing 100 mM DTT and 2% (v/v) IPG buffer was added and incubated at room temperature for 10 min. The final volume for all preparations was adjusted to a total of 340 μL with rehydration buffer (7 M urea, 2 M thiourea, 1% IPG buffer, 50 mM DTT, 4% CHAPS, and a trace amount of bromophenol blue). A reciprocal labeling experiment was also performed. The labeling protocols for the 2D DIGE experiments are shown in Table 1.

Two dimensional gel electrophoresis

Two dimensional gel electrophoresis of Cy dye labeled proteins was done as described already [78] with the following modifications. Eighteen cm IPG strips of pH 4–7 (GE Healthcare, Uppsala, Sweden) were employed in the first dimension. Labeled proteins were focused for a total of 80,000 Vhs at a constant temperature (20°C) under linear voltage ramp after an active IPG rehydration at 30 V in a IPGPhor III (GE Healthcare, Uppsala,

Sweden) apparatus with following IEF conditions 500 V step-n-hold for 1 h, 1000 V gradient for 1 h, 8000 V gradient for 3 h and 8000 V step-n-hold for 8 h. Following IEF, each IPG strip was placed in the equilibration buffer containing 2% DTT first followed by incubation in another buffer in which the DTT was replaced by 2.5% iodoacetamide. The second dimension PAGE (12.5%) was carried out in an Ettan DaltSix systems (GE Healthcare, Uppsala, Sweden) at 1 W/gel for 1 hr and 13 W/gel for 5 hr. All experimental procedures were performed in dim light or in the dark.

Protein Visualisation and DeCyder image analysis

After second dimension electrophoresis, the gels were scanned with Typhoon TRIO Variable Mode Imager (GE Healthcare, Uppsala, Sweden). All laser power adjustments and image acquisition were done using default settings of the Typhoon Scanner Control program. Cy2, Cy3 & Cy5 images were captured using the settings recommended by the manufacturer. The scanned gels were saved as modified 16-bit.gel format which gave good gray-scale representation covering the dynamic range of protein spots. Prior to analysis, all gel images were cropped to identical size in ImageLoader module of DeCyder version 7.0 (GE Healthcare, Uppsala, Sweden) and then transferred to the

Table 4. Identified tear proteins and their function.

Spot ID	Identified Tear proteins	Database/ Accession no.	Mowse score[a]	X & Y coordinate in DIGE gel	Mr/pI 2-D[b]	Mr/pI data base[c]	Peptides Matched[d]	Sequence Coverage (%)[e]	Function
10	cystatin SA-III = potential precursor of acquired enamel pellicle [human, Peptide, 121 aa]	NCBI/gi|235948	182(38)	484,835	16/5.4	14.1/4.7	R.IIPGGIYDADLNDEWVQR.A R.RPLQVLR.A K.SQPNLDTCAFHEQPELQK.K K.SQPNLDTCAFHEQPELQK.K	35	Cysteine protease inhibitor
19	Haptoglobin OS = Homo sapiens GN = HP PE = 1 SV = 1- α2 chain (M)	Swissprot/ HPT_HUMAN	212 (35)	555,724	20/5.9	45.8/6.1	K.NYYKLR.T K.LRTEGDGVYTLNNEK.Q R.TEGDGVYTLNNEK.Q R.TEGDGVYTLNNEKQWINK.A	6	Haeme binding protein
24	Lacrimal lipocalin precursor	MSDB/LCHUL	112 (36)	174,733	19/4.4	19.2/5.39	K.NNLEALEDFEK.A R.GLSTESILIPR.Q	12	Lipid scavenging and transport to outer tear layer
30	Lacritin Precursor	NCBI/gi|15187164	62 (38)	244,622	26/4.8	14.2/5.43	K.SILLTEQALAK.A K.KFSLLKPWA	14	Secretion, renewal of lacrimal & ocular surface epithelia
32	Pro Apolipoprotein	NCBI/gi|178775	204 (27)	367,575	30/5.2	28.9/5.45	K.LLDNWDSVTSTFSK.L R.THLAPYSDELRQR.L K.ATEHLSTLSEK.A K.AKPALEDLR.Q	18	Lipid profile regulator
38	Zn-alpha2-glycoprotein [Homo sapiens]	NCBI/gi|38026	607 (36)	293,317	51/4.8	34.7/5.71	R.YSLTYIYTGLSK.H K.SQPMGLWR.Q R.QVEGMEDWK.Q R.QVEGMEDWKQDSQLQK.A K.AREDIFMETLK.D R.EDIFMETLK.D K.YYYDGKDYIEFNK.E K.QKWEAEPVYVQR.A K.WEAEPVYVQR.A K.AYLEEECPATLR.K K.AYLEEECPATLRK.Y R.QDPPSVVVTSHQAPGEK.K K.CLAYDFYPGK.I	37	Stimulates lipid degradation
40	Haptoglobin precursor – β chain	NCBI/gi|306882	182(35)	379,336	39/5.6	45.1/6.24	R.ILGGHLDAK.G K.GSFPWQAK.M K.DIAPTLTLYVGK.K K.QLVEIEK.V R.VGYVSGWGR.N K.FTDHLK.Y K.VTSIQDWVQK.T	15	Haeme binding protein
52	Lactoferrin	NCBI/gi|2104522	222 (38)	800,269	50/7	53.6/7.09	K.CGLVPVLAENYK.S R.SDTSLTWNSVK.G R.CLAENAGDVAFVK.D	9	Antimicrobial activity
58	Serum albumin, chain A	MSDB/1AO6A	639 (36)	550,131	66/5.1	65.6/5.63	R.FKDLGEENFK.A K.LVNEVTEFAK.T K.KYLYEIAR.R18 K.YLYEIAR.R K.VHTECCHGDLLECADDR.A K.VHTECCHGDLLECADDRADLAK.Y K.QNCELFEQLGEYK.F K.FQNALLVR.Y K.KVPQVSTPTLVEVSR.N K.VPQVSTPTLVEVSR.N K.QTALVELVK.H K.AVMDDFAAFVEK.C	9	Regulation of the colloidal osmotic pressure of blood
63	Alpha-1-antitrypsin	Swissprot/ A1AT_HUMAN	76 (28)	269,210	45/5.2	46.8/5.3	K.TDTSHHDQDHPTFNK.I K.IVDLVK.E K.FLENEDRR.S K.LSITGTYDLK.S	9	Inhibitor of serine proteases

[a]MOWSE scores greater than the values given in the parenthesis are considered to be significant ($p<0.05$). All proteins were also searched across multiple databases to confirm their identity.
[b]Apparent/experimental molecular weight and pI of protein spot on 2-DE gels.
[c]Theoretical molecular weight and pI of the identified protein in database.
[d]Represents the peptides matched.
[e]Sequence coverage (SC) represents the % aminoacid sequence covered in the protein by the matched peptides. 18R, 19M and 20L of α2 isoforms are labeled according to Gupta[22] et al., 2007.

Table 5. Differentially Expressed Proteins in Tears of keratitis patients.

Spot.ID	Protein Name	Gene ID	Pattern of regulation	Fold Variation	One way ANOVA p value	T – test p value
63	Alpha-1-antitrypsin	SERPINA1	Up regulation	12.04	0.00074	2.8e-005
19	Haptoglobin α2 chain (M)	HP	Up regulation	4.93	0.0030	0.00050
38	Zinc-alpha-2-glycoprotein	AZGP1	Up regulation	4.37	0.043	0.0032
32	Apolipoprotein	APOA2	Up regulation	5.19	0.023	0.0014
58	Albumin	ALB	Up regulation	4.56	0.041	0.0059
40	Haptoglobin precursor - β chain	HP	Up regulation	10.96	0.0053	0.00024
52	Lactoferrin	LTF	Up regulation	5.35	0.0098	0.00088
24	Lacrimal lipocalin precursor	LCN1	Down regulation	−4.04	0.037	0.0038
10	Cystatin SA III Precursor	CST4	Down regulation	−3.22	0.0066	0.00029
30	Lacritin Precursor	LACRT	Down regulation	−9.64	0.00025	0.00036

DeCyder Differential Analysis Software,version 7.0. The standardized spot volume (the sum of pixel values within a detected spot boundary) was calculated as the ratio between the absolute volume of the individual spot and the total volume of all spots in the gel. The internal standard (Cy2) on each gel intrinsically linked all gel images (Cy3 and Cy5) within the same gels and across all the gels in the specific set of an experiment. A DeCyder differential in-gel analysis (DIA) module was used for image analysis between samples within the same gel while a DeCyder biological variation analysis (BVA) module was performed for pairwise image analysis among multiple gels. Ratios of differentially expressed proteins were shown as "fold" changes between the spots of keratitis tears and the control tears. An increase of protein abundance in the keratitis tear was expressed as a positive value while a negative value denoted a decrease in the protein abundance. Protein spot

has been normalized using the corresponding spot on the pooled internal standard on every gel. Student's t-test and ANOVA were used to compare the average spot volume and differences of protein abundance for all detectable spots between the keratitis and control groups. Reciprocal dye labeling was performed to normalize bias in labeling.

Protein Identification and Mass Spectrometry

Pooled proteins (300 μg) from control tear group were separated on 18 cm IPG strips of pH 4–7 in the first dimension. First and second dimension electrophoresis were done as given under 2D DIGE method. The second dimension gels were stained with colloidal coomassie blue G-250 [79] and gel spots from this preparative gel were excised manually for in-gel trypsin digestion [15], and LC-MS/MS was performed. The resulting peptides were

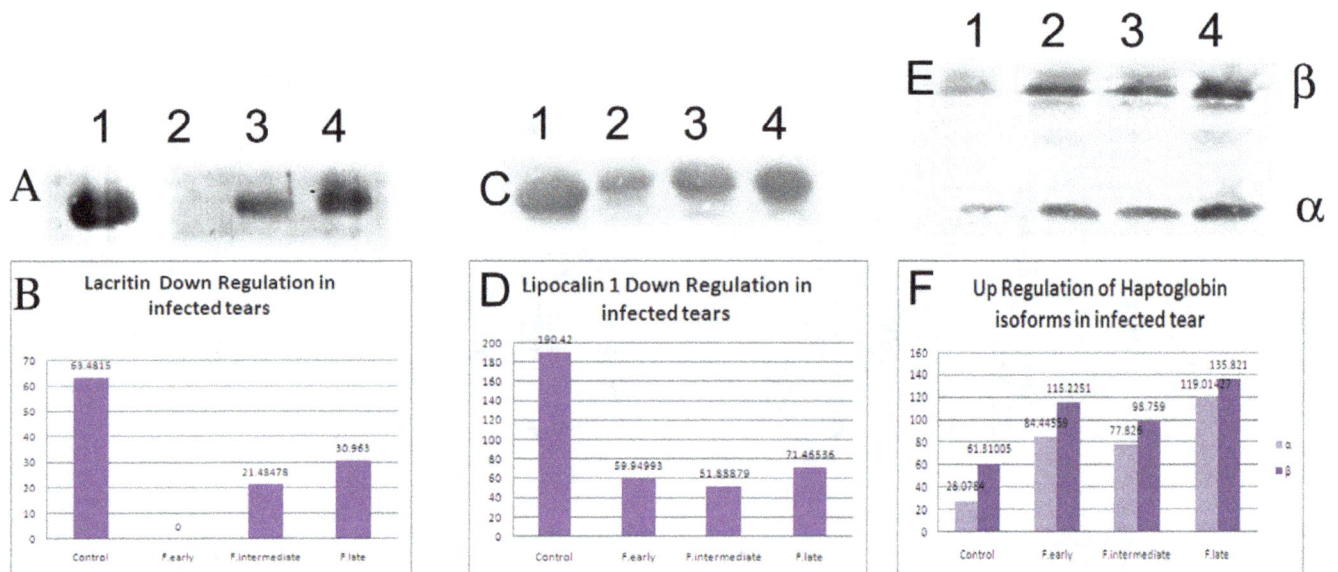

Figure 9. 1-DE Immunoblot of keratitis patients tear proteins separated on 1D PAGE; control subject (1) and tears of fusarium keratitis early stage (2), intermediate stage (3) and late stage (4) patients. Forty μg tear proteins were separated on 13.5% SDS PAGE. Tear proteins were transferred to nitrocellulose membranes for subsequent immunodetection with appropriate primary antibody. Secondary antibody used was HRP labeled and the images were scanned using a Typhoon Trio scanner as described under materials and methods. B, D and F are histograms showing the spot intensities.

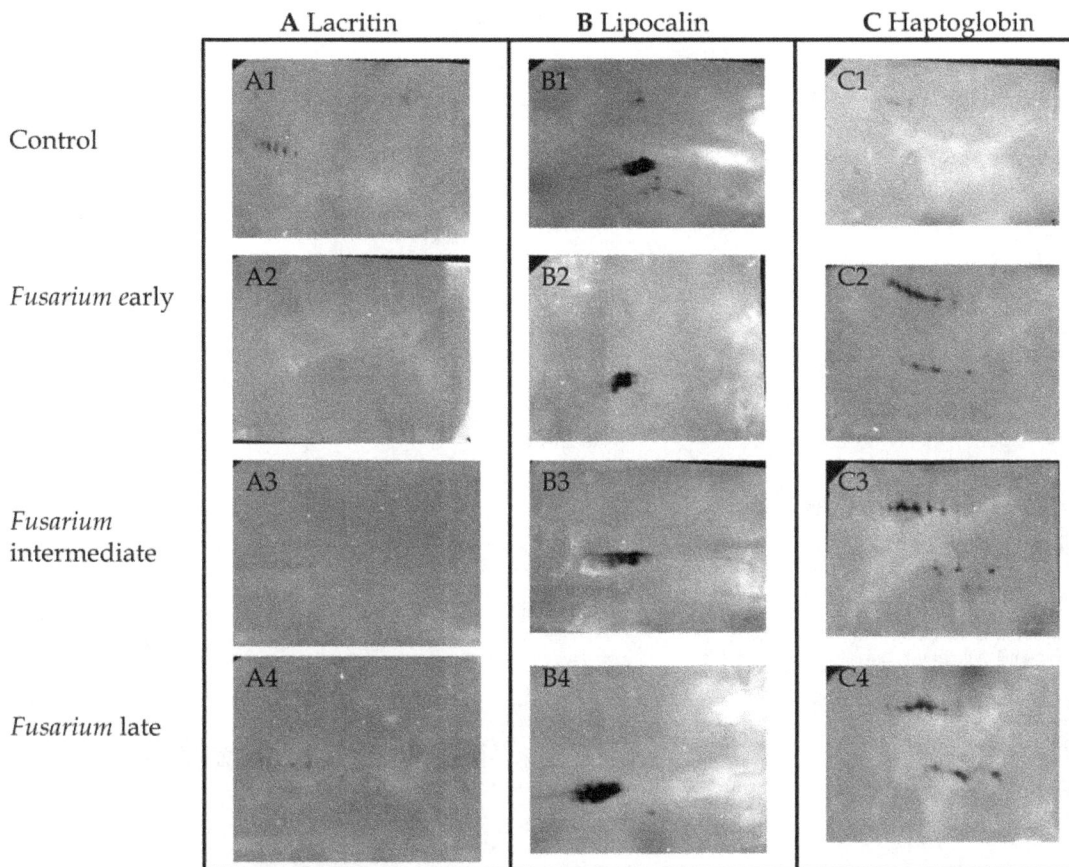

Figure 10. Immunoblot of tear proteins from control & keratitis patients separated on 2D PAGE. For 2-DE western blotting, 40 μg tear proteins was separated on pH 4–7 strip (7 cm), followed by second dimension separation on a 13.5% polyacrylamide gel. Tear proteins were transferred to nitrocellulose membranes for subsequent immunodetection with appropriate primary antibodies as described already.

separated by an electrospray ionisation (ESI) quadrupole time-of-flight (Q-TOF) Bruker MicrOTOF Q (Bruker Daltonics) coupled with a nano liquid chromatography system (Ultimate 3000, Dionex, Hongkong). After data acquisition, the generated XML files were used to perform database searches using the MASCOT software v. 2.2 (Matrix Science, London, UK) using the following parameters: peptide tolerance, 0.2 Da; MS/MS ion mass tolerance, 0.1 Da; one missed cleavage; variable modifications used were methionine oxidation and cysteine carboxyamidomethylation.

Gene Ontology by DAVID software

Analysis of functional enrichment of differentially regulated proteins was performed in DAVID 6.7 software [34] http://david.abcc.ncifcrf.gov/ according to the standard protocol [80]. The combined list of official gene symbols corresponding to the identified proteins was used for input.

1-D and 2-D Western Blot Analysis

Proteins (40 μg) were resolved either by SDS-PAGE or 2-DE and transferred onto a nitrocellulose membrane (GE Healthcare, Uppsala, Sweden) by semidry blotting using a Trans-Blot SD Semi-Dry Electrophoretic Transfer Cell (Bio-Rad Laboratories). Membrane was presoaked and equilibrated in Towbin transfer buffer [25 mM Tris, 192 mM glycine (20% methanol)]. Nonspecific binding was blocked with 5% skim milk in phosphate buffered saline (PBS). Primary antibodies used for immunodetection were given in Figure legends. They were obtained from the following

sources Dako Denmark A/S, Denmark; Santa Cruz,USA; kindly provided by Robert McKown, James Madison University and Gordon Laurie, University of Virginia.

Immunodetection was performed by incubating the membranes in antibody solutions; The list of antibodies used include the following- Polyclonal rabbit anti-human haptoglobin (Dako Denmark A/S, Denmark), polyclonal rabbit anti lipocalin 1 (Santa Cruz,USA) and polyclonal rabbit anti lacritin (kindly provided by Robert McKown, James Madison University and Gordon Laurie, University of Virginia). The antibodies were diluted in 1% BSA prepared in Tween PBS (TPBS) and used for incubation with the membrane at RT for 2 h. After three washes with 0.5% TPBS, the membrane was exposed to secondary antibody conjugated with horseradish peroxidase Goat anti Rabbit Ig G (Jackson ImmunoResearch Laboratories, USA) diluted 1:2000 in 0.5% TPBS for one hour at RT. The membranes were then incubated with 4Chloro-Naphthol substrate for 30 minutes. The membranes were rinsed with water thrice and documented using Typhoon Trio variable mode scanner (with TAMRA, Alexaflour 546) (GE Healthcare, Uppsala, Sweden) and Image analysis was done using ImageQuantTL software (GE Healthcare, Uppsala, Sweden) was used for image analysis.

Supporting Information

Table S1 Differentially Expressed Proteins in Tears of keratitis patients.

Table S2 Identified Tear proteins and their functions.

Table S3 Classification of differentially regulated proteins according to biological process, cellular & molecular.

Table S4 Tear sample details used in this study.

Acknowledgments

We thank T. Parameswari & G. Reka for sample collection & lab assistance.

Author Contributions

Conceived and designed the experiments: SA NVP PL KD. Performed the experiments: SA MV. Analyzed the data: SA NVP PL KD. Wrote the paper: SA NVP PL KD.

References

1. Whitcher JP, Srinivasan M (1997) Corneal ulceration in the developing world-a silent epidemic. The British Journal of Ophthalmology 81:622–623.
2. Gonzales CA, Srinivasan M, Whitcher JP, Smolin G (1996) Incidence of corneal ulceration in Madurai district, South India. Ophthalmic Epidemiology 3:159–166.
3. Erie JC, Nevitt MP, Hodge DO, Ballard DJ (1993) Incidence of ulcerative keratitis in a defined population from 1950 through 1988. Archives of Ophthalmology 111:1665–1671.
4. Srinivasan M, Gonzales CA, George C, Cevallos V, Mascarenhas JM, et al. (1997) Epidemiology and aetiological diagnosis of corneal ulceration in Madurai, south India. The British Journal of Ophthalmology 81:965–971.
5. Hagan M, Wright E, Newman M, Dolin P, Johnson G (1995) Causes of suppurative keratitis in Ghana. The British Journal of Ophthalmology 79:1024–1028.
6. Poole TRG, Hunter DL, Maliwa EMK, Ramsay ARC (2002) Aetiology of microbial keratitis in northern Tanzania. The British Journal of Ophthalmology 86:941–942.
7. Upadhyay MP, Karmacharya PC, Koirala S, Tuladhar NR, Bryan LE, et al. (1991) Epidemiologic characteristics, predisposing factors, and etiologic diagnosis of corneal ulceration in Nepal. American Journal of Ophthalmology 111:92–99.
8. Thomas PA, Geraldine P (2007) Infectious keratitis. Current Opinion in Infectious Diseases 20:129–141.
9. Srinivasan M (2004) Fungal keratitis. Current Opinion in Ophthalmology 15:321–327.
10. Levin LA, Avery R, Shore JW, Woog JJ, Baker AS (1996) The spectrum of orbital aspergillosis: a clinicopathological review. Survey of Ophthalmology 41:142–154.
11. Yohai RA, Bullock JD, Aziz AA, Markert RJ (1994) Survival factors in rhino-orbital-cerebral mucormycosis. Survey of Ophthalmology 39:3–22.
12. Jones BR (1975) Principles in the management of oculomycosis. XXXI Edward Jackson memorial lecture. American Journal of Ophthalmology 79:719–75.
13. Kuriakose T, Thomas PA (1991) Keratomycotic malignant glaucoma. Indian Journal of Ophthalmology 39:118–121.
14. Vasanthi M, Prajna NV, Lalitha P, Mahadevan K, Muthukkaruppan V (2007) A pilot study on the infiltrating cells and cytokine levels in the tear of fungal keratitis patients. Indian Journal of Ophthalmology 55:27–31.
15. Ananthi S, Chitra T, Bini R, Prajna NV, Lalitha P, et al. (2008) Comparative analysis of the tear protein profile in mycotic keratitis patients. Molecular Vision 14:500–507.
16. de Souza GA, Godoy LMF, Mann M (2006) Identification of 491 proteins in the tear fluid proteome reveals a large number of proteases and protease inhibitors. Genome Biology 7:R72.
17. Zhou L, Beuerman RW, Foo Y, Liu S, Ang LPK, Tan DTH (2006) Characterisation of human tear proteins using high-resolution mass spectrometry. Annals of the Academy of Medicine, Singapore 35:400–407.
18. Li N, Wang N, Zheng J, Liu XM, Lever OW, et al. (2005) Characterization of human tear proteome using multiple proteomic analysis techniques. Journal of Proteome Research 4:2052–2061.
19. Koo BS, Lee DY, Ha HS, Kim JC, Kim CW (2005) Comparative analysis of the tear protein expression in blepharitis patients using two-dimensional electrophoresis. Journal of Proteome Research 4:719–724.
20. Herber S, Grus FH, Sabuncuo P, Augustin AJ (2001) Two-dimensional analysis of tear protein patterns of diabetic patients. Electrophoresis 22:1838–1844.
21. Righetti PG, Castagna A, Antonucci F, Piubelli C, Cecconi D, et al. (2005) Proteome analysis in the clinical chemistry laboratory: myth or reality? Clinica Chimica Acta; International Journal of Clinical Chemistry 357:123–139.
22. Gupta N, Shankernarayan NP, Dharmalingam K (2007) Serum proteome of leprosy patients undergoing erythema nodosum leprosum reaction: regulation of expression of the isoforms of haptoglobin. Journal of Proteome Research 6:3669–3679.
23. Gupta N, Shankernarayan NP, Dharmalingam K (2010) Alpha1-acid glycoprotein as a putative biomarker for monitoring the development of the type II reactional stage of leprosy. Journal of Medical Microbiology 59:400–407.
24. Zolg W (2006) The proteomic search for diagnostic biomarkers: lost in translation? Molecular & Cellular Proteomics 5:1720–1726.
25. Lescuyer P, Hochstrasser D, Rabilloud T (2007) How shall we use the proteomics toolbox for biomarker discovery? Journal of Proteome Research 6:3371–3376.
26. Good DM, Thongboonkerd V, Novak J, Bascands JL, Schanstra JP, et al. (2007) Body fluid proteomics for biomarker discovery: lessons from the past hold the key to success in the future. Journal of Proteome Research 6:4549–4555.
27. Tomosugi N, Kitagawa K, Takahashi N, Sugai S, Ishikawa I (2005) Diagnostic potential of tear proteomic patterns in Sjogren's syndrome. Journal of Proteome Research 4:820–825.
28. Molloy MP, Bolis S, Herbert BR, Ou K, Tyler MI, et al. (1997) Establishment of the human reflex tear two-dimensional polyacrylamide gel electrophoresis reference map: new proteins of potential diagnostic value. Electrophoresis 18:2811–2815.
29. Unlu M, Morgan ME, Minden JS (1997) Difference gel electrophoresis: a single gel method for detecting changes in protein extracts. Electrophoresis 18:2071–2077.
30. Alban A, David SO, Bjorkesten L, Andersson C, Sloge E, et al. (2003) A novel experimental design for comparative two-dimensional gel analysis: two-dimensional difference gel electrophoresis incorporating a pooled internal standard. Proteomics 3:36–44.
31. Marouga R, David S, Hawkins E (2005) The development of the DIGE system: 2D fluorescence difference gel analysis technology. Analytical and Bioanalytical Chemistry 382:669–678.
32. Tonge R, Shaw J, Middleton B, Rowlinson R, Rayner S, et al. (2001) Validation and development of fluorescence two-dimensional differential gel electrophoresis proteomics technology. Proteomics 1:377–396.
33. Dennis G Jr, Sherman BT, Hosack DA, Yang J, Gao W, et al. (2003) DAVID: Database for Annotation, Visualization, and Integrated Discovery. Genome Biology 4:P3.
34. Saijyothi AV, Angayarkanni N, Syama C, Utpal T, Shweta A, et al. (2010) Two dimensional electrophoretic analysis of human tears: collection method in dry eye syndrome. Electrophoresis 31:3420–3427.
35. Zhou L, Huang LQ, Beuerman RW, Grigg ME, et al. (2004) Proteomic analysis of human tears: defensin expression after ocular surface surgery. J Proteome Res 3: 410–416.
36. Green-Church KB, Nichols KK, Kleinholz NM, Zhang L, Nichols JJ (2008) Investigation of the human tear film proteome using multiple proteomic approaches. Mol Vis 7:14:456–470.
37. Gachon AM, Verrelle P, Betail G, Dastugue B (1979) Immunological and electrophoretic studies of human tear proteins. Experimental Eye Research 29:539–553.
38. Fullard RJ (1988) Identification of proteins in small tear volumes with and without size exclusion HPLC fractionation. Current Eye Research 7:163–179.
39. Kijlstra A, Kuizenga A (1994) Analysis and function of the human tear proteins. Advances in Experimental Medicine and Biology 350:299–308.
40. Gachon A, Lacazette E (1998) Tear lipocalin and the eye's front line of defence. The British Journal of Ophthalmology 82:453–455.
41. Sitaramamma T, Shivaji S, Rao GN (1998) HPLC analysis of closed, open, and reflex eye tear proteins. Indian Journal of Ophthalmology 46:239–245.
42. Twining SS, Fukuchi T, Yue BY, Wilson PM, Boskovic G (1994) Corneal synthesis of alpha 1-proteinase inhibitor (alpha 1-antitrypsin). Investigative Ophthalmology & Visual Science 35:458–462.
43. Abrahamson M, Barrett AJ, Salvesen G, Grubb A (1986) Isolation of six cysteine proteinase inhibitors from human urine. Their physicochemical and enzyme kinetic properties and concentrations in biological fluids. The Journal of Biological Chemistry 261:11282–11289.
44. Barka T, Asbell PA, van der Noen H, Prasad A (1991) Cystatins in human tear fluid. Current Eye Research 10:25–34.
45. Isemura S, Saitoh E, Sanada K, Minakata K (1991) Identification of full-sized forms of salivary (S-type) cystatins (cystatin SN, cystatin SA, cystatin S, and two phosphorylated forms of cystatin S) in human whole saliva and determination of phosphorylation sites of cystatin S. Journal of Biochemistry 110:648–654.
46. Reitz C, Breipohl W, Augustin A, Bours J (1998) Analysis of tear proteins by one- and two-dimensional thin-layer iosoelectric focusing, sodium dodecyl sulfate electrophoresis and lectin blotting. Detection of a new component: cystatin C. Graefe's Archive for Clinical and Experimental Ophthalmology 236:894–899.
47. Ananthi S, Santhosh RS, Nila MV, Prajna NV, Lalitha P, et al. (2011) Comparative proteomics of human male and female tears by two-dimensional electrophoresis. Experimental Eye Research 92:454–463.
48. ter Rahe BS, van Haeringen NJ (1998) Cystatins in tears of patients with different corneal conditions. Ophthalmologica 212:34–36.

49. Ma P, Wang N, McKown RL, Raab RW, Laurie GW, et al. (2006) Heparanase deglycanation of syndecan-1 is required for binding of the epithelial-restricted prosecretory mitogen lacritin. The Journal of Cell Biology 174:1097–1106.

50. Sanghi S, Kumar R, Lumsden A, Dickinson D, Klepeis V, et al. (2001) cDNA and genomic cloning of lacritin, a novel secretion enhancing factor from the human lacrimal gland. Journal of Molecular Biology 310:127–139.

51. Samudre S, Lattanzio FA Jr, Lossen V, Hosseini A, Sheppard JD Jr, et al. (2011) Lacritin, a novel human tear glycoprotein, promotes sustained basal tearing and is well tolerated. Invest Ophthalmol Vis Sci 5: 52(9):6265–6270.

52. Nichols JJ, Green-Church KB (2009) Mass spectrometry-based proteomic analyses in contact lens-related dry eye. Cornea 28:1109–1117.

53. Breit SN, Wakefield D, Robinson JP, Luckhurst E, Clark P (1985) The role of alpha 1-antitrypsin deficiency in the pathogenesis of immune disorders. Clinical Immunology and Immunopathology 35:363–380.

54. Chevance LG, Causse JR, Bergès J (1976) Alpha 1-antitrypsin activity of perilymph. Occurrence during progression of otospongiosis. Arch Otolaryngol 102(6):363–364.

55. Kyaw-Myint TO, Howell AM, Murphy GM, Anderson CM (1975) Alpha-1-antitrypsin in duodenal fluid and gallbladder bile. Clin Chim Acta 22:59(1):51–54.

56. Talamo RC (1975) Basic and clinical aspects of the alpha1-antitrypsin. Pediatrics 56(1):91–9.

57. Sharp HL (1976) The current status of alpha-1-antityrpsin, a protease inhibitor, in gastrointestinal disease. Gastroenterology 70(4):611–621.

58. Arora PK, Miller HC, Aronson LD (1978) Alpha1-Antitrypsin is an effector of immunological stasis. Nature 274:589–590.

59. Berman MB, Barber JC, Talamo RC, Langley CE (1973) Corneal ulceration and the serum antiproteases. I. Alpha 1-antitrypsin. Investigative Ophthalmology 12:759–770.

60. Gupta AK, Sarin GS, Mathur MD, Ghosh B (1988) Alpha 1-antitrypsin and serum albumin in tear fluids in acute adenovirus conjunctivitis. The British Journal of Ophthalmology 72:390–393.

61. Prause JU (1983) Serum albumin, serum antiproteases and polymorphonuclear leucocyte neutral collagenolytic protease in the tear fluid of patients with corneal ulcers. Acta Ophthalmologica 61:272–282.

62. Sen DK, Sarin GS (1986) The preocular tear film in health, disease and contact lens wear. Texas: Lubbock. Dry Eye Institute. pp 192–199.

63. Sharp HL (1975) Modern trends in gastroenterology. 5th ed. London: Butterworths. 140 p.

64. Langlois MR, Delanghe JR (1996) Biological and clinical significance of haptoglobin polymorphism in humans. Clin Chem 42:1589–1600.

65. Mii S, Nakamura K, Takeo K, Kurimoto S (1992) Analysis of human tear proteins by two-dimensional electrophoresis. Electrophoresis 13:379–382.

66. Tseng CF, Lin CC, Huang HY, Liu HC, Mao SJT (2004) Antioxidant role of human haptoglobin. Proteomics 4:2221–2228.

67. Tada T, Ohkubo I, Niwa M, Sasaki M, Tateyama H (1991) Immunohisto-chemical localization of Zn-alpha 2-glycoprotein in normal human tissues. The Journal of Histochemistry and Cytochemistry: Official Journal of the Histochemistry Society 39:1221–1226.

68. Hirai K, Hussey HJ, Barber MD, Price SA, Tisdale MJ (1998) Biological evaluation of a lipid-mobilizing factor isolated from the urine of cancer patients. Cancer Res 1:58(11):2359–2365.

69. Russell ST, Zimmerman TP, Domin BA, Tisdale MJ (2004) Induction of lipolysis in vitro and loss of body fat in vivo by zinc-alpha2-glycoprotein. Biochimica Et Biophysica Acta 1636:59–68.

70. Baker GRC, Morton M, Rajapaska RS, Bullock M, Gullu S, et al. (2006) Altered tear composition in smokers and patients with graves ophthalmopathy. Archives of Ophthalmology 124:1451–1456.

71. Kawai S, Nakajima T, Hokari S, Komoda T, Kawai K (2002) Apolipoprotein A-I concentration in tears in diabetic retinopathy. Annals of Clinical Biochemistry 39:56–61.

72. Kolte RA, Kolte AP, Kohad RR (2010) Quantitative estimation and correlation of serum albumin levels in clinically healthy subjects and chronic periodontitis patients. Journal of Indian Society of Periodontology 14:227–230.

73. Metz-Boutigue MH, Jollès J, Mazurier J, Schoentgen F, Legrand D, et al. (1984) Human lactotransferrin: amino acid sequence and structural comparisons with other transferrins. European Journal of Biochemistry/FEBS 145:659–676.

74. Kanyshkova TG, Buneva VN, Nevinsky GA (2001). Lactoferrin and Its biological functions. Biochemistry (Moscow) 66 p1-7-7.

75. Birgens HS (1985) Lactoferrin in plasma measured by an ELISA technique: evidence that plasma lactoferrin is an indicator of neutrophil turnover and bone marrow activity in acute leukaemia. Scandinavian Journal of Haematology 34:326–331.

76. Brock JH (2002) The physiology of lactoferrin. Biochemistry and Cell Biology 80:1–6.

77. Bradford MM (1976) A rapid and sensitive method for the quantitation of microgram quantities of protein utilizing the principle of protein-dye binding. Analytical Biochemistry 72:248–254.

78. Ramachandran B, Dikshit KL, Dharmalingam K (2012) Recombinant E.coli expressing Vitreoscilla haemoglobin prefers aerobic metabolism under micro-aerobic conditions: A proteome level study. J Biosci 37: 617–633.

79. Neuhoff V, Stamm R, Eibl H (1985) Clear background and highly sensitive protein staining with Coomassie Blue dyes in polyacrylamide gels: A systematic analysis. Electrophoresis 6:427–448.

80. Huang DW, Sherman BT, Lempicki RA (2009) Systematic and integrative analysis of large gene lists using DAVID bioinformatics resources. Nature Protocols 4:44–57.

12

Vision-Related Quality of Life in Herpetic Anterior Uveitis Patients

Lisette Hoeksema[1,2]*, Leonoor I. Los[1,2]

1 Department of Ophthalmology, University Medical Center Groningen, University of Groningen, Groningen, the Netherlands, **2** W.J. Kolff Institute, Graduate School of Medical Sciences, University of Groningen, Groningen, the Netherlands

Abstract

We investigated the vision-related quality of life (VR-QOL) and the prevalence and severity of depression in patients with herpetic anterior uveitis (AU). This study was conducted in 2012 at the ophthalmology department of the University Medical Center of Groningen (tertiary referral center). We selected patients from an existing uveitis database, all eligible patients were approached. Thirty-six of 66 (55%) patients with herpetic AU (herpes simplex virus or varicella zoster virus) participated, patients were 18 years or older. The diagnosis was made by clinical presentation or a positive anterior chamber tap. All patients received an information letter, informed consent form, National Eye Institute Visual Functioning Questionnaire-25 (NEI VFQ-25), Beck Depression Inventory (BDI-II), Social Support List – Interactions (SSL-I), Social Support List – Discrepancies (SSL-D) and an additional questionnaire for gathering general information. Medical records were reviewed for clinical characteristics. Analyses were conducted on various patient and ocular characteristics. We compared our NEI VFQ-25 scores with those previously found in the literature. Our main outcome measures were VR-QOL, prevalence and severity of depression, social support and various patient and ocular characteristics that could influence the VR-QOL. We found that the NEI VFQ-25 mean overall composite score (OCS) was 88.1 ± 10.6. Compared with other ocular diseases our OCS is relatively high, but lower than that found in a normal working population. The mean general health score was 59.0 ± 19.0; this score is lower than in patients with other ocular diseases, except for untreated Behçet's patients. Depression was scarce, with only one patient (2.8%) having a moderate depression (BDI-II score of 21). We concluded that herpetic AU affects the VR-QOL in a moderate way. The prevalence of depression in our group of herpetic AU patients was low and therefore does not seem to indicate a need for specific screening and intervention measures in these patients.

Editor: Deepak Shukla, University of Illinois at Chicago, United States of America

Funding: Professor Mulder Stichting, Stichting Nederlands Oogheelkundig Onderzoek, Stichting Blindenhulp. The funders had no role in study design, data collection and analysis, decision to publish, or preparation of the manuscript.

Competing Interests: Dr. Los has received personal fees paid by Abbott for giving lectures on uveitis. These fees consisted of travel expenses and hotel costs for lectures given in June 2010 and 2011. There are no further financial or other relations between Dr. Los and Abbott or any other commercial company.

* E-mail: l.hoeksema@umcg.nl

Introduction

Anterior uveitis (AU) is the predominant form of uveitis and herpetic AU is the most frequently observed form of infectious AU. [1] Characteristics like dermatitis, keratitis, elevated intraocular pressure (IOP) and iris sector atrophy are seen in herpetic AU. [2] Also secondary complications, like glaucoma and cataract are reported. [3] Complications of uveitis can lead to irreversible loss of visual functioning. [4] Previous studies showed that 35% of uveitis patients in the Western society are significantly visually impaired or blind [5].

Uveitis is seen in all age groups, and a substantial proportion of patients is of working age. During active uveitis, the inflammation and its treatment may – temporarily – affect visual functioning in such a way that it interferes with reading, computer work, driving, etc. Some patients may lose their job because of – recurrent – uveitis. Fear of a recurrence may cause increased stress levels, even when the uveitis is quiet. This may result in a decreased vision-related quality of life (VR-QOL) and an increased risk of developing a depression.

The purpose of this study is to evaluate the VR-QOL and the prevalence and severity of depression in a group of patients with a specific type of uveitis, i.e. herpetic AU (including herpes simplex virus (HSV) or varicella zoster virus (VZV) related AU). Previous research on a large group of uveitis patients found that uveitis patients reported a markedly poorer visual functioning and general health status than healthy subjects. [6] That study evaluated a non-homogeneous group of uveitis patients with different causes and manifestations of the disease. Since each cause and manifestation of uveitis may differ with regard to clinical characteristics and residual symptoms, it would also be of interest to examine the VR-QOL in the different uveitis entities separately. This may give valuable information for entity-related counseling of patients and may indicate the entity-related need for developing intervention strategies.

Methods

Ethics Statement

The Medical Ethical Committee of the University Medical Center of Groningen ruled that approval was not required for this study. The study was conducted according to the tenets of the Declaration of Helsinki.

Patients

The patients included in this study were selected from an existing database, containing uveitis patients who had been treated or are currently being treated for uveitis at the ophthalmology department of the University Medical Center of Groningen, which is a tertiary referral center. We included 66 patients with herpetic AU. All patients were 18 years or older. The diagnosis was made by clinical presentation (keratitis - dendritic herpes branch - followed by AU, elevated intraocular pressure at presentation, iris sector atrophy developing over time and/or clear facial varicella zoster infection (ophthalmic nerve) with subsequent kerato-uveitis) or a positive anterior chamber tap for local antibody production or the presence of virus DNA by PCR. Patients with other forms or possible causes of uveitis were excluded.

Data

All 66 patients received an information letter and an informed consent form by mail. Included in this letter, they received the following questionnaires; the National Eye Institute Visual Functioning Questionnaire-25 (NEI VFQ-25), the Beck Depression Inventory (BDI-II), Social Support List – Interactions (SSL-I), Social Support List – Discrepancies (SSL-D) and an additional questionnaire for gathering general information. The patients were asked to complete the questionnaires at home, to sign the informed consent form and to return them by mail.

For measuring the VR-QOL, we used the validated Dutch version of the NEI VFQ-25. The NEI VFQ-25 has been developed by the National Eye Institute. This validated [7,8] self-administered questionnaire consists of 25 questions, with a total score and subscores ranging from 0–100. In this questionnaire, the score of 0 corresponds to the lowest and of 100 to the highest VR-QOL. There are 12 subscales, each consisting of one or more questions. These subscales are general health, general vision, ocular pain, near activities, distance activities, vision specific social functioning, vision specific mental health, vision specific role difficulties, vision specific dependency, driving, color vision and peripheral vision.

The BDI-II is a validated [9] self-administered questionnaire consisting of 21 questions on how the patient feels and experiences things. Each question can be answered on a four-point scale ranging from 0 to 3. Subscores are added to create a total score. A total score of 0 to 13 corresponds with no depression, of 14 to 19 with a mild depression, of 20 to 28 with a moderately severe depression and of 29 to 63 with a severe depression. The SSL-I and SSL-D are questionnaires developed and validated by the University of Groningen (RUG). These questionnaires measure (1) social interactions between patients and persons with whom they interact and (2) if the received social support corresponds with the desired social support. They each consist of 34 four-choice questions, resulting in scores ranging from 1–4. A high SSL-I score corresponds with sufficient social support. A high SSL-D score corresponds with a deficiency in desired social support. The maximum score of the SSL-I is 136 and of the SSL-D it is 102.

The following information was gathered by the additional questionnaire: present activity of the uveitis, presence of other chronic diseases or diseases with a large impact (recent or in the past), medication use (ocular and other medication), history of depression and/or treatment, and need for visual revalidation. By reviewing medical records, we gathered the following information: present age, sex, unilateral or bilateral AU, systemic disease, follow-up time (defined as time between the start of the first uveitis episode and the end of the last uveitis episode), total time of active disease, total number of uveitis episodes, remission time (defined as time between the end of the last uveitis episode and the date on the questionnaire), Snellen visual acuity (VA), ocular complications in history (elevated IOP, glaucoma, cataract, secondary cataract, keratitis, dry eyes, cystoid macular edema (CME), papillitis, scleritis and herpes zoster ophthalmicus (HZO)) and presence of active uveitis at the time of completing the questionnaire.

Active uveitis was defined as $\geq 0.5+$ cells in the anterior chamber. [10] Transiently elevated IOP was defined as a measured IOP>20 mmHg without pressure reducing medication. Glaucoma was defined as the presence of visual field defects typical for glaucoma that were reproducible and could not be explained by other pathology, with or without glaucomatous disc abnormalities. Dry eyes were defined as the presence of dry eye symptoms and need for artificial tears.

Statistics

Data were statistically analyzed using SPSS Statistics 20.0.0.1. For the comparison of continuous variables of two groups, we used the Mann-Whitney U test. For comparison of continuous variables of more than two groups, we used the Kruskal–Wallis one-way analysis and the Mann-Whitney U test for post hoc analysis with a Bonferroni correction, using a critical value of 0.05 divided by the number of tests conducted. Correlations were assessed with the Spearman's Rank Correlations test. For analyzing, Snellen VA was converted to the logarithm of the minimum angle of resolution (logMAR) equivalent. Statistical significance level was set at 0.05.

Results

Thirty-six of 66 (55%) patients participated by filling out the questionnaires and returning them by mail. Table 1 summarizes the clinical characteristics of the 27 HSV and nine VZV AU patients. Males were slightly overrepresented in relation to females (58 versus 42%). Mean age of the HSV patients was 55.7 ± 17.5 years and of VZV patients it was 63.7 ± 15.1 years (p = 0.201). Complications most frequently observed (in % of patients) were elevated IOP (69%), keratitis (64%), dry eyes (42%) and cataract (36%). We checked and confirmed that all complications developed after the diagnosis of AU. The mean ($\pm$ SD) of the NEI VFQ-25, BDI-ll, SSL-I and SSL-D scores are given in Table 1. Only one patient had a moderate depression (BDI-II score of 21) at the time of completing the questionnaires, for which he already received medical treatment.

Tables 2 and 3 give information on the mean ($\pm$ SD) of the overall composite score (OCS) and the subscales of the NEI VFQ-25 in the total group. Also, differences herein related to various patient characteristics and ocular variables are presented. The mean OCS in the total group was 88.1 ± 10.6 and the mean general health score was 59.0 ± 19.0.

Female patients scored significantly lower on ocular pain (indicating that they experienced more pain or discomfort around or in the eye). VZV patients scored lower on all subscales and on the OCS compared to HSV patients, but only the difference in scores on vision specific mental health reached significance. Patients with active uveitis had significantly lower vision specific social functioning and vision specific dependency scores. They also had lower distance activities scores, but this did not reach significance. Patients who experienced just one uveitis episode had significantly lower ocular pain scores (more pain) than patients who experienced multiple uveitis episodes. Dry eye patients scored significantly lower on ocular pain (more pain) and on the OCS. Patients with transiently or persistently elevated IOP had

Table 1. Clinical characteristics of herpetic AU patients and overall scores on questionnaires (N and (%) or Mean ± SD (range)).

Number of patients	36
HSV/VZV	27 (75%)/9 (25%)
Female/male	15 (42%)/21 (58%)
Unilateral/bilateral	36 (100%)/0 (0.0%)
Age at completing questionnaire (yrs)	57.7±17.1 (25–88)
Follow-up time (yrs)	8.7±12.4 (0.04–41.3)
Number of uveitis episodes	4.7±5.4 (1–27)
Time of active uveitis (months)	5.1±4.3 (1–17)
Remission time (yrs)	3.6±2.5 (0.02–10.7)
Depression in past[a]	4 (11%)
Complications[b]	
- Elevated IOP	25 (69%)
- Keratitis	23 (64%)
- Dry eyes[c]	15 (42%)
- Cataract	13 (36%)
- HZO	8 (22%)
- Glaucoma	5 (14%)
- Secondary cataract	4 (11%)
- CME	2 (6%)
- Scleritis	0 (0%)
- Papillitis	0 (0%)
NEI VFQ-25 OCS[d]	88.1±10.6 (51.7–97.6)
BDI-II score	3.7±4.5 (0–21)
SSL-I score	74.0±17.8 (34–105)
SSL-D score	45.3±16.1 (34–102)

AU: anterior uveitis, HSV: Herpes Simplex Virus, VZV: Varicella Zoster Virus, IOP: Intraocular Pressure, CME: Cystoid Macular Edema, HZO: Herpes Zoster Ophthalmicus, OCS: Overall Composite Score, BDI: Beck Depression Inventory, SSL-I: Social Support List - Interactions, SSL-D: Social Support List - Discrepancies.
[a]Diagnosed by a physician and medically treated.
[b]Developed during follow-up AU.
[c]Medication needed.
[d]Average of vision-targeted subscale scores, without general health subscore.

significantly lower distance activities scores. Patients with a Snellen VA of less than 0.5 in at least one eye, scored lower on the OCS and on all subscales, but only the scores on general vision, near activities and peripheral vision reached significance.

Age, keratitis and uveitis treatment showed no significant correlation with any of the NEI VFQ-25 outcomes. Also, patients with or without other chronic diseases (in our group: diabetes, respiratory diseases, hypercholesterolemia, hypertension and back pain) or diseases with a large impact (in our group: multiple brain infarcts, cancer, psoriasis vulgaris, depression, antithrombin III deficiency, polymyalgia-rheumatica, hypothyroidism and cardiovascular diseases (recent or in the past)) did not score significantly different on the NEI VFQ-25 scales, including the general health subscale.

Table 4 shows the results of the Spearman's Rank Correlations tests between studied variables and NEI VFQ-25 subscale scores and OCS. Age at completing the questionnaire and general vision, near activities and vision specific role difficulties were negatively correlated. LogMAR VA of the uveitic eye was negatively

correlated with near activities and peripheral vision. Remission time was positively correlated with peripheral vision and central vision. The BDI score was negatively correlated with general health, vision specific social functioning, vision specific mental health, vision specific role difficulties, vision specific dependency, driving and OCS. There was no significant correlation between the subscale scores and OCS and logMAR VA of the healthy eye, duration of active uveitis, total of uveitis episodes, follow-up time, SSL-I score and SSL-D score. There was no significant correlation between the BDI-II score and the SSL-I score or the SSL-D score.

Discussion

We found that in general NEI VFQ-25 subscale scores and the OCS were reasonably high in herpetic AU patients. We found a mean OCS of 88.1 which means that the majority of patients scored between the best possible (100.0) and the second best score (75.0). General health is the only subscale that is not included in the OCS. The mean general health score was lower than the means of the other subscales, namely 59.0. However, this still means that the majority of patients scored their general health between 'good' (50.0) and 'very good' (75.0). Depression was scarce in our study group, with only one patient having a moderate depression.

To give an overall idea of the height of the scores in our patient group in relation to those previously found in healthy persons and in patients with ocular disease, we constructed Table 5. Interestingly, Hirneiss et al. who obtained NEI VFQ-25 scores in a normal working population as well as in subpopulations thereof with and without ocular disease, found that general health scores were lower in the subgroup with ocular disease. [11] The general health scores of his total group and subpopulations were higher than in our patient group. Studies on patients with noninfectious ocular inflammatory disease and Birdshot chorioretinopathy showed general health scores comparable with our general health score. [12,13] Highest general health scores were achieved in patients with acute posterior vitreous detachment. [14] Untreated Behçet's disease patients had the lowest general health scores, which is not surprising because of the commonly associated systemic manifestations in this entity [15].

The overall composite score (OCS) is low in untreated Behçet's disease and Birdshot chorioretinopathy. [13,15] Unfortunately, OCS was not given in the study on bilateral age-related macular degeneration patients, but from the subscale scores, it can be derived that it will have been lowest in this patient group. [16] Schiffman et al. also found a relatively low OCS (±63.0) in a large group of uveitis patients. Their data was presented graphically and therefore it is difficult to derive exact values on NEI VFQ-25 scores. Because of this, we did not include that study in Table 5. [6] In our patient group, OCS was relatively high, but lower than those in the working population and in acute posterior vitreous detachment patients. [11,14] A possible explanation for the relatively high OCS in our study is that all our patients had a unilateral disease.

Looking at subgroup analyses in our study group (Tables 2, 3 and 4), age at the moment of completing the questionnaires seemed to be of no influence on total NEI VFQ-25 scores. When evaluating correlations between age and the NEI VFQ-25 subscales, it seems that general vision, near vision and performing tasks nearby become more difficult with age. Also, older patients more often indicate that accomplishing things is getting more difficult because of reduced vision and they feel limited because of their vision. Surprisingly, a history of keratitis seemed to have no effect on VR-QOL, whereas we would expect that residuals of

Table 2. NEI VFQ-25 subscale scores and overall composite score (OCS), Mean ± SD.

		GH	GV	OP	NA	DA	VSSF	VSMH	VSRD	VSD	D	CV	PV	OCS[a]
		(n=36)	(n=36)	(n=36)	(n=36)	(n=36)	(n=35)	(n=36)	(n=36)	(n=36)	(n=30)	(n=35)	(n=34)	(n=36)
Total group (n=36)		59.0±19.0	76.1±9.3	73.3±22.8	87.7±16.7	92.6±12.6	97.1±8.1	84.9±14.4	84.0±21.9	97.7±7.1	87.1±16.2	97.1±10.1	91.2±20.3	88.1±10.6
Sex	- Male (n=21)	61.9±23.2	78.1±8.7	81.5±17.1	87.7±18.0	92.5±11.8	96.3±9.2	85.4±11.4	88.1±12.8	97.6±6.0	88.3±15.4	96.3±12.2	91.3±23.3	89.4±10.3
	- Female (n=15)	55.0±10.4	73.3±9.6	61.7±25.2	87.8±15.4	92.8±14.0	98.3±6.5	84.2±18.3	78.3±30.1	97.8±8.6	84.6±18.2	98.3±6.5	91.1±15.8	86.2±11.1
		p=0.19	p=0.14	p=0.02	p=0.99	p=0.54	p=0.30	p=0.61	p=0.58	p=0.35	p=0.50	p=0.71	p=0.59	p=0.24
Present age (yrs)	- <45 (n=8)	56.3±17.7	80.0±0.0	75.0±16.4	96.9±6.2	97.9±3.9	100.0±0.0	88.3±5.2	96.9±5.8	100.0±0.0	95.8±7.0	100.0±0.0	96.4±9.4	93.3±3.1
	- 45-65 (n=14)	62.5±19.0	75.7±11.6	73.2±28.1	83.3±22.2	89.3±17.7	96.4±10.3	81.3±19.1	82.1±22.8	97.0±7.0	85.8±19.2	94.6±14.5	88.5±30.0	86.2±14.7
	- >65 (n=14)	57.1±20.6	74.3±9.4	72.3±21.5	86.9±13.0	92.9±8.6	96.4±7.6	86.6±12.5	78.6±24.7	97.0±9.0	84.0±15.7	98.2±6.7	91.1±12.4	87.1±7.9
		p=0.68	p=0.35	p=0.93	p=0.15	p=0.39	p=0.44	p=0.83	p=0.04[b]	p=0.40	p=0.25	p=0.53	p=0.51	p=0.24
HSV/VZV	- HSV (n=27)	61.1±20.0	77.0±9.1	76.4±22.3	89.2±14.6	93.5±11.4	98.6±5.4	87.3±13.1	87.5±18.0	98.8±5.0	88.7±16.2	98.1±6.8	93.0±13.5	89.8±8.9
	- VZV (n=9)	52.8±15.0	73.3±10.0	63.9±22.9	83.3±22.4	89.8±16.0	93.1±12.7	77.8±16.6	73.6±29.6	94.4±11.0	80.6±15.5	94.4±16.7	86.1±33.3	83.0±14.0
		p=0.23	p=0.31	p=0.12	p=0.59	p=0.44	p=0.06	p=0.03	p=0.07	p=0.06	p=0.14	p=0.70	p=0.98	p=0.09
Activity uveitis	- Active (n=4)	56.3±12.5	75.0±10.0	71.9±21.3	75.0±28.9	79.2±21.0	87.5±17.7	76.6±19.3	78.1±18.8	95.8±4.8	75.0±16.7	87.5±25.0	68.8±47.3	79.6±19.6
	- Inactive (n=32)	59.4±19.8	76.3±9.4	73.4±23.3	89.3±14.5	94.3±10.5	98.4±5.3	85.9±13.7	84.8±22.4	97.9±7.3	88.4±15.6	98.4±6.2	94.2±12.6	89.2±8.9
		p=0.70	p=0.82	p=0.78	p=0.22	p>0.05	p=0.03	p=0.23	p=0.30	p=0.04	p=0.11	p=0.18	p=0.14	p=0.27
Uveitis episodes[c]	- 1 episode (n=11)	61.4±17.2	74.5±12.9	61.4±21.3	86.4±15.5	95.5±7.8	96.6±8.1	85.8±12.8	75.0±28.5	96.2±10.1	88.4±13.8	95.5±10.1	95.0±10.5	86.2±8.7
	- >1 episode (n=22)	56.8±20.7	77.3±7.0	77.8±22.5	88.6±18.6	90.9±14.8	97.6±8.5	84.7±16.1	89.2±17.8	98.5±5.5	87.3±18.1	97.6±10.9	90.5±24.3	89.2±12.1
		p=0.65	p=0.36	p=0.04	p=0.52	p=0.47	p=0.51	p=0.92	p=0.06	p=0.44	p=0.96	p=0.26	p=0.95	p=0.11

NEI VFQ-25: National Eye Institute Visual Functioning Questionnaire-25, GH: General Health, GV: General Vision, OP: Ocular Pain, NA: Near Activities, DA: Distance Activities, VSSF: Vision Specific Social Functioning, VSMH: Vision Specific Mental Health, VSRD: Vision Specific Role Difficulties, VSD: Vision Specific Dependency, D: Driving, CV: Color Vision, PV: Peripheral Vision, OCS: Overall Composite Score, HSV: Herpes Simplex Virus, VZV: Varicella Zoster Virus. Mean scores ± one standard deviation are given.
[a] Average of vision-targeted subscale scores, without GH. [b] Bonferroni correction, significance level p<0.017. [c] Missing data in three patients.

Table 3. NEI VFQ-25 subscale scores and overall composite score (OCS), Mean ± SD.

		GH (n=36)	GV (n=36)	OP (n=36)	NA (n=36)	DA (n=36)	VSSF (n=35)	VSMH (n=36)	VSRD (n=36)	VSD (n=36)	D (n=30)	CV (n=35)	PV (n=34)	OCS[a] (n=36)
Dry eyes	- No (n=21)	58.3±19.9	77.1±9.6	79.2±21.8	89.7±16.9	93.3±12.3	97.5±6.5	86.0±14.6	88.1±18.7	98.4±5.7	89.4±15.7	97.5±7.7	94.7±13.4	90.1±9.9
	- Yes (n=15)	60.0±18.4	74.7±9.2	65.0±22.3	85.0±16.7	91.7±13.4	96.7±10.0	83.3±14.5	78.3±25.2	96.7±8.8	82.5±16.9	96.7±12.9	86.7±26.5	85.3±11.3
		p=0.88	p=0.46	*p=0.04*	p=0.12	p=0.61	p=0.93	p=0.39	p=0.08	p=0.38	p=0.16	p=0.78	p=0.25	*p=0.04*
Elevated IOP	- No (n=11)	68.2±16.2	80.0±8.9	73.9±21.3	94.7±8.6	98.5±3.4	98.9±3.8	89.8±5.8	92.0±12.8	99.2±2.5	93.8±12.4	97.7±7.5	95.5±10.1	92.1±5.6
	- Yes (n=25)	55.0±19.1	74.4±9.2	73.0±23.8	84.7±18.6	90.0±14.2	96.4±9.4	82.8±16.6	80.5±24.2	97.0±8.3	84.7±16.9	96.9±11.2	89.1±23.6	86.3±11.8
		p=0.05	p=0.11	p=0.99	p=0.11	*p=0.04*	p=0.52	p=0.40	p=0.10	p=0.55	p=0.09	p=0.97	p=0.55	p=0.12
Keratitis	- No[b] (n=20)	53.8±16.8	75.0±8.9	71.9±16.5	89.2±16.5	92.1±11.9	96.1±9.4	85.0±13.5	81.9±23.8	97.1±7.8	85.3±16.1	97.4±11.5	90.3±24.5	87.4±10.8
	- Yes[c] (n=16)	65.6±20.2	77.5±10.0	75.0±27.4	85.9±17.4	93.2±13.7	98.4±6.3	84.8±16.0	86.7±19.6	98.4±6.3	88.9±16.6	96.9±8.5	92.2±15.1	88.9±10.7
		p=0.08	p=0.46	p=0.37	p=0.58	p=0.38	p=0.24	p=0.87	p=0.47	p=0.27	p=0.42	p=0.50	p=0.87	p=0.39
Other disease[d]	- No (n=17)	61.8±17.9	76.5±7.9	74.3±22.3	88.7±13.5	96.1±6.0	99.2±3.1	85.3±11.5	83.8±24.1	96.1±9.8	91.3±9.1	100.0±0.0	95.0±10.4	89.5±6.7
	- Yes (n=19)	56.6±20.1	75.8±10.7	72.4±23.8	86.8±19.5	89.5±15.9	95.4±10.4	84.5±17.0	84.2±20.3	99.1±2.6	83.8±19.6	94.7±13.4	88.2±25.5	86.8±13.2
		p=0.42	p=0.77	p=0.86	p=0.76	p=0.26	p=0.20	p=0.56	p=0.96	p=0.48	p=0.51	p=0.10	p=0.57	p=0.79
Visual acuity[e,f]	- <0.5 (n=10)	67.5±16.9	70.0±10.5	68.8±29.0	75.8±21.0	85.0±20.0	93.8±13.5	75.6±22.9	68.8±32.9	95.8±10.6	80.6±20.8	92.5±16.9	77.5±32.2	80.3±16.4
	- ≥0.5 (n=22)	54.5±19.9	78.2±8.5	74.4±20.6	90.9±13.1	94.7±7.1	98.2±4.5	88.1±7.9	89.2±13.0	98.1±5.7	89.6±14.2	98.8±5.5	96.3±9.2	90.6±5.4
		p=0.082	*p=0.027*	p=0.649	*p=0.021*	p=0.230	p=0.552	p=0.174	p=0.053	p=0.607	p=0.256	p=0.174	*p=0.031*	p=0.149
Treatment uveitis[g]	- No (n=16)	62.5±18.3	77.5±10.0	74.2±19.6	91.7±12.5	95.8±7.5	97.7±6.8	87.1±11.3	86.7±26.8	97.4±8.5	91.7±12.7	96.9±8.5	96.9±8.5	90.2±8.5
	- Yes (n=20)	56.3±19.7	75.0±8.9	72.5±25.5	84.6±19.2	90.0±15.2	96.7±9.2	83.1±16.6	81.9±17.4	97.9±6.0	83.6±18.0	97.4±11.5	86.1±26.0	86.4±12.0
		p=0.32	p=0.96	p=0.96	p=0.25	p=0.21	p=0.79	p=0.65	p=0.05	p=0.87	p=0.14	p=0.50	p=0.14	p=0.20

NEI VFQ-25: National Eye Institute Visual Functioning Questionnaire-25, GH: General Health, GV: General Vision, OP: Ocular Pain, NA: Near Activities, DA: Distance Activities, VSSF: Vision Specific Social Functioning, VSMH: Vision Specific Mental Health, VSRD: Vision Specific Role Difficulties, VSD: Vision Specific Dependency, D: Driving, CV: Color Vision, PV: Peripheral Vision, OCS: Overall Composite Score, IOP: Intraocular Pressure. Mean scores ± one standard deviation are given.

[a] Average of vision-targeted subscale scores, without GH. [b] No keratitis in history or keratitis in history without residuals. [c] Keratitis with residuals. [d] Medical chronic condition or medical condition with large impact, recent or in the past, except for uveitis. [e] At least one eye with Snellen visual acuity <0.5. [f] Measured with Snellen chart within six months before or after completing the NEI VFQ-25. [g] Treatment of the uveitis and/or complications at the moment of completing the NEI VFQ-25.

Table 4. Spearman's Rank Correlations between studied variables and NEI VFQ-25 subscale scores and OCS.

	GH	GV	OP	NA	DA	VSSF	VSMH	VSRD	VSD	D	CV	PV	OCS[a]
Age at completing questionnaire	-0.035	**-0.360**	0.097	**-0.371**	-0.220	-0.192	0.057	**-0.407**	-0.113	-0.325	-0.008	-0.206	-0.267
	p=0.84	**p=0.03**	p=0.57	**p=0.03**	p=0.20	p=0.27	p=0.74	**p=0.01**	p=0.51	p=0.08	p=0.96	p=0.24	p=0.12
LogMAR VA uveitic eye	0.115	-0.273	-0.099	**-0.352**	-0.201	0.029	-0.206	-0.218	-0.116	-0.085	-0.090	**-0.383**	-0.219
	p=0.53	p=0.12	p=0.59	**p=0.04**	p=0.26	p=0.87	p=0.25	p=0.22	p=0.52	p=0.67	p=0.63	**p=0.03**	p=0.22
LogMAR VA fellow eye	-0.107	-0.261	0.139	-0.243	-0.003	0.049	-0.138	-0.164	-0.122	-0.079	0.173	0.042	-0.130
	p=0.56	p=0.15	p=0.45	p=0.18	p=0.99	p=0.80	p=0.45	p=0.37	p=0.51	p=0.70	p=0.35	p=0.82	p=0.48
Number of uveitis episodes	-0.008	0.110	0.170	-0.045	-0.271	-0.005	-0.051	0.185	0.142	0.030	0.084	-0.244	0.098
	p=0.97	p=0.54	p=0.34	p=0.81	p=0.13	p=0.98	p=0.78	p=0.30	p=0.43	p=0.88	p=0.65	p=0.19	p=0.59
Duration of active uveitis	-0.028	0.099	0.143	0.009	-0.193	0.036	0.107	0.011	0.056	-0.058	0.070	-0.155	0.054
	p=0.88	p=0.58	p=0.43	p=0.96	p=0.28	p=0.85	p=0.55	p=0.95	p=0.76	p=0.77	p=0.71	p=0.41	p=0.76
Follow-up time	0.115	0.144	0.145	0.013	-0.201	0.086	0.061	0.185	0.123	0.068	0.164	-0.250	0.139
	p=0.51	p=0.41	p=0.41	p=0.94	p=0.25	p=0.63	p=0.73	p=0.29	p=0.48	p=0.72	p=0.35	p=0.16	p=0.43
Remission time	-0.092	0.061	-0.071	0.294	0.291	0.274	0.092	0.046	0.283	-0.075	**0.387**	**0.429**	0.107
	p=0.59	p=0.72	p=0.68	p=0.08	p=0.09	p=0.11	p=0.59	p=0.79	p=0.09	p=0.69	**p=0.02**	**p=0.01**	p=0.53
BDI-II score	**-0.433**	-0.255	-0.261	-0.131	-0.134	**-0.485**	**-0.493**	**-0.348**	**-0.414**	**-0.558**	-0.066	-0.175	**-0.456**
	p=0.01	p=0.15	p=0.14	p=0.46	p=0.45	**p=0.004**	**p=0.003**	**p=0.04**	**p=0.02**	**p=0.002**	p=0.71	p=0.32	**p=0.007**
SSL-I score	-0.081	-0.211	0.065	-0.143	0.184	0.091	0.088	0.059	0.105	0.237	0.003	0.179	-0.006
	p=0.67	p=0.25	p=0.73	p=0.44	p=0.32	p=0.63	p=0.64	p=0.75	p=0.57	p=0.24	p=0.99	p=0.34	p=0.97
SSL-D score	-0.024	0.046	-0.060	0.022	-0.066	-0.143	-0.174	-0.197	0.021	-0.356	-0.018	-0.077	-0.130
	p=0.90	p=0.81	p=0.75	p=0.91	p=0.73	p=0.45	p=0.35	p=0.29	p=0.91	p=0.07	p=0.93	p=0.69	p=0.49

NEI VFQ-25: National Eye Institute Visual Function Questionnaire-25, GH: General Health, GV: General Vision, OP: Ocular Pain, NA: Near Activities, DA: Distance Activities, VSSF: Vision Specific Social Functioning, VSMH: Vision Specific Mental Health, VSRD: Vision Specific Role Difficulties, VSD: Vision Specific Dependency, D: Driving, CV: Color Vision, PV: Peripheral Vision, OCS: Overall Composite Score, VA: Visual Acuity, BDI: Beck Depression Inventory, SSL-I: Social Support List - Interactions, SSL-D: Social Support List - Discrepancies.
[a]Average of vision-targeted subscale scores, without GH.

Table 5. NEI VFQ-25 subscale scores and OCS compared with literature.

Study	Mean age ± SD (yrs)	Group composition	GH	GV	OP	NA	DA	VSSF	VSMH	VSRD	VSD	D	CV	PV	OCS[a]
								Mean (SD)							
Hoeksema	58±17	Herpetic anterior uveitis	59.0	76.1	73.3	87.7	92.6	97.1	84.9	84.0	97.7	87.1	97.1	91.2	88.1
n=36			(19.0)	(9.3)	(22.8)	(16.7)	(12.6)	(8.1)	(14.4)	(21.9)	(7.1)	(16.2)	(10.1)	(20.3)	(10.6)
Hirmeiss 2010 [11]	42±9	Normal working population - Total group	73.0	78.6	85.4	91.9	91.8	97.9	87.4	92.8	98.4	88.7	97.9	93.3	91.1
n=619			(18.1)	(15.7)	(16.6)	(13.1)	(11.3)	(9.0)	(10.5)	(13.8)	(5.6)	(10.6)	(9.3)	(15.0)	(7.4)
Hirmeiss 2010 [11]	42±9	Normal working population - Without ocular disease	79.9	79.0	87.6	92.3	92.1	98.1	87.8	93.4	98.5	88.8	98.0	93.4	91.6
n=511			(17.4)	(15.9)	(15.1)	(13.0)	(11.4)	(8.2)	(10.0)	(13.3)	(5.5)	(10.6)	(8.7)	(14.6)	(7.1)
Hirmeiss 2010 [11]	43	Normal working population - Only with ocular disease	68.6	79.1	75.1	90.2	90.6	96.8	85.3	89.7	97.9	88.4	97.3	92.5	88.8
n=108			(20.7)	(15.9)	(19.2)	(13.6)	(10.7)	(12.3)	(12.5)	(15.6)	(5.8)	(10.4)	(11.6)	(16.7)	(8.3)
Qian 2011 [12]	41	Noninfectious ocular inflammatory disease	60.3	72.8	73.9	79.2	78.8	89.9	70.8	74.2	84.9	77.4	94.9	81.3	79.7
n=104			–	–	–	–	–	–	–	–	–	–	–	–	–
Sakai 2013 [15]	45±14	Behçet uveitis untreated	31.3	48.0	78.8	53.3	60.6	69.6	43.4	53.2	77.3	58.3	82.5	75.0	63.6
n=20			(13.8)	(10.1)	(12.9)	(4.9)	(6.8)	(10.2)	(15.3)	(14.0)	(12.7)	(12.2)	(11.8)	(16.2)	(8.9)
Sakai 2013 [15]	45±14	Behçet uveitis infliximab[b]	77.5	82.0	98.1	87.4	85.2	90.0	92.6	92.6	95.4	85.0	92.5	93.8	90.3
n=20			(11.2)	(11.1)	(4.6)	(11.9)	(10.8)	(12.6)	(13.7)	(10.2)	(9.9)	(18.5)	(11.8)	(11.1)	(8.7)
Kuiper 2013 [13]	59.5 (median)	Birdshot chorioretinopathy	61.6	63.8	75.1	68.6	70.3	84.5	71.2	64.5	84.2	66.8	80.2	67.6	71.0
n=105			–	–	–	–	–	–	–	–	–	–	–	–	–
Cahill 2005 [16]	76.4±5.6	Bilateral severe AMD	–	31.4	81.8	29.4	38.8	58.4	34.1	38.2	42.7	16.1	67.5	66.8	–
n=70			–	(15.8)	(20.3)	(18.6)	(24.7)	(28.1)	(25.1)	(27.1)	(29.7)	(31.3)	(27.7)	(25.1)	–
Schweitzer 2011 [14]	Males: 64.5±6.6	Acute posterior vitreous detachment[c]	80.56	85.77	89.58	89.58	94.43	99.11	91.78	95.68	99.40	87.87	99.11	95.53	93.47
n=84	Females: 62.1±7.6		(15.95)	(10.94)	(12.85)	(10.89)	(8.27)	(3.43)	(9.75)	(8.62)	(3.01)	(14.56)	(6.07)	(11.09)	(6.20)

NEI VFQ-25: National Eye Institute Visual Function Questionnaire-25. GH: General Health, GV: General Vision, OP: Ocular Pain, NA: Near Activities, DA: Distance Activities, VSSF: Vision Specific Social Functioning, VSMH: Vision Specific Mental Health, VSRD: Vision Specific Role Difficulties, VSD: Vision Specific Dependency, D: Driving, CV: Color Vision, PV: Peripheral Vision, OCS: Overall Composite Score. [a]Average of vision-targeted subscale scores, without GH. [b] 12 months after receiving infliximab. [c] Six week follow-up visit.

keratitis would influence visual functioning and thereby some of the vision related subscales of the NEI VFQ-25. Also, any medical chronic condition or medical condition (other than ophthalmologic) with a large impact seemed to have no influence on the NEI VFQ-25 scores. Our study and studies summarized in Table 5 seem to suggest that ophthalmic disease itself may influence general health scores.

In our study, significantly more pain or discomfort in or around the eye was reported by female patients and patients who experienced only one uveitis episode. Previous clinical and epidemiological studies show that women are at an increased risk of developing chronic pain and some evidence suggests that women may experience more severe pain. Multiple biopsychosocial mechanisms may contribute to these gender differences in experienced pain, including sex hormones, endogenous opioid function, genetic factors, pain coping and catastrophizing and gender roles. [17] A possible explanation for the difference in reported pain between patients with one versus multiple uveitis episodes, could be the fact that herpes viruses are neurotrophic, and can destroy sensible nerve fibers. This is well-known for corneal sensibility [18] but may also apply to other structures within the eye. Presumably, repeated herpes activity will have a cumulative effect. Another possibility is that coping strategies may change with a longer duration of the disease.

VZV patients scored somewhat lower on all subscales and OCS compared with HSV patients, and this was not due to age or VA. Eight out of nine (89%) VZV patients had had HZO, and it is therefore possible that the lower scores are at least partly due to the occurrence of dermatitis or post-herpetic neuralgia in these patients. Lukas et al. showed that herpes zoster, and especially post-herpetic neuralgia, is associated with increased levels of pain that have a significant impact on QOL scores. [19] In our study, dry eye patients had a lower OCS, which was mainly due to more ocular pain. Li et al. also reported that VR-QOL in dry eye patients can be impaired [20].

Patients with a Snellen VA of less than 0.5 in at least one eye, were more likely to have lower VR-QOL scores, compared to patients with a Snellen VA of more than 0.5 at both eyes. Of these, only the scores on the subscales general vision, near activities and peripheral vision reached significance. The VA of the uveitic eye was correlated with near activities and peripheral vision scores (Table 4). The VA in the fellow eye does not seem to have any influence on the VR-QOL. The fact that we did not find major

significant differences based on VA, was possibly due to the fact that most patients had a relatively good VA in both eyes.

In our study, we identified only one patient (2.8%) with a moderate depression. By comparison, de Graaf et al. found a 12–month prevalence of any mood disorder (i.e. depression and other mood disorders) of 6.1% in the Netherlands between 1996 and 2009. [21] Qian et al. reported that 28/104 (26.9%) of patients with ocular inflammatory disease screened positive for depression, using the BDI-II questionnaire. These depressed patients scored far lower on the composite VFQ-25 score than non-depressed patients. [12] In our study, patients with a higher BDI-II score were also likely to score lower on the VR-QOL. We found that a higher BDI-II score was negatively correlated with general health, vision specific social functioning, vision specific mental health, vision specific role difficulties, vision specific dependency, driving and OCS. A possible explanation for the higher prevalence of depression in the study of Qian et al., is that they included patients with severe posterior and panuveitis in addition to AU patients. Qian et al. also mention that inadequate emotional support is a predictor of depression. In our study, the amount of social support appeared to have no influence on VR-QOL or depression.

The main shortcoming of our study is its modest sample size. Our sample size is considered adequate for overall analyses [22], but it may be too limited for all subgroup analyses, resulting in an underreporting of possibly relevant associations. Also, only 55% of herpetic uveitis patients participated in the present study, which may have resulted in a selection bias. Furthermore, our patients were seen at a tertiary referral center and therefore this population may not represent the general uveitis population.

In conclusion, herpetic AU affects the VR-QOL, but only in a moderate way. The NEI VFQ-25 subscale scores and OCS are reasonably good. The prevalence of depression in our group of herpetic AU patients was low and therefore does not seem to indicate a need for specific screening and intervention measures in this specific patient group.

Author Contributions

Conceived and designed the experiments: LH LL. Performed the experiments: LH. Analyzed the data: LH. Wrote the paper: LH LL. Drafting the article: LH. Revising the article critically for important intellectual content: LL. Final approval of the version to be published: LH LL.

References

1. Jakob E, Reuland MS, Mackensen F, Harsch N, Fleckenstein M, et al. (2009) Uveitis subtypes in a German interdisciplinary uveitis center–analysis of 1916 patients. J Rheumatol 36: 127–136.
2. Jap A, Chee SP (2011) Viral anterior uveitis. Curr Opin Ophthalmol 22: 483–488.
3. Wensing B, Relvas LM, Caspers LE, Valentincic NV, Stunf S, et al. (2011) Comparison of rubella virus- and herpes virus-associated anterior uveitis: clinical manifestations and visual prognosis. Ophthalmol 118: 1905–1910.
4. Huang JJ, Gaudio PA (2010) Ocular inflammatory disease and uveitis manual: diagnosis and treatment. Philadelphia, Wolters Kluwer, Lippincott Williams & Wilkins 41–60.
5. Rothova A, Suttorp van Schulten MS, Frits Treffers W, Kijlstra A (1996) Causes and frequency of blindness in patients with intraocular inflammatory disease. Br J Ophthalmol 80: 332–336.
6. Schiffman RM, Jacobsen G, Whitcup SM (2001) Visual functioning and general health status in patients with uveitis. Arch Ophthalmol 119: 841–849.
7. Mangione CM, Lee PP, Pitts J, Gutierrez P, Berry S, et al. (1998) Psychometric properties of the National Eye Institute Visual Function Questionnaire (NEI-VFQ). NEI-VFQ Field Test Investigators. Arch Ophthalmol 116: 1496–1504.
8. Mangione CM, Lee PP, Gutierrez PR, Spritzer K, Berry S, et al. (2001) National Eye Institute Visual Function Questionnaire Field Test Investigators. Development of the 25-item National Eye Institute Visual Function Questionnaire. Arch Ophthalmol 119: 1050–1058.
9. Arnau RC, Meagher MW, Norris MP, Bramson R (2001) Psychometric evaluation of the Beck Depression Inventory-II with primary care medical patients. Health Psychol 20: 112–119.
10. Jabs DA, Nussenblatt RB, Rosenbaum JT (2005) Standardization of Uveitis Nomenclature (SUN) Working Group. Standardization of uveitis nomenclature for reporting clinical data. Results of the First International Workshop. Am J Ophthalmol 140: 509–516.
11. Hirneiss C, Schmid-Tannwald C, Kernt M, Kampik A, Neubauer AS (2010) The NEI VFQ-25 vision-related quality of life and prevalence of eye disease in a working population. Graefes Arch Clin Exp Ophthalmol 248: 85–92.
12. Qian Y, Glaser T, Esterberg E, Acharya NR (2012) Depression and visual functioning in patients with ocular inflammatory disease. Am J Ophthalmol 153: 370–378.
13. Kuiper JJ, Missotten T, Baarsma SG, Rothova A (2013) Vision-related quality of life in patients with birdshot chorioretinopathy. Acta Ophthalmol 91: e329–331.
14. Schweitzer KD, Eneh AA, Hurst J, Bona MD, Rahim KJ, et al. (2011) Visual function analysis in acute posterior vitreous detachment. Can J Ophthalmol 46: 232–236.
15. Sakai T, Watanabe H, Kuroyanagi K (2013) Health- and vision-related quality of life in patients receiving infliximab therapy for Behcet uveitis. Br J Ophthalmol 97: 338–342.
16. Cahill MT, Banks AD, Stinnett SS, Toth CA (2005) Vision-related quality of life in patients with bilateral severe age-related macular degeneration. Ophthalmol 112: 152–158.

17. Bartley EJ, Fillingim RB (2013) Sex differences in pain: a brief review of clinical and experimental findings. Br J Anaesth 111: 52–58.
18. Pavan-Langston D (1995) Herpes zoster ophthalmicus. Neurology 45: S50–51.
19. Lukas K, Edte A, Bertrand I (2012) The impact of herpes zoster and post-herpetic neuralgia on quality of life: patient-reported outcomes in six European countries. Z Gesundh Wiss 20: 441–451.
20. Li M, Gong L, Chapin WJ, Zhu M (2012) Assessment of vision-related quality of life in dry eye patients. Invest Ophthalmol Vis Sci 53: 5722–5727.
21. de Graaf R, Ten Have M, van Gool C, van Dorsselaer S (2012) Prevalence of mental disorders, and trends from 1996 to 2009. Results from NEMESIS-2. Tijdschr Psychiatr 54: 27–38.
22. Mangione CM (2000) NEI-VFQ Scoring Algorithm. Version 2000.

13

Cortisol Biosynthesis in the Human Ocular Surface Innate Immune Response

Radhika Susarla[1⦾], Lei Liu[1⦾], Elizabeth A. Walker[2], Iwona J. Bujalska[2], Jawaher Alsalem[1], Geraint P. Williams[1], Sreekanth Sreekantam[1], Angela E. Taylor[2], Mohammad Tallouzi[1], H. Susan Southworth[1], Philip I. Murray[1], Graham R. Wallace[1], Saaeha Rauz[1]*

1 Academic Unit of Ophthalmology, Centre for Translational Inflammation Research, College of Medical and Dental Sciences, University of Birmingham, Birmingham, United Kingdom, 2 Centre for Endocrinology, Diabetes and Metabolism, College of Medical and Dental Sciences, University of Birmingham, Birmingham, United Kingdom

Abstract

Innate immune responses have a critical role in regulating sight-threatening ocular surface (OcS) inflammation. While glucocorticoids (GCs) are frequently used to limit tissue damage, the role of intracrine GC (cortisol) bioavailability via 11-beta-hydroxysteroid dehydrogenase type 1 (11β-HSD1) in OcS defense, remains unresolved. We found that primary human corneal epithelial cells (PHCEC), fibroblasts (PHKF) and allogeneic macrophages (M1, GM-CSF; M2, M-CSF) were capable of generating cortisol (M1>PHKF>M2>PHCEC) but in corneal cells, this was independent of Toll-like receptor (TLR) activation. While Polyl:C induced maximal cytokine and chemokine production from both PHCEC (IFNγ, CCL2, CCL3, and (CCL4), IL6, CXCL10, CCL5, TNFα) and PHKF (CCL2, IL-6, CXCL10, CCL5), only PHKF cytokines were inhibited by GCs. Both Poly I:C and LPS challenged-corneal cells induced M1 chemotaxis (greatest LPS-PHKF (250%), but down-regulated M1 11β-HSD1 activity (30 and 40% respectively). These data were supported by clinical studies demonstrating reduced human tear film cortisol:cortisone ratios (a biomarker of local 11β-HSD1 activity) in pseudomonas keratitis (1:2.9) versus healthy controls (1:1.3; p<0.05). This contrasted with putative TLR3-mediated OcS disease (Stevens-Johnson Syndrome, Mucous membrane pemphigoid) where an increase in cortisol:cortisone ratio was observed (113.8:1; p<0.05). In summary, cortisol biosynthesis in human corneal cells is independent of TLR activation and is likely to afford immunoprotection under physiological conditions. Contribution to ocular mucosal innate responses is dependent on the aetiology of immunological challenge.

Editor: James T. Rosenbaum, Oregon Health & Science University, United States of America

Funding: Funding: Guide Dogs for the Blind (UK registered Charity in England and Wales (209617) and Scotland (SC038979)) ref 2006-01b; Action Medical Research (UK Registered Charity in England & Wales (208701) and in Scotland (SC039284)) ref SP4215; Henry Smith Charity (UK Registered Charity 230102); Wellcome Trust (UK): GPW, SR. The funders had no role in study design, data collection and analysis, decision to publish, or preparation of the manuscript.

Competing Interests: The authors have declared that no competing interests exist.

* E-mail: s.rauz@bham.ac.uk

⦾ These authors contributed equally to this work.

Introduction

Ocular surface (OcS) pathology is a leading cause of worldwide blindness and represents a major proportion of ophthalmological emergencies in the developed world. The OcS provides an intricate mucosal barrier against infectious pathogens and immune-mediated processes that trigger innate responses. Unlike other mucosal surfaces the cornea is avascular and optically clear, and supports a highly complex tear film that is vital for lubrication, nutrition and immunological defence of the eye. The tear film ultrastructure comprises (i) a negatively charged, hydrophilic mucinous glycocalyx that limits adhesion of foreign debris or pathogens to the OcS, (ii) a more superficial nutritive aqueous phase consisting of a range of electrolytes, carbohydrates, antioxidants, vitamins, proteins, immunoglobulins, hormones, growth factors and cytokines that support epithelial cell proliferation, maturation and movement across the ocular surface, and (iii) a complex triplex lipid layer consisting of outer non-polar lipids, inner polar lipids with intercalated proteins together with a novel long chain (O-acyl)-ω-hydroxy fatty acid functioning as an intermediate surfactant lipid interface [1]. Immunological damage of the OcS results in mucosal inflammatory cell invasion, angiogenesis and ultimately a blinding keratopathy.

The tissue-specific regulation of the active glucocorticoid (GC), cortisol, is a purported mechanism for determining the length and type of inflammatory response [2–4]. The actions of GCs are largely mediated via the glucocorticoid receptor (GRα) that acts as a nuclear transcription factor for a variety of GC responsive genes and has been implicated in the pathogenesis of disease [5–8]. Systemic regulation of cortisol levels are controlled by the hypothalamic-pituitary-adrenal axis, but local regulation is mediated via the 11β-hydroxysteroid dehydrogenases (11β-HSDs). Two isoforms control the cortisol-cortisone shuttle [9]: 11β-HSD2 inactivating cortisol to cortisone [10,11] in sodium and water secreting tissues protecting the mineralocorticoid receptor from GC excess, and 11β-HSD1 inducing GRα through activation of cortisol. 11β-HSD1 exhibits bidirectional enzyme activity *in vitro*, but *in vivo*, functions as an oxo-reductase, converting cortisone to cortisol - a reaction which is dependent on the delivery of co-factor NADPH via hexose-6-phosphate dehydrogenase (H6PD) and the glucose-6-phosphate transporter [12]. In the eye, our earlier work has localised 11β-HSD1 to the basal cells of the central corneal (differentiated) epithelium, and serum and glucocorticoid-regulated kinase 1 (SGK1, a GR mediated target gene) to the actively proliferating peripheral limbal region [13,14]. The importance of GCs in maintaining the integrity of the corneal epithelium is further supported by analyses of cultured rabbit corneal epithelial cells (CECs)[3]. More recently we have shown that synthetic GCs, such as dexamethasone, are able to change the global gene and miR profile of corneal fibroblasts down-regulating inflammatory genes and inducing expression of anti-angiogenic and anti-inflammatory genes [15].

During pathogen-driven processes, the recognition of pathogen products occurs via receptors such as Nod-Like Receptors (NLR), NALPS/inflammasomes, RIG-I-like receptors (RLR) and Toll like Receptors (TLR) [16]. Several TLR have been shown to be expressed in the cornea with TLR 1–6 and TLR 9–10 in human conjunctival and limbal epithelial cells [17], and TLR3 in primary human corneal epithelial cells (PHCEC) [18]. The absence of expression of TLR7 and TLR8 in primary cells is of interest, as this suggests that PHCEC and primary human corneal fibroblasts (PHKF) do not respond to ssDNA and dsDNA through these receptors. TLR induction in these cells produce cytokines (IL-6, IL-8 and TNFα) but data are limited as no studies have examined a wider cytokine profile in order to interrogate disease signaling pathways in more detail. This is particularly relevant as TLR recognition of pathogen-derived products is also known to trigger an activating signal for the innate immune system during not only ocular infections, but also dry eye disease states and immune-mediated OcS disease such as Stevens-Johnson Syndrome/Toxic epidermal necrolysis (SJS-TEN) where ongoing sub-clinical inflammation remains a therapeutic challenge [16,19–23].

In addition, macrophages and immature dendritic cells (iDCs) also respond to pathogens. Response may be direct via receptors such as the TLR or indirect, through cytokines and chemokines released by barrier cells under threat of the originating innate immune challenge agent. The autocrine regulation of 11β-HSD1 is pivotal; balancing the cortisol and cortisone shuttle appears to be a contributory driver of monocyte maturation, immune-cell function and down-regulation of tissue damaging inflammation [24,25]. This could be particularly relevant in ocular disease where the optically clear media are paradoxically compromised by the innate immune response that is vital for eradication of the triggering agent.

In this study, we used a combination of in vitro and clinical studies to examine the interplay between TLR and GCs in the context of OcS health, and when the OcS is actively threatened by microbial insult or immune-mediated disease, to determine whether the local provision of GCs contributes to the innate immunity of the OcS in health and in disease.

Materials and Methods

Human corneal cells

Ethics Statement. The study was undertaken after formal ethics approval from the Black Country Research Ethics Committee (incorporating the Dudley Research Ethics Committee (LREC 06/Q2702/44)), and all experiments were carried out in accordance with the Tenets of the Declaration of Helsinki.

Donor peripheral corneal rims and central corneal buttons (transplant waste) from penetrating and lamellar keratoplasty surgical procedures, where the donor had given written informed consent for research were used for the culture of primary human corneal epithelial cells (PHCEC) and corneal fibroblasts (PHKF). According to United Kingdom Guidelines for Organ Donation, only those patients with normal eyes in the absence of absolute

exclusion criteria including active transmissible disease or infection, Creuzfeldt-Jakob Disease, intravenous drug abuse, and neurodegenerative disorders, are suitable to donate organs and tissues for transplantation. Additional exclusions include previous ocular surgery, inflammation and tumors such as retinoblastoma.

The average age of the corneal donors was 69.1 (range 18–81.2) years. The corneal–scleral rims were incubated for 2 h at 37°C with 1.2 IU/ml neutral protease (Dispase II, Roche). Using a surgical 'hockey stick', the epithelium was stripped off with gentle scraping radially from the limbus towards the corneal apex in phosphate buffered saline (PBS). PHCEC were maintained in keratinocyte serum-free medium (KSFM) supplemented with 0.05 mg/mL bovine pituitary extract, 5 ng/mL human recombinant epidermal growth factor (Invitrogen, CA), 50 000 U/l penicillin and 50 000 µg/l streptomyocin, and 5% fetal calf serum (FCS) (Sigma, UK). Cells were grown at 37°C in a humid environment containing 5% CO_2 and the cell culture media was changed every 2 to 3 days.

PHKF were generated from corneal tissue excised from the corneoscleral rims. The corneal epithelial layer was removed from the stroma using dispase enzyme digestion, and the endothelial layer stripped under direct visualisation with the aid of trypan blue. The remaining corneal stroma was chopped into small pieces and cultured in a 25 cm^2 flask with 2 mL Fibro-medium. Cells were grown at 37°C in a humid environment containing 5% CO_2 and the cell culture media was changed every 2 to 3 days. Confluent cells were trypsinised and only cells up to 4 generations were used for subsequent experiments.

The identity of the cell types were confirmed by immunocytochemical analyses for cytokeratin 3, anti-vimentin and anti-5B5 as previously described [15]. The PHCEC were identified by their hexagonal morphology and CK3$^+$/vimentin$^+$/5B5$^-$ staining characteristics, whereas PHKF exhibited an elongated morphology and CK3$^-$/vimentin$^+$/5B5$^+$.

Monocyte-derived macrophages

Homogenous macrophage populations were generated by isolating peripheral blood mononuclear cells cells (PBMC) from the venous blood of healthy volunteers incubating pellets for at least 15 minutes in 20 µl of CD14$^+$ beads (Miltenyi Biotech, UK) and 80 µl of MACS buffer (Miltenyi Biotech) per 1×10^7/ml PBMC. Cells were then washed twice using MACS buffer and passed through a MACS column inserted into a magnetic holder. Negative subsets were excluded in the run through of column. The column was then removed from the holder and CD14$^+$ cells were collected by washing and set up in complete media at an appropriate concentration. To grow M1 or M2 macrophages either 10 ng/ml of recombinant human GM-CSF (PeproTech, UK) or 50 ng/ml recombinant human M-CSF (PeproTech, UK), respectively, was added to purified monocytes in complete medium; RPMI 1640 media supplemented with 10 mM L-Glutamine, and 5000 U/ml penicillin with 10 mg/ml Streptomycin (GPS) with 10% heated inactivated fetal calf serum (HIFCS) (all Sigma UK) and 4% human serum (HD Supplies UK) and incubated at 37°C in a humidified atmosphere of 5% CO2 for 6–7 days and harvested for use.

11β-HSD enzyme assays

Cells grown to confluence were pre-treated with 10 ng/ml of cytokines (IL-1, IL6, IL-8, TNFα, IL-4, IL-10, IL-13; Peprotech,UK) for 24 h and 1 µg/ml LPS (Sigma UK) for 48 h in serum containing KSFM before the start of the assay. Dehydrogenase activity (cortisol to cortisone conversion) was assessed using 100 nM unlabelled cortisol (Sigma, UK) diluted in growth medium and tracer amounts (1.5 nM) of [³H]cortisol (specific activity 74.0 Ci/mmol; NEN, USA) at 37°C for 24 h. Conversion of cortisone to cortisol (oxo-reductase activity) was analysed by incubating cells with 100 nM cortisone and tracer amounts of [³H]cortisone (50000 cpm synthesised in-house) with or without cytokines. After 24 h incubation, steroids were extracted from the medium with ten volumes of dichloromethane, separated by thin-layer chromatography with chloroform:ethanol (92:8) as a mobile phase and the fractional conversion of steroids was calculated after scanning analysis using a Bioscan 2000 radioimaging detector (Bioscan, Washington, DC, USA). Following enzyme assay, cell monolayers were lysed in 1 ml water for subsequent protein assays. Total protein in each well was determined using a standard protein assay reagent (Bio-Rad), and enzyme activities were expressed as pmol/mg/h.

RNA isolation and reverse-transcription (RT)

Total RNA was extracted from cells according to the manufacturer's instructions (Tri reagent, Sigma, UK) using. Total RNA was DNase I treated to remove any genomic DNA contamination (Invitrogen, CA). The quantity and quality of mRNA was assessed spectrophotometrically at and optical density of 260 /280 nm and by electrophoresis of 2 µl on a 1% agarose gel. Total RNA (100 ng-1 µg) in a total volume of 50 µl was reverse-transcribed using Multiscribe reverse transcriptase and random hexamers according to manufacturer's protocol (Applied Biosystems, UK). cDNA (50 ng) was used for conventional polymerase chain reaction (PCR) to define the expression of the genes of interest.

Polymerase chain reaction (PCR)

RT was performed as above and 2 µl cDNA (PHCEC, PHKF) was used in subsequent PCR reactions for the following genes: 11β-HSD1; 11β-HSD2, GR, H6PD (PHCEC, PHKF, M1 and M2). The primer sequences, annealing temperatures and the PCR product sizes are detailed in **Table S1**. For the glucocorticoid signaling genes, the PCR cycling conditions consisted of 94°C for 5 mins followed by 35 cycles of denaturation at 94°C for 30 sec, annealing step for 30 sec, extension step 72°C for 30 sec and followed by heating at 72°C for 5 mins and storage at 4°C. The PCR products were analyzed on 2% agarose gel in 1xTBE buffer (0.089 M Tris-base, 0.089 M boric acid, 0.002 M EDTA, pH 8.3) and the DNA was stained with ethidium bromide and visualized with UV light.

Cytokine analysis

PHCEC and PHKF cells at 90% confluence were treated with TLR1-9 ligands (Invivogen) (San Diego, CA, USA) for 16 h with cell culture medium only as negative control. The various TLR ligands and their concentrations used were: TLR1/2 (Pam3CSK 4 1µg/ml), TLR2 (HKLM 10⁸ cells/ml), TLR3 ((Poly(I:C) 10 µg/ml), TLR4 (LPS 1µg/ml), TLR5 (Flagellin 1 µg/ml), TLR6 (FSL1 1 µg/ml), TLR7 (Imiquimod 1 µg/ml), TLR8 (ssRNA40 1µg/ml) and TLR9 (ODN2006 5 µM).

Cell supernatants were collected and multiplex bead assay analyzer (Luminex 100; Luminex Corporation, Austin, TX) was performed with a human cytokine 30-Plex kit (Invitrogen, Camarillo, CA) according to manufacturer's protocol and as previously described [26]. The panel included EGF, Eotaxin, FGF-basic, G-CSF, GM-CSF, HGF, IFN-α, IFN-γ, IL-1RA, IL-1β, IL-2, IL-2R, IL-4, IL-5, IL-6, IL-7, IL-8, IL-10, IL-12p40/p70, IL-13, IL-15, IL-17, CCL2, CXCL9, CCL3, CCL4, CCL5, TNF-α, and VEGF.

Monocyte migration assays

PBMC were prepared from fresh whole blood sample from healthy volunteers by Ficoll-Paque PLUS (GE Healthcare Life Sciences, Amersham, UK). Briefly, whole blood was diluted by mixing with equal volume of RPMI containing 50 000 U/L penicillin, 50 000 µg/L streptomycin and 1% (v/v) Hepes. Diluted blood sample was carefully layered onto the Ficoll-Paque PLUS and centrifuged at 1200 rpm for 30 min at 20°C. PBMC was carefully collected at the interface between the Ficoll-Paque PLUS and sample layers. PBMC was washed with RPMI for 5 times.

Migration assays were performed with a 48-well Microchemo-taxis Chamber (Neuro Probe, Inc., Gaithersburg,USA). The supernatants of LPS and Poly I:C treated PHKF and PHCEC at volume of 26 µL were loaded in the bottom wells. A slight positive meniscus formed to prevent air bubbles from being trapped when the filter membrane was applied. PBMC suspension of 50 µL volume at concentration of 1×10^6 cells/mL was loaded in the upper wells. The Chamber was incubated at 37°C in humidified air with 5% CO_2 for 90 min. The non-migrated cells on the top side of the filter were wiped off and washed with PBS in a container. The filter was stained in Diff-Quick staining kit (IMEB, San. Marcos, CA) and mounted in immersion oil on a slide. Migrated cells were counted in three random 400× fields by two observers and averages of migrated cell number were calculated.

Immunohistochemistry

Immunohistochemical analyses for the expression of TLR3, TLR4 and CD68 were performed on formalin-fixed, paraffin-embedded tissue sections of normal human anterior segments enucleated for posterior segment pathologies, and from herpetic keratitis and gram-negative keratitis tissue sections (6 µm). Antigen retrieval was performed by heating the slides at 95°C for 1 h in 10 mM sodium citrate buffer, pH 6.0 and subsequent cooling in cold sodium citrate buffer for 20 min. Sections were incubated with primary antibodies at 1;100 for anti-human TLR3, TLR4 and CD68 in 1% normal donkey serum overnight at 4°C. Following washing in PBS, biotin-conjugated secondary antibody was diluted in 1% blocking serum and and added to sections for 45 min at room temperature at dilutions of 1:250 (donkey anti-sheep HRP conjugate) and 1:150 (anti-rabbit). The detection was carried using DAB substrate (Dako, Cambridge, UK) and nuclei were counterstained using Meyer's Haemalum (Lamb Ltd, UK). Sections incubated in secondary antibody alone were used as controls.

Quantification of hormones in human ocular biofluids

Tears (10 µl), aqueous humor (AqH −50 µl) and serum samples (100 µl) were collected from 43 healthy subjects prior to cataract surgery, and tears and serum from patients with either culture positive gram negative bacterial (pseudomonas) keratitis (n = 6) or PCR confirmed herpes simplex viral epithelial keratitis (n = 7) presenting to the Accident & Emergency Department at the Birmingham & Midland Eye Centre before initiation of treatment or instillation of eye drops. Tears and serum were also collected from patients with clinically quiescent chronic immune-mediated ocular surface disease (OcSD) for a minimum of 3 months who were not using therapeutic glucocorticoids (OcSD: Ocular Mucous Membrane Pemphigoid (OcMMP; n = 8); SJS-TEN; n = 5). Steroids were identified and quantified using liquid chromatography with tandem mass spectrometry (LC/MS/MS) which combines the physical separation capabilities of liquid chromatography with the sensitivity of mass spectrometry (Waters Xevo with Acquity uPLC), as previously described [27,28]. Each steroid was extracted by liquid/liquid extraction and quantified by comparison to a calibration series with respect an internal standard, yielding quantification of unbound 'free' steroid hormone. Data were converted to ng/ml and presented in nM.

All human samples were taken after written informed consent approved by the Birmingham East, North and Solihull (BENS) Research Ethics Committee (LREC 08/H1206/165) and from the Black Country Research Ethics Committee (incorporating the Dudley Research Ethics Committee (LREC 06/Q2702/63).

Statistical analysis

Statistical analysis was performed using the software package SigmaStat (Systat Software, USA.) and Prism for Windows version 4.03c (GraphPad Software, Inc., San Diego, CA, USA). One-way ANOVA with Dunnett's multiple comparisons post-test (for comparisons between untreated control and treatments) and Two-way ANOVA with Bonferroni post-test (for comparisons between groups of treatments) for analyses involving primary culture data. Due to donor variability in the cytokine production, the data have been normalized to respective untreated control values and presented as Mean ± SE, n = 3 donors. For biofluid hormone levels, the data are presented as median and ranges and analysed using two-tailed Mann-Whitney post–test for comparisons between group, and nonparametric Spearman-Rank correlation. P values <0.05 were accepted as statistically significant.

Results

Human corneal epithelial cells and corneal fibroblasts produce cortisol

All cell types (PHCEC, PHKF, M1 and M2 macrophages) showed expression of 11β-HSD1, H6PD and GRα mRNA, whereas no cell type expressed 11β-HSD2 (**Figure 1A**). To confirm whether cells were capable of generating cortisol, oxo-reductase activity assays were performed by incubating cells with tritiated cortisone and conversion to cortisol was measured by using thin-layer radio-chromatography. All cell types produced active cortisol (**Figure 1B**), but activity was greatest for M1 macrophages (38.1±10.1 pmol/mg/h) followed by PHKF (16.3±3.1 pmol/mg/h), M2 macrophages (10.2±3.3 pmol/mg/h) then PHCEC (2.3±0.6 pmol/mg/h). There was no dehydrogenase activity in each of the cell types. Although expression of TLR mRNA was confirmed in these cells (**Figure S1**) as previously reported, TLR 1-9 agonism did not affect 11β-HSD1 mediated cortisol production in either of the corneal cell types (**Figure 1C**).

TLR induction of cytokines by human corneal epithelial cells and fibroblasts

As previous literature had analyzed only specific cytokine production by these cells after TLR stimulation, we wished to address a wider cytokine profile using multiplex technology in order to interrogate GR signaling pathways in more detail. Cells were incubated with TLR ligands 1–9 and a "30-plex" multiplex analysis for cytokine and chemokine production was performed. Although synthesis of TNFα increased after TLR 1, 4, 7, and 9 stimulation of PHCEC this was not significant (**Figure S2**), and the epithelial cells were relatively specific to TLR3 challenge only, producing a large spectrum of cytokines and chemokines (CCL2, IL6, CXCL-10, IL12, CCL3, CCL4, IFNγ, IFNβ, and CCL5) (**Figure 2A**). By contrast, PHKF were weakly responsive to TLR stimulation showing increased expression of CCL2, IL-6, CXCL8, G-CSF CCL5 and CXCL-10. However none of these responses reached significance. (**Figure S2**).

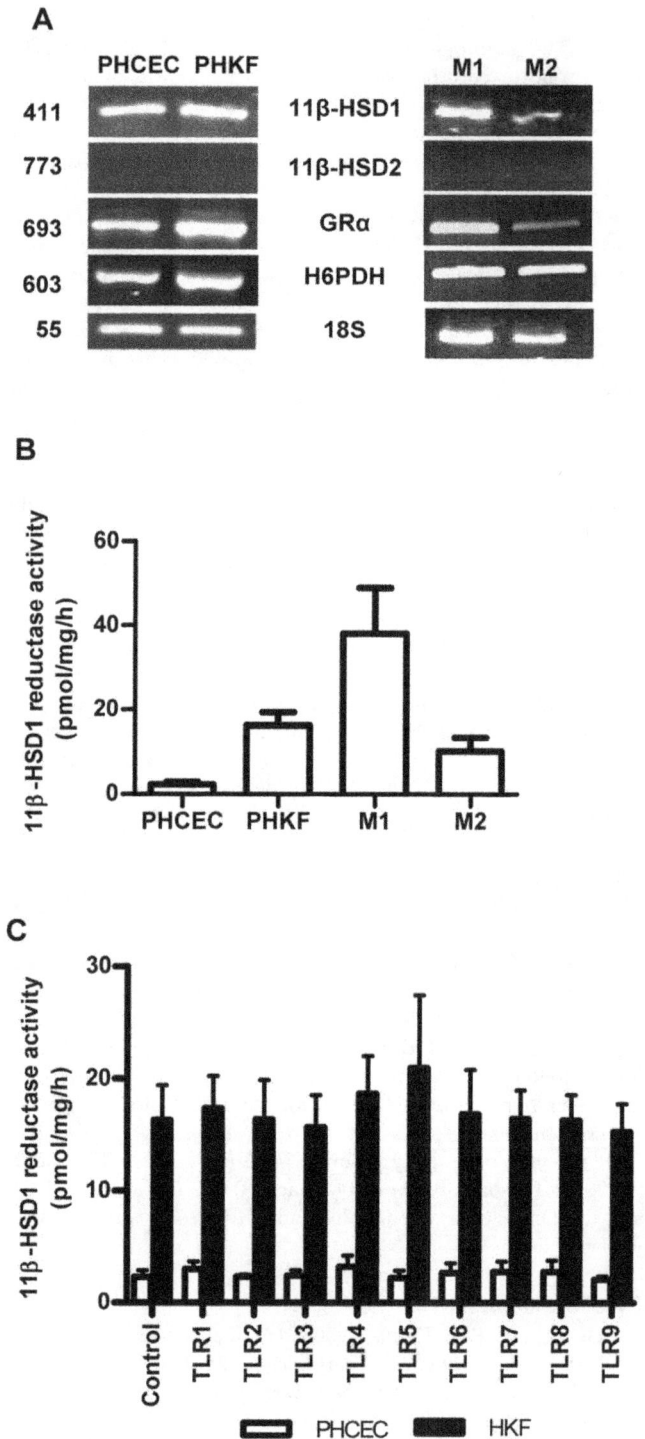

Figure 1. Pre-receptor regulation of glucocorticoids and TLR expression in human corneal cells. (A) RT-PCR of PHCEC, PHKF showing expression of the major genes for the pre-receptor regulation of glucocorticoids: 11β-HSD1, 11β-HSD2, H6PD and GR. Macrophages, M1 and M2, also express 11β-HSD1 but not 11β-HSD2. All cell types demonstrate 11β-HSD1 oxo-reductase activity (B), most marked in M1 macrophages. (C) TLR 1–9 induction did not alter 11β-HSD1 activity in either PHCEC or PHKF after stimulation for 16 h.

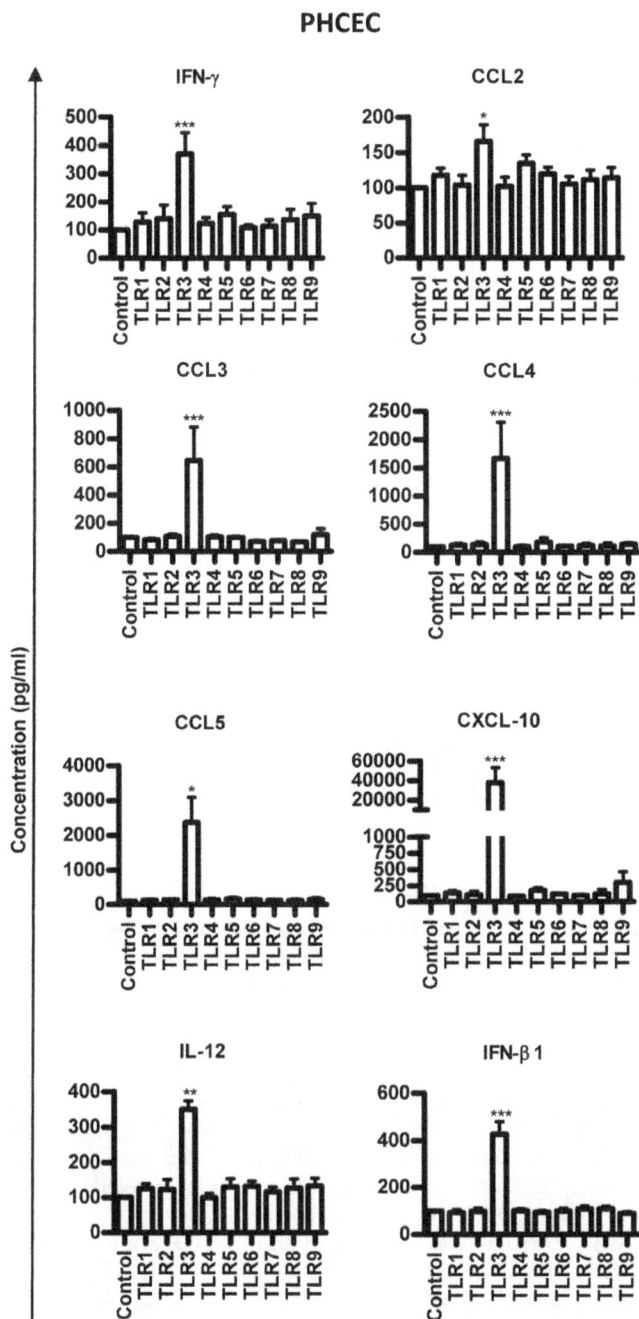

Figure 2. Human corneal cells respond to TLR stimulation by producing cytokines. Multiplex bead ELISA analysis (Plex-30) of cytokine production in response to TLR 1–9 stimulation for 16 hours is shown. Cytokines analysed included: IL-1β, IL-1Rα, IL-2, IL-4, IL-5, IL-6, IL-7, IL-8, IL-9, IL-10, IL-12(p70), IL-13, IL-15, IL-17, Eotaxin, Basic FGF, G-CSF, GM-CSF, IFN-γ, CXCL-10, CCL2, CCL3, CCL4, PDGF-BB, CCL5, TNF-α, VEGF. Induction of a range of cytokines and chemokines was seen after TLR 3 challenge (CCL2, CCL3, CCL4, CCL5, CXCL10, IL1, IFNγ and IFNβ). Values = Mean+SE, n = 3, Statistical analysis was carried using One-way ANOVA and comparisons were drawn with untreated control Vs TLR stimulated cells. * $p<0.05$, ** $p<0.01$, *** $p<0.001$.

Glucocorticoid control of cytokine production by corneal cells

Having identified that TLR3 and TLR4 stimulation of PHCEC and PHKF produced maximal production of most cytokines and chemokines we went on to assess the effects of natural and synthetic glucocorticoids (cortisol and dexamethasone respectively) on this process using multiplex bead analysis. The results are expressed as fold change to compare the two treatments with controls. Both cortisol and dexamethasone inhibited VEGF, CCL5, IFNγ, CXCL-10, CXCL8 and G-CSF production by PHKF (**Figure 3**) but no change in the other cytokines measured. There was no change any of the measured cytokines in PHCEC. (**Figure S3**)

Monocyte/Macrophage infiltration in human keratitis

The interplay between infiltrating monocytes/macrophages and corneal cells was examined. Immunohistochemistry of the normal human central corneal tissue showed no evidence of CD68+ve resident macrophages, and only basal TLR3 or no TLR4 expression. Stromal infiltration of CD68+ve positive cells was seen in both herpetic and gram-negative keratitis sections (**Figure 4A**), associated with TLR3 and TLR4 expression in the corneal epithelium, respectively. The response was most pronounced in gram-negative keratitis.

To determine if inflammatory cell infiltration into infected corneas was mediated by PHCEC and PHKF cytokines after TLR3 and TLR4 ligation, migration assays were performed. Supernatants from three different donor PHCEC cultures treated with TLR3 ligand poly I:C, induced migration of human monocytes generated from (i) one PBMC donor ((127±19% (mean±SE) increase in migration compared with control **Figure 4B**: PHCEC-S), and (ii) with one culture supernatant from one corneal donor tested on 4 different monocyte donors (127±24% increase **Figure 4C**: PHCEC-D). A similar effect was seen when PHKF were stimulated by poly I:C (**Figure 4D**: PHKF-S and - **Figure 4E**: PHKF-D (117±7% and 114±11% respectively)). Importantly, LPS (TLR4) stimulation of PHKF produced supernatants that induced potent monocyte migration in both experiments (**Figure 4D and E** 254±41% for PHKF-S and 242±10.8% for PHKF-D p<0.01) supporting immunohistochemistry data, while the effect on PHCEC was weaker (**Figure 4B and C** - 87±13% for PHCEC-S and 87±16% for PHCEC-D respectively). These results show a differential chemotactic potential to TLR induction between PHCEC and PHKF.

Corneal cell supernatant control of macrophage cortisol production

As TLR stimulation of corneal cells induced differential rates of monocyte chemotaxis, we investigated whether the cumulative inflammatory response was a candidate for regulating macrophage intracrine cortisol bioavailability. There was a marked depletion of macrophage cortisol synthesis after TLR3 challenge of both PHCEC (−30%) and PHKF (−40%) (supernatants taken from the migration experiments described above), and after TLR4 challenge (PHCEC −10%; PHKF −20%) (**Figure 4F**). These data indicate that net cortisol biosynthesis is attenuated after activation of innate signaling pathways in the ocular surface.

Relationship between glucocorticoid hormone metabolites in human ocular biofluids, in health and disease

Having demonstrated that corneal cells in vitro have 11β-HSD1 oxoreductase activity and that macrophage cortisol bioavailability was inhibited following incubation with TLR stimulated corneal cell supernatant, which could occur during chemotaxis, we sought to investigate whether the human OcS, in vivo, was capable of synthesizing cortisol from cortisone in healthy eyes and during

A   PHKF

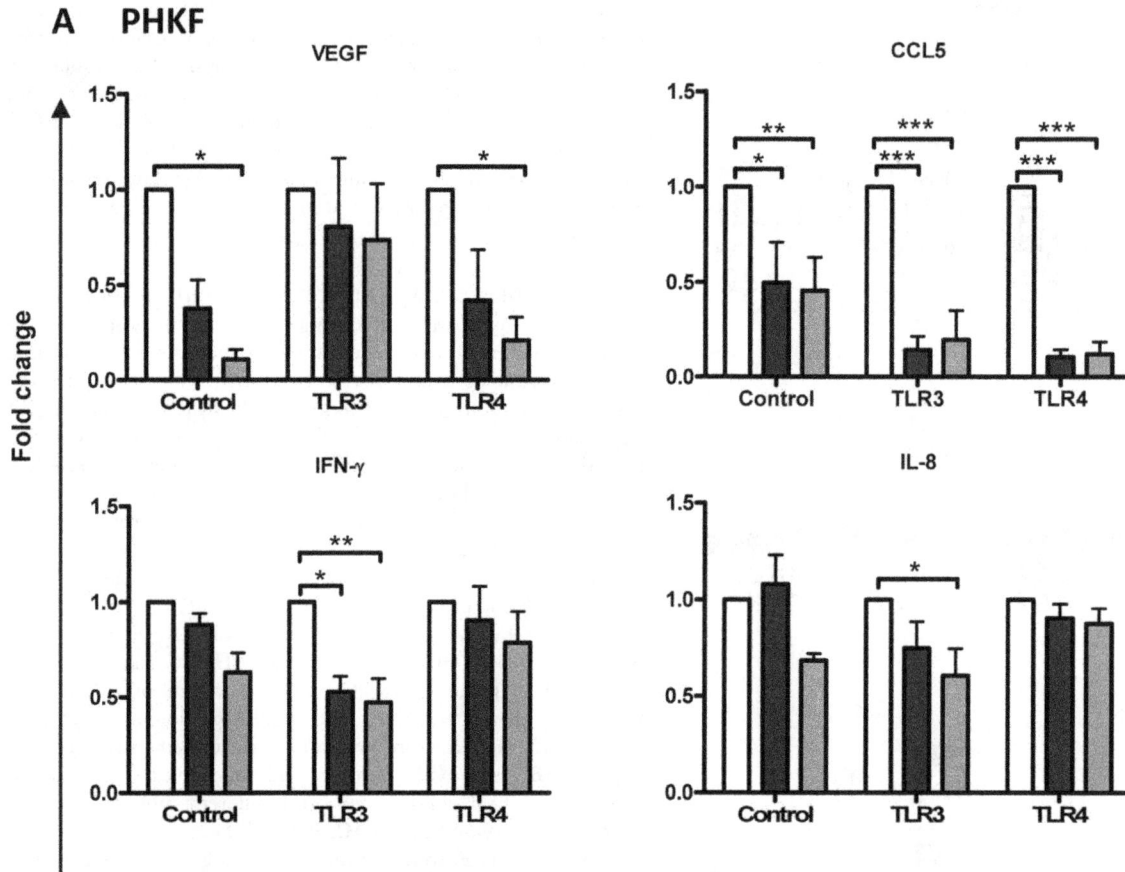

Figure 3. Regulation of cytokine production with Cortisol/Dexamethasone on TLR3 or TLR4 stimulated Primary Human Corneal Fibroblasts (PHKF). Both cortisol (■, black square) and dexamethasone (■, gray square) reduced cytokines: VEGF, CCL5, IFN-γ, CXCL-10, IL-8 and GCSF (B) after either or both TLR 3 and 4 stimulation of PHKF. (Values = Mean+SE, normalising to No Cortisol/Dexamethasone (□, white square) for each treatment n = 3; Statistical analysis 2-way ANOVA with Bonferroni post-test; *p<0.05, **p<0.01, ***p<0.001).

active infective keratitis or putative TLR 3 mediated OcSD disease. We used a highly sensitive technique of LC/MS/MS and quantified GC metabolites in human ocular biofluid compartments as surrogates for OcS (tears) and intraocular (AqH) steroidogenesis, versus peripheral blood (serum).

(i) Normal healthy eyes. Both cortisone and cortisol were detected in all three bio-fluid compartments in the proportion serum = tears>AqH   and   serum>tears = AqH,   respectively (**Figure 5 A–B**). No gender difference was observed. Both ocular biofluids showed positive correlation between cortisone and cortisol levels, AqH (r = 0.98, p<0.0001, **Figure 5C**) and tears (r = 0.79, p<0.001, **Figure 5D**), but there was no correlation between serum cortisol and cortisone versus that found in tears or AqH (**Figure 5E–H**) indicating that simple diffusion from the peripheral circulation into the tear film and AqH was not likely to be the main source of these hormones. Cortisone and cortisol levels were consistently higher in tears versus AqH where a positive correlation was observed between tear cortisol vs AqH cortisol (r = 0.79, p<0.003) (**Figure 5I–J**), suggesting that the tear film may be the driver for AqH cortisol, delivering either active cortisol into the anterior chamber or substrate (cortisone) for intraocular 11β-HSD1. The cortisol:cortisone ratio (a marker of 11β-HSD1 oxo-reductase activity) showed cortisol:cortisone ratios in AqH (3:1) exceeded those in tears (1:1) in healthy individuals (**Figure 5K**). These data suggest greater 11β-HSD1 activity

within the eye than on the surface of the eye in normal physiological states. There was no relationship between age or gender on cortisol or cortisone levels, or cortisol:cortisone ratios, in each of the ocular bio-fluids (**Figure S4A (cortisol), S4B (cortisone), S4C (cortisol:cortisone)**).

(ii) Infective keratitis and immune-mediated ocular surface disease. Having established that the healthy human OcS is capable of generating cortisol from cortisone *in vivo*, and that *in vitro* induction of TLR3 and TLR4 in PHCEC and PHKF triggered pro-inflammatory cytokine production with subsequent macrophage migration and abrogation of immune-cells cortisol biosynthesis, we sought to establish whether the tear film glucocorticoid profile was altered in patients with untreated herpetic and pseudomonas keratitis presenting to the emergency room, and those patients with chronic immune-mediated ocular surface inflammatory disease. These data showed that the mean (±SEM) free cortisol in healthy volunteer tear film 85.6(0–1306.2) nM/L was lower than in patients with acute herpes simplex keratitis (288.1(136.5–434.1) nM/L) and pseudomonas keratitis (223.0 (154.9–418.6) nM/L). These data equated to cortisol:cortisone ratios of 1.33(0.39–131.3) in the healthy tear film versus 0.33(0.0–0.50) (p<0.01) in patients with pseudomonas keratitis and 1.42(0.12–6.44) (p = 0.42) in herpes simplex keratitis (**Figure 6**), confirming an attenuation of OcS cortisol biosynthesis (and 11β-HSD1 activity) *in vivo* during active OcS pseudomonas

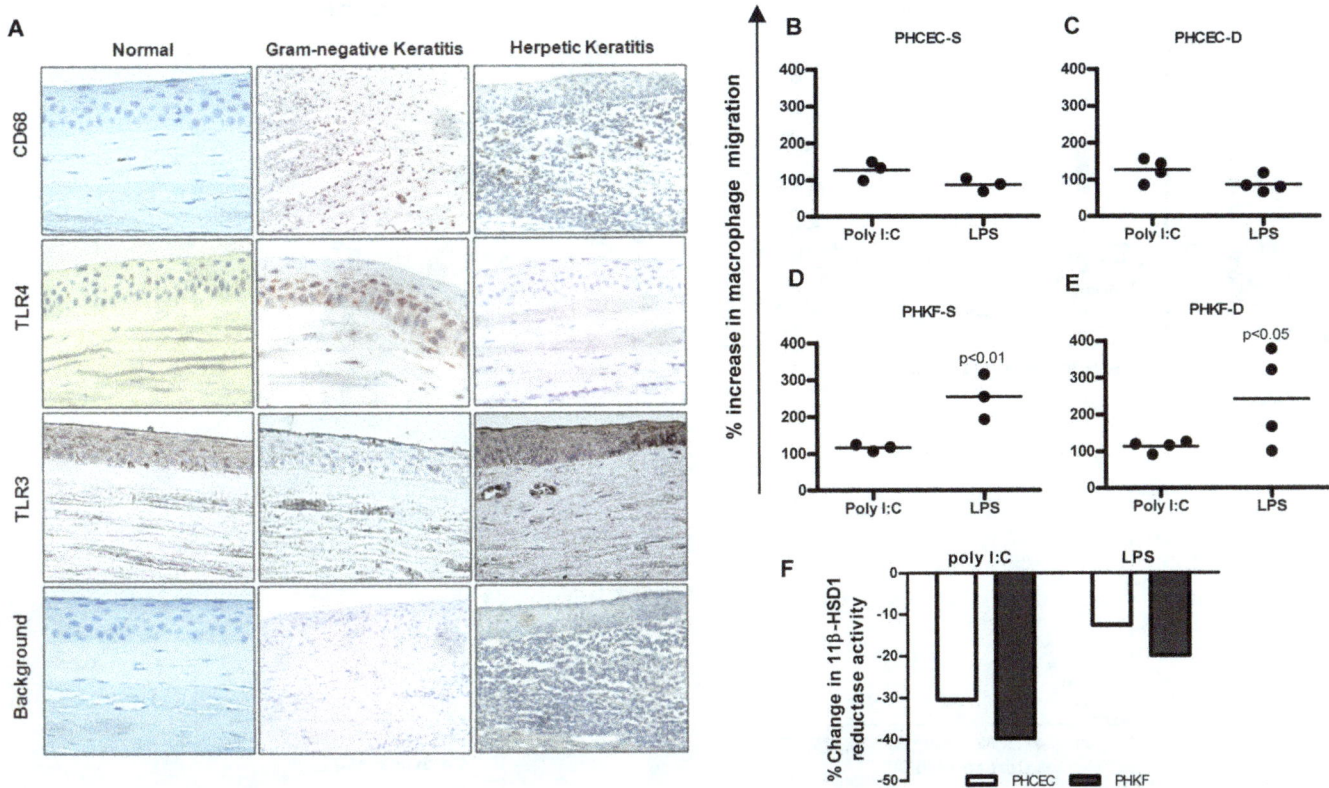

Figure 4. Macrophage infiltration in human keratitis. (A) Immunohistochemistry of the normal human central corneal epithelium showed no evidence of CD68 positive resident macrophages or basal TLR4 expression, although there was some basal TLR3 expression. Corneal stromal infiltration of CD68 positive cells is seen in both herpetic and gram negative keratitis associated with increased TLR3 and TLR4 expression in the corneal epithelium, respectively. (B–E) Migration assay showing culture supernatants of corneal cells having chemotactic potential on monocytes. Cell supernatants from PHCEC/PHKF stimulated with TLR3 (poly I:C) or TLR4 (LPS) ligands for 16 h were tested for the ability to induce monocyte migration. 'S' denotes culture supernatants from PHCEC/PHKF cultures generated from 3 corneal donors, tested on a single allogenic PBMC donor. 'D' denotes 3 different PBMC donors subjected to culture supernatant from a single donor derived PHCEC/PHKF treated with TLR3 and TLR4 ligands. Data show that both LPS and Poly I:C stimulation of corneal cells induce monocyte migration but LPS stimulation of PHKF has the greatest chemotactic potential. (Panels D and E). (F) Culture supernatants from experiments A–D (TLR3 and TLR4 induction of PHCEC/PHKF for 16 h) downregulates M1 macrophage 11β-HSD1 activity. Statistical analysis was carried using one-way ANOVA and comparisons were drawn with untreated control cells vs. TLR3/TLR4 treated cells.

infection (supporting *in vitro* data (**Figure 4E**)). By contrast, cortisol:cortisone ratios were increased in patients with chronic (putative TLR 3 regulated) immune-mediated OcS disease states (OcMMP, 9.05(0.9–20.7); SJS/TEN, 113.8(11.73–1070.0 ($p<0.01$) (**Figure 6**).

Discussion

In the human eye, the ocular surface provides the first line of defense to potential exogenous triggers, but is also a target for autoimmune disease. The surface is a non-keratinized mucosa with a unique avascular component known as the cornea, critical for refracting light and for sight. The cornea is considered to be an immune privileged site exhibiting both immunological ignorance, but also a range of active immunosuppression mechanisms [29] that infer a 90% 5 year survival rate of low risk corneal allografts [30,31]. Several pathways have been purported to be involved in the immune-privileged status of the eye including a range of systemic and neural factors, in addition to local intraocular mechanisms such as soluble immunosuppressive agents in the aqueous humour [α-melanocyte stimulating hormone (αMSH), vasoactive intestinal peptide (VIP), transforming growth factor-β2 (TGF-β2), IL-1Rα, somatostatin, cortisol][32–34] or cell surface

molecules (CD95-L, B7H1, MHC Class Ib, CD46, CD55, CD59) [35].

Adrenal hormones are known to be regulators of ocular surface health and dry eye induced inflammation [36–40]. Our previous work has indicated that endogenous production of GCs mediated by the isozyme 11β-HSD1 may also be a contributing factor, specifically ocular surface renewal and putative barrier function [3,15]. 11β-HSD1 is involved in several disease processes including insulin resistance, osteoporosis, obesity, idiopathic intracranial hypertension, glaucoma, orbital adipogenesis, inflammation and immune cell function [3,28,32,41–43].

While a small resident population of myeloid cells populate the central cornea [44], critical to clearing infection is the recruitment of phagocytes (macrophages and iDCs) to the site of infection and these cells too, appear to be mediated in part, by local cortisol. There is an enhanced ability of myeloid-derived immune cells to produce cortisol after TLR-induced maturation signals. This is associated with an increased expression of MHC class I and class II, CD40L and synthesis of pro-inflammatory cytokines, leading to inflammation at the site of infection [20]. Conversely, maturation of iDCs induced by CD40 ligation not only leads to a fall in the ability of DCs to produce cortisol, differentiation of DCs from

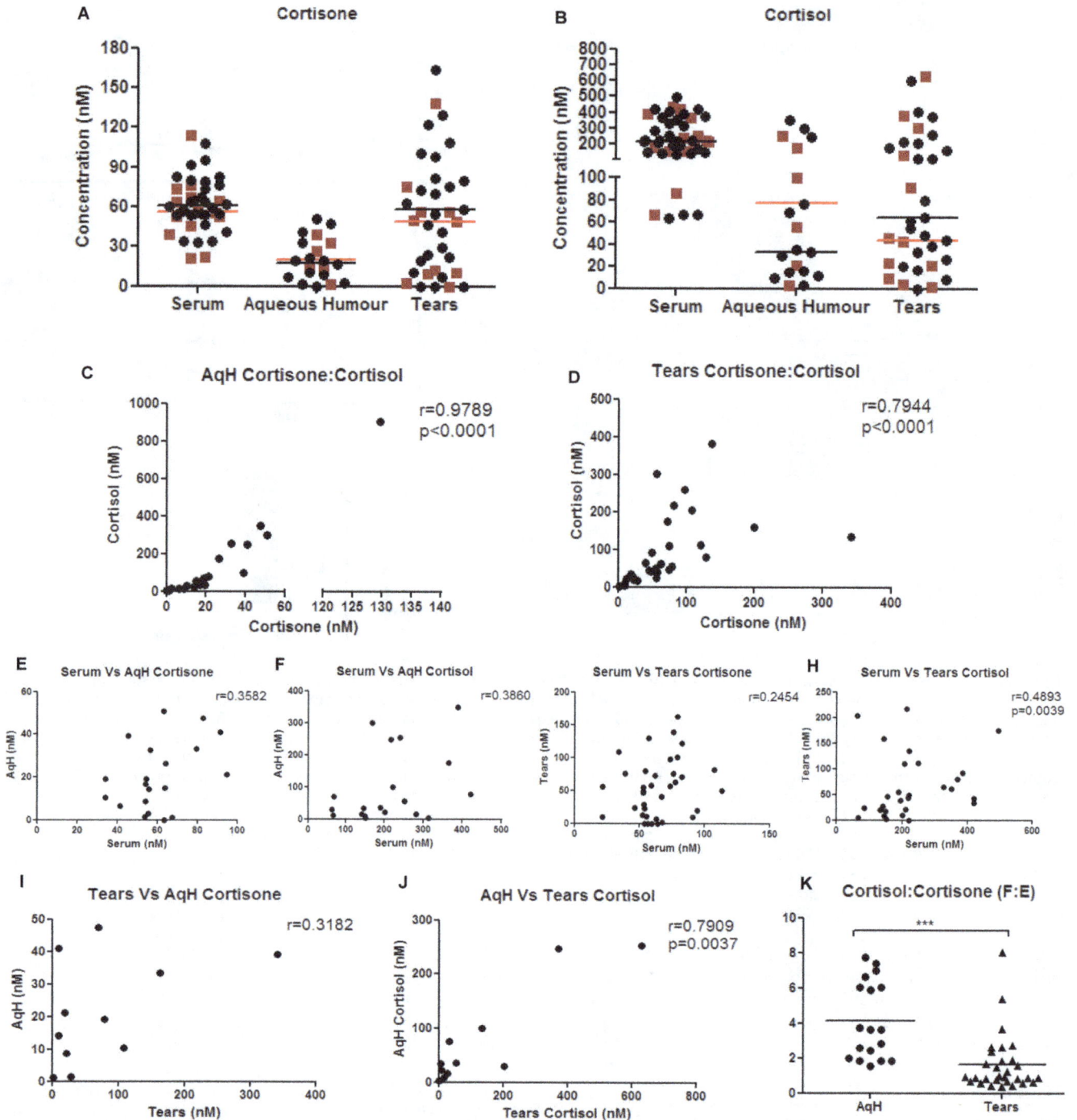

Figure 5. Hormones detected in human ocular biofluids versus serum. A) Cortisone and (B) cortisol levels in the tear film and AqH. There was no gender dependency for any of the analyte (● black circle, Male and (■ red square, Female)). There was a positive correlation between cortisol and cortisone in both ocular biofluids (C–D), but concentrations were largely independent of those found in serum (E–H). There was an association between AqH and Tear film cortisone (I) and cortisol (J), and cortisol:cortisone (F:E) ratios were consistently higher in AqH versus the tear film (K).

monocyte precursors is inhibited by physiological concentrations of cortisone, indicating that inactive GC acts as an autocrine-negative regulator of DC maturation thereby imposing a checkpoint on differentiation of monocytes to mature DCs [24,25].

In this study, we examined the tissue-specific cortisol regulation by human corneal cells in the context of immune responses to TLR ligation, and how this could have impact on clinical disease.

Both PHCEC and PHKF cells were shown to express major components of the glucocorticoid pre-receptor signaling pathways consistent with earlier human and rabbit studies [3,14]. These cells were capable of producing cortisol, although the rate of conversion was less than that of M1 and M2 macrophages. In our study, TLR ligation in vitro did not alter cortisol bioavailability but elicited cell-specific cytokine and chemokine release, including TNFα only

Tears Cortisol:Cortisone

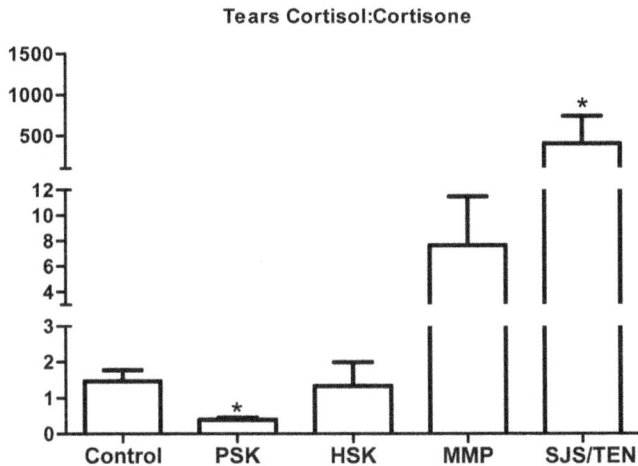

Figure 6. Ocular surface glucocorticoid bioavailability in health and disease. Evaluation of tear film glucocorticoid profiles as surrogate readouts of net ocular surface glucocorticoid bioavailability, defines cortisol depletion (reduced cortisol:cortisone (F:E ratio, mean±SE) during active untreated pseudomonas keratitis (PSK) but not herpes simplex keratitis (HSK), and amplification during chronic clinically quiescent immune-mediated disease (MMP, mucous membrane pemphigoid; SJS/TEN, Stevens-Johnson Syndrome/Toxic-epidermal Necrolysis). Statistical analysis performed using t-test with two-tailed Mann Whitney post -test. * = P<0.05.

after TLR 1, 4, 7, and 9 stimulation of PHCEC; and CCL2, IL-6, CXCL8, G-CSF after TLR 1–8 stimulation of PHKF. Cytokine induction however, was regulated by the presence of synthetic (dexamethasone) and natural (cortisol) GCs in PHKF only, but only TNFα in PHCEC. This dichotomy is of interest, and the relative resistance of PHCEC to glucocorticoids is the focus of future study.

Stimulation of PHCEC with TLR ligands showed that only poly I:C could induce multi-cytokine synthesis. The range of molecules produced, include proinflammatory cytokines IL-12 and IFNγ indicative of a Th1 mediated adaptive response, chemokines CCL3, CCL4, and CCL5 that are associated with mononuclear cell recruitment, and IFNβ that has both antiviral and immunosuppressive function. There is a particularly strong increase in CXCL10 production after ligation of TLR 3 in both cell types and also TLR4 in HKF. This is of interest as this cytokine has pleiotropic function including angiostasis due to its lacking an ELR motif (Glu-Leu-Arg tripeptide sequence). In CXCL10 deficient mice, an increase in liver fibrosis is seen due to inhibition of natural killer cells (NK) which target hepatic stellar cells [45]. In murine corneal infection with Herpes simplex virus, depletion of NK cells leads to loss of viral control [46]. As TLR3 recognizes double-stranded RNA these data support an inductive role for PHCEC in response to infection or possibly TLR3 related immune-mediated disease e.g. SJS-TEN, dry eye disease states, may induce an increase in CXCL10 and a reduction in NK cells exacerbating infection or persistence of inflammation. With the exception of TNFα, the failure of other TLR ligands to induce cytokines by PHCEC has been suggested to be due to the intracellular expression of TLR2 and TLR4 in PHCEC, receptors that are normally expressed on the cell surface [47]. It is also possible that PHCEC do not have the co-receptors necessary for TLR signaling, although CD14 expression has been reported [48]. This relative inertness of the corneal epithelium may be a contributory factor to barrier function, and it is possible that

breaches of this barrier are required to trigger resident stromal keratocytes to differentiate into an activated fibroblast phenotype with subsequent wider cytokine response, as shown in our study. Activated fibroblasts may therefore represent sentinels for ocular surface inflammation. Regardless, the stimulation of TLR3 strongly suggests and supports the concept that the human OcS produces a vigorous immune response possibly underpinning reactivation of viral keratitis and exacerbations of inflammation in chronic OcS immune-mediated disease [18,21–23].

Responses in PHKF to TLR ligands were inhibited by the addition of exogenous glucocorticoids. Unlike monocyte–derived cells [24,49]. TLR stimulation had no effect on cortisol biosynthesis by PHCEC or PHKF. By comparison, blood-derived macrophages, particularly M1 cells showed 3-fold greater production of cortisol compared to ocular cells. These data suggest that infiltrating inflammatory (M1) macrophages are capable of controlling not only their own inflammatory processes, but also ocular surface cytokine production via paracrine cortisol control. While endogenous cortisol has been shown in several studies to down-regulate MHC class II, co-stimulatory molecules (CD80, CD86) and the ability to activate allogeneic cells, inhibition of endogenous cortisol can also lead to a reduction in IL-1 and TNFα. A recent study has shown that IL-17 may orchestrate resolution of innate inflammation, whereas IFN-γ and IL-4 may represent major determinants of IL-10 and glucocorticoid resistance [50].

The potential role of cortisol produced by corneal cells versus that produced by infiltrating macrophages is of considerable interest [51–54]. The differing response to TLR induction between ocular surface epithelial cells and macrophages may be an element of silencing induced by coexistent protective commensal bacteria, a mechanism seen in the gut vital intestinal homeostasis [55]. Breaches in intestinal epithelial cell cross-communication with gut flora provide the basis of inflammatory bowel disease and this may be relevant in driving ocular surface disease pathogenesis.

Using the novel technique of LC/MS/MS we have been able to detect cortisol and cortisone levels in human ocular bio-fluids as functional readouts of tissue specific regulation of cortisol. Overall, cortisol levels were greater than those reported in other bio-fluids such as CSF [28], saliva [56] and skin microdialysis [57]. Cortisol concentrations at the ocular surface consistently exceeded those in the intraocular aqueous humor amongst healthy human subjects in a consistent pattern of expression (serum>tears>AqH) with no gender variations observed. Correlations of cortisol in ocular bio-fluids versus those found in serum, confirmed that ocular cortisol was potentially independent of circulatory cortisol. By contrast, intraocular cortisol and cortisone correlated with that on the ocular surface (consistently tears>AqH). Cortisol:cortisone (F:E) ratios (an in vivo biomarker of 11β-HSD1 enzyme activity) were greater within aqueous humor than in the tear film. These data indicate that the OcS cortisol-cortisone shuttle may be the driver for intraocular cortisol, either by delivering cortisol directly into the anterior chamber of the eye or substrate for 11β-HSD1. In patients with acute presentation of pseudomonas keratitis, the net ocular surface cortisol:cortisone ratios were significantly reduced, suggesting either an abrogation of cortisol is required to allow inflammatory cell migration to eradicate infection, or an increased utilization of cortisol in an acute bacterial disease state. These data supported our in vitro findings that demonstrated a reduction in macrophage 11β-HSD1 oxo-reductase activity when challenged by a cytokine cocktail produced by either PHCEC or PHKF induced by TLR4 ligation. It would be interesting to interrogate longitudinal tear film glucocorticoid profiles during clinical disease

A: Normal

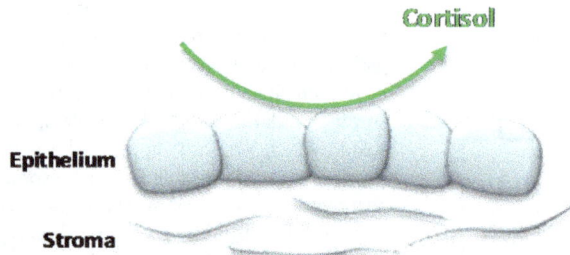

B: TLR3

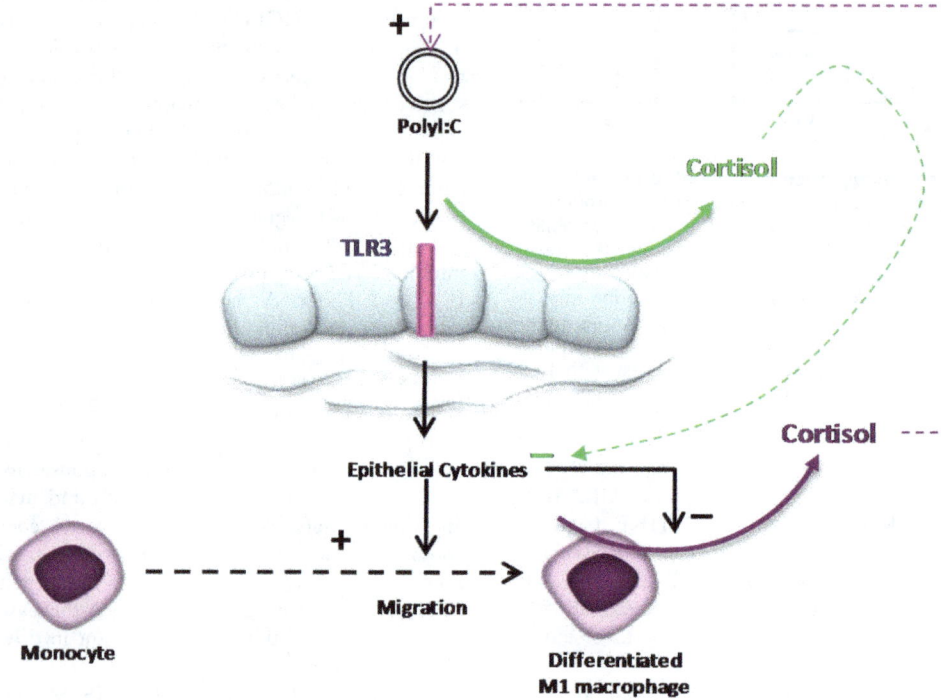

C: TLR4

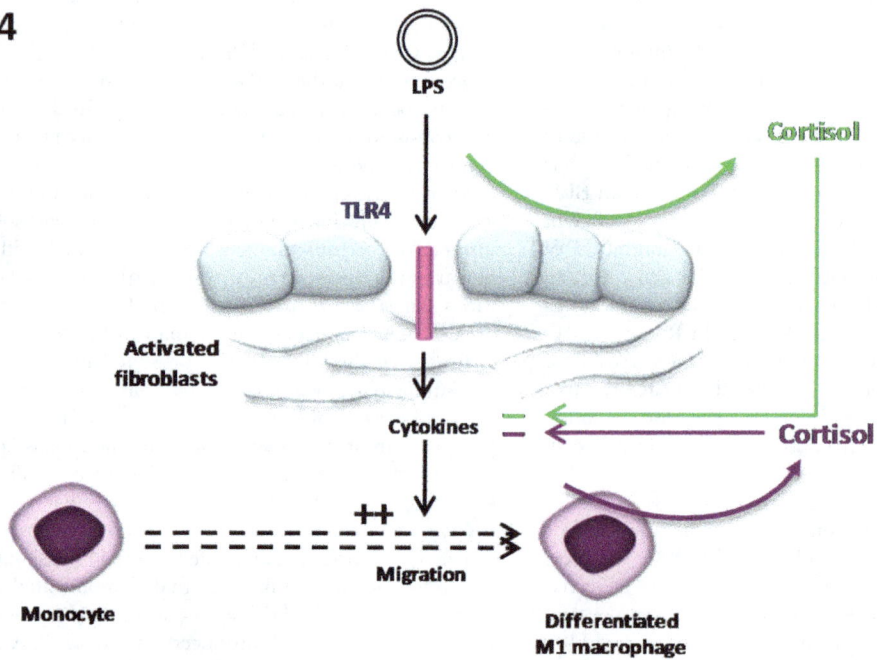

Figure 7. Putative interaction of TLR signaling and local regulation of cortisol in the human cornea. (A) Under physiological conditions, autocrine synthesis of cortisol in corneal epithelial cells contributes to the immunoprotection of the ocular surface mucosa. During induction of ocular surface TLRs cytokines are released in a ligand and cell specific manner. (B) On TLR3 ligation such as chronic immune -mediated disease e.g. SJS-TEN, synthesis of a diverse spectrum of cytokines primarily from the corneal epithelial cells, induces weak monocyte chemotaxis and differentiation to M1 macrophages. These cytokines potently attenuate M1 cortisol biosynthesis leading to a net reduction of ocular surface cortisol levels, promoting recruitment of inflammatory cells necessary for resolving the initial trigger. By contrast, on TLR4 ligation (C) activation of keratocytes to a fibroblast phenotype, form the first line of defense producing chemokines that potently induce monocyte migration to the site of infection for rapid eradication of bacterial invasion. Attenuation of M1 cortisol production is less pronounced and this facilitates resolution of the inflammatory response, limiting tissue damage thereby preserving optical clarity (and sight).

course, to determine whether specific profile patterns correlate with the sterilization and healing phases of infective corneal disease. Although there appeared to be no change in net tear film cortisol:cortisone ratios in patients with untreated herpes simplex keratitis, there was a marked intensification of cortisol compared to cortisone in patients with chronic immune-mediated disease states not using local or systemic therapeutic glucocorticoids. TLR3 is an integral player in chronic SJS-TEN [23], experimental inflammatory dry eye [19] and hypersensitivity responses in the conjunctiva [58]. While the local regulation of cortisol is clearly important in physiological and innate immune responses in the eye, the role is multifaceted and the mechanisms underpinning therapeutic glucocorticoid use is highly complex. The data though intriguing is based on small numbers of patients with each disease and further investigation is necessary to explore these data further, with the potential for longitudinal studies an important consideration

In summary, we have shown that intracrine cortisol biosynthesis in human corneal cells is independent of TLR activation and is likely to afford immuno-protection under physiological conditions (**Figure 7A**). During microbial or immune-mediated challenge, release of cytokines from these cells, trigger migration of monocytes and differentiation to macrophages that in turn are capable of generating large quantities of cortisol that contribute to resolution of the local inflammatory response thereby maintaining optical clarity (**Figures 7B and C**). Nevertheless, *in vivo*, the net OcS cortisol measured in the tear film is dependent on the nature of the OcS disease and a reduction in acute infection or an increase during chronic immune-mediated disease, is observed. These data indicate that OcS generation of cortisol contributes to ocular mucosal innate responses, but its role is complex and dependent on the cell type and nature of the underlying immunological challenge.

Supporting Information

Figure S1 Expression of TLRs in Primary Corneal Cells. PHCEC expressed TLR1, TLR2, TLR3, TLR4 and TLR10 mRNA, while PHKF expressed mRNA for TLR 1–4, and TLR9-10. GAPDH was used as a housekeeping gene and distilled water (DW) alone as the negative control.

Figure S2 Cytokine Expression after TLR Stimulation of Primary Corneal Cells. Multiplex bead ELISA analysis (Plex-30) of cytokine production in PHCEC and PHKF in response to TLR 1–9 stimulation for 16 hours is shown. Cytokines analysed included: IL-1β, IL-1Rα, IL-2, IL-4, IL-5, IL-6, IL-7, IL-8, IL-9, IL-10, IL-12(p70), IL-13, IL-15, IL-17, Eotaxin, Basic FGF, G-CSF, GM-CSF, IFN-γ, CXCL-10, CCL2, CCL3, CCL4, PDGF-BB, CCL5, TNF-α, VEGF. TNFα increased after TLR 1, 4, 7, and 9 stimulation of PHCEC and IL6 after TLR 3. (B) PHKF were variably responsive to TLRs 1–8 producing non-significant induction of G-CSF, CCL2, IL-6, IL-8, CXCL10 and CCL5. Values = Mean+SE, n = 3, Statistical analysis was carried using One-way ANOVA and comparisons were drawn with untreated control Vs TLR stimulated cells.

Figure S3 Effect of Glucocorticoids on the Production of Corneal Cell Cytokine Production. Both Dexamethasone (■, grey square) and cortisol (■, black square) had no effect on the production of the cytokines (VEGF, CCL2, IL-6, IL-12, GCSF, IFN-Y,CXCL10, IL-8) after TLR 3 and 4 stimulation in PHCEC. However, for PHKF, the cytokines MCP-1 and Il-6 were over the detection limit and TNF-α and IL-12 were below the detection limit and the effect of cortisol or dexamethasone could not be verified on these cytokines. (Values = Mean+SE, n = 3 normalized to no Cortisol/Dexamethasone □, white).

Figure S4 Correlation studies of glucocorticoid bio-availability in the human eye with age. There was no correlation between cortisol and cortisone and their ratios in both ocular biofluids (Tears or AqH) with age or gender (A–C).

Table S1 Oligonucleotide sequences of PCR primers.

Author Contributions

Conceived and designed the experiments: RS LL GRW EAW PIM SR. Performed the experiments: RS LL JA AET HSS SS. Analyzed the data: RS LL AET SR GRW. Contributed reagents/materials/analysis tools: EAW IJB GPW SS MT PIM SR. Wrote the paper: RS LL GRW SR. Consented patients; anonymized and collected samples: HSS SS.

References

1. Nichols KK, Foulks GN, Bron AJ, Glasgow BJ, Dogru M, et al. (2011) The International Workshop on Meibomian Gland Dysfunction: Executive Summary. Investigative Ophthalmology and Visual Science 52: 1922–1929.
2. Hardy R, Filer A, Cooper M, Parsonage G, Raza K, et al. (2006) Differential expression, function and response to inflammatory stimuli of 11beta-hydroxy-steroid dehydrogenase type 1 in human fibroblasts: a mechanism for tissue-specific regulation of inflammation. Arthritis Research & Therapy 8: R108.
3. Onyimba CU, Vijapurapu N, Curnow SJ, Khosla P, Stewart PM, et al. (2006) Characterisation of the Prereceptor Regulation of Glucocorticoids in the Anterior Segment of the Rabbit Eye. Journal of Endocrinology 190: 483–493.
4. Flammer JR, Rogatsky I (2011) Minireview: Glucocorticoids in Autoimmunity: Unexpected Targets and Mechanisms. Molecular Endocrinology: 1075–1086.
5. Fujishima S-i, Takeda H, Kawata S, Yamakawa M (2009) The relationship between the expression of the glucocorticoid receptor in biopsied colonic mucosa and the glucocorticoid responsiveness of ulcerative colitis patients. Clinical Immunology 133: 208–217.
6. Li X, Zhang F-S, Zhang J-H, Wang J-Y (2010) Negative Relationship Between Expression of Glucocorticoid Receptor-α and Disease Activity: Glucocorticoid Treatment of Patients with Systemic Lupus Erythematosus. The Journal of Rheumatology 37: 316–321.

7. Yakirevich E, Matoso A, Sabo E, Wang LJ, Tavares R, et al. (2011) Expression of the glucocorticoid receptor in renal cell neoplasms: an immunohistochemical and quantitative reverse transcriptase polymerase chain reaction study. Human Pathology In Press, Corrected Proof.

8. Gross KL, Oakley RH, Scoltock AB, Jewell CM, Cidlowski JA (2011) Glucocorticoid Receptor-α Isoform-Selective Regulation of Antiapoptotic Genes in Osteosarcoma Cells: A New Mechanism for Glucocorticoid Resistance. Molecular Endocrinology 25: 1087–1099.

9. Tomlinson JW, Walker EA, Bujalska IJ, Draper N, Lavery GG, et al. (2004) 11β-Hydroxysteroid Dehydrogenase Type 1: A Tissue-Specific Regulator of Glucocorticoid Response. Endocrine Reviews 25: 831–866.

10. Stewart PM (1996) 11β-hydroxysteroid dehydrogenase: implications for clinical medicine. Clinical Endocrinology 44: 493–499.

11. White PC, Mune T, Agarwal AK (1997) 11β-hydroxysteroid dehydrogenase and the syndrome of mineralocorticoid excess. Endocrine Reviews 18: 135–156.

12. Draper N, Walker EA, Bujalska IJ, Tomlinson JW, Chalder SM, et al. (2003) Mutations in the genes encoding 11beta-hydroxysteroid dehydrogenase type 1 and hexose-6-phosphate dehydrogenase interact to cause cortisone reductase deficiency. Nature Genetics 34: 434–439.

13. Rauz S, Walker EA, Murray PI, Stewart PM (2003) Expression and distribution of the serum and glucocorticoid regulated kinase and epithelial sodium channel subunits in the human cornea. Experimental Eye Research 77: 101–108.

14. Rauz S, Walker EA, Shackleton CHL, Hewison M, Murray PI, et al. (2001) Expression and putative role of 11β-hydroxysteroid dehydrogenase isozymes within the human eye. Investigative Ophthalmology and Visual Science 42: 2037–2042.

15. Liu L, Walker EA, Kissane S, Khan I, Murray PI, et al. (2011) Gene Expression and miR Profiles of Human Corneal Fibroblasts in Response to Dexamethasone. Investigative Ophthalmology and Visual Science 52: 7282–7288.

16. Williams GP, Tomlins PJ, Denniston AK, Southworth HS, Sreekantham S, et al. (2013) Elevation of conjunctival epithelial CD45INTCD11b+CD16+CD14-neutrophils in Ocular Stevens-Johnson Syndrome and Toxic Epidermal Necrolysis. Investigative Ophthalmology and Visual Science: doi:10.1167/iovs.1113–11859

17. Li J, Shen J, Beuerman RW (2007) Expression of toll-like receptors in human limbal and conjunctival epithelial cells Molecular Vision 13: 813–822.

18. Ueta M, Hamuro J, Kiyono H, Kinoshita S (2005) Triggering of TLR3 by polyI:C in human corneal epithelial cells to induce inflammatory cytokines. Biochemical and Biophysical Research Communications 331: 285–294.

19. Redfern RL, Patel N, Hanlon S, Farley W, Gondo M, et al. (2013) Toll-Like Receptor Expression and Activation in Mice with Experimental Dry Eye. Investigative Ophthalmology and Visual Science 54: 1554–1563.

20. Carpenter S, O'Neill LAJ (2009) Recent insights into the structure of Toll-like receptors and post-translational modifications of their associated signalling proteins. Biochemical Journal 422: 1–10.

21. Ueta M, Kinoshita S (2010) Innate immunity of the ocular surface. Brain Research Bulletin 81: 219–228.

22. Ueta M, Sotozono C, Inatomi T, Kojima K, Tashiro K, et al. (2007) Toll-like receptor 3 gene polymorphisms in Japanese patients with Stevens-Johnson syndrome. British Journal of Ophthalmology 91: 962–965.

23. Ueta M, Tokunaga K, Sotozono C, Sawai H, Tamiya G, et al. (2012) HLA-A*0206 with TLR3 Polymorphisms Exerts More than Additive Effects in Stevens-Johnson Syndrome with Severe Ocular Surface Complications. PLoS ONE 7: e43650.

24. Freeman L, Hewison M, Hughes SV, Evans KN, Hardie D, et al. (2005) Expression of 11{beta}-hydroxysteroid dehydrogenase type 1 permits regulation of glucocorticoid bioavailability by human dendritic cells. Blood 106: 2042–2049.

25. Gilmour JS, Coutinho AE, Cailhier J-F, Man TY, Clay M, et al. (2006) Local Amplification of Glucocorticoids by 11beta-Hydroxysteroid Dehydrogenase Type 1 Promotes Macrophage Phagocytosis of Apoptotic Leukocytes. J Immunol 176: 7605–7611.

26. Curnow SJ, Falciani F, Durrani OM, Cheung CMG, Ross EJ, et al. (2005) Multiplex Bead Immunoassay Analysis of Aqueous Humor Reveals Distinct Cytokine Profiles In Uveitis. Invest Ophthalmol Vis Sci 46: 4251–4259.

27. Krone N, Hughes BA, Lavery GG, Stewart PM, Arlt W, et al. (2010) Gas chromatography/mass spectrometry (GC/MS) remains a pre-eminent discovery tool in clinical steroid investigations even in the era of fast liquid chromatography tandem mass spectrometry (LC/MS/MS). The Journal of Steroid Biochemistry and Molecular Biology 121: 496–504.

28. Sinclair AJ, Walker EA, Burdon MA, van Beek AP, Kema IP, et al. (2010) Cerebrospinal Fluid Corticosteroid Levels and Cortisol Metabolism in Patients with Idiopathic Intracranial Hypertension: A Link between $11\hat{I}^2$-HSD1 and Intracranial Pressure Regulation? Journal of Clinical Endocrinology and Metabolism 95: 5348–5356.

29. Streilein JW (2003) Ocular immune privilege: therapeutic opportunities from an experiment of nature. Nat Rev Immunol 3: 879–889.

30. Niederkorn JY, Larkin DFP (2010) Immune Privilege of Corneal Allografts. Ocular Immunology and Inflammation 18: 162–171.

31. Hori J (2008) Mechanisms of immune privilege in the anterior segment of the eye: what we learn from corneal transplantation. J Ocul Biol Dis Infor 1: 94–100.

32. Rauz S, Cheung CMG, Wood PJ, Coca-Prados M, Walker EA, et al. (2003) Inhibition of 11β-hydroxysteroid dehydrogenase type 1 lowers intraocular pressure in patients with ocular hypertension. Quarterly Journal of Medicine 96: 481–490.

33. Denniston AK, Kottoor SH, Khan I, Oswal K, Williams GP, et al. (2011) Endogenous Cortisol and TGF-β in Human Aqueous Humor Contribute to Ocular Immune Privilege by Regulating Dendritic Cell Function. The Journal of Immunology 186: 305–311.

34. Denniston AK, Tomlins P, Williams GP, Kottoor S, Khan I, et al. (2012) Aqueous Humor Suppression of Dendritic Cell Function Helps Maintain Immune Regulation in the Eye during Human Uveitis. Investigative Ophthalmology and Visual Science 53: 888–896.

35. Hori J, Vega JL, Masli S (2010) Review of Ocular Immune Privilege in the Year 2010: Modifying the Immune Privilege of the Eye. Ocular Immunology and Inflammation 18: 325–333.

36. Barabino S, Chen Y, Chauhan S, Dana R (2012) Ocular surface immunity: Homeostatic mechanisms and their disruption in dry eye disease. Progress in Retinal and Eye Research Epub ahead of print.

37. Cascallana JL, Bravo A, Page A, Budunova I, Slaga TJ, et al. (2003) Disruption of eyelid and cornea development by targeted overexpression of the glucocorticoid receptor. International Journal of Developmental Biology 47: 59–64.

38. Forsblad-d'Elia H, Carlsten H, Labrie F, Konttinen YT, Ohlsson C (2009) Low Serum Levels of Sex Steroids Are Associated with Disease Characteristics in Primary Sjogren's Syndrome; Supplementation with Dehydroepiandrosterone Restores the Concentrations. Journal of Clinical Endocrinology and Metabolism 94: 2044–2051.

39. Mantelli F, Moretti C, Micera A, Bonini S (2007) Conjunctival mucin deficiency in complete androgen insensitivity syndrome (CAIS). Graefe's Archive for Clinical and Experimental Ophthalmology 245: 899–902.

40. Mostafa S, Seamon V, Azzarolo AM (2012) Influence of sex hormones and genetic predisposition in Sjogren's syndrome: A new clue to the immunopatho-genesis of dry eye disease. Experimental Eye Research 96: 88–97.

41. Tomlinson JW, Bujalska I, Stewart PM, Cooper MS (2000) The role of 11β-hydroxysteroid dehydrogenase in central obesity and osteoporosis. Endocrine Research 26: 711–722.

42. Thieringer R, Grande CBL, Carbin L, Cai T, Wong B, et al. (2001) 11β-hydroxysteroid dehydrogenase type 1 is induced in human monocytes upon differentiation to macrophages. Journal of Immunology 167: 30–35.

43. Tomlinson JW, Durrani OM, Bujalska IJ, Gathercole LL, Tomlins PJ, et al. (2010) The Role of 11β-Hydroxysteroid Dehydrogenase 1 in Adipogenesis in Thyroid-Associated Ophthalmopathy. Journal of Clinical Endocrinology and Metabolism 95: 398–406.

44. Cruzat A, Witkin D, Baniasadi N, Zheng L, Ciolino JB, et al. (2011) Inflammation and the Nervous System: The Connection in the Cornea in Patients with Infectious Keratitis. Investigative Ophthalmology and Visual Science 52: 5136–5143.

45. Hintermann E, Bayer M, Pfeilschifter JM, Luster AD, Christen U (2010) CXCL10 promotes liver fibrosis by prevention of NK cell mediated hepatic stellate cell inactivation. Journal of Autoimmunity 35: 424–435.

46. Frank GM, Buela K-AG, Maker DM, Harvey SAK, Hendricks RL (2012) Early Responding Dendritic Cells Direct the Local NK Response To Control Herpes Simplex Virus 1 Infection within the Cornea. The Journal of Immunology 188: 1350–1359.

47. Zhang J, Xu K, Ambati B, Yu F-SX (2003) Toll-like Receptor 5-Mediated Corneal Epithelial Inflammatory Responses to Pseudomonas aeruginosa Flagellin. Invest Ophthalmol Vis Sci 44: 4247–4254.

48. Song PI, Abraham TA, Park Y, Zivony AS, Harten B, et al. (2001) The Expression of Functional LPS Receptor Proteins CD14 And Toll-Like Receptor 4 in Human Corneal Cells. Invest Ophthalmol Vis Sci 42: 2867–2877.

49. Chapman KE, Gilmour JS, Coutinho AE, Savill JS, Seckl JR (2006) 11[beta]-Hydroxysteroid dehydrogenase type 1—A role in inflammation? Molecular and Cellular Endocrinology 248: 3–8.

50. Zizzo G, Cohen PL (2013) IL-17 Stimulates Differentiation of Human Anti-Inflammatory Macrophages and Phagocytosis of Apoptotic Neutrophils in Response to IL-10 and Glucocorticoids. The Journal of Immunology 190: 5237–5246.

51. Piemonti L, Monti P, Allavena P, Sironi M, Soldini L, et al. (1999) Glucocorticoids Affect Human Dendritic Cell Differentiation and Maturation. The Journal of Immunology 162: 6473–6481.

52. Pan J, Ju D, Wang Q, Zhang M, Xia D, et al. (2001) Dexamethasone inhibits the antigen presentation of dendritic cells in MHC class II pathway. Immunology Letters 76: 153–161.

53. Xia CQ, Peng R, Beato F, Clare-Salzler MJ (2005) Dexamethasone Induces IL-10-Producing Monocyte-Derived Dendritic Cells with Durable Immaturity. Scandinavian Journal of Immunology 62: 45–54.

54. Ishii T, Masuzaki H, Tanaka T, Arai N, Yasue S, et al. (2007) Augmentation of 11[beta]-hydroxysteroid dehydrogenase type 1 in LPS-activated J774.1 macrophages - Role of 11[beta]-HSD1 in pro-inflammatory properties in macrophages. FEBS Letters 581: 349–354.

55. Goto Y, Kiyono H (2012) Epithelial barrier: an interface for the cross-communication between gut flora and immune system. Immunological Reviews 245: 147–163.

14

Extracellular Matrix Protein Lumican Promotes Clearance and Resolution of *Pseudomonas aeruginosa* Keratitis in a Mouse Model

Hanjuan Shao[1]¤, Sherri-Gae Scott[1], Chiaki Nakata[2], Abdel R. Hamad[2], Shukti Chakravarti[1,3,4]*

1 Department of Medicine, Johns Hopkins School of Medicine, Baltimore, Maryland, United States of America, 2 Department of Pathology, Johns Hopkins School of Medicine, Baltimore, Maryland, United States of America, 3 Department of Cell Biology, Johns Hopkins School of Medicine, Baltimore, Maryland, United States of America, 4 Department of Ophthalmology, Johns Hopkins School of Medicine, Baltimore, Maryland, United States of America

Abstract

Lumican is an extracellular protein that associates with CD14 on the surface of macrophages and neutrophils, and promotes CD14-TLR4 mediated response to bacterial lipopolysaccharides (LPS). Lumican-deficient ($Lum^{-/-}$) mice and macrophages are impaired in TLR4 signals; raising the possibility that lumican may regulate host response to live bacterial infections. In a recent study we showed that *in vitro* $Lum^{-/-}$ macrophages are impaired in phagocytosis of gram-negative bacteria and in a lung infection model the $Lum^{-/-}$ mice showed poor survival. The cornea is an immune privileged barrier tissue that relies primarily on innate immunity to protect against ocular infections. Lumican is a major component of the cornea, yet its role in counteracting live bacteria in the cornea remains poorly understood. Here we investigated Pseudomonas aeruginosa infections of the cornea in $Lum^{-/-}$ mice. By flow cytometry we found that 24 hours after infection macrophage and neutrophil counts were lower in the cornea of $Lum^{-/-}$ mice compared to wild types. Infected $Lum^{-/-}$ corneas showed lower levels of the leukocyte chemoattractant CXCL1 by 24–48 hours of infection, and increased bacterial counts up to 5 days after infection, compared to $Lum^{+/-}$ mice. The pro-inflammatory cytokine TNF-α was comparably low 24 hours after infection, but significantly higher in the $Lum^{-/-}$ compared to $Lum^{+/-}$ infected corneas by 2–5 days after infection. Taken together, the results indicate that lumican facilitates development of an innate immune response at the earlier stages of infection and lumican deficiency leads to poor bacterial clearance and resolution of corneal inflammation at a later stage.

Editor: Alexander V. Ljubimov, Cedars-Sinai Medical Center, United States of America

Funding: NIH grant EY11654. The funders had no role in study design, data collection and analysis, decision to publish, or preparation of the manuscript.

* E-mail: schakra1@jhmi.edu

¤ Current address: Anatomy & Neurobiology, School of Medicine, University of California Irvine, Irvine, California, United States of America

Introduction

Lumican is an extracellular matrix proteoglycan that is known to regulate collagen fibril structure and corneal transparency [1,2]. Our recent work and those of others suggest that lumican regulates wound healing and innate immune responses [3–7]. The lumican core protein carries tandem repeats of leucine rich motifs, a feature shared by pathogen recognition receptors [8], that prompted us to investigate recognition of pathogen associated molecular patterns (PAMPs) by lumican [3]. We found that lumican interacts with bacterial lipopolysaccharide (LPS) endotoxins and facilitates host response to LPS. Mice deficient in lumican ($Lum^{-/-}$) were hypo responsive to LPS and compared to wild types showed improved survival in a septic shock model induced by intraperitoneal injection of LPS [3]. LPS sensing is mediated by toll-like receptor (TLR) 4; the sequence of events upon LPS encounter involves its binding to LBP (LPS-binding protein), subsequent binding to CD14, a glycosylphosphatidyl inositol linked adaptor protein, which delivers LPS to MD-2, a soluble protein, complexed to TLR4, causing a conformational change in TLR4, recruitment of cytoplasmic adaptor proteins and signal transduction [8]. We identified binding between lumican and CD14, and determined

that recombinant lumican could rescue LPS signaling in $Lum^{-/-}$ peritoneal macrophages [3,5]. Peritoneal macrophages from lumican knockout mice were also impaired in *in vitro* phagocytosis of gram-negative bacteria in a CD14-dependent mechanism. These LPS signaling deficiencies raise the possibility that challenged with live bacteria, the lumican-null mice may manifest specific host defense susceptibilities.

We have minimally examined lumican functions in a live bacterial infection setting in a lung infection model where the $Lum^{-/-}$ mice showed increased bacterial persistence and poor host survival [5]. In the cornea lumican may have a particularly important and unique role in bacterial defense for two reasons. First, lumican, together with other small leucine-rich repeat proteoglycans (SLRPs), decorin, biglycan, keratocan and collagen types I, III and V, is a major component of the cornea [9]. Second, the cornea relies heavily on innate immune functions for barrier protection as adaptive immunity is restricted to ensure its immune privileged status, limit inflammation and maintain clarity [10,11]. TLR4 and 5 are active regulators of innate immunity in the cornea, and shown to promote infiltration of polymorphonuclear leukocytes or neutrophils (PMN) and macrophages into the stroma, to up regulate cytokines and chemokines, but unabated TLR signals can cause inflammation-associated opacity [12,13]. While lumican has been investigated in the context of sterile LPS keratitis [14,15], its role in host response to live bacterial challenge remains poorly understood.

In the current study we investigated the role of lumican in bacterial keratitis. We selected gram-negative *Pseudomonas aeruginosa* as the bacterium of choice as it is frequently an opportunistic pathogen that causes an ulcerative and vision debilitating keratitis in humans [16]. Predisposing risk factors for bacterial keratitis vary with geographic location; in developing countries it is primarily linked to non-surgical traumas [17], whereas, in the United States it is associated with extended-wear contact lenses [18,19], photorefractive keratectomy and keratoplasty [20–22]. Disruptions in the mucus barrier of the cornea allow *P.aeruginosa* to enter and traverse the corneal epithelium, and reach the stroma. Bacterial encounter elicits an innate immune response from the host that involves toll-like receptor (TLR) 4, 5 and 9 to bacterial lipopolysaccharide endotoxins, flagellin and bacterial DNA, respectively [8,13,23–25]. In *P.aeruginosa* infections of the cornea, tissue damage ensues initially from bacterial activities [26–28], and subsequently from host inflammatory response, inflammatory cell infiltrates, release of proteinases and extracellular matrix (ECM) degradation [16,29]. While many components of the host innate and adaptive immune responses are being investigated in *P.aeruginosa*-keratitis [10], the role of stromal ECM components in this regard is just beginning to be elucidated. Our findings show increased survival of bacteria and un-resolved inflammation with associated bystander corneal tissue damage in infected *Lum*$^{-/-}$ corneas.

Materials and Methods

P. aeruginosa Strains and Growth Conditions

The *P. aeruginosa* strain 19660 (ATCC, Manassas, VA) was used for the murine keratitis model. *P. aeruginosa* strain 808 (gift from Dr. David P. Speert, University of British Columbia and BC Children's Hospital, Canada), which is taken up by the host in a CD14 dependent manner, was used in the *in vitro* killing assays. The *P. aeruginosa* strains were incubated overnight in Cetrimide agar (Fluka Analytical, Sigma-Aldrich) at 37°C. Colonies were washed with 1xPBS and centrifuged at 5000 rpm for 10 minutes, and then resuspended in 1xPBS. Colony forming units (CFU) were quantified by plating dilutions onto Cetrimide agar.

Infection of the Cornea

Lum$^{+/-}$ and *Lum*$^{-/-}$ mice on a C57BL/6J background, 8–10 weeks of age, were generated as we described before [1]. All animals were housed in a specific pathogen-free mouse facility at Johns Hopkins University, according to protocols approved by the Animal Care and Use Committee. Animals were treated in adherence to the ARVO Statement. The *P. aeruginosa* strain 19660 was used for the murine keratitis model. Anesthetized mice (350 mg/Kg bodyweight of 2-2-2 Tribromoethanol or Avertin®, Sigma-Aldrich, St. Louis, MO), were placed under the microscope, and the cornea of the right eye was wounded with three 1 μm incisions with a sterile 26-gauge needle such that the scratches had invaded the top 1/10th of the stroma [30]. We have previously examined incision wounds of the wild type and *Lum*$^{-/-}$ corneas exposed to saline only and found no increase in inflammatory cell infiltration, and basal levels of the cytokines

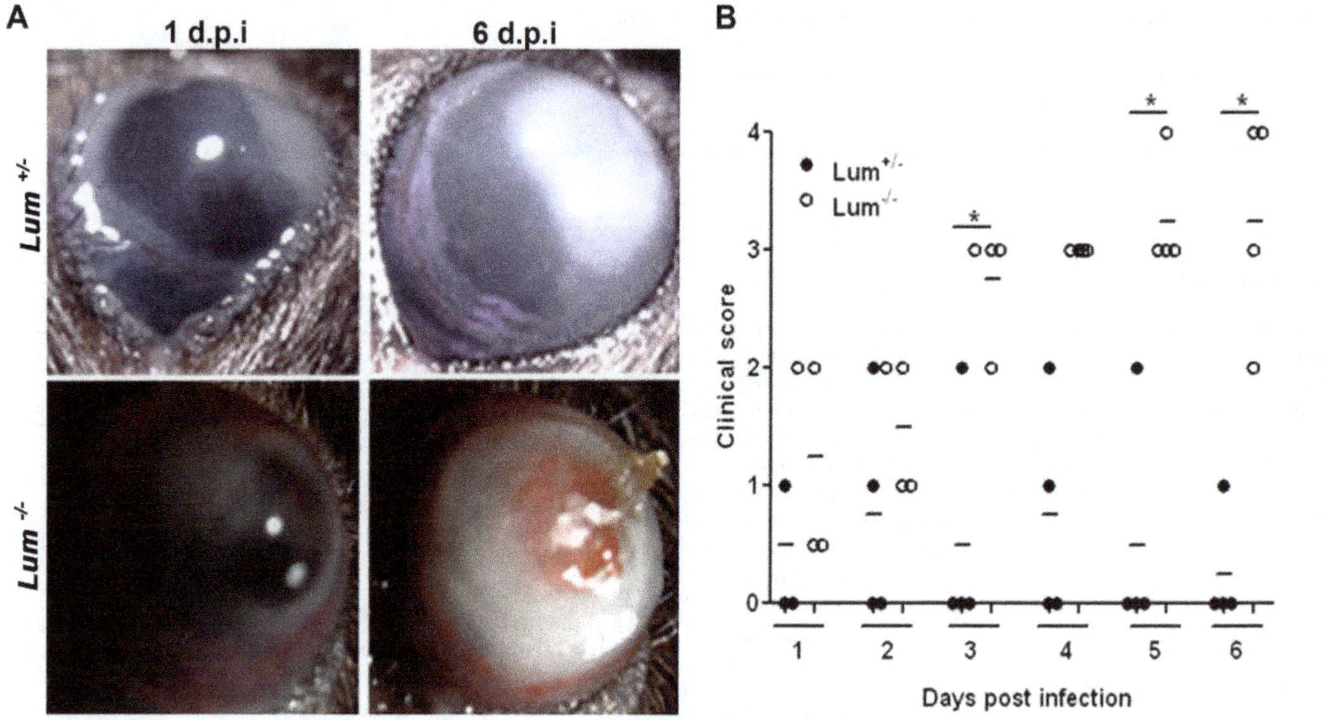

Figure 1. Increased clinical score in *P.aeruginosa* infected *Lum*$^{-/-}$ mice. Mice were infected with 2×10^4 CFU *P.aeruginosa* ATCC19660 in one eye and scored in a blinded manner for 6 days. A representative image of infected eyes 1 and 6 days post infection (d.p.i) shown for each genotype indicates relatively similar severity on day 1 but increased opacity and damage in the *Lum*$^{-/-}$ cornea on 6 d.p.i (A). Daily disease scores (B) of individual animals shows increased average scores for infected *Lum*$^{-/-}$ corneas.* $p\leq0.05$.

A

B

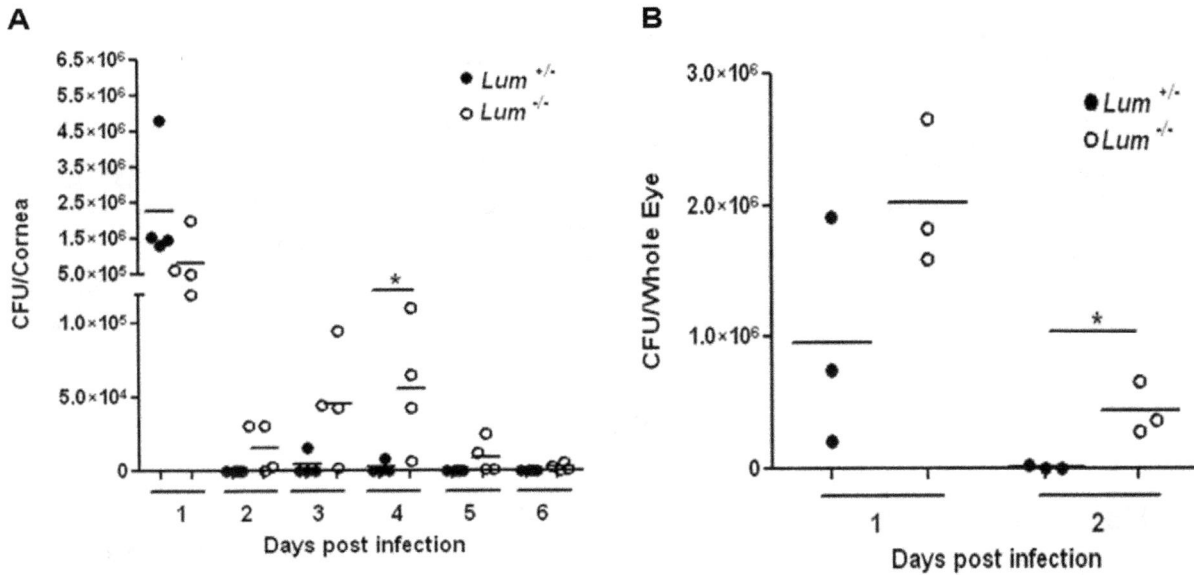

Figure 2. Poor clearance of *P.aeruginosa* in infected *Lum* $^{-/-}$ corneas. Viable bacterial CFU were quantified from infected *Lum* $^{+/-}$ and *Lum* $^{-/-}$ corneas. CFU were higher in ocular surfaces sampled with filter lifts (A) and whole eye homogenates (B) during the infection. Both methods yielded significantly higher CFU counts from *Lum* $^{-/-}$ corneas as shown at day 4 (cornea surface lift) and day 2 (whole eye homogenate). *$p \leq 0.05$.

IL-1β, TNFα and IL-6 [31]in the saline controls. An aliquot of 2×10^4 CFU of *P. aeruginosa* in 5 μL PBS was applied to the scarified cornea, and the mice were undisturbed for 30 min. Mice without any treatment were set as controls. The eyes were inspected microscopically and photographed using a Nikon Eclipse E400 Microscope with a Nikon Digital DXM 1200 Camera.

Corneal disease was scored daily in a blinded manner for 6 days after *P. aeruginosa* infection for each group of mice (3–4 mice for each group) using a scoring mechanism described earlier [32]. Score 0: eye identical with the uninfected contra lateral control eye; Score 1: faint opacity partially covering the pupil; Score 2: dense opacity covering the pupil; Score 3: dense opacity covering the entire anterior segment; Score 4: perforation of the cornea, phthisis bulbi, or both. Slit lamp photography was used to illustrate the disease.

Quantification of Bacteria

Whole eyes were homogenized in 0.5 ml PBS on ice and serial dilutions were plated on Cetrimide Agar plates. After overnight incubation at 37°C, the number of individual colonies on plates was counted and presented as CFU per ml.

Alternatively, the surface of the cornea was sampled for the presence of bacteria in the following way. A sterile filter (2 mm diameter) was placed over the central cornea of anesthetized mice and then resuspended in 300 μL of sterile PBS. Serial 10-fold dilutions of the filter washes were plated to obtain CFU per ml.

Quantitative RT-PCR

Whole corneas from uninfected and infected mice (n = 4 per time point) were harvested and homogenized in 800 μl TRIzol with 5 mm stainless steel beads in a TissueLyser LT small bead mill (Qiagen, Valencia, CA) at 4°C and total RNA was isolated using the Qiagen RNeasy Miniprep Kit. One microgram of each RNA sample was reverse transcribed to cDNA using Superscript II Reverse Transcriptase Kit (Applied Biosystems Life Technologies, Carlsbad, CA). Quantitative RT-PCR was performed with

SYBR Green PCR Master Mix Taqman 7900HT System (Applied Biosystems). We designed the following primers (IDT Integrated DNA Technologies, Coralville, IA) using Primer 3 software for mouse *Cxcl1* 5′-ACTGCACCCAAACCGAAGTC-3′ forward and 5′- CAAGGGAGCTTCAGGGTCAA-3′ reverse, *Lum* 5′-TCGAGCTTGATCTCTCCTAT-3′ forward and 5′-TGGTCCCAGGTCTTACAGAA-3′ reverse, 18S 5′-GTAACCCGTTGAACCCCATT-3′ forward and 5′-CCATC-CAATCGGTAGTAGCG-3′ reverse. Target genes were amplified in 25 μl reaction volume for 1 min at 95°C followed by 40 cycles of 30 seconds at 95°C, 30 seconds at 58°C and 1 min at 72°C and a final extension for 10 min at 72°C. PCR reactions were analyzed in quadruplicate, using the SDS 2.3 software (Applied Biosystems) and mRNA fold changes were calculated after normalizing to 18S RNA.

ELISA Analysis of Cytokines

Total protein was extracted from individual corneas by homogenization using a TissueLyser LT small bead mill for 30 min in 200 μL T-PER (Thermo Scientific Pierce Protein Biology Products, Rockford, IL) and centrifuged at 13,000 rpm for 10 min. Protein concentration of the supernatant was determined by BCA assay (Thermo Fisher Scientific) and the samples were stored in aliquots at −80°C until use. TNF-α, IL-12, IL-1β and CXCL1 concentrations were measured by ELISA (R & D Systems; Minneapolis, MN) according to manufacturer's instructions.

Histology

Whole mouse eyes were harvested and fixed for 48 hrs in fresh 4% Methanol-free Formaldehyde Solution (Thermo Scientific) at room temperature (RT), paraffin – embedded and sectioned. The slides were stained with H&E by the Johns Hopkins Pathology Core. Images were taken in a Zeiss AXIO Observer A1 Microscope (Carl Zeiss) with an Olympus DP72 Camera (Olympus Imaging America).

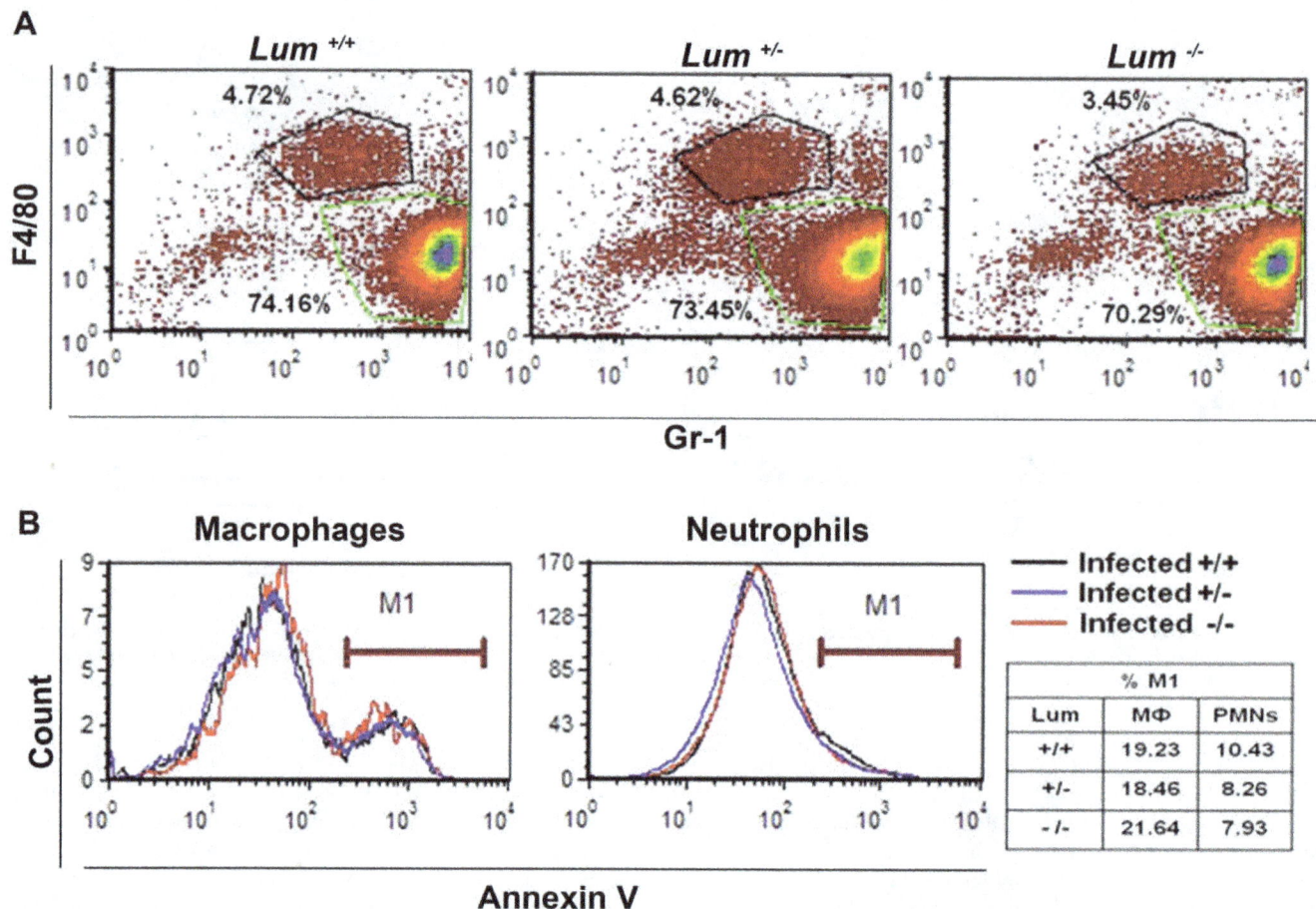

Figure 3. Flow cytometry of 24 hrs infected corneas shows reduced inflammatory cell percentages in $Lum^{-/-}$ corneas. Total cells from control and infected corneas per genotype (n = 5) were subjected to FACS analysis. Cells were immunostained with F4/80 (macrophage or MΦ marker), Gr-1 (neutrophil or PMN marker) (A) and with APC-Annexin V for detecting apoptotic cells (B). The percentage of MΦs and PMNs with respect to total cells was reduced in the $Lum^{-/-}$ pool to 3.45% and 70.29% respectively, compared to the $Lum^{+/+}$ and $Lum^{+/-}$ controls. There was a decrease in the percentage of AnnexinV$^+$cells in the $Lum^{-/-}$ PMN population.

Flow Cytometry

Five whole eyes from infected and control mice were harvested and rinsed in cold PBS. Corneal cells were isolated using a modified protocol described previously (Sun et. al., 2010). Residual iris material was removed and five corneas were rinsed, pooled, minced and incubated at 37°C in 500 μl of Collagenase L/PBS (Sigma-Aldrich) for 75 mins with shaking at 125 rpm. The released cells were centrifuged, washed and resuspended in 1 ml FACS buffer (Ca^{2+}/Mg^{2+} free 1x PBS and 1% FBS), and viable cell count was established by Trypan Blue exclusion. The cells were blocked and immunostained for 30 minutes on ice using the following antibodies: PE-F4/80 (eBioscience, San Diego, CA), PerCP-Gr-1(eBioscience) and APC-Annexin V (eBioscience). Flow cytometry was performed on a FACS Calibur (Becton Dickinson &Co., San Jose, CA), using the FCS Express Version 3 software.

In vitro Killing by Peritoneal Neutrophils

Mice were injected with 1 ml of 9% Casein solution (Sigma), and PMNs were harvested by peritoneal lavage 3 hours after the second injection and stored in cold 1xPBS and 0.02% EDTA as described earlier [4]. The PMNs were purified by Histopaque 1077 and 1119 (Sigma-Aldrich) density gradient cell separation as previously described [4]. The PMNs were plated in serum - free RPMI (Invitrogen) in 96 well plates (Corning) at a concentration

of 2×10^5 cells/ml in 100 μl and incubated overnight at 37°C. The concentration of *P. aeruginosa* was adjusted to 1×10^4 CFU/3.3 μL in PBS and added to each well without prior opsonization and incubated for 30, 60 and 120 minutes. Viable CFU at the time of the experiment was determined by plating dilutions of the bacterial suspension onto Cetrimide agar plates. Bacterial killing was measured as viable CFU recovered and quantified on Cetrimide agar plates from lysed PMNs and the supernatant.

Statistical Analysis

P values were ascertained using unpaired, two-tailed student's *t*-tests using the GraphPad Prism 4 software. Data were considered as significantly different at $p \le 0.05$.

Results

Increased Disease Score and Bacterial Load in $Lum^{-/-}$ Mice

The course of *P. aeruginosa* keratitis in the $Lum^{-/-}$ was compared to $Lum^{+/-}$ mice, used as a lumican expressing control group. There were no major differences in the appearance of $Lum^{+/-}$ and $Lum^{-/-}$ infected eyes one day after infection; after 6 days the $Lum^{-/-}$ infected eye became suppurative and opaque in most animals (Fig. 1A). By contrast, visible signs of infection subsided by

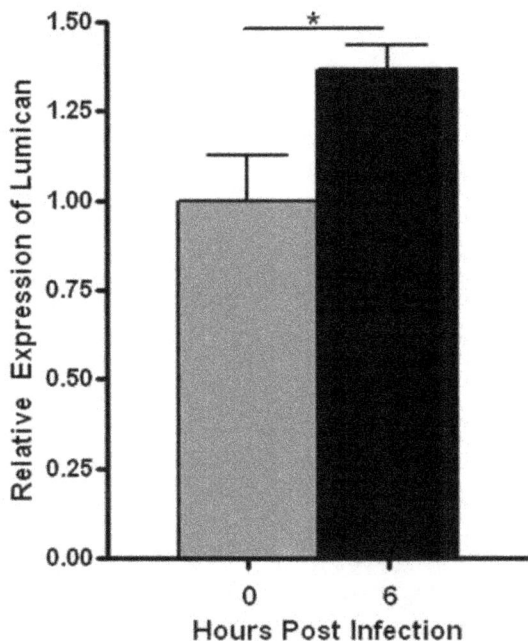

Figure 4. Increased lumican expression in Lum$^{+/-}$ corneas 6 hr post infection. Lumican transcript relative to18S RNA was significantly increased in Lum$^{+/-}$ corneas 6 hrs after infection as determined by qRT-PCR (n = 4). * $p \leq 0.05$.

2–5 days in the Lum$^{+/-}$ group. The mice were scored in a blinded manner every 24 hours (hrs) for six days for clinical appearance of disease (Fig. 1B). We should point out that the Lum$^{-/-}$ mice have diffused cloudy corneas resulting from increased backscattering of light due to collagen fibril disorganization, detectable by slit lamp biomicroscopy or high resolution confocal microscopy [1,2], however, this does not interfere with scoring the mice for infection-associated corneal opacity. Clinical disease scores were generally similar in Lum$^{-/-}$ and Lum$^{+/-}$ around 24 hrs of infection. Over time however, the Lum$^{-/-}$ mice showed higher disease scores and poor resolution of corneal opacity.

We examined bacterial load per infected eye using two different approaches. In the first, we sampled bacterial counts at the ocular surface using small circular filters, daily for 6 days (Fig. 2A). Viable bacterial yield from filters lifted off the surface 24 hrs after infection was comparable between Lum$^{+/-}$ and Lum$^{-/-}$ animals. However, by 48 hrs, three of the four Lum$^{+/-}$ mice had cleared the infection while the Lum$^{-/-}$ mice continued to yield viable bacteria for up to 6 days after infection. Second, we harvested whole eyes, 24 and 48 hrs after infection, and obtained viable bacterial counts by plating serial dilutions of whole eye homogenates. The results showed significantly higher bacterial counts from the Lum$^{-/-}$ whole eye homogenates (Fig. 2B).

Inflammatory Cell Infiltration in Infected Corneas

Increased survival of the bacterium in the Lum$^{-/-}$ cornea could be due to impaired functions of macrophages and neutrophils and/or poor recruitment of inflammatory cells. We used flow cytometry to obtain a total count of PMNs and macrophages from 5 animals after 24 hrs infection. Total cells from 5 pooled corneas per genotype were immunostained with F4/80 (macrophage marker), Gr-1 (PMN marker) and binding of AnnexinV as an indicator of apoptotic cells. Five uninfected corneas per genotype used as controls showed minimal infiltrates and no genotype-

dependent differences (data not shown). After infection, the total cell count was similar in heterozygous (164×10^4/ml) and wild types (186×10^4/ml), but lower in the knockout (84×10^4/ml) pool. We quantified the F4/80^{high} Grl^{low} (macrophages) and the F4/80^{low} Gr1^{high} (PMNs) cells in each pool and expressed these as a percentage of total cells. The percentages of PMNs and macrophages were comparable in the wild type and heterozygous pool, but markedly reduced in the infected Lum$^{-/-}$ pool (Fig. 3A). To determine if leukocyte apoptosis was affected by lumican-deficiency, we quantified AnnexinV$^+$ cells in the total cell population and cells gated for F4/80 and GR-1 (Fig. 3B). There was a slight reduction in the percentage of AnnexinV$^+$ cells in the PMN population, and no significant difference in the macrophage population in Lum$^{-/-}$ compared to the heterozygous and wild type pool.

We showed previously that CD14-dependent phagocytosis and bacterial clearance by macrophages in vitro was reduced in Lum$^{-/-}$ mice [5]. To determine if Lum$^{-/-}$ PMNs were also defective in bacterial killing, we incubated peritoneal PMNs and bacteria together and measured viable CFU recovered from lysed cells and the supernatant. We used the P. aeruginosa strain 808 to assay in vitro killing, as this strain is known to be taken up by the host in a CD14 dependent manner and our study with Lum$^{-/-}$ macrophages showed its dependence on lumican [5]. The yield of viable CFU was similar from Lum$^{+/-}$ and Lum$^{-/-}$ PMNs at each time point (Fig. S1). Thus, in vitro killing by peritoneal neutrophils was not adversely affected by lumican deficiency. Taken together, increased bacterial yield in the infected Lum$^{-/-}$ corneas could be due to a combination of reduced macrophage and PMN infiltration and phagocytosis deficiency in macrophages, even though bacterial killing by PMNs was not affected.

Lumican Expression in P. aeruginosa Infected Corneas

We have previously shown that lumican expression is up regulated during inflammation in the colon and in vitro in fibroblasts after treatment with LPS or IL-1β [3,33]. We questioned whether expression of lumican is similarly up regulated during P. aeruginosa infections of the cornea. By qRT-PCR we detected increased lumican transcript in Lum$^{+/-}$ corneas by 6 hrs after infection, indicating up regulation of lumican expression in resident corneal cells before inflammatory cell infiltrations, underscoring a role for lumican during the development of host response to pathogenic bacteria (Fig. 4).

Induction of Inflammation Mediators after Infection

To determine if induction of pro-inflammatory cytokines and chemokines in response to P. aeruginosa infection was affected adversely by lumican-deficiency, we measured selected cytokines and chemokines in total protein extracts of control and infected corneas. Three hours after infection, when neutrophils have yet to infiltrate the cornea, TNF-α concentration was close to baseline in infected corneas of both genotypes (Fig. 5A). By 24 hrs after infection the level of TNF-α had increased to similar extents in Lum$^{+/-}$ and Lum$^{-/-}$ corneas (94 and 84 pg/ml on average, respectively). However, by 2 days after infection the TNF-α level in Lum$^{-/-}$ infected corneas was significantly higher - 930 pg/ml versus 210 pg/ml, and by 5 days it was 1607 pg/ml in infected Lum$^{-/-}$ versus 963 pg/ml in wild type corneas (Fig. 5B).

IL-1β, a pro-inflammatory cytokine activated by NLRP inflammosome signals, has been shown to be elevated in P. aeruginosa keratitis [34,35]. Mature IL-1β was undetectable before corneal infection, and induced comparably to 1200–1600 pg/ml in the Lum$^{+/-}$ and the Lum$^{-/-}$ infected corneas for up to 5 days after infection (Fig. 5C). IL-12 is produced by macrophages and

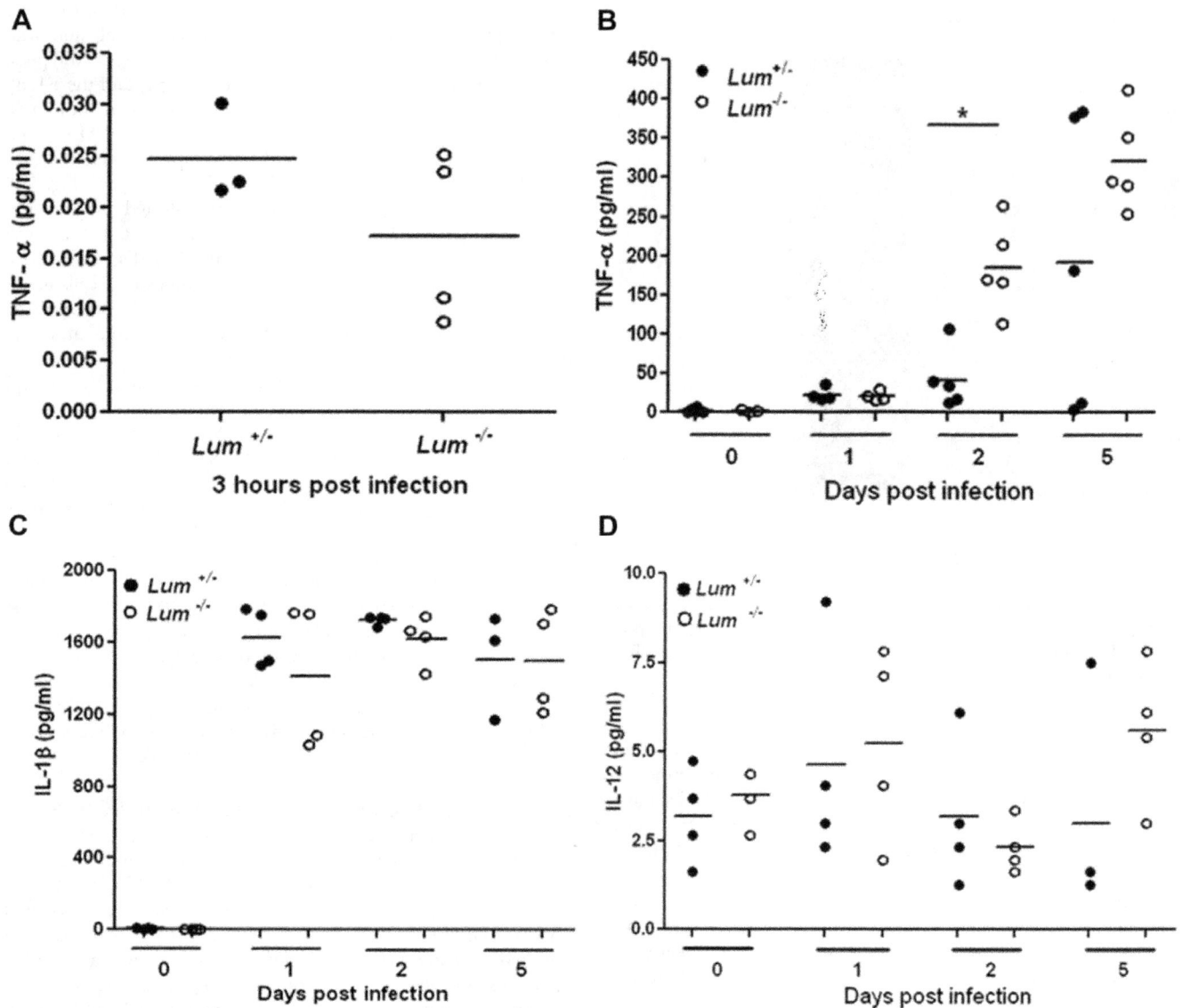

Figure 5. Proinflammatory cytokines measured by ELISA in *P.aeruginosa* infected corneas. TNF-α level was low and comparable in Lum$^{+/-}$ and Lum$^{-/-}$ corneal protein extracts 3 hrs after infection (A) but significantly higher in Lum$^{-/-}$ infected corneas 2 days after infection (B). IL-1β was induced comparably in Lum$^{+/-}$ and Lum$^{-/-}$ infected corneas for up to 5 days after infection (C) and IL-12 (D) was detected at very low levels in infected corneas of both genotypes. * $p \leq 0.05$.

NK cells in some bacterial and viral infections and facilitates the development of T$_H$1 differentiation [36]. We tested the induction of IL-12 after infection. Using the IL-12 p70 ELISA, which recognizes the IL-12 p35/p40 heterodimer specifically, we detected very low levels of the IL-12 heterodimer in infected corneas of all genotypes (Fig. 5D), while measuring the p40 subunit, common to IL-12 and IL-23, another study reported a small increase in *P. aeruginosa* infected B6 mouse corneas [37].

The CXC chemokine ligand 1 (CXCL1/GRO-α), produced by fibroblasts and macrophages, is a key chemoattractant for neutrophils in inflamed corneas [38,39]. CXCL1 was elevated within 24 hrs of infection in both genotypes; however, its level was consistently lower in infected Lum$^{-/-}$ corneas compared to Lum$^{+/-}$ corneas. Average levels in Lum$^{+/-}$ and Lum$^{-/-}$ infected corneas were 717 and 566 pg/ml after one day, 705 and 500 pg/ml after 2 days, and 408 and 377 pg/ml after 5 days of infection, respectively (Fig. 6A). Three hours after infection, CXCL1 was slightly

increased in both genotypes without significant differences (Fig. 6B). To determine if the decrease in CXCL1 at the later stages of infection was due to transcriptional differences in regulation in the absence of lumican, we determined *Cxcl1* expression by real time qRT-PCR in total RNA extracted from Lum$^{+/-}$ and Lum$^{-/-}$ infected corneas. Six hrs after infection *Cxcl1* expression was higher in the Lum$^{+/-}$ compared to Lum$^{-/-}$ corneas. However, 24 and 48 hrs after infection *Cxcl1* transcript levels were significantly higher in the knockout infected corneas - a trend that was just the opposite of final chemokine levels measured by ELISA (Fig. 6C). This dichotomy between protein and transcript levels, suggesting translational regulation of *Cxcl1* as a function of lumican is discussed later.

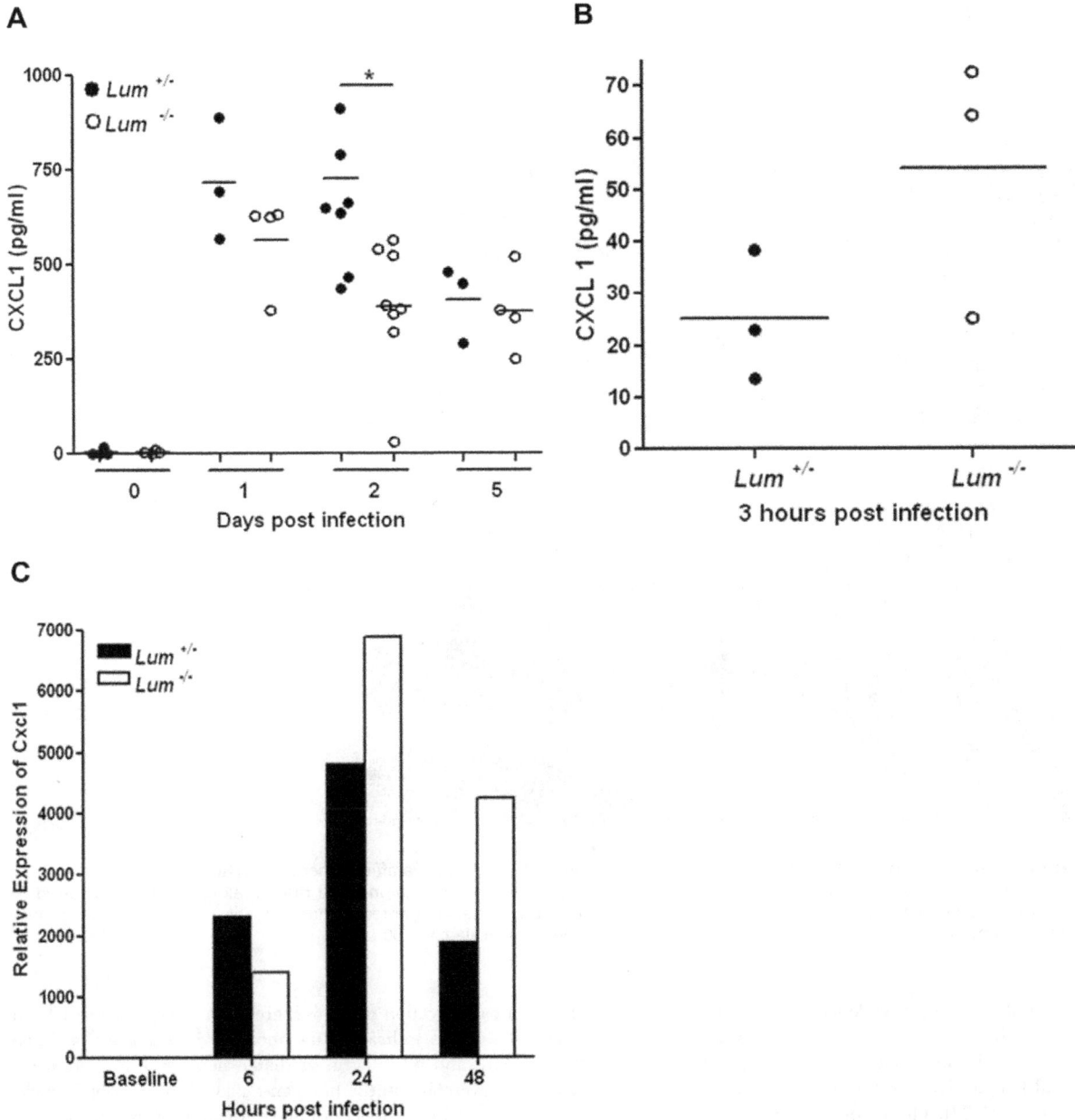

Figure 6. Differential regulation of CXCL1 in infected Lum $^{+/-}$ and Lum $^{-/-}$ corneas. CXCL1 measured by ELISA increased 24 hrs after infection in both genotypes, with its level being consistently lower in the Lum $^{-/-}$ corneal extracts - the difference being statistically significant at the 2 d.p.i time point (A). Three hours after infection CXCL1 levels were comparably low in both genotypes (n = 3) (B). The Cxcl1 transcript measured by qRT-PCR in quadruplicates/animal was increased over baseline 6 hrs post infection; by 24–48 hrs post infection Lum $^{-/-}$ corneas showed higher levels of Cxcl1 compared to Lum $^{+/-}$ (C). * $p \leq 0.05$.

Inflammatory Cell Infiltration and Tissue Damage in Infected Lum $^{-/-}$ Corneas

To specifically examine tissue damage in infected Lum $^{+/-}$ and Lum $^{-/-}$ mice by histology, we harvested mice 24 and 48 hrs after infection with disease scores of 2 and 3, respectively. Tissue damage at the 24 hrs time point was similar in Lum $^{+/-}$ and Lum $^{-/-}$ corneas (Fig. 7A). By 48 hrs the Lum $^{-/-}$ corneas showed large areas of epithelial ulcerations, and increased damage of the stroma (Fig. 7B). Also, there was very little damage of the corneal endothelium and no obvious edema in infected corneas of either genotype, further underscoring lumican involvement in bacterial infections of the stroma directly.

Discussion

Here we showed that in a *P. aeruginosa* keratitis model, the Lum $^{-/-}$ mice responded differently from control mice in a number of ways such that their recovery from keratitis was compromised. The Lum $^{-/-}$ mice showed poor resolution of keratitis, increased bacterial survival, and differences in pro-inflammatory cytokines, chemokine ligands and inflammatory cell infiltrates. Our previous studies show that lumican is a structural extracellular matrix protein that also interacts with macrophage and neutrophil cell surfaces and regulates TLR4 mediated LPS sensing specifically [3–5,33]. Several aspects of keratitis, such as poor bacterial clearance,

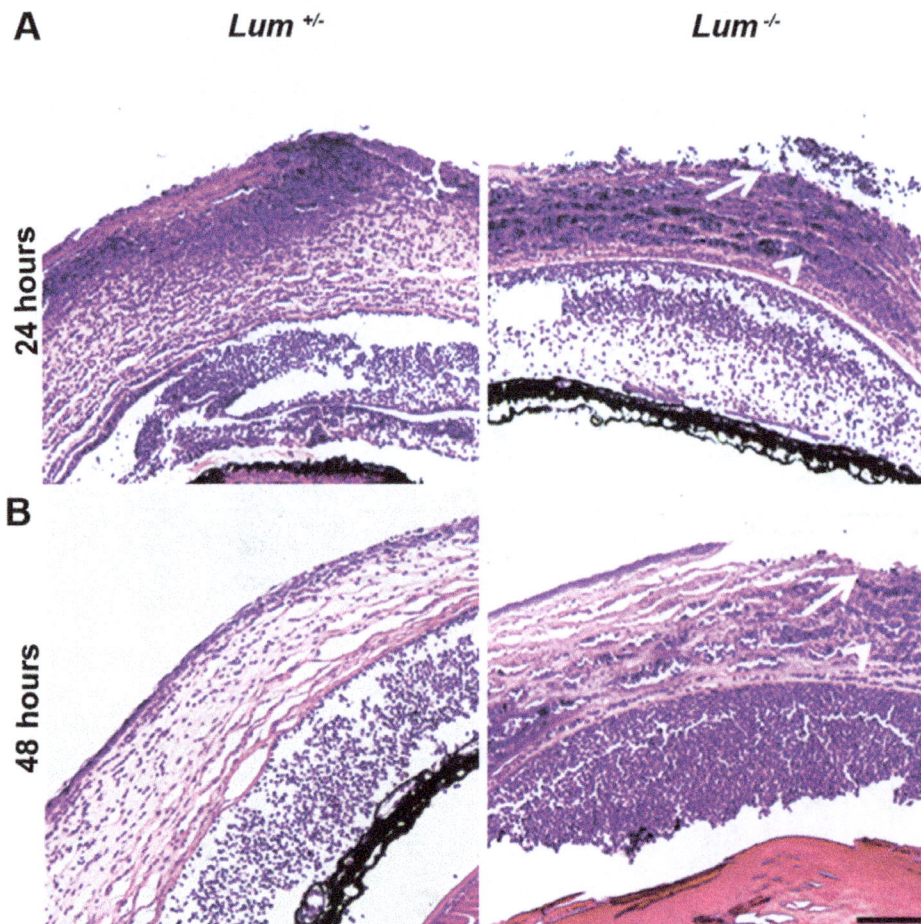

Figure 7. Increased tissue damage in infected corneas of Lum^{+/−} and Lum^{−/−} mice. Paraffin-embedded sections of eyes 24 hrs (A) and 48 hrs (B) after infection were stained with H and E. To examine tissue damage in mice with comparable disease all infected animals used for histology had an initial disease score of 2 to 3 and showed PMN infiltrations in the cornea and anterior chamber. The Lum^{−/−} infected corneas showed large areas of epithelial ulcerations (arrow) and stromal damage (arrowhead). Scale bar, 100 μm.

induction of pro-inflammatory cytokines and poor disease resolution manifested by *Lum*^{−/−} mice are features shared by, and more pronounced in mice lacking major LPS signaling intermediates, TLR4 or MyD88 or transgenic Mafia mice after macrophage depletion [13,28]. This is consistent with our findings that lumican is a modulator of the LPS response.

TNF-α is a pro-inflammatory cytokine produced by a variety of antigen presenting cells of innate immunity, and by CD4+ T_H1 cells of adaptive immunity [40]. As TNF-α also leads to further activation of NF-κB and amplification of inflammatory responses, it can contribute to harmful corneal damages if uncontrolled. Three hrs after infection TNF-α was close to baseline in both genotypes, indicating that early innate immune response from resident corneal cells was not affected by lumican-deficiency. However, TNF-α was significantly higher in the *Lum*^{−/−} corneas by 2 days after infection. In our earlier study, we reported that in a LPS-stimulated septic shock model the *Lum*^{−/−} mice produced lower levels of TNF-α, and isolated macrophages stimulated with LPS *in vitro* also produced lower levels of TNF-α due to poor LPS sensing. The answer to why we see an increase in TNF-α in *Lum*^{−/−} corneas at the later stages of infection with live bacteria may not be a simple one. One explanation for this difference in the *Lum*^{−/−} mouse response to LPS versus live *P. aeruginosa* is the fact that host response to live bacteria involves multiple PAMPs and not LPS

alone. The observation that this increase in TNF-α occurs later in disease by 48 hrs indicates that once the initial delay in TLR4 signals [3,5], and β2 integrin mediated neutrophil migration [4], have been overcome in the lumican-deficient mice, poor bacterial clearance contributes to continued induction of innate immune responses via other TLRs, such as TLR5 mediated response to flagellin [41], resulting in elevated pro-inflammatory cytokines.

The CXC chemokine ligand 1, CXCL1 or keratinocyte-derived chemokine, KC, produced by epithelial cells, fibroblasts, PMNs and macrophages, is a major chemoattractant for PMNs. CXCL1 was shown to be temporally up regulated in an LPS treated sterile keratitis model in the mouse [38], but its increase in lumican-deficient corneas was lower than that of wild types. It has been shown by others that in the sterile LPS-keratitis model, CXCL1 is up regulated within 3 hrs of injury, with maximum induction 24 hrs after injury and subsiding by 72 hrs [38]. In agreement with these sterile keratitis findings, after infection with *P. aeruginosa*, we also noted a rapid increase in CXCL1. Furthermore, by 48 hrs of infection the increase in CXCL1 levels in *Lum*^{−/−} infected corneas was much lower than *Lum*^{+/−}. However, *Cxcl1* expression was higher in the *Lum*^{−/−} corneas at the later stages of infection, suggesting that reduced CXCL1 levels in the *Lum*^{−/−} infected corneas may contribute to a feedback up regulation of gene expression. Similarly, CXCL1 levels in the sterile LPS-keratitis model was reportedly increased in the anterior chamber of mice deficient in lumican and keratocan, another corneal proteoglycan. It was proposed that in the absence of these proteoglycans, the chemokine is not retained in the cornea and accumulates in the anterior chamber [14]. Thus, our observation that the $Lum^{-/-}$ infected corneas harbored lower levels of the chemokine compared to $Lum^{+/-}$ corneas could be due to poor retention, or increased degradation of the chemokine.

Another important pro-inflammatory cytokine induced during infections is IL-1β; its expression is induced by NF-κB transcription factors. At the protein level, pro-IL-1 β is cleaved to release the mature IL-1β by caspase-1 activated by NLRP inflammosome signals in the presence of bacterial toxins [42]. Mature IL-1β had increased dramatically in the cornea by 24 h of infection, and this was not significantly affected by lumican deficiency. Thus, it appears that lumican may not regulate inflammosome mediated elevation of mature IL-1β. Overall, $Lum^{+/-}$ and $Lum^{-/-}$ infected corneas showed comparable increases in IL-1β. While TNFα and CXCL1 had increased in both genotypes by 48 hrs, coinciding with the timing of inflammatory cell influx, the increase in these two cytokines were significantly lower in $Lum^{-/-}$ infected corneas compared to their wild type allele carrying counter parts.

The increased severity of keratitis seen in the $Lum^{-/-}$ mice with P. aeruginosa ATCC19660 may be most closely linked to poor bacterial clearance by phagocytosis in the $Lum^{-/-}$ mice. Thus, failure to clear the bacteria in the $Lum^{-/-}$ cornea is likely to contribute to increased bacterial toxins, increased host innate immune response and production of TNF-α and tissue damaging proteases by the host. Interestingly, we also found poor bacterial clearance in the $Lum^{-/-}$ mice in an earlier lung infection model; however lung tissue TNF-α level was comparable to wild types [5]. This may be partly due to intrinsic differences between the cornea as a naturally macrophage poor tissue, and the lungs rich in resident alveolar macrophages. In vitro, we have shown previously that the P. aeruginosa ATCC19660 and the 808 strain were not

taken up and killed by $Lum^{-/-}$ peritoneal macrophages as effectively as wild types [5]. By contrast, here when we examined in vitro killing by PMNs, we found no major difference between $Lum^{-/-}$ and $Lum^{+/-}$ mice. So why is there an increased bacterial load in $Lum^{-/-}$ keratitis? Several factors may be at play here. First, by flow cytometry we found that 24 hrs after infection, macrophage and PMN percentages were lower in $Lum^{-/-}$ corneas. Second, while $Lum^{-/-}$ PMNs are competent in bacterial killing, $Lum^{-/-}$ macrophages are phagocytosis-impaired. This must impact bacterial clearance, as well as antigen presentation, recruitment/proliferation of other lymphocytes and corneal immune privilege. Future temporal analyses of these cell populations in the infected cornea will address these questions.

In conclusion, lumican deficiency leads to poor clearance of P. aeruginosa infections of the cornea, continued production of pro-inflammatory cytokines and inefficient resolution of inflammation.

Supporting Information

Figure S1 *In vitro* **killing by peritoneal PMNs.** *In vitro* killing was determined by measuring viable CFU in the supernatant and cell lysate of $Lum^{+/-}$ and $Lum^{-/-}$ PMNs. There was no significant difference in the killing capabilities of PMNs from both genotypes.

Acknowledgments

We thank Randall Gunther and Anthony Sin for technical assistance with the qRT-PCR assays.

Author Contributions

Performed the keratitis experiments: HJS. Performed the flow cytometry experiments: CN HJS S-GS. Conceived and designed the experiments: SC HJS ARH. Analyzed the data: SC ARH. Wrote the paper: SC HJS S-GS.

References

1. Chakravarti S, Magnuson T, Lass JH, Jepsen KJ, LaMantia C, et al. (1998) Lumican regulates collagen fibril assembly: skin fragility and corneal opacity in the absence of lumican. J Cell Biol 141: 1277–1286.

2. Chakravarti S, Petroll WM, Hassell JR, Jester JV, Lass JH, et al. (2000) Corneal opacity in lumican-null mice: defects in collagen fibril structure and packing in the posterior stroma. Invest Ophthalmol Vis Sci 41: 3365–3373.

3. Wu F, Vij N, Roberts L, Lopez-Briones S, Joyce S, et al. (2007) A novel role of the lumican core protein in bacterial lipopolysaccharide-induced innate immune response. J Biol Chem 282: 26409–26417.

4. Lee S, Bowrin K, Hamad AR, Chakravarti S (2009) Extracellular matrix lumican deposited on the surface of neutrophils promotes migration by binding to beta2 integrin. J Biol Chem 284: 23662–23669.

5. Shao H, Lee S, Gae-Scott S, Nakata C, Chen S, et al. (2012) Extracellular matrix lumican promotes bacterial phagocytosis and Lum−/− mice show increased Pseudomonas aeruginosa lung infection severity. J Biol Chem.

6. Kao WW, Funderburgh JL, Xia Y, Liu CY, Conrad GW (2006) Focus on molecules: lumican. Exp Eye Res 82: 3–4.

7. Saika S, Shiraishi A, Liu CY, Funderburgh JL, Kao CW, et al. (2000) Role of lumican in the corneal epithelium during wound healing. J Biol Chem 275: 2607–2612.

8. Kawai T, Akira S (2010) The role of pattern-recognition receptors in innate immunity: update on Toll-like receptors. Nat Immunol 11: 373–384.

9. Hassell JR, Birk DE (2010) The molecular basis of corneal transparency. Exp Eye Res 91: 326–335.

10. Hazlett LD, Hendricks RL (2010) Reviews for immune privilege in the year 2010: immune privilege and infection. Ocul Immunol Inflamm 18: 237–243.

11. Streilein JW (2003) Ocular immune privilege: therapeutic opportunities from an experiment of nature. Nat Rev Immunol 3: 879–889.

12. Johnson AC, Heinzel FP, Diaconu E, Sun Y, Hise AG, et al. (2005) Activation of toll-like receptor (TLR)2, TLR4, and TLR9 in the mammalian cornea induces MyD88-dependent corneal inflammation. Invest Ophthalmol Vis Sci 46: 589–595.

13. Sun Y, Karmakar M, Roy S, Ramadan RT, Williams SR, et al. (2010) TLR4 and TLR5 on corneal macrophages regulate Pseudomonas aeruginosa keratitis

by signaling through MyD88-dependent and -independent pathways. J Immunol 185: 4272–4283.

14. Carlson EC, Lin M, Liu CY, Kao WW, Perez VL, et al. (2007) Keratocan and lumican regulate neutrophil infiltration and corneal clarity in lipopolysaccharide-induced keratitis by direct interaction with CXCL1. J Biol Chem 282: 35502–35509.

15. Carlson EC, Sun Y, Auletta J, Kao WW, Liu CY, et al. (2010) Regulation of corneal inflammation by neutrophil-dependent cleavage of keratan sulfate proteoglycans as a model for breakdown of the chemokine gradient. J Leukoc Biol 88: 517–522.

16. Hazlett LD (2004) Corneal response to Pseudomonas aeruginosa infection. Prog Retin Eye Res 23: 1–30.

17. Jeng BH, McLeod SD (2003) Microbial keratitis. Br J Ophthalmol 87: 805–806.

18. Willcox MD (2007) Pseudomonas aeruginosa infection and inflammation during contact lens wear: a review. Optom Vis Sci 84: 273–278.

19. Robertson DM, Cavanagh HD (2008) The Clinical and Cellular Basis of Contact Lens-related Corneal Infections: A Review. Clin Ophthalmol 2: 907–917.

20. Vajpayee RB, Sharma N, Sinha R, Agarwal T, Singhvi A (2007) Infectious keratitis following keratoplasty. Surv Ophthalmol 52: 1–12.

21. Karimian F, Baradaran-Rafii A, Javadi MA, Nazari R, Rabei HM, et al. (2007) Bilateral bacterial keratitis in three patients following photorefractive keratectomy. J Refract Surg 23: 312–315.

22. Wroblewski KJ, Pasternak JF, Bower KS, Schallhorn SC, Hubickey WJ, et al. (2006) Infectious keratitis after photorefractive keratectomy in the United States army and navy. Ophthalmology 113: 520–525.

23. Khatri S, Lass JH, Heinzel FP, Petroll WM, Gomez J, et al. (2002) Regulation of endotoxin-induced keratitis by PECAM-1, MIP-2, and toll-like receptor 4. Invest Ophthalmol Vis Sci 43: 2278–2284.

24. Huang X, Barrett RP, McClellan SA, Hazlett LD (2005) Silencing Toll-like receptor-9 in Pseudomonas aeruginosa keratitis. Invest Ophthalmol Vis Sci 46: 4209–4216.

25. Kumar A, Hazlett LD, Yu FS (2008) Flagellin suppresses the inflammatory response and enhances bacterial clearance in a murine model of Pseudomonas aeruginosa keratitis. Infect Immun 76: 89–96.

26. O'Callaghan RJ, Engel LS, Hobden JA, Callegan MC, Green LC, et al. (1996) Pseudomonas keratitis. The role of an uncharacterized exoprotein, protease IV, in corneal virulence. Invest Ophthalmol Vis Sci 37: 534–543.

27. Fleiszig SM, Evans DJ (2002) The pathogenesis of bacterial keratitis: studies with Pseudomonas aeruginosa. Clin Exp Optom 85: 271–278.

28. Sun Y, Karmakar M, Taylor PR, Rietsch A, Pearlman E (2012) ExoS and ExoT ADP Ribosyltransferase Activities Mediate Pseudomonas aeruginosa Keratitis by Promoting Neutrophil Apoptosis and Bacterial Survival. J Immunol 188: 1884–1895.

29. Hazlett LD (2005) Role of innate and adaptive immunity in the pathogenesis of keratitis. Ocul Immunol Inflamm 13: 133–138.

30. Lee EJ, Evans DJ, Fleiszig SM (2003) Role of Pseudomonas aeruginosa ExsA in penetration through corneal epithelium in a novel in vivo model. Invest Ophthalmol Vis Sci 44: 5220–5227.

31. Vij N, Roberts L, Joyce S, Chakravarti S (2005) Lumican regulates corneal inflammatory responses by modulating Fas-Fas ligand signaling. Invest Ophthalmol Vis Sci 46: 88–95.

32. Zaidi TS, Zaidi T, Pier GB (2010) Role of neutrophils, MyD88-mediated neutrophil recruitment, and complement in antibody-mediated defense against Pseudomonas aeruginosa keratitis. Invest Ophthalmol Vis Sci 51: 2085–2093.

33. Wu F, Chakravarti S (2007) Differential Expression of Inflammatory and Fibrogenic Genes and Their Regulation by NF-{kappa}B Inhibition in a Mouse Model of Chronic Colitis. J Immunol 179: 6988–7000.

34. Cole N, Hume E, Khan S, Madigan M, Husband AJ, et al. (2005) Contribution of the cornea to cytokine levels in the whole eye induced during the early phase of Pseudomonas aeruginosa challenge. Immunol Cell Biol 83: 301–306.

35. Huang X, Du W, McClellan SA, Barrett RP, Hazlett LD (2006) TLR4 is required for host resistance in Pseudomonas aeruginosa keratitis. Invest Ophthalmol Vis Sci 47: 4910–4916.

36. Vignali DA, Kuchroo VK (2012) IL-12 family cytokines: immunological playmakers. Nat Immunol 13: 722–728.

37. Hazlett LD, Rudner XL, McClellan SA, Barrett RP, Lighvani S (2002) Role of IL-12 and IFN-gamma in Pseudomonas aeruginosa corneal infection. Invest Ophthalmol Vis Sci 43: 419–424.

38. Lin M, Carlson E, Diaconu E, Pearlman E (2007) CXCL1/KC and CXCL5/LIX are selectively produced by corneal fibroblasts and mediate neutrophil infiltration to the corneal stroma in LPS keratitis. J Leukoc Biol 81: 786–792.

39. Spandau UH, Toksoy A, Verhaart S, Gillitzer R, Kruse FE (2003) High expression of chemokines Gro-alpha (CXCL-1), IL-8 (CXCL-8), and MCP-1 (CCL-2) in inflamed human corneas in vivo. Arch Ophthalmol 121: 825–831.

40. Aggarwal BB (2003) Signalling pathways of the TNF superfamily: a double-edged sword. Nat Rev Immunol 3: 745–756.

41. Kumar A, Gao N, Standiford TJ, Gallo RL, Yu FS (2010) Topical flagellin protects the injured corneas from Pseudomonas aeruginosa infection. Microbes Infect 12: 978–989.

42. Elinav E, Strowig T, Henao-Mejia J, Flavell RA (2011) Regulation of the antimicrobial response by NLR proteins. Immunity 34: 665–679.

15

Contribution of Corneal Neovascularization to Dendritic Cell Migration into the Central Area during Human Corneal Infection

Mari Narumi[1]*, Yoshiko Kashiwagi[2], Hiroyuki Namba[1], Rintaro Ohe[3], Mitsunori Yamakawa[3], Hidetoshi Yamashita[1]

1 Department of Ophthalmology and Visual Sciences, Yamagata University Faculty of Medicine, Yamagata, Japan, 2 Department of Health and Nutrition, Yamagata Prefectural Yonezawa Women's Junior College, Yamagata, Japan, 3 Department of Pathological Diagnostics, Yamagata University Faculty of Medicine, Yamagata, Japan

Abstract

Compared with the peripheral corneal limbus, the human central cornea lacks blood vessels, which is responsible for its immunologically privileged status and high transparency. Dendritic cells (DCs) are present in the central avascular area of inflamed corneas, but the mechanisms of their migration to this location are poorly understood. Here, we investigated the contribution of vessel formation to DC migration into the central cornea, and analyzed the DC chemotactic factors produced by human corneal epithelial (HCE) cells. Using human eyes obtained from surgical procedures, we then assessed vessel formation, DC distribution, and activin A expression immunohistochemically. The results demonstrated increased numbers of vessels and DCs in the central area of inflamed corneas, and a positive correlation between the number of vessels and DCs. Activin A was expressed in the subepithelial space and the endothelium of newly formed blood vessels in the inflamed cornea. In infected corneas, DCs were present in the central area but no vascularization was observed, suggesting the presence of chemotactic factors that induced DC migration from the limbal vessels. To test this hypothesis, we assessed the migration of monocyte-derived DCs toward HCE cell supernatants with or without lipopolysaccharide (LPS) stimulation of HCE cells and inflammatory cytokines (released by HCE cells). DCs migrated toward tumor necrosis factor alpha (TNF-α), interleukin (IL)-6, and activin A, as well as LPS-stimulated HCE cell supernatants. The supernatant contained elevated TNF-α, IL-6, and activin A levels, suggesting that they were produced by HCE cells after LPS stimulation. Therefore, vessels in the central cornea might constitute a DC migration route, and activin A expressed in the endothelium of newly formed vessels might contribute to corneal vascularization. Activin A also functions as a chemotactic factor, similar to HCE-produced TNF-α and IL-6. These findings enhance our understanding of the pathophysiology of corneal inflammation during infection.

Editor: Alexander V. Ljubimov, Cedars-Sinai Medical Center; UCLA School of Medicine, United States of America

Funding: This study was supported by Grants-in-Aid for Scientific Research from Japan Society for the Promotion of Science. The funder had no role in study design, data collection and analysis, decision to publish, or preparation of the manuscript.

Competing Interests: The authors have declared that no competing interests exist.

* Email: mari.narumi1101@gmail.com

Introduction

Unlike most other organs, the central part of the human cornea lacks blood vessels and lymphatic vessels. This anatomical feature is necessary for high transparency and good visual acuity, and it contributes to its immunologically privileged status. As in other tissues, antigen-presenting cells (APCs) such as macrophages, Langerhans cells (LCs), and dendritic cells (DCs) are present in the human cornea, and participate in corneal immunity [1–3].

Hamrah and Dana [4] demonstrated that corneal LCs upregulate the expression of co-stimulatory molecules such as CD80 and CD86 in inflamed corneas. Mayer [5] described the characteristics of DCs in corneal buttons that were enucleated for transplantation purposes, and demonstrated the presence of LCs and immature DCs (imDCs) in the human corneal epithelium, and DC-SIGN-positive (i.e., CD209+) DCs in the stroma. These studies also reported that the number of APCs in the central part of the cornea was lower than that in the paracentral and peripheral regions.

In general, the recruitment of APCs in inflamed organs occurs through vessels, and the cells then migrate back to draining lymph nodes to accelerate the T-cell responses [6]. In terms of protecting the cornea from infection, its avascularity and small numbers of distributed APCs in the central part could be limiting factors. Prolonged inflammation often induces the formation of novel vessels in the central region of the cornea; however, this leads to a poor prognosis for visual acuity. A certain amount of APC recruitment and vessel formation is necessary to combat a corneal infection. Thus, understanding both the pathophysiology of APC movements in the cornea and their relationship with vessel formation might help identify therapeutic targets for regulating the corneal inflammatory response to infection.

In this study, we characterized DCs in the human cornea using infected and uninfected corneal tissues obtained from surgical units. We first analyzed the relationship between the distribution of DCs and the newly formed vessels, and found that the number of DCs in the central cornea increased during infection and/or vessel formation. In addition, DCs were detected in the central cornea in the absence of vascularization in some infected samples. Accordingly, we performed additional experiments with chemotactic factors that induce the migration of DCs into the central part of the cornea, and found that interleukin 6 (IL-6), tumor necrosis factor alpha (TNF-α), and activin A, which are produced by corneal epithelial cells and/or DCs, are involved in DC migration.

Materials and Methods

Materials

This study was performed in compliance with the tenets of the Declaration of Helsinki. All experiments were performed after approval from the Ethical Committee of Yamagata University Faculty of Medicine. After securing written informed consent from the subjects, we obtained corneal tissues surgically. The sample tissues in this study consisted of 28 eyes from 27 patients (13 males and 14 females) aged between 34 and 94 years (mean, 75 years). Six eyes were obtained by enucleation, and 22 corneal buttons were obtained during penetrating keratoplasty (PKP). The cases included seven infectious corneal ulcers and/or corneal perforation, six corneal degenerative diseases, six graft failures due to endothelial dysfunction, five herpetic keratitis infections, two choroidal malignant melanomas, one corneal perforation due to an autoimmune ulcer, and one corneal perforation from trauma. The precise sample data are shown in Table 1. Any cases with a history of herpetic keratitis were excluded from the cases of graft failure because of endothelial dysfunction. All five cases of herpetic keratitis showed typical epithelial keratitis (dendritic) when treatment was started. These cases included two corneal perforations. Cases 24 and 25 were tissues from the same patients as previous samples because of the recurrence of herpetic keratitis after PKP.

Seven cases were defined as infected because of clinical findings that supported corneal infection, including focus in the cornea (7/7) and the presence of hypopyon (5/7), in slit-lamp examinations. The infection-causing pathogens were confirmed by cultures in three out of the seven infectious corneal ulcer and/or corneal perforation cases. The patient with autoimmune disease had corneal perforation 1 week after cataract surgery. Although the location of the ulcer was the epicenter, a slit-lamp examination showed the formation of a focus. This patient had discharge, hypopyon, and injection of the conjunctiva, which also strongly suggested the presence of infection. The infiltration of neutrophils in the subepithelial area and stroma of the cornea was confirmed histopathologically in all infected samples, as well as by reactivity to antibiotics and antifungal treatments.

Immunohistochemistry (IHC)

IHC analyses were performed using paraffin-embedded corneal tissues and primary antibodies against CD1a (MTB1; mouse IgG1, κ; 1:30 dilution; Novocastra; Newcastle-upon-Tyne, UK), DC-SIGN (CD209; H-200; rabbit polyclonal; 1:400; Santa Cruz Biotechnology; Santa Cruz, CA, USA), langerin (CD207; 12D6; mouse IgG2b; 1:100; Ylem S.R.L.; Rome, Italy), and CD83 (1H4b; mouse IgG1, κ; 1:40; Novocastra). The expression of MHC-class II molecules on DCs was analyzed using anti-s-100 (rabbit polyclonal; ready to use; Nichirei, Tokyo, Japan) and anti-MHC-class II antibodies (mouse IgG2a; 1:80; Abcam; Cambridge, UK). Corneal blood vessel formation was analyzed using anti-CD31 antibodies (JC70A; mouse IgG1, κ; 1:50; Abcam), and anti-von Willebrand factor (factor VIII; rabbit polyclonal; 1:1000; Dako; Carpinteria, California, USA). Lymphatic vessel formation was studied using anti-D2-40 (mouse IgG1, κ, 1:50, Dako) and

anti-vascular endothelium growth factor receptor-3 (VEGFR-3) antibodies (D1–D7; rabbit polyclonal; 1:40; Abcam). VEGFR-3 is the specific receptor for VEGF-C and VEGF-D, which induce lymphangiogenesis [7,8]. The presence of activin A, a chemotactic factor in DCs [9,10], was confirmed using anti-activin A antibodies (goat polyclonal; 1:50; R&D Systems; Minneapolis, MN, USA).

Formalin-fixed, paraffin-embedded (FFPE) tissues were sliced into 3-μm-thick sections. The sections were then deparaffinized, and endogenous peroxidase activity was blocked using methanol containing 0.3% hydrogen peroxide. Antigen retrieval was performed using ethylenediamine tetraacetic acid (antigen retrieval solution, pH 9; Nichirei Biosciences; Tokyo, Japan) in an autoclave (2 atm, 121°C, 20 min). After washing in phosphate-buffered saline (0.01 M, pH 7.4), tissue sections were incubated with primary antibodies at room temperature overnight. The labeled streptavidin-biotin peroxidase method (Ultra Tech HRP Streptavidin-Biotin Detection system, PN IM2391; Immunotech; Marseille, France) was used. Positive reactions were detected as brown coloration after incubation with 3,3′-diaminobenzidine tetrahydrochloride. The sections were counterstained with hematoxylin, and then observed using light microscopy.

Multiple Immunofluorescence Staining

Multiple immunofluorescence staining of FFPE tissue sections was carried out as described previously [11]. Antigen retrieval was performed using the same method as described above in the IHC section. A cocktail of primary antibodies was applied to the tissue sections, which were incubated at room temperature overnight. A fluorescein-conjugated AffiniPure goat anti-rabbit IgG (H+L) antibody (Jackson ImmunoResearch Laboratories; West Grove, PA, USA) and a rhodamine-conjugated AffiniPure donkey anti-mouse IgG (H+L) antibody (Jackson ImmunoResearch Laboratories) were used as secondary antibodies, and the samples were mounted using Fluoromount (Diagnostic Biosystems Inc.; Pleasanton, CA, USA). Staining was observed using a fluorescent microscope.

Evaluation of IHC Staining

The distribution of DCs and vessels in the central area of the corneas was evaluated. A NanoZoomer (Hamamatsu Photonics; Hamamatsu, Japan) was used to determine the central area and evaluate the size of the cornea. The type and density (per mm^2 of a section) of infiltrating APCs, the number of blood and lymphatic vessels, and the expression of activin A in the corneal buttons (6–7 mm in diameter) obtained from PKP were observed using IHC. The anatomical limbus and the central area were determined in enucleated eyes. Cell counting was performed five times by two blinded observers, and the mean numbers were used.

Isolation of Dendritic Cells

Peripheral blood samples were collected from healthy donors after securing written permission from the subjects. Peripheral blood mononuclear cells were isolated using Ficoll-Paque PLUS (GE Healthcare Life Science; Little Chalfont, Buckinghamshire, UK). After removing T and B cells using a DynaMag-15 Magnet with pan-T (CD2) and pan-B Dynabeads (CD19; Veritas; Tokyo, Japan), the eluted monocytes (1.0×10^6 cells/well in 24-well tissue culture plates) were incubated in RPMI1640 medium supplemented with 10% fetal bovine serum, 50 ng/mL GM-CSF, and 20 ng/mL IL-4 (Primmune Inc.; Kobe, Japan) at 37°C and in a humidified incubator with 5.0% CO_2, according to previously reported methods [12].

Table 1. Number of dendritic cells (DCs) and vessels in the central cornea.

Case	Age	Sex	Cause	Culture	Operation	CD1a	Langerin	DC-SIGN	CD83	Lymphatic vessels	Blood vessels
1	78	F	Malignalt choroidal melanoma	N.P	enucleation	N.D	N.D	N.D	N.D	N.D	N.D
2	37	M	Malignat choroidal melanoma	N.P	enucleation	N.D	0.34	N.D	N.D	N.D	N.D
3	64	M	Bullous keratopathy	N.P	PKP	1.05	0.53	0.53	1.05	N.D	1.05
4	34	M	Keratoconus	N.P	PKP	N.D	N.D	N.D	N.D	N.D	N.D
5	77	F	Bullous keratopathy	N.P	PKP	0.25	N.D	0.12	N.D	N.D	0.86
6	74	F	Bullous keratopathy	N.P	PKP	N.D	0.52	N.D	N.D	0.26	N.D
7	68	F	Bullous keratopathy	N.P	PKP	N.D	N.D	N.D	N.D	N.D	N.D
8	90	F	Bullous keratopathy	N.P	PKP	N.D	N.D	N.D	N.D	0.45	0.56
9	63	M	Trauma, Corneal perforation	N.P	PKP	N.D	N.D	N.D	N.D	2.45	2.45
10	78	F	Graft failure	N.P	PKP	N.D	N.D	0.3	N.D	N.D	N.D
11	78	F	Graft failure	N.P	PKP	0.78	0.39	N.D	0.39	0.98	7.23
12	75	F	Graft failure	N.P	PKP	0.18	0.18	N.D	N.D	0.18	N.D
13	70	M	Graft failure	N.P	PKP	2.58	3.23	N.D	3.23	2.58	2.58
14	79	F	Graft failure	N.P	PKP	0.65	N.D	N.D	N.D	N.D	N.D
15	58	M	Graft failure	N.P	PKP	N.D	N.D	0.31	N.D	N.D	N.D
16	92	F	Bacterial keratitis Corneal perforation	N.D	enucleation	N.D	0.42	0.42	N.D	1.68	N.D
17	64	M	Bacterial endophthalmitis, Bacterial keratitis	N.D	PKP	6.83	1.25	4.21	2.62	3.08	9.57
18	94	F	Bacterial corneal ulcer	N.D	PKP	1.31	0.49	18.23	17.73	0.66	3.61
19	85	F	Bacterial endophthalmitis	P. aeurginosa	enucleation	0.33	0.5	4.33	0.5	2.5	7.67
20	78	F	Bacterial keratitis, Corneal perforation, Autoimmune ulcer	N.D	PKP	0.3	0.3	0.3	0.3	2.11	N.D
21	72	M	Fungal keratitis, Corneal perforation	filamentous fungi	PKP	0.14	0.29	0.29	0.29	0.14	N.D
22	69	M	Trauma, Cornel perforation, Post PKP, Bacterial infection	N.D	enucleation	0.91	0.54	2.36	0.18	1.99	1.45
23	76	M	Fungal keratitis, Corneal perforation	filamentous fungi	PKP	0.38	0.19	1.5	2.63	0.75	N.D

Table 1. Cont.

Case	Age	Sex	Cause	Culture	Operation	CD1a	Langerin	DC-SIGN	CD83	Lymphatic vessels	Blood vessels
24	67	M	Herpetic keratitis, Corneal perforation	N.P	PKP	0.00	0.44	2.22	0.59	2.63	0.00
25	70	M	Post PKP, Herpetic keratitis	N.P	PKP	3.01	0.91	0.78	0.00	0.00	24.31
26	68	F	Herpetic keratitis	N.P	PKP	2.58	0.86	3.23	0.00	0.00	2.58
27	59	M	Herpetic keratitis	N.P	PKP	0.00	0.00	0.00	0.00	0.00	5.61
28	72	M	Herpetic keratitis, Graft failure	N.P	PKP	0	0	0.31	0	0	0

M, male; F, female; N.P., not performed; N.D., not detected; PKP, penetrating keratoplasty.

Monocyte-derived imDCs were harvested after 3–5 days of culture. After 3 days in culture, imDCs were stimulated with 1.5-µg/mL lipopolysaccharide (LPS; derived from *Escherichia coli* serotype O-157: B8; Sigma-Aldrich; St. Louis, MO, USA) to obtain mature DCs (mDCs). The purity of the population of isolated DCs was determined using immunocytochemistry.

Immunocytochemical analyses were performed using antibodies against CD1a, DC-SIGN, CD83, CD40 (11E9; mouse IgG2b; dilution titer, 1:25; Novocastra), CD14 (7; mouse IgG2a; dilution titer, 1:50; Novocastra), and MHC-class II (the same antibodies described above in the IHC section). The slides were fixed in 10% formalin for 10 min. Endogenous peroxidase activity was then blocked with methanol containing 0.3% hydrogen peroxide. Samples were incubated with primary antibodies overnight at room temperature. The method used for immunocytochemistry was the same as that described above for the IHC method. Approximately 80% of the imDCs used in this study expressed DC-SIGN, CD1a, and CD14, and approximately 90% expressed MHC-class II; however, only ~10% expressed CD83 and CD40. Approximately 80% of the mDCs expressed CD83 and CD40, but only ~10% expressed DC-SIGN, CD1a, and CD14.

Culture of HCE Cells and Sampling of Supernatants

HCE cells (Ocucell; Corneal epithelial cells, Kurabo; Osaka, Japan) were cultured in a 28-cm^2 dish according to the product manual. HCE cells at passage (P)3 or P4 were used in all experiments. Supernatants were collected from four treatment groups: (A) HCE cells, (B) HCE cells stimulated with 5 µg/mL LPS, (C) HCE cells co-cultured with imDCs (10^5/well), and (D) HCE cells co-cultured with imDCs and stimulated with LPS. The co-culture of HCE cells and DCs was performed as described previously [13]. All samples were collected after centrifuging at 220×*g* for 10 min to remove cells, and were stored at −80°C for a maximum of 1 month.

Migration Assays

DCs isolated from healthy donors (N = 5) were used in the migration assays. The migration of imDCs and mDCs was quantified using the Boyden chamber method. Migration assays were performed to assess for the movement of imDCs and mDCs into the supernatants of HCE cells from groups A and B described above. Migration assays were also performed in the presence of the following inflammatory cytokines: TNF-α, TGF-β$_1$, IL-6, and activin A (R&D Systems), as described previously [14–16]. ImDCs and mDCs (2.0–3.0×10^5/mL, 30 µL) were placed in the upper chamber, and supernatants A and B and the cytokine preparations were placed in the lower chamber. Membranes with 8-µm pores were used to trap the migrating DCs. The assays were performed in a humidified incubator at 37°C with 5% CO$_2$ for 2 h. After incubation, the membranes were gently removed, and the migrating cells were visualized using Giemsa staining. The migration assays were repeated three times. The number of migrating cells was counted five times by one observer, and the mean numbers were calculated.

Suppression of DC Migration by Neutralization with Anti-Activin A Antibodies

DCs isolated from healthy donors (N = 5) were used in migration assays. HCE cells were incubated with 1 µg/mL anti-activin A antibody (goat polyclonal; R&D Systems) for 12 h. The HCE cells were then stimulated with 5 µg/mL LPS, and supernatants (group E) were collected. Supernatants from group B HCE cells stimulated with 5 µg/mL LPS were also collected as a

Table 2. Numbers of dendritic cells and vessels (per mm²) in the central area of the cornea.

Dendritic cells/vessels	Non-infected (N = 15)	Infected (N = 7)	P value^A)
CD1a⁺ DCs	0.37	1.28	0.06
Langerin⁺ DCs	0.35	0.50	0.02*
DC-SIGN⁺ DCs	0.08	3.96	0.00*
CD83⁺ DCs	0.31	3.03	0.01*
Lymphatic vessels	0.46	1.61	0.01*
Blood vessels	0.98	2.79	0.32

A)Mann-Whitney U test,
*$p < 0.05$.
There were statistically significant differences in the numbers of langerin⁺ DCs, DC-SIGN⁺ DCs, CD83⁺ DCs, and lymphatic vessels between infected and non-infected cases. Herpetic keratitis cases were excluded from the statistical analyses. This is because they were all in chronic states without neutrophil infiltration; therefore, infections could not be defined.

control. The migration of imDCs toward these supernatants was quantified using a CytoSelect™96-well Cell Migration kit (Cell Biolabs, Inc.; San Diego, CA, USA) and the experiment was repeated three times.

Enzyme-Linked Immunosorbent Assay (ELISA) in HCE Cell Supernatants

The concentrations of TNF-α, TGF-β₁, IL-6, and activin A in HCE cell supernatants were quantified using ELISA kits (R&D Systems). The following supernatants were analyzed: (A) HCE cells, (B) HCE cells stimulated with LPS, (C) HCE cells co-cultured with imDCs, and (D) HCE cells co-cultured with imDCs and stimulated with LPS. ImDCs were isolated from the peripheral blood of healthy donors (N = 7). Cells were incubated in a 28-cm² dish for 1.5 h, 3 h, or 6 h at 37°C in an incubator with 5% CO_2 and a humidified atmosphere. The ELISAs were repeated four times to ensure consistent results.

Statistical Analysis

Statistical analyses were performed using SPSS ver. 18.00 (IBM; Chicago, IL, USA). The numbers of DCs and vessels, and expression of activin A were analyzed using Mann-Whitney U tests with Spearman's rank correlation coefficients. The cytokine levels in supernatants were analyzed using analysis of variance (ANOVA) with Bonferroni correction. The numbers of DCs in the migration assays were analyzed using Mann-Whitney U tests. Differences with $p < 0.05$ were considered statistically significant. In addition, stepwise multiple regression analysis was used to analyze the factors relevant to the distribution of DCs (Table 2). The independent variable was the number of DCs, and the

dependent variables included regraft, the number of blood and lymphatic vessels, and the presence of infection.

Results

IHC

Distribution of DCs and vascularization of the cornea. The infiltration of inflammatory cells, including neutrophils, was observed in seven cases of infectious corneal ulcer or corneal perforations. CD1a⁺ DCs were observed mainly in the epithelium and the subepithelial space. Langerin⁺ DCs (LCs) were observed in the epithelium. DC-SIGN⁺ DCs were observed in the subepithelial space and in the stroma. CD83⁺ DCs were found in the subepithelial space and in the upper layers of the stroma. Each type of DC was present simultaneously with inflammatory cells (Fig. 1). In inflamed corneas, the mean percentage of expression of MHC-class II molecules on the DCs was 64.3%, compared with 75.0% in non-inflamed corneas.

Blood vessels, lymphatic vessels, and corneal inflammation were more abundant in cases of infection and graft failure than choroidal tumors and degenerative diseases. Blood vessels were found in the stroma and the subepithelial space. Lymphatic vessels were mainly present in the subepithelial space (Fig. 2). VEGF-R3 was observed in the endothelium of the lymphatic vessels, and DCs were observed around these newly formed vessels (Fig. 3).

Correlations between DCs and vessels. The numbers of DCs were compared between the infected and uninfected cases. The five cases with herpetic keratitis were excluded from the present statistical analysis because clinical and histopathological evaluation revealed that the corneas were in a chronic state. Neutrophil infiltration was not detected and the presence of infection could not be confirmed in these cases. The numbers of

Table 3. Multiple regression analysis.

Dependent variable	Independent variable	Regression coefficient β	P value^A)
DC-SIGN (immature DCs)	Infection	0.537	0.01*
CD1a (immature DCs)	Blood vessels	0.683	0.00*
CD83 (mature DCs)	Infection	0.471	0.02*
Langerin (Langerhans cells)	Lymphatic vessels	0.557	0.00*

A)Mann-Whitney U test,
*$p < 0.05$.

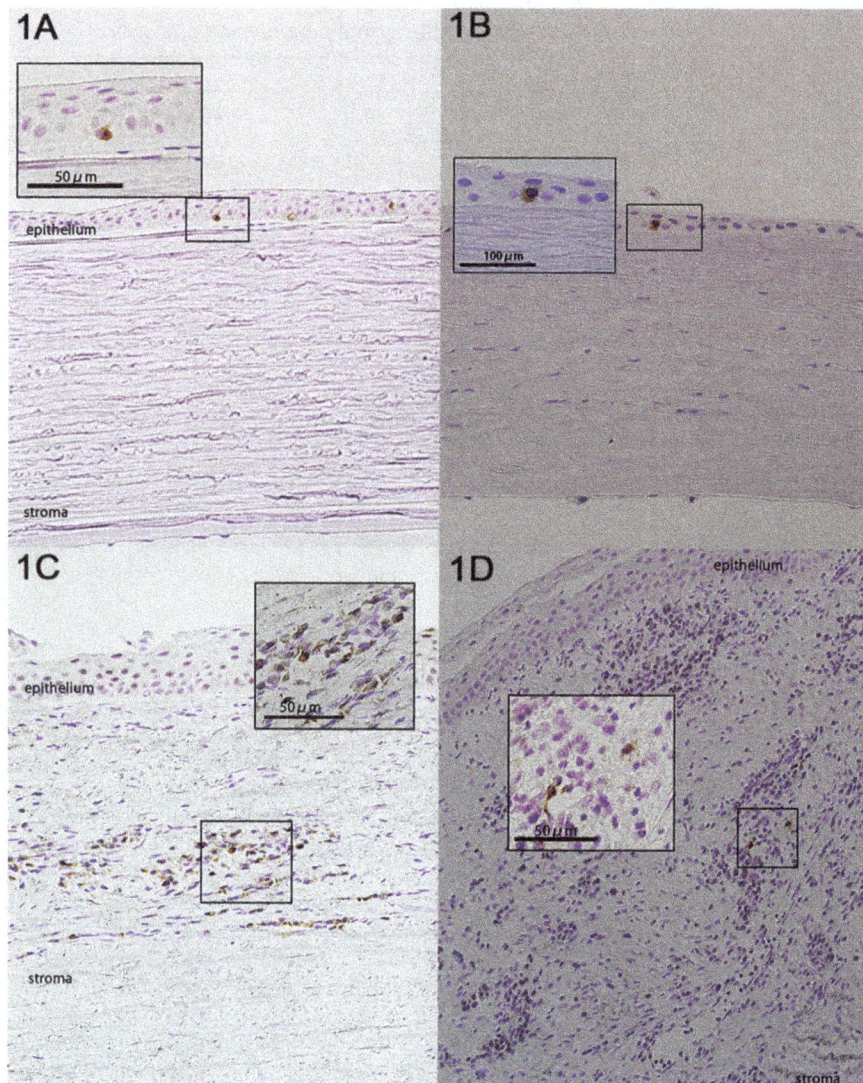

Figure 1. Distribution of dendritic cells (DCs). DCs were observed under a light microscope. Primary antibodies against CD1a (MTB1; mouse IgG1, κ; 1:30 dilution; Novocastra; Newcastle-upon-Tyne, UK), DC-SIGN (CD209; H-200; rabbit polyclonal; 1:400; Santa Cruz Biotechnology; Santa Cruz, CA, USA), langerin (CD207; 12D6; mouse IgG2b; 1:100; Ylem S.R.L.; Rome, Italy), and CD83 (1H4b; mouse IgG1, κ; 1:40; Novocastra) were used to observe DCs. **A.** Case 17; infected endophthalmitis. CD1a$^+$ DCs were observed mainly in the epithelium and the subepithelial space of an inflamed cornea. **B.** Case 17; infected endophthalmitis. Langerin$^+$ DCs were observed in the epithelium. **C.** Case 18; infected keratitis. DC-SIGN$^+$ DCs were observed in the stroma. **D.** Case 22; corneal perforation, post PKP. CD83$^+$ DCs were observed in the subepithelial space together with lymphocytic infiltration.

langerin$^+$ DCs, DC-SIGN$^+$ DCs, and CD83$^+$ DCs were significantly greater in the cases with infection compared with those without infection (Table 2).

There were statistically significant correlations between the numbers of blood vessels and lymphatic vessels ($p = 0.002$; Spearman's rank correlation coefficient). There were also statistically significant correlations between the numbers of blood vessels and DCs expressing CD1a ($p = 0.001$), langerin ($p = 0.01$), and CD83 ($p = 0.002$; Spearman's rank correlation coefficient). Additional statistically significant correlations were observed between the numbers of lymphatic vessels and of DCs expressing CD1a ($p = 0.023$), langerin ($p = 0.002$), and CD83 ($p = 0.004$; Spearman's rank correlation coefficient). Large numbers of lymphatic vessels were observed in cases of infection ($p = 0.01$), but there was no significant difference in the numbers of blood

vessels between the infected and the non-infected cases (Mann-Whitney U test, $p = 0.318$; Table 2).

Expression of activin A. Activin A was detected in the cytoplasm of epithelial cells in both the infected and the non-infected corneas. Activin A in the subepithelial space and stroma was observed in all the cases of infection, but not in the cases without infection. Inflammatory cells and DCs were simultaneously present along with activin A in the subepithelial space (Fig. 3A, B). In two of the seven infected cases (cases 19 and 22), activin A was detected in the endothelium of blood vessels (Fig. 3B).

Activin A expression in the subepithelial space (N = 8), large numbers of DCs expressing CD1a ($p = 0.002$), DC-SIGN ($p = 0.002$), and CD83 ($p = 0.007$, Mann-Whitney U test) were detected. There was no significant difference in the numbers of blood vessels and lymphatic vessels between cases with and without the expression of activin A in the subepithelial space.

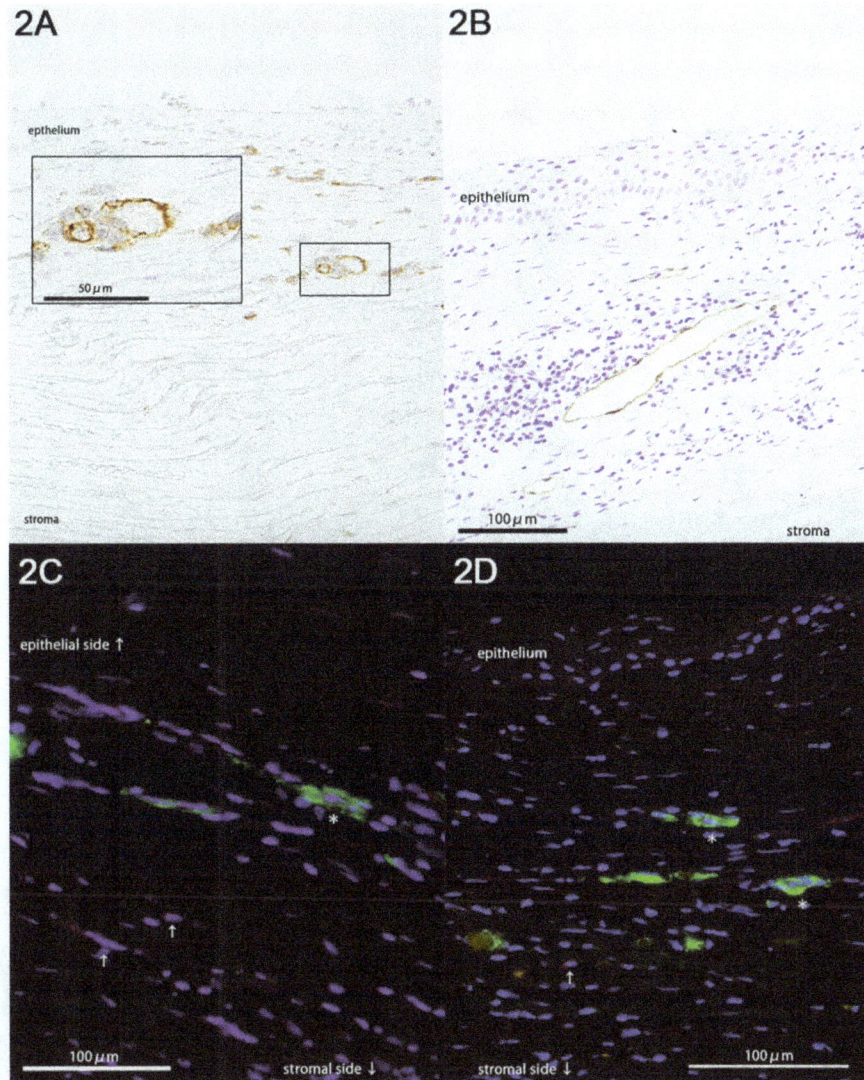

Figure 2. Vessel formations and DCs. A. Case 18; infected keratitis. Blood vessel formation was observed in the upper stroma. Blood vessels were determined by staining with anti-CD31 antibodies (JC70A; mouse IgG1,κ; 1:50; Abcam). **B.** Case 17; infected endophthalmitis. Lymphatic vessel formation was assessed using anti-D2-40 antibodies (mouse IgG1, κ, 1:50, Dako). Lymphatic vessel formation was observed in the subepithelial space. **C.** Case 18; infected keratitis. Lymphatic vessel was determined using anti-D2-40 (mouse IgG1, κ, 1:50, Dako) antibodies, and immature DCs were identified using anti-DC-SIGN antibodies (CD209; H-200; rabbit polyclonal; 1:400; Santa Cruz Biotechnology; Santa Cruz, CA, USA). A merged image of immunofluorescence staining for D2-40 (green), DC-SIGN (red), and DAPI (blue) captured using a fluorescence microscope. DC-SIGN$^+$ DCs (arrows) were observed around a lymphatic vessel (*). **D.** Case 17; infected endophthalmitis. Blood vessels were determined using anti-von Willebrand factor staining (factor VIII (rabbit polyclonal; 1:1000, Dako; Carpinteria, California, USA), and mature DCs were identified using anti-CD83 antibodies (1H4b; mouse IgG1, κ; 1:40; Novocastra). A merged image of immunofluorescence staining for factor 8 (green), CD83 (red), and DAPI (blue) was captured using a fluorescence microscope. CD83$^+$ DCs (arrow) were observed around the blood vessels (*).

Multiple Regression Analysis

Data revealed an increased number of DC-SIGN$^+$ imDCs and CD83$^+$ mDCs in the infected cases. The large number of CD1a$^+$ imDCs was related to the increase in the number of blood vessels, whereas the large number of langerin$^+$ DCs was related to the increase in the formation of lymphatic vessels. The regraft status was not related either to the increased numbers of any specific type of DC or to the increased number of blood vessels and/or lymphatic vessels (Table 3).

Migration Assay

ImDCs migrated toward LPS-stimulated HCE cell supernatant (group B), but not toward that from HCE cells only (group A),

whereas few mDCs migrated toward either supernatant. ImDCs, but few mDCs, also migrated toward all preparations of TNF-α, TGF-β$_1$, IL-6, and activin A (Table 4).

Suppression of imDC Migration by anti-Activin A

The migration of ImDCs for 1.5 h toward LPS-stimulated HCE cell supernatants with (group E) or without (group B) neutralization with anti-activin A antibodies was evaluated using relative fluorescent units (RFU). Neutralization with anti-activin A antibodies reduced the migration of imDCs toward LPS-stimulated HCE cell supernatants by ~40%. However, there was no statistically significant difference between the two treatment

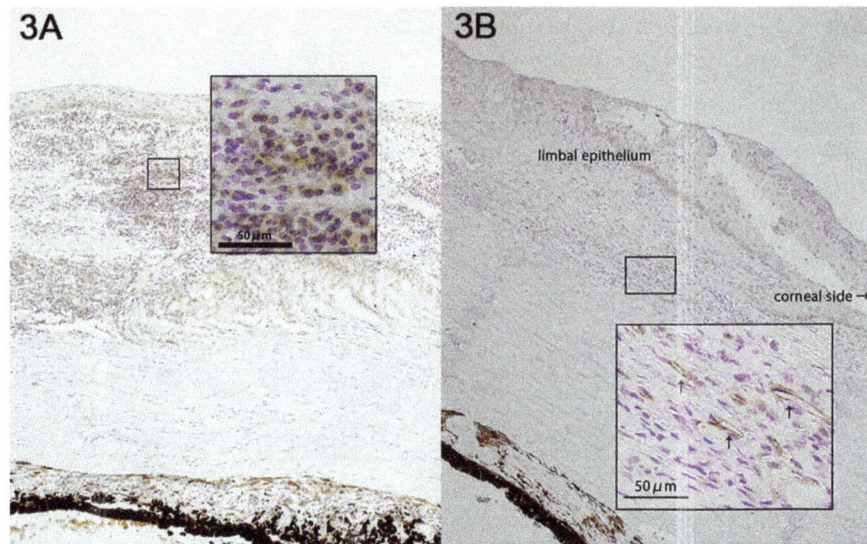

Figure 3. Expression of activin A. Activin A expression was determined using anti-activin A antibodies (goat polyclonal; 1:50; R&D Systems; Minneapolis, MN, USA). **A.** Case 17; infected endophthalmitis. Activin A was expressed in the corneal epithelial and the subepithelial space with inflammatory cells. **B.** Case 19; bacterial endophthalmitis. Activin A was expressed in the endothelium of newly formed blood vessels, which suggests the presence of vessel formation in the central cornea.

groups (group B [N = 19], 7.49 RFU vs. group E [N = 30], 4.39 (RFU); Mann-Whitney U test, $p = 0.850$].

ELISA

TGF-β_1 was not detected in any of the supernatant samples. The results of ELISAs for activin A, IL-6, and TNF-α are shown in Fig. 4. TNF-α was not detected in HCE cell supernatants from groups A, B, or C. In the supernatants from group D (LPS-stimulated HCE cells co-cultured with imDCs), elevated levels of TNF-α were observed in a time-dependent manner. IL-6 was detected in all supernatant samples. The elevation in IL-6 concentrations occurred in a time-dependent manner, except in supernatants from untreated HCE cells (group A). There were no significant differences in the IL-6 concentrations in the supernatants from groups B, C, or D after 6 h. Activin A was detected in all supernatants, but the increase in activin A concentrations was only time-dependent in HCE cells supernatants stimulated with LPS (group B).

Discussion

This study revealed that an increased number of DCs that expressed CD1a, langerin, DC-SIGN, and CD83 were distributed in the central cornea in cases with acute inflammatory cell infiltration and vessel formation. DC-SIGN is also expressed on M2 macrophages. Therefore the DC-SIGN$^+$ DCs that were observed in the stroma might include macrophages. Mayer et al. [5] revealed the presence of some types of DCs in the central human cornea, consistent with the observations in the current study. In addition, Yamagami et al. reported the presence of DCs in the corneal epithelium of human donors, which were MHC-class II positive and from the myeloid lineage [17]. Mastropasqua et al. showed the presence of DCs in normal and inflamed corneal epithelium using confocal microscopy [18], as well as an increased number of distributed DCs in inflammatory states. Although the study by Masropasqua et al. might have included both dendritic cells and macrophages because they defined DCs only using morphological findings, the results of these studies [5,17–18] are supportive of the current observations. Therefore, it is possible that the DCs present in the human cornea could induce the recruitment of additional migrating DCs for protection.

The current study revealed that vessel formation contributed to the migration of DCs into the central cornea. Large numbers of vessels in the central area could potentially induce a much faster recruitment of DCs than could the peripheral limbal vessels.

Table 4. Numbers of dendritic cells (DCs) that migrated toward the supernatants of human corneal epithelial cells that were either stimulated or not stimulated with lipopolysaccharide (LPS).

	N	Immature DCs	Mature DCs	P value[A]
LPS (−)	7	2.6	3.6	1.000
LPS (+)	7	106.1	3.3	0.00*
P value[A]		0.00*	0.45	

[A]Mann-Whitney U test,
*p<0.05.
The numbers of migratory dendritic cells in each well of the Boyden chamber are shown. LPS (−), supernatants from human corneal epithelial cells without LPS stimulation. LPS (+), supernatants from human corneal epithelial cells stimulated with LPS for 1.5 hours.

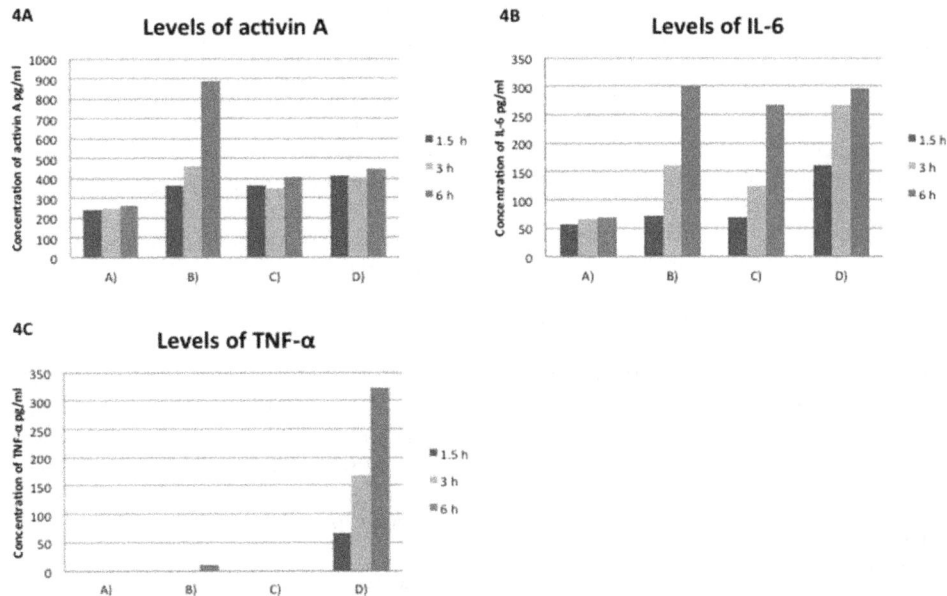

Figure 4. Increasing levels of cytokines in the supernatant of human corneal epithelial (HCE) cells. A. Levels of activin A in the supernatants from group A (HCE cells), B (HCE cells stimulated with 5 μg/mL LPS), C (HCE cells co-cultured with 10^5/well, and D (HCE cells co-cultured with imDCs and stimulated with LPS for 1 hour, 3 hours, and 6 hours). The levels of activin A increased in a time-dependent manner in supernatants from group B. After 6 hours, they were higher in groups B and D than in group C ($p<0.01$, Uni-ANOVA with a Bonferroni correction). **B.** Levels of IL-6 in the supernatants of the groups described in **A.** The levels of IL-6 increased in a time-dependent manner in groups B, C, and D. The levels of IL-6 increased after 6 hours in supernatants from groups B, C, and D, but were undetectable in those from group A. There were no significant differences in the levels of IL-6 among the supernatants from groups B, C, and D after 6 hours. **C.** Levels of TNF-α in supernatants from the groups described in **A.** TNF-α was not detectable in those from group A. TNF-α levels increased significantly only in group D, and the increase was time-dependent ($p<0.01$, Uni-ANOVA with a Bonferroni correction).

Vessel formation was observed in cases with infection, herpetic keratitis, and graft failure. Most cases of corneal perforation after trauma injury are emergencies, and vascularization is rarely observed in the cornea. However, in the current study vessel formation was observed in case 9, which exhibited corneal perforation due to trauma. This is because the patient had a history of medically treated corneal perforation before the trauma episode.

The five cases of herpetic keratitis were diagnosed according to the guidelines for herpetic keratitis from the AAO PPP Committee (Secretary for Quality of Care, Hoskins Center for Quality Eye Care). These cases were excluded from the statistical analysis of the number of distributed DCs and vessels between infected and non-infected cases (Table 2). This is because clinical and histopathological evaluations revealed that they were in the chronic state, and no neutrophils were detected. In addition, corneal perforation occurred in two of the five cases, and another two cases had recurrence of herpes virus epithelial keratitis after PKP. Therefore, we determined that these complicated backgrounds might have affected the results. In all herpetic keratitis cases, increased numbers of DCs were observed in the central area. In three of these, the herpetic keratitis resulted in significant vessel formation that might have contributed to DC migration. However, there were no statistical correlations between any types of DC and blood vessels or lymphatic vessels. Nevertheless, a study analyzing large numbers of herpetic keratitis cases from different phases is necessary to clarify the distribution of DCs during viral infection.

Activin A is a diametric glycoprotein that belongs to the TGF-β superfamily. The activin family promotes the secretion of follicle-stimulating hormone (FSH). Many additional studies have revealed that activin A is a wide-ranging cytokine and proliferative factor that functions in the reproductive system, during DC chemotaxis [9–10,19–20], and in developmental processes such as the developing nervous system [21]. In eyes, it plays roles in retinal development and inhibiting the proliferation of retinal pigment cells. In addition, the activin A receptor has been identified in the cornea (corneal epithelial cells, stromal cells, and endothelial cells), the epithelium of the ciliary body, in epithelial cells of the lens, and in retinal pigment cells [22]. However, the function of activin A in the human cornea has not yet been fully investigated. In the current study, activin A was expressed in the endothelium of newly formed blood vessels in infected corneas. Activin A promotes neovascularization in the cornea [23]; therefore, this observation suggests that activin A might promote blood vessel formation in infected and inflamed corneas. VEGFR-3 was expressed in the endothelium of the newly formed lymphatic vessels in the central part of infected corneas. It is a specific receptor for VEGF-C and VEGF-D, which induce lymphangiogenesis [7,8]; therefore, the expression of VEGFR-3 is suggestive of the lymphatic vessel formation. As such, vessel formation in infected and inflamed corneas accelerates in the central area, and these vessels form an accelerated pathway for migratory DCs to enter the central cornea and protect it from infection.

IHC data in the current study revealed activin A expression in the subepithelial space of infected corneas (N = 7). In three of seven cases (cases 20, 21, and 23), the number of DCs increased significantly without blood vessel formation (Table 1). In addition, migration assays confirmed the migration of imDCs toward activin A and supernatants from LPS-stimulated HCE cells. ELISA also demonstrated constant production of activin A by HCE cells and DCs with or without stimulation by LPS. From these findings, we concluded that, at the early stage of infection without vessel formation in the central area, activin A induced the rapid recruitment of DCs into the central cornea from the peripheral limbal vessels. It is already known that the corneal limbus is vessel-rich, and that larger numbers of DCs are present there than in the central area [5,17–18]. The recruitment of DCs from the limbus is another key pathway by which DCs enter the central cornea. Similar to the observations for activin A, our data also suggest the possible involvement of TNF-α and IL-6 in DC recruitment (Fig. 4). Although the production of cytokines by corneal cells has been studied widely [14–16] ours is the first report to demonstrate that some of these cytokines function as chemotactic factors to induce the migration of DCs into the central cornea. The results of migration assays in the presence of neutralizing anti-activin A antibodies revealed no statistically significant difference in the migration of imDCs toward the supernatants of HCE cells with or without stimulation with LPS. This suggests that activin A might be a chemotactic factor for DCs, but that it is not the only factor that stimulates the migration of DCs into the central cornea. As such, the function of activin A in the human cornea needs to be investigated further.

ELISA results in the current study showed that HCE cells stimulated with LPS produced IL-6, but not TNF-α; HCE cells only produced TNF-α when they were co-cultured with DCs and LPS. These results suggest that these two cytokines act at different stages of corneal infection. It also suggests that the secondary migration of DCs was induced by both the production of IL-6 by HCE cells during the early phase, which led to the recruitment of DCs into the central area, as well as the production of TNF-α as a result of the interaction between HCE cells and migratory DCs. Additional future studies would help clarify the mechanisms underlying the interactions between HCE cells and DCs.

Generally, dominant infiltration of neutrophils is a typical pathological finding in infected tissues. In this study it was very difficult to discuss the presence of infection based only on clinical findings because the detection rate of the pathogens was ~40%. Therefore, we hypothesized that the use of topical antibiotics before the culture affected the detection rate. However, the rate was similar to that reported previously when corneal cultures were formed from 9934 patients [24]. Therefore to confirm infection we defined infected cases according to both clinical and pathological findings. For example, a corneal ulcer due to autoimmune disease is a non-infected ulcer. In the current study the patient with autoimmune disease (case 20) had corneal perforation 1 week after cataract surgery, and she was using topical steroid and antibiotics. She had symptoms of discharge and ocular pain. The slit lamp examination showed ulceration in the epicenter, hypopyon, injection of the conjunctiva, and focus formation, which together strongly suggested infection. However, a bacterial examination did not detect any causative pathogens. IHC revealed that the discharge was neutrophil-dominant and there was significant

neutrophil infiltration into the ulcer; therefore, the patient was diagnosed with an infectious ulcer.

A limitation of this study is that we only used corneas from individuals with diseased states (Table 1); therefore, it is challenging to make rigorous comparisons of the numbers of DCs in these cases. Nevertheless, it was clear that fewer DCs were observed in cases from degenerative diseases or choroidal malignant melanomas, and no inflammatory cells were detected in the central cornea of these cases. In samples from patients with choroidal tumors, the cornea was intact, and the expression of activin A and the distribution of DCs in these cases were used as the control cases. Another limitation is that the subjects included those with a variety of diseases, past histories, and treatments. Therefore, not only infection, but also patients' backgrounds might have affected the distribution of DCs in the cornea. Multiple regression analyses suggested that the number of DC-SIGN+ and CD83+ DCs increased with inflammatory cell infiltration, and that CD1a+ and langerin+ increased with vessel formation. It is likely that these are important for the recruitment of DCs.

Conclusion

In inflamed human corneas, the number of migratory DCs increased in the avascular central area, probably to protect against infection. Newly formed corneal blood vessels and lymphatic vessels in the central cornea constitute faster paths for the migration of DCs into the central area. Activin A accelerates blood vessel formation and functions as a chemotactic factor for DCs in infected corneas. Similar to the inflammatory cytokines IL-6 and TNF-α, activin A (produced by HCE cells and imDCs) participates in the recruitment of DCs from the peripheral vessels. Therefore, the recruitment of DCs into the central cornea is orchestrated by vessel formation and the production of chemotactic factors from epithelial cells and inflammatory cells. Understanding the mechanism by which DCs migrate into the cornea will lead to the identification of therapeutic targets for corneal inflammation during corneal infection.

Acknowledgments

H. Takamura, H. Konno, and K. Nishitsuka helped with the sampling of corneas during the surgical procedures. H. Suzuki provided technical support for the immunohistochemical analysis. T. Narumi supported the sampling of peripheral blood from donors.

Author Contributions

Conceived and designed the experiments: MN. Performed the experiments: MN YK RO. Analyzed the data: MN YK HN MY. Contributed reagents/materials/analysis tools: HN RO. Wrote the paper: MN MY HY.

References

1. Knickelbein JE, Watkins SC, MacMenamin PG, Hendricks RL (2009) Stratification of antigen-presenting cells within the normal cornea. Ophthalmol Eye Dis 1: 45–54.

2. Ueta M, Kinoshita S (2010) Innate immunity of the ocular surface. Brain Res Bull 81: 219–228. DOI:10.1016/j.brainresbull.2009.10.001.

3. Forrester JV, Xu H, Kuffov L, Dick AD, McMenamin PG (2010) Dendritic cell physiology and function in the eye. Immunol Rev. 234: 282–304. DOI:10.1111/j.0105-2896.2009.00873.x.

4. Hamrah P, Dana MR (2007) Corneal antigen-presenting cells. Chem Immunol Allergy 92: 58–70.

5. Mayer WJ, Irschick UM, Moser P, Wurm M, Huemer HP, et al. (2007) Characterization of antigen presenting cells in fresh and cultured human corneas using novel dendritic cell markers. Invest Ophthalmol Vis Sci 48: 4459–4467.

6. Abbas A, Lichtman A (2008) Antigen processing and presentation to T lymphocytes. Cellular and Molecular Immunology. 5th ed. Tokyo, Japan: Elsevier Japan. 94–95.

7. Regina M, Zimmerman R, Malik G, Gausas R (2007) Lymphangiogenesis concurrent with haemangiogenesis in the human cornea. Clin Exp Ophthalmol. 35: 541–544.

8. Nakao S, Hafezi-Moghadam A, Ishibashi T (2012) Lymphatics and lymphangiogenesis in the eye. J Opthalmol DOI:10.1155/2012/783163. Epub 2012 Mar 5.

9. Salogni L, Musso T, Bosisio D, Mirolo M, Jala VR, et al. (2009) Activin A induces dendritic cell migration through the polarized release of CXC chemokine ligands 12 and 14. Blood 113: 5848–5856. DOI:10.1182/blood-2008-12-194597.

10. Robson NC, Phillips DJ, McAlpine T, Shin A, Svobodova S, et al. (2008) Activin A: a novel dendritic cell-derived cytokine that potently attenuates CD40 ligand-specific cytokine and chemokine production. Blood 111: 2733–2743.

11. Namimatsu S, Ghazizadeh M, Sugisaki Y (2005) Reversing the effects of formalin fixation with citraconic anhydride and heat: a universal antigen retrieval method. J Histochem Cytochem. 53: 3–11.

12. Romani N, Reider D, Heuer M, Ebner S, Kämpgen E, et al. (1996) Generation of mature dendritic cells from human blood. An improved method with special regard to clinical applicability. J Immunol Methods 196: 137–151.

13. Gibbs S, Spiekstra S, Corsini E, McLeod J, Reinders J (2012) Dendritic cell migration assay: A potential production model for identification of contact allergens. Toxicol In Vitro. 27(3): 1170–1179. DOI:10.1016/j.tiv.2012.05.016.

14. Zhang J, Wu XY, Yu FS (2005) Inflammatory responses of corneal epithelial cells to Pseudomonas aeruginosa infection. Curr Eye Res 30: 527–534.

15. Lu JM, Song XJ, Wang HF, Li XL, Zhang XR (2012) Murine corneal stroma cells inhibit LPS-induced dendritic cell maturation partially through TGF-β2 secretion in vitro. Mol Vision 18: 2255–2264.

16. Ebihara N, Matsuda A, Nakamura S, Matsuda H, Murakami A (2011) Role of the IL-6 classic- and trans-signaling pathways in corneal sterile inflammation and wound healing. Invest Ophthalmol Vis Sci 52: 8549–8557. DOI:10.1167/iovs.11-7956.

17. Yamagami S, Yokoo S, Usui T, Yamagami H, Amano S, et al. (2005) Distinct populations of dendritic cells in the normal human donor corneal epithelium. Invest Ophthalmol Vis Sci 46: 4489–4495.

18. Mastropasqua L, Nubile M, Lanzini M, Carpineto P, Ciancaglini M, et al. (2006) Epithelial dendritic cell distribution in normal and inflamed human cornea: in vivo confocal microscopy study. Am J Ophthalmol 142: 736–744.

19. Poulaki V, Mitsiades N, Kruse FE, Radetzky S, Ilaki E, et al. (2004) Activin a in the regulation of corneal neovascularization and vascular endothelial growth factor expression. Am J Pathol 164: 1293–1302.

20. Scutera S, Riboldi E, Daniele R, Elia AR, Fraone T, et al. (2008) Production and function of activin A in human dendritic cells. Eur Cytokine Netw 19: 60–68. DOI:10.1684/ecn.2008.0121.

21. Davis AA, Matzuk MM, Reh TA (2000) Activin A promotes progenitor differentiation into photoreceptors in rodent retina. Mol Cell Neurosci 15: 11–21.

22. Yamashita H (1997) Function of the transforming growth factor-β superfamily in eyes. Jpn J Ophthalmol 101(12): 927–947.

23. Luisi S, Florio P, Reis FM, Petraglia F (2001) Expression and secretion of activin A: possible physiological and clinical implications. Eur J Endocrinol 145: 225–236.

24. Henry RC, Flynn WH Jr, Miller D, Forster KR, Alfonso CE (2012) Infectious keratitis progressing to endophthalmitis: A 15-year study of microbiology, associated factors, and clinical outcomes. Ophthalmol 119: 2443–2449.

16

Early Keratectomy in the Treatment of Moderate *Fusarium* Keratitis

Hsin-Chiung Lin[1]*****, **Ja-Liang Lin**[2], **Dan-Tzu Lin-Tan**[2], **Hui-Kang Ma**[1], **Hung-Chi Chen**[1]

1 Department of Ophthalmology, Chang Gung Memorial Hospital, Chang Gung University College of Medicine, Taoyuan, Taiwan, **2** Department of Internal Medicine, Chang Gung Memorial Hospital, Chang Gung University College of Medicine, Taoyuan, Taiwan

Abstract

Purpose: To evaluate the treatment outcomes and costs of early keratectomy in the management of moderate *Fusarium* keratitis.

Methodology/Principal Findings: Consecutive cases of culture proven *Fusarium* keratitis treated at our hospital between January 2004 to December 2010 were included in this retrospective study. There were 38 cases of moderate keratitis with infiltrates between 3 to 6 mm in diameter and depth of infiltration not exceeding the inner 1/3 of the cornea. After excluding 5 patients with incomplete follow-up data, 13 patients who received early keratectomy within 1 week of admission were compared with a group of 20 patients treated medically. The significance of the association between early keratectomy and visual acuity, progression to perforation, secondary glaucoma and cataract formation, adjuvant therapy, hospitalization days and cost were assessed. There were no differences between the keratectomy and medication groups in regards to age, sex, presence of systemic diseases, and hypopyon formation on presentation. The early keratectomy group had a shorter hospital stay than the medical therapy group. Disease duration was significantly lower in the early keratectomy group (median: 29.0 vs. 54.5 days, $P<0.001$). Median hospitalization costs per patient were lower with early keratectomy (mean ward fee: 15175.4 vs. 44159.5 NTD, $P<0.001$; mean donor fee: 0 vs. 900.0 NTD, $P<0.001$), primarily because of reductions in hospital stay. More patients in the medication group developed perforations than in the keratectomy group (20% vs. 0%, respectively) and the perforation-free rate was higher in those with early keratectomy, but the results were not statistically significant.

Conclusions/Significance: Early keratectomy in moderate *Fusarium* keratitis may reduce length of hospital stay, hospital costs, and perforation rates.

Editor: Suzanne Fleiszig, University of California, Berkeley, United States of America

Funding: These authors have no support or funding to report.

Competing Interests: The authors have declared that no competing interests exist.

* E-mail: hclinn@adm.cgmh.org.tw

Introduction

The treatment of fungal keratitis can be challenging because the typical feathery, fluffy infiltration and endothelial plaque formation are not evident at the early stage of the disease, and the infection is often advanced on presentation due to inherent delays in arriving at an accurate diagnosis. Medical management is normally employed for the initial management of fungal keratitis, especially in mild cases where the infiltrates are located superficially, and surgical intervention is performed when medical management has failed. In advanced fungal keratitis with imminent perforation, surgical intervention in the form of therapeutic penetrating keratoplasty, conjunctival flap, or cryotherapy is often required [1–5].

Fungal infection has a relatively silent early phase in the cornea as compared with bacterial keratitis, as a few weeks are usually required before the infiltrate becomes evident and the stroma becomes inflamed [6,7]. The lack of marked inflammation in the surrounding stroma permits direct visualization of the delicate, feathery branching hyphae and facilitates debulking of the fungal elements by keratectomy; there is concern regarding an increased

risk of corneal perforation after early keratectomy; however, because *Fusarium* keratitis appears to be the most virulent and most common form of fungal keratitis in tropical and subtropical regions, it might be valuable to figure out the effectiveness and risk of complications of performing early keratectomy in moderate *Fusarium keratitis*.

The objectives of this study were to compare treatment outcomes, costs of care, and long-term complications in patients with moderate *Fusarium* keratitis that received early keratectomy as compared to those treated medically.

Methods

Patients and Treatments

The study protocol adhered to the tenets of the Declaration of Helsinki, and was approved by the Human Research Ethics Committee at Chang Gung Memorial Hospital, Taiwan (99-0576B). Based on our previous report on the treatment of *Fusarium solani* keratitis [8], corneal smears were cultured for bacteria and fungi on chocolate, 5% sheep blood, anaerobic blood agar, inhibitory mold agar (IMA), IMA supplemented with chloramphenicol and gentamicin (ICG) agar, and thioglycollate medium. External eye photographs were documented weekly, and reculture was performed in cases of progression or poor medical response after the cessation of empiric topical antibiotics for 24 hours. At the initial encounter all patients were informed about the possibility of ulcer progression and that an operation may be needed during the disease process. In some cases, keratectomy was suggested for the purpose of obtaining a diagnostic biopsy in culture negative cases. Other patients with moderate severity disease were given the option of surgical or medical management.

Inclusion criterion was culture proven *Fusarium* infection of the cornea in patients seen between January 2004 and December 2010. Severity of keratitis was graded prospectively according to a modification of that described by Jones [1] (Table 1). The ulcer was graded as severe if the area of suppuration was >6 mm in diameter, involved the inner third of the cornea, or if perforation was imminent. Because the progression of *Fusarium* keratitis is relatively slow as compared with bacterial keratitis, we further divided non-severe keratitis into mild and moderate. Study cases were included if the corneal infiltrate was ≥3 mm but <6 mm in diameter, and the depth of involvement was not more than the inner 1/3 of the corneal thickness. Cases were excluded from analysis if <16 years of age, severe ocular surface disease was present such as Stevens-Johnson syndrome, chemical burn, or neurotrophic keratitis [9]. Subjects were followed-up for a minimum of 3 months.

Data collected from the medical records included age, sex, presence of systemic diseases, inciting factors, presenting symptoms, location and size of the infiltrate, presence of anterior chamber reaction, hypopyon, endothelial plaque, significant progressive pain, visual acuity (initial visual acuity was assessed at the initial patient visit, and final visual acuity was assessed upon healing of the epithelial defect), antibiotics chosen for outpatient therapy, initial medical treatment and surgical procedures after admission, length of hospital stay, disease duration, readmission, subsequent adjuvant therapy or surgery, and secondary complications.

Areas of keratitis were debrided with a No. 15 blade for microbial culture and sensitivity testing before initiation of therapy. Empiric broad-spectrum antibiotics, such as an aminoglycoside and cefazolin, ciprofloxacin, or levofloxacin were administered before culture results were obtained. Subsequent modifications in antibiotic choice and dosage depended on results of culture and sensitivity testing and clinical response. *Fusarium* keratitis was treated with topical 5% natamycin drops (Alcon Labs, Texas, USA). Superficial keratectomy was performed with a No. 57 Beaver blade, and the stromal infiltrate was removed as completely as possible. The maximum depth of keratectomy was approximately 1/2 to 2/3 of the cornea depth. In cases of severe keratitis, a corneal patch graft or amniotic membrane transplan-

tation was used as adjuvant therapy as previously described [8,10]. Supportive therapy included cycloplegics, analgesics, and anti-glaucoma medications whenever required.

The patients were monitored until the ulcer healed, which was considered the absence of symptoms and corneal infiltrate, with decreased ciliary congestion and healed epithelial defect. Follow-up visits for a minimum of 3 months after ulcer healing were scheduled to ensure there was no recurrence of *Fusarium* keratitis.

Cost Analysis

Component costs were estimated by reviewing the cost of treatment of a series of cases of microbial keratitis at a tertiary referral hospital. This analysis yielded values for components of treatment, i.e., hospital bed days, operating room time, and surgical team.

Statistical Analysis

Continuous data are presented as median and inter-quartile range (IQR) except for cost data, which are presented as mean and standard deviation. The differences between groups were tested with the non-parametric Wilcoxon rank-sum test except for cost data that were tested with the independent two samples test. Categorical data are presented as the number and percentage, and the differences between groups were tested with Fisher's exact test. The primary outcome measure, perforation-free rate, was determined by the Kaplan-Meier estimates and tested with the log-rank test. As visual acuity data are not linear, they were converted to LogMAR for statistical analysis [11]. In brief, Log $20/2000 = 2 =$ counting fingers, and Log $20/20000 = 3 =$ hand motion. Cost analysis data are reported in New Taiwan Dollars (NTDs). All hypothesis tests were 2-tailed, and a value of $P<0.05$ was considered to indicate statistical significance. All statistical analyses were performed using Stat View (Abacus Concepts, Inc).

Results

A total of 38 patients with moderate keratitis (involving 1/3 to 2/3 the stromal depth, and 3 to 6 mm in diameter) were seen during the study period. Of the 38 patients, 13 received superficial keratectomies within 1 week of admission, 20 patients received medical therapy only, and 5 patients were excluded due to follow-up of <3 months (Table 2). There were no significant differences between the two groups with respect to age, sex, involved eyes, location (central or periphery), baseline chronic diseases, smoking, and severity of the corneal ulcer. However, the baseline visual acuity of the medication group was statistically significantly worse than that of the surgery group.

Outcomes of the two groups are shown in Table 3, and specific data of the keratectomy group are presented in Table 4. In the keratectomy group, two patients had resolution of the corneal ulcer after keratectomy without the application of natamycin. In

Table 1. Clinical grading and treatment of fungal keratitis*.

Grade	Clinical Findings	Treatment
Mild	Infiltration not exceeding anterior 1/3 stroma, <3 mm in diameter	Debridement and topical antifungal medication
Moderate	Infiltration of 1/3 to 2/3 of the stroma, 3–6 mm in diameter	Debridement or superficial keratectomy, topical/with or without oral antifungal medication
Severe	Infiltration deep to inner 1/3 stroma, or >6 mm in diameter	Therapeutic keratoplasty, topical/with or without oral antifungal medication

*As described by Jones [1], with modifications.

Table 2. Baseline characteristics of patients with moderate severe *Fusarium* keratitis.

		Keratectomy group (*n*=13)	Medication group (*n*=20)	*P*-value
Age (year)		57.0 (48.0, 59.0)	62.0 (54.5, 67.0)	0.060
Sex	Female	8 (61.5)	7 (35.0)	0.169
	Male	5 (38.5)	13 (65.0)	
Infected Eye	OD	4 (30.8)	9 (45.0)	0.485
	OS	9 (69.2)	11 (55.0)	
Diabetes mellitus		3 (23.1)	6 (30.0)	>0.999
Hypertension		4 (30.8)	7 (35.0)	>0.999
Smoking		2 (15.4)	2 (10.0)	>0.999
Initial VA (log Mar)		1.2 (1.0, 2.0)	2.0 (1.6, 2.0)	0.033*
Area of keratitis (mm^2)		12.5 (11.9, 16.0)	12.6 (9.5, 13.9)	0.319
Hypopyon formation		5 (38.5)	6 (30.0)	0.714

Data are presented as median (interquartile range) or number (percentage).
*Indicates a signficant difference between the two groups.

these patients the keratitis healed with re-epithelialization before the culture grew *Fusarium* sp. Topical antibiotics were switched to natamycin after culture results were available. Five patients had progression of keratitis after keratectomy that was successfully controlled with natamycin, and no patients experienced perforation or glaucoma.

In the medication group, eight patients exhibited stationary recovery of keratitis with medical therapy and 12 patients had progression of keratitis. Of the 12 patients with progression, four received amniotic membrane grafts as adjuvant therapy and four experienced microperforations and focal peripheral anterior synechiae and patch grafts were needed to seal the perforations. Increased intraocular pressure occurred in four patients due to inflammation of the disease process. Three patients had recurrence of keratitis that required readmission within 30 days.

Length of stay and clinical outcomes

The median hospital stay in the keratectomy and medication groups was 11.0 vs. 31.5 days (*P*<0.001). Significantly more patients were discharged home within 10 days after superficial keratectomy; five patients in the keratectomy group had a hospital stay of <10 days, but all patients in the medication group had a hospital stay >10 days (38.5% vs. 0%, respectively, *P*=0.005). Disease duration and hospital bed fee were significantly lower in the study group (Table 3). The costs for adjuvant surgical procedures (amniotic membrane or patch grafts) were significantly lower in the keratectomy group (mean 0 vs. 900 NTD, *P* <0.001). The ward fee was also significantly lower in the keratectomy group (mean 15175.4 vs. 44159.5 NTD, *P*<0.001). Expenses for the operating room and surgical team were comparable between the groups.

Table 3. Comparison of treatment methods, outcomes, and complications.

	Keratectomy group (*n*=13)	Medication group (*n*=20)	*P*-value
Hospital stay (d)	11.0 (9.0, 14.0)	31.5 (19.5, 49.0)	<0.001*
Disease duration (d)	29.0 (24.0, 33.0)	54.5 (37.0, 70.0)	<0.001*
Hospital cost†			
Ward fee	15175.4±7062.7	44159.5±25926.9	<0.001*
Operation room	3479.0±0	4068.3±4642.7	0.577
Donor fee	0±0	900.0±923.4	<0.001*
AMG	0 (0.0%)	4 (20.0%)	0.136
Patch graft	0 (0.0%)	4 (20.0%)	0.136
Glaucoma	0 (0.0%)	4 (20.0%)	0.136
Final VA (log Mar)	0.4 (0.2, 1.1)	2.0 (0.9, 3.0)	<0.001*
Perforation	0 (0.0%)	4 (20.0%)	0.136
Recurrence	0 (0.0%)	3 (15.0%)	0.261
Follow-up time (month)	6.0 (5.0, 12.0)	10.0 (6.0, 23.5)	0.083

Hospital stay, disease duration, final VA, and follow-up time were presented as median with IQR. Hospital costs were presented by mean ± standard deviation. Other categorical data are presented by count with percentage.
AMG, amniotic membrane graft; VA, visual acuity.
*Indicates a signficant difference between the two groups.
†New Taiwan Dollars (NTD).

Table 4. Data of patients treated with early keratectomy.

Case	Foreign body	Gender/age/eye/systemic disease/smoking	Keratectomy (days after admission)	Hospital stay (d)	Size of ulcer/depth	Hypopyon	Medications/culture before referral	Adjuvant therapy*	Initial VA/Final VA	Complications/follow-up time (months)
1	Vegetable	F/64/OS/H	3	9	3×4 mm	No	Gentamicin/No	No	0.1/0.4	None/6
2	UFB	F/77/OS/smoking	6	14	3.5×3 mm	Yes	Norfloxacin/No	No	CF 40 cm/0.06	None/6
3	UFB	F/62/OS/DM	3	11	4×4 mm	No	Acyclovir, Ciprofloxacin/No	No	CF 30 cm/0.08	None/7
4	NA	F/39/OS/H	2	3	4.5×3.8 mm	Yes	NA	No	CF 50 cm/0.06	None/5
5	Iron dust	M/41/OS	3	9	4×6 mm	No	Gentamicin/No	No	HM 10 cm/0.7	None/4
6	NA	M/48/OD	4	10	3.6×3.3 mm	Yes	NA	No	0.8/1.0	None/36
7	Dirt	F/37/OS	5	8	3×3 mm	No	Ciprofloxacin/No	No	0.3/0.7	None/4
8	Flower	F/56/OD	2	4	3×3 mm	No	Levofloxacin/No	No	0.4/0.5	None/3
9	Dirt	M/57/OS/H	6	23	6×4 mm	Yes	Norfloxacin/no growth	No	0.1/0.3	None/12
10	Plastic	F/57/OD/DM	6	14	3.5×3.5 mm	No	Oral famciclovir, dexan, ciprofloxacin/No	No	CF 30 cm/0.7	None/5
11	Vegetable	M/53/OS	3	20	4.5×3 mm	No	Norfloxacin/No	No	CF 1 m/0.4	None/6
12	UFB	F/59/OS	4	16	2.5×5 mm	Yes	Gentamicin/No	No	0.1/0.05	None/14
13	UFB	M/57/OD/DM, HTN/smoking	3	11	4×4 mm	No	NA/No	No	0.05/0.1	None/12

F, female; M, male; DM, diabetes mellitus; HTN, hypertension; UFB, unknown foreign body; CF, counting finger visual acuity; NA, not applicable.
*Adjuvant therapy other than early keratectomy. Disease duration: healing of epithelial defect. Final visual VA: determined upon healing of the epithelial defect.

Initial visual acuity ranged from hand motion to 1.0 in both groups, but final visual acuity was significantly decreased in the medication group (median log MAR 0.4 vs. 2.0, $P<0.001$). To account for the difference in baseline visual acuity, a linear regression model using the bootstrapping method with 60 repetitions was performed which showed that the final visual acuity of the keratectomy group was significantly better than the medication group (difference in logMAR = 1.05, ($P = 0.001$), a result similar to the unadjusted analysis. More patients in the medication group developed perforations than in the keratectomy group (20% vs. 0%, respectively) and the perforation-free rate was higher in those with early keratectomy, but the results did not obtain statistical significance ($P = 0.093$ by log-rank test) (Fig. 1). Four patients experienced secondary glaucoma and three had recurrence of *Fusarium* keratitis within 30 days in the medical treatment group, while no patients in the keratectomy group developed secondary glaucoma or recurrence.

Discussion

The management of keratitis varies depending on the severity at presentation. Ophthalmologists treat suspected infectious keratitis differently with various antibiotics, debridement, and/or keratectomy, and are more likely to forgo scrapings for Gram-staining and cultures when ulcers appear less severe [1–4,12–13]. Less severe *Fusarium* keratitis cases are treated initially with antibiotics before culture results are available, and some may resolve before the application of antifungal medications because of the resolution of the superficial lesion from scraping and the possible antifungal effects of some antibiotics [14–17].

In moderate *Fusarium* keratitis, the infiltrate usually cannot be removed by scraping alone, and a superficial keratectomy with a Beaver blade or phototherapeutic keratectomy is needed in order to remove the stromal infiltrate as completely as possible [8,18]. Debate about the treatment of moderate *Fusarium* keratitis centers around concern over the increased risk of corneal perforation after early keratectomy. Despite this concern, there are a number of reasons for performing early keratectomy in moderate *Fusarium* keratitis. There are few commercially available antifungal medications (as compared to the number available for bacterial keratitis), clinical drug sensitivity testing is not widely available,

and the growth of fungi tends to be slower as compared to bacterial growth, making clinical judgment surrounding medication efficacy less efficient. The disease duration is longer in *Fusarium* keratitis, making the length of treatment and related drug toxicity a concern in the medical management of moderate *Fusarium* keratitis. In moderate *Fusarium* keratitis, the corneal infiltrates usually appear rough and dry in texture with distinct margins and little surrounding inflammation, making superficial keratectomy easy to perform. Lastly, the risk of progression of moderate to severe keratitis may occur within a few days in *Fusarium* keratitis, the most virulent species (Figure 2), leading to secondary cataract formation, glaucoma and perforation.

Fusarium keratitis most frequently occurs in tropical areas [19,20]; however, an increasing prevalence has been noted in temperate climates, partly due to contact lens usage [9]. Most patients with superficial keratitis due to fungal origin respond to medical therapy, several antifungals have been found effective, and natamycin and voriconazole appear to forestall the need for surgical intervention [21,22]. In contrast, almost 70% of patients with *Fusarium* keratitis with deep lesions do not respond to medical therapy alone. *Fusarium solani* is able to destroy an eye completely within a few weeks since the infection is usually severe; perforation, deep extension, and malignant glaucoma may supervene [8]. Rosa et al. [19] treated patients with superficial keratitis due to *Fusarium solani* with topical natamycin and those with deep lesions received topical natamycin and systemic antifungal medication. The average duration of treatment was 38 days and 22 (28%) patients ultimately required penetrating keratoplasty and enucleation was required in 1 patient. Alexandrakis et al. [23] reported that diagnostic corneal biopsy contributed significantly to the diagnosis, treatment, and outcome of patients with progressive infectious keratitis. A microorganism was isolated from 27 (82%) of 33 corneal biopsies, and *Fusarium spp* was one of the most common isolates in progressive keratitis.

The progression of *Fusarium* keratitis depends on the host as well as pathogenic factors [9,24–30]. In this study, patients who received early keratectomy had shorter hospitalization stays and disease duration compared to those who did not. In moderate *Fusarium* keratitis, superficial keratectomy may aid in medical management by increasing drug penetration, by removing infected corneal tissue and subsequently reducing or eliminating the microbial load. In the present study, 13 study cases showed decreased inflammation after keratectomy at an early stage of moderate keratitis, without progression of ulcer or perforation or secondary glaucoma. Strategies for reducing perforation from fungal keratitis are important in Taiwan, where fungal keratitis accounts for 50% of corneal transplantations [31].

Surgery may be necessary when *Fusarium* keratitis responds poorly, or not at all, to medical therapy or when perforation is imminent [32,33]. In the medical treatment group, four patients experienced microperforations and focal peripheral anterior synechiae and patch graft or therapeutic penetrating keratoplasty (PK) was needed to seal the perforation more than 2 weeks after admission, and three patients required readmission due to recurrence of *Fusarium* keratitis. Those complications of keratitis were primarily due to fungal keratitis refractory to treatment, leading to progression of a moderate *Fusarium* keratitis to a severe form. *Fusarium* keratitis is notorious for its recurrence after therapeutic PK [30,34]. Furthermore, performance of early superficial keratectomy for moderate *Fusarium* keratitis, in lieu of corneal transplant surgery, could reduce the chance of intraocular extension during the acute infectious stage, and enable subsequent optical keratoplasty to be more successful.

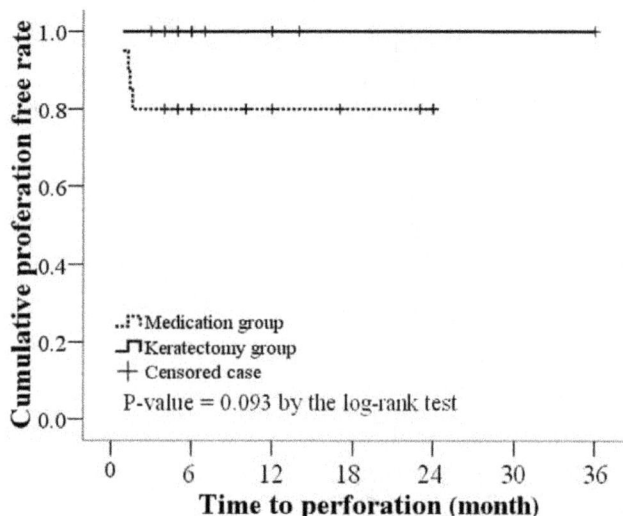

Figure 1. Kaplan-Meier survival analysis of corneal perforation.

2.1

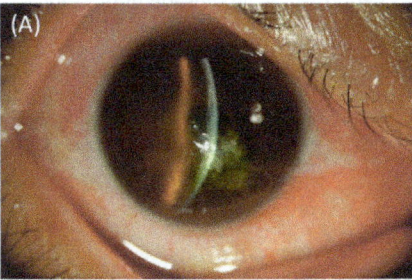
(A)

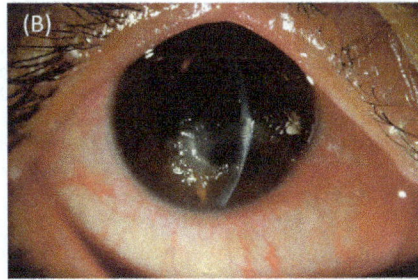
(B)

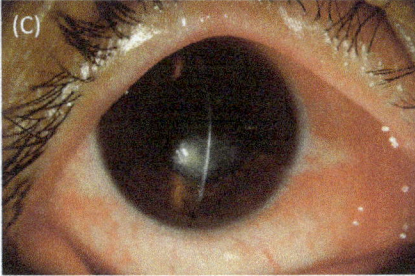
(C)

2.2

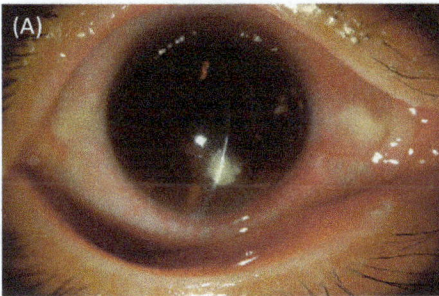
(A)

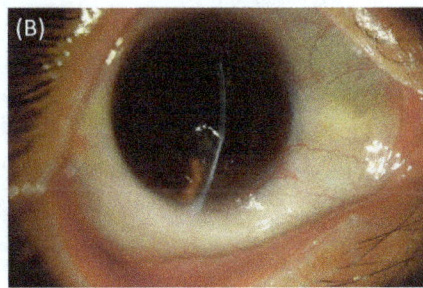
(B)

2.3

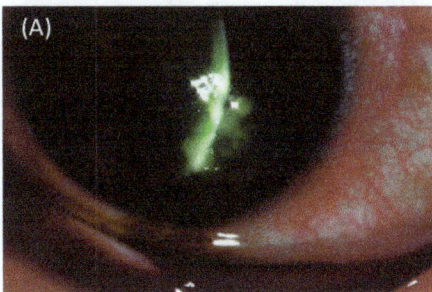
(A)

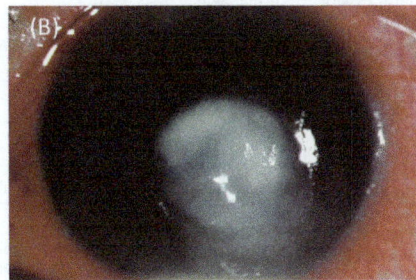
(B)

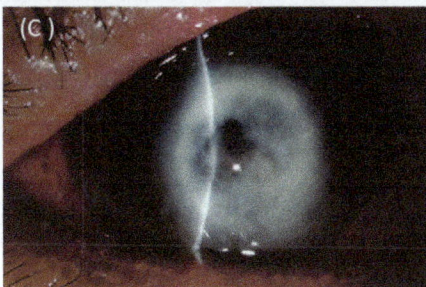
(C)

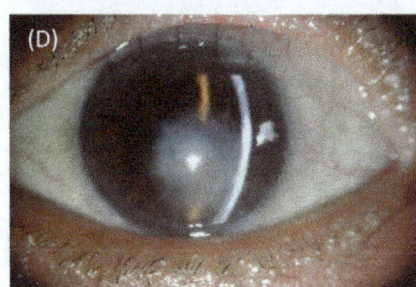
(D)

Figure 2. Clinical photography. 1. Clinical photographs of 57-year-old female. A) On presentation a corneal infiltrate with a feathery margin and anterior chamber inflammation were noted. Initial visual acuity was CF 30 cm. Initial debridement was performed. B) Progression of the keratitis 7 days later despite initial debridement. C) One month after superficial keratectomy and treatment with natamycin suspension. The ulcer was healed and best-corrected visual acuity was 0.7. 2. A 56-year-old female who presented with right eye pain 10 days after a foreign body injury. A) The paracentral corneal lesion appeared dry, rough, and elevated. Visual acuity 0.4. The other cornea was not inflamed. B) One week after superficial keratectomy, the lesion was healed and appeared thinned. Visual acuity 0.5. 3. A 66-year-old male. A) Central, fluffy corneal infiltration was noted on presentation. Visual acuity was hand motion. B) Three days later the infiltration had progressed with descementocele formation (C) despite topical natamycin therapy. He then received amniotic membrane transplantation as adjuvant therapy for the imminent perforation. D) Eleven months later a cataract surgery was performed and visual acuity remained counting fingers due to central scarring.

Keay et al. [35] reported the major cost of treating microbial keratitis was hospital visits and hospital bed days and treating fungal keratitis is more expensive than treating bacterial keratitis. Hospital direct expenses were significantly lower in the early keratectomy group in the current study, mainly due to the decreased number of hospital days.

Possible biases and limitations of this study include that the data were examined retrospectively and that the study was conducted in a subspecialty clinic at a university hospital. Treatment was based on the personal preferences of the physicians (there were up to 8 specialty physicians treating patients during the study period) and whether or not the patient consented to surgery.

Conclusions

In this population of Taiwanese with moderate *Fusarium* keratitis, early keratectomy was associated with decreased short-term and long-term complication rates, and required fewer financial resources to treat fungal keratitis. Early keratectomy may be useful in the treatment of patients with moderate severity *Fusarium* keratitis.

Acknowledgments

The authors would like to thank Dr. Kwan-Wu Chen, Chang Gung University and College of Technology, for his assistance with the statistical analysis.

Author Contributions

Conceived and designed the experiments: HCL. Performed the experiments: HCL HKM HCC. Analyzed the data: DTLT. Contributed reagents/materials/analysis tools: HCL HKM HCC. Wrote the paper: HCL KWC. Statistic assistance: KWC JLL.

References

1. Jones DB (1981) Decision-making in the management of microbial keratitis. Ophthalmology 88: 814–820.
2. Forster RK, Rebell G (1975) The Diagnosis and Management of Keratomycoses II. Medical and Surgical Management. Arch Ophthalmol 93: 1134–1136.
3. Meleod S, DeBacker C, Viana M (1996) Differential care of corneal ulcers in the community based on apparent severity. Ophthalmology 103: 479–484.
4. Loh AR, Hong K, Lee S, Mannis M, Acharya NR (2009) Practice Patterns in the Management of Fungal Corneal Ulcers. Cornea 28: 856–859.
5. Thomas P (2003) Current Perspectives on Ophthalmic Mycoses. Clin Microbiol Rev 16: 730–797.
6. Alfonso E, Rosa RJ, Miller D (2005) Fungal keratitis. In: Krachmer JH, Mannis MJ, Holland EJ Cornea 2nd Ed Elsevier. Mosby 1 (86): 1101.
7. Srinivasan M (2004) Fungal keratitis. Curr Opin Ophthalmol 15: 321–327.
8. Lin HC, Chu PH, Kuo YH, Shen SC (2005) Clinical experience in managing Fusarium solani keratitis. Int J Clin Pract 59: 549–554.
9. Jurkunas U, Behlau I, Colby K (2009) Fungal keratitis: changing pathogens and risk factors. Cornea 28: 638–643.
10. Chen H, Tan HY, Hsiao CH, Huang SCM, Lin KK, et al. (2006) Amniotic membrane transplantation for persistent corneal ulcers and perforations in acute fungal keratitis. Cornea 25: 564–572.
11. Journal of Refractive Surgery (2009) Visual Acuity Conversion Chart/Masthead. J Cataract Refract Surg 2009;35:A4.
12. Vajpayee RB, Dada T, Saxena R, Vajpayee M, Taylor HR, et al. (2000) Study of the first contact management profile of cases of infectious keratitis: a hospital-based study. Cornea 19: 52–56.
13. Tananuvat N, Suwanniponth M (2008) Microbial keratitis in Thailand: a survey of common practice patterns. J Med Assoc Thai 91: 316–322.
14. Day S, Lalitha P, Haug S, Fothergill AW, Cevallos V, et al. (2009) Activity of antibiotics against Fusarium and Aspergillus. Br J Ophthalmol 93: 116–119.
15. Lin HC, Hsiao CH, Ma DHK, Yeh LK, Tan HY, et al. (2009) Medical treatment for combined Fusarium and Acanthamoeba keratitis. Acta Ophthalmol 2009 87: 199–203.
16. Bhartiya P, Daniell M, Constantinou M, Islam F, Taylor H (2007) Fungal keratitis in Melbourne. Clin Experiment Ophthalmol 35: 124–130.
17. Munir W, Rosenfeld S, Udell I, Miller D, Karp C, et al. (2007) Clinical response of contact lens-associated fungal keratitis to topical fluoroquinolone therapy. Cornea 26: 621–624.
18. Lin CP, Chang CW, Su CY (2005) Phototherapeutic keratectomy in treating keratomycosis. Cornea 24: 262–268.
19. Rosa RH Jr, Miller D, Alfonso EC (1994) The changing spectrum of fungal keratitis in south Florida. Ophthalmology 101: 1005–1013.
20. Wang L, Sun S, Jing Y, Han L, Zhang H, et al. (2009) Spectrum of fungal keratitis in central China. Clin Experiment Ophthalmol 37: 763–771.
21. Tanure MA, Cohen EJ, Sudesh S, Rapuano CJ, Laibson PR (2000) Spectrum of fungal keratitis at Wills Eye Hospital, Philadelphia, Pennsylvania. Cornea 19: 307–312.
22. Hariprasad SM, Mieler WF, Lin TK, Sponsel WE, Graybill JR (2008) Voriconazole in the treatment of fungal eye infections: a review of current literature. Br J Ophthalmol 92: 871–878.
23. Alexandrakis G, Haimovici R, Miller D, Alfonso EC (2000) Corneal biopsy in the management of progressive microbial keratitis. Am J Ophthalmol 129: 571–576.
24. Bharathi MJ, Ramakrishnan R, Meenakshi R, Shivakumar C, Raj DL (2009) Analysis of the risk factors predisposing to fungal, bacterial & Acanthamoeba keratitis in south India. Indian J Med Res 130: 749–757.
25. Doczi I, Gyetvai T, Kredics L, Nagy E (2004) Involvement of Fusarium spp. in fungal keratitis. Clin Microbiol Infect 10: 773–776.
26. Furlanetto R, Andreo EG, Finotti IG, Arcieri ES, Ferreira MA, et al. (2010) Epidemiology and etiologic diagnosis of infectious keratitis in Uberlandia, Brazil. Eur J Ophthalmol.
27. Galarreta DJ, Tuft SJ, Ramsay A, Dart JK (2007) Fungal keratitis in London: microbiological and clinical evaluation. Cornea 26: 1082–1086.
28. Green M, Apel A, Stapleton F (2008) Risk factors and causative organisms in microbial keratitis. Cornea 27: 22–27.
29. Vemuganti GK, Garg P, Gopinathan U, Naduvilath TJ, John RK, et al. (2002) Evaluation of agent and host factors in progression of mycotic keratitis: A histologic and microbiologic study of 167 corneal buttons. Ophthalmology 109: 1538–1546.
30. Shi W, Wang T, Xie L, Li S, Gao H, et al. (2010) Risk Factors, Clinical Features, and Outcomes of Recurrent Fungal Keratitis after Corneal Transplantation. Ophthalmology 117: 890–896.
31. Chen WL, Hu FR, Wang IJ (2001) Changing indications for penetrating keratoplasty in Taiwan from 1987 to 1999. Cornea 20: 141–144.
32. Xie L, Dong X, Shi W (2001) Treatment of fungal keratitis by penetrating keratoplasty. Br J Ophthalmol 85: 1070–1074.
33. Xie L, Shi W, Liu Z, Li S (2002) Lamellar keratoplasty for the treatment of fungal keratitis. Cornea 21: 33–37.
34. Gupta G, Feder RS, Lyon AT (2009) Fungal keratitis with intracameral extension following penetrating keratoplasty. Cornea 28: 930–932.
35. Keay L, Edwards K, Naduvilath T, Taylor H, Snibson G, et al. (2006) Microbial keratitis predisposing factors and morbidity. Ophthalmology 113: 109–116.

17

A Simple Isothermal DNA Amplification Method to Screen Black Flies for *Onchocerca volvulus* Infection

Andy Alhassan[1], Benjamin L. Makepeace[2], Elwyn James LaCourse[3], Mike Y. Osei-Atweneboana[4], Clotilde K. S. Carlow[1]*

1 Division of Genome Biology, New England Biolabs, Ipswich, Massachusetts, United States of America, 2 Institute of Infection & Global Health, University of Liverpool, Liverpool, United Kingdom, 3 Liverpool School of Tropical Medicine, Liverpool, United Kingdom, 4 Council for Scientific and Industrial Research, Water Research Institute, Accra, Ghana

Abstract

Onchocerciasis is a debilitating neglected tropical disease caused by infection with the filarial parasite *Onchocerca volvulus*. Adult worms live in subcutaneous tissues and produce large numbers of microfilariae that migrate to the skin and eyes. The disease is spread by black flies of the genus *Simulium* following ingestion of microfilariae that develop into infective stage larvae in the insect. Currently, transmission is monitored by capture and dissection of black flies and microscopic examination of parasites, or using the polymerase chain reaction to determine the presence of parasite DNA in pools of black flies. In this study we identified a new DNA biomarker, encoding *O. volvulus* glutathione *S*-transferase 1a (*OvGST1a*), to detect *O. volvulus* infection in vector black flies. We developed an *OvGST1a*-based loop-mediated isothermal amplification (LAMP) assay where amplification of specific target DNA is detectable using turbidity or by a hydroxy naphthol blue color change. The results indicated that the assay is sensitive and rapid, capable of detecting DNA equivalent to less than one microfilaria within 60 minutes. The test is highly specific for the human parasite, as no cross-reaction was detected using DNA from the closely related and sympatric cattle parasite *Onchocerca ochengi*. The test has the potential to be developed further as a field tool for use in the surveillance of transmission before and after implementation of mass drug administration programs for onchocerciasis.

Editor: Henk D. F. H. Schallig, Royal Tropical Institute, Netherlands

Funding: CKSC and AA received funding from New England Biolabs. The funders had no role in study design, data collection and analysis, decision to publish, or preparation of the manuscript.

Competing Interests: CKSC and AA have received funding from and are employed by New England Biolabs.

* Email: carlow@neb.com

Introduction

Onchocerciasis, or River Blindness, is a neglected tropical disease caused by the parasitic worm *Onchocerca volvulus*. The parasite is transmitted to humans through exposure to repeated bites of infected black flies of the genus *Simulium*. The disease is a major public health concern, and has severe social and economic impact. Recent estimates indicate that, more than 30.4 million people are infected, mostly in sub-Saharan Africa [1,2]. Over 700,000 people are visually impaired and another 265,000 are blinded by the disease [3]. There is no vaccine against infection or suitable macrofilaricidal drug that kills the adult stage of *O. volvulus*. Current control is based on annual or semi-annual distribution of the larvicidal compound ivermectin (Mectizan, Merck) to the population irrespective of infection status [4–6]. In the absence of an adulticide, it is recommended that these mass drug administration (MDA) campaigns should be continued for 10–15 years [7].

MDA programs have now progressed for several years in many areas, and careful monitoring of infection levels in human populations, as well as vectors, is required to evaluate their success, certify elimination and guide the decision to stop MDA.

Definitive diagnosis of infection with *O. volvulus* in humans involves identification of subcutaneous nodules or observation of microfilariae in skin snips using microscopy. The detection of microfilariae in skin can be a challenge when parasite densities are low, which is often the case when MDA programs are underway. Several serological methods exist involving antibody detection to *O. volvulus*-specific antigens. The most widely used assays are based on the detection of IgG4 responses to the Ov-16 antigen in children [8–11]. Of all the methods developed thus far for diagnosis of infection in humans, the highest levels of sensitivity have been achieved in skin snip/scratch analyses using the polymerase chain reaction (PCR) targeting the O-150 repeat sequence [12–14]. Infection rates in black flies are rapid and sensitive indicators of the change in community microfilarial load that results from ivermectin distribution, and correlate well with the percentage coverage of the community [7]. Importantly, they are also an important indicator of when MDA is succeeding in breaking transmission of *O. volvulus*. In addition, from logistical and ethical perspectives, monitoring infections in the vector offers some advantages over repeated blood examinations of the human population [15,16]. For detection of *O. volvulus* infection in black flies, the World Health Organization (WHO) recommends the use of PCR-based methods [7]. To date, these assays have been performed using the O-150 repeat sequence identified more than 20 years ago [17–22], where the amplification products are subsequently detected by several methods including an enzyme-linked immunosorbent assay (PCR-ELISA) [23–26].

In sub-Saharan Africa, cattle are frequently infected with *Onchocerca ochengi*, a species that exclusively parasitizes Bovidae. This is the closest extant relative of *O. volvulus* and is transmitted in West Africa by the same species complex of black fly vectors, *Simulium damnosum sensu lato* [27]. Discrimination between these two species requires an additional step of hybridization of the PCR amplified products with an *O. volvulus*-specific DNA probe [17,19,28,29]. Since the complexity of a test can be a technical barrier, a simpler method for the specific detection of human parasites in the vector would be a significant advance. In addition for low-resource settings, PCR can be a challenge as it requires skilled personnel and expensive equipment [30]. Therefore a new molecular method for the detection of *O. volvulus* that circumvents some of the current limitations would be a useful tool to aid onchocerciasis control and elimination efforts [31].

Loop-mediated isothermal amplification (LAMP) is an alternative technique which amplifies DNA with high specificity, sensitivity and rapidity under isothermal conditions [32]. The LAMP reaction includes two sets of primers that hybridize to six sites on the target DNA, and a third set of primers (loop primers) to accelerate the reaction [33]. The mixture of stem-loops containing alternately inverted repeats of the target sequence and cauliflower-like structures that are generated result in exponential amplification of the target sequence (>10 μg,>50× PCR yield) [32–34]. Using three primer sets recognizing eight sites in the target DNA engenders the specificity to discriminate between genomic DNA at both genus and species specific levels [35,36]. In recent years this technology has been explored for the diagnosis of several infectious diseases including those caused by parasitic protozoa [37,38] and the filarial parasites *Brugia malayi* [39], *Wuchereria bancrofti* [40] and *Loa loa* [41,42]. The simplicity, rapidity, and versatility in readout options available for LAMP, offer a distinct advantage over other molecular diagnostic methods. LAMP test kits for use in resource-limited settings are now commercially available for the detection of *Mycobacterium tuberculosis* complex [43,44] and human African trypanosomiasis [45].

In the present study we report on the identification of a new DNA biomarker, encoding *O. volvulus* glutathione *S*-transferase 1a (*OvGST1a*), and the development of a simple, single-step, LAMP assay that easily distinguishes between *O. volvulus* and *O. ochengi* DNA. Our results demonstrate that the test represents a significant technical advance, and has the potential to be used as a new field tool for surveillance of parasite transmission and evaluation of MDA programs for onchocerciasis.

Materials and Methods

Reagents

O. ochengi DNA was extracted from adult worms obtained from cattle skin nodules after normal processing at the Ngaoundéré abattoir, Adamawa Region, Cameroon. *L. loa* DNA was prepared from infective stage larvae isolated from *Chrysops silacea* collected in the Southwest Region of Cameroon. Genomic DNA was extracted using DNAzol reagent (Invitrogen) according to the manufacturer's instructions. *Onchocerca volvulus* genomic DNA was prepared from adult female worms as described [46]. Bovine DNA and human DNAs were obtained from Millipore, USA.

Black flies

Uninfected, laboratory reared female *Simulium vittatum* were obtained from the Black fly Rearing and Bioassay Laboratory, University of Georgia, USA. Pools containing varying numbers of black flies (50, 100, 150 and 200 each) were prepared according to established protocols [21,23].

Spiking and DNA extraction

Each pool of black flies was placed in a 1.5 mL micro centrifuge tube and the insects were crushed in 500 μL extraction buffer (100 mM NaCl, 10 mM Tris-HCl, pH 8.0, 1 mM EDTA, 0.1% sodium dodecyl sulfate, 100 μg/mL of proteinase K) using a blunted glass pipette. An additional 500 μL extraction buffer containing either no DNA, or purified *O. volvulus* genomic DNA (1.0 ng, 0.1 ng, or 0.01 ng) was added to the homogenized pool. DNAs were then purified from the individual pool preparations using the Qiagen Tissue and Blood Kit [Qiagen, Valencia, CA, USA] according to the manufacturer's instructions, or extracted by boiling at 95°C for 15 min and used directly as template in both PCR and LAMP reactions. DNA extracted from non-spiked pools of black flies and purified *O. ochengi* DNA were included as negative controls. Purified *O. volvulus* genomic DNA was used as a positive control. All experiments were performed in duplicate at least 3 times.

Sequence analysis

O. ochengi sigma-class GST sequences were obtained from predicted coding nucleotide sequences available at http://www.nematodes.org/genomes/onchocerca_ochengi (Nematode genomes from the Blaxter lab, University of Edinburgh). Putative homologous protein sequences to *O. ochengi* sigma-class GSTs with relevant predicted domains [cd03039 (GST_N_Sigma_like) and cd03192 (GST_C_Sigma_like), available at the Conserved Domain Database at NCBI (http://www.ncbi.nlm.nih.gov/cdd/) [47] were identified via BLAST analysis (http://blast.ncbi.nlm.nih.gov/Blast.cgi; [48,49] using the non-redundant database at NCBI (http://www.ncbi.nlm.nih.gov/; non-redundant GenBank CDS translations + PDB + SwissProt + PIR + PRF, excluding those in env_nr). Organisms for GST sequence comparison were selected using the following rationale: (a) nematode taxonomy – including 'shared family Filariidae' [*Onchocerca volvulus* {AAG44696.1, AAG44695.1}, *Brugia malayi* {XP_001901855.1} *and Loa loa* {003139665.1}]; 'shared nematode Clade III' [*Ascaris suum* {ERG83753.1, ERG81431.1}]; 'different nematode Clade V' [*Caenorhabditis elegans* {NP_508625.1, NP_509652.2}]; (b) mammalian definitive host-relatedness [*Homo sapiens* {NP_055300.1}, *Bos taurus* {XP_002688181.1}, *Rattus norvegicus* {NP_113832.1} and *Mus musculus* {NP_062328.3}]; (c) insect intermediate host-relatedness [*Musca domestica* {NP_001273827.1}, *Drosophila melanogaster* {NP_725653.1}, *Pediculus humanus corporis* {XP_002426887.1} and *Tribolium castaneum* {XP_970714.1}]. BLAST hits of putative GST sigma-class protein homologues were subjected to multiple sequence alignment using ClustalX Version 2.1 [50,51]. Phylogenetic bootstrap neighbor-joining trees were produced as PHYLIP output files according to the neighbour-joining method [52]. ClustalX default settings for alignments were accepted using the GONNET protein weight matrices with PHYLIP tree format files viewed within the TREEVIEW program [53].

For comparative analysis of sigma GST genomic sequences, *OvGST1a* and *OvGST1b* and the *O. ochengi* homologue g09064 were aligned over the complete gene sequence (total distance, 3,870 bp) using Kalign [54,55] at http://www.ebi.ac.uk/Tools/msa/kalign/with ClustalW output. Parameters comprised a gap open

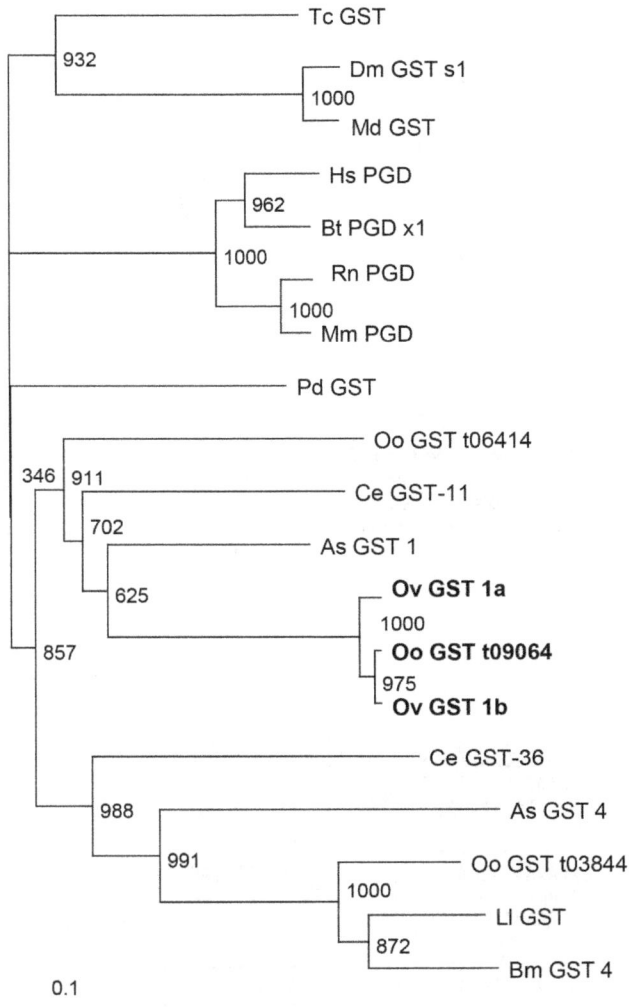

Figure 1. Phylogenetic neighbour-joining tree showing the relationship of the sigma-class GSTs of *Onchocerca ochengi* **to similar enzymes of nematodes, mammals and insects.** Numbers shown alongside branches are bootstrap values of 1,000 replications. The key for protein sequence accession numbers and organisms displayed in the tree is as follows: <u>Nematodes:</u> Oo_GST_t09064, Oo_GST_t03844 and Oo_GST_t06414 glutathione transferase [*Onchocerca ochengi*]; Ov_GST_1b AAG44696.1 glutathione *S*-transferase Ia [*Onchocerca volvulus*]; Ov _GST_1a AAG44695.1 glutathione *S*-transferase Ia [*Onchocerca volvulus*]; Ll_GST XP_003139665.1 hypothetical protein LOAG_04080 [*Loa loa*]; Bm_GST_4 XP_001901855.1 glutathione *S*-transferase 4 [*Brugia malayi*]; As_GST_1 ERG83753.1 glutathione *S*-transferase 1 [*Ascaris suum*]; As_GST_4 ERG81431.1 glutathione s-transferase 4 [*Ascaris suum*]; Ce_GST-11 NP_508625.1 protein GST-11 [*Caenorhabditis elegans*]; Ce_GST-36 NP_509652.2 protein GST-36 [*Caenorhabditis elegans*]. <u>Mammals:</u> Hs_PGD NP_055300.1 hematopoietic prostaglandin D synthase [*Homo sapiens*]; Bt_PGD_x1 XP_002688181.1 PREDICTED: hematopoietic prostaglandin D synthase isoform X1 [*Bos taurus*]; Rt_PGD NP_113832.1 hematopoietic prostaglandin D synthase [*Rattus norvegicus*]; Mm_PGD NP_062328.3 hematopoietic prostaglandin D synthase [*Mus musculus*]. <u>Insects:</u> Md_GST_ NP_001273827.1 glutathione *S*-transferase [*Musca domestica*]; Dm_GST_s1 NP_725653.1 glutathione *S*-transferase S1, isoform A [*Drosophila melanogaster*]; Ph_GST XP_002426887.1 glutathione *S*-transferase, putative [*Pediculus humanus corporis*]; Tc_GST XP_970714.1 PREDICTED: glutathione *S*-transferase [*Tribolium castaneum*]. The GSTs from *O. volvulus* and their closest relative in *O. ochengi* are shown in bold.

penalty of 11, a gap extension penalty of 0.85, terminal gap penalties of 0.45, and a bonus score of zero.

Primer design

To design specific primers for *O. volvulus*, glutathione *S*-transferase-1 gene, sequences from *O. volvulus* [*OvGST1a*, GenBank: AF265556.1; *OvGST1b*, GenBank: AF265557.1] and *O. ochengi* [locus tag: nOo.2.0.1.go9064, http://www.nematodes.org/genomes/onchocerca_ochengi/] were aligned using ClustalW [50]. Regions specific for *O. volvulus* were identified in *OvGST1a* and LAMP primers were designed to target the gene using Primer Explorer V4 [http://primerexplorer.jp/e/]. Two sets of primers comprising two outer (F3 and B3), and two inner (FIP and BIP) were selected. FIP contained F1c (complementary to F1), and the F2 sequence. BIP contained the B1c sequence (complementary to B1) and the B2 sequence. Additional loop primers, forward loop primer (FLP) and backward loop primer (BLP) were included in the reaction.

The outer LAMP primer pair F3 and B3 was also used for specific amplification of *OvGST1a* by PCR. PCR primers for amplification of actin were as previously described [39]. The forward and reverse primer sequences are (5′ GCTCAGTCBAA-GAGAGGTAT 3′) and (5′ACAGCYTGGATDGCAACGTACA 3′), respectively, where B = C, G or T; Y = C or T, and D = A, G or T. PCR and LAMP primers were synthesized by Integrated DNA Technologies (Coralville, IA, USA).

LAMP assay

LAMP reactions were performed in a final volume of 25 µL reaction buffer [10 mM Tris–HCl (pH 8.8), 50 mM KCl, 10 mM $(NH_4)_2SO_4$, 8 mM $MgSO_4$, and 0.1% Tween 20], 8 U *Bst* 2.0 DNA polymerase (New England Biolabs, Ipswich, MA, USA), (1.4 mM) of each deoxynucleoside triphosphate (dNTP), 1.6 mM of each FIP and BIP primer, 0.2 mM of each F3 and B3 primer, 0.4 mM of FLP and BLP, and 2 µL of target DNA. The mixture was incubated at 63°C for 60 min, then heated at 80°C for 2 min to terminate the reaction. Reactions were carried out using either a Loop Amp Realtime Turbidimeter (LA-320c, Eiken Chemical Co, Japan) or a 2720 Thermocycler (Applied Biosystems, USA) set at a constant temperature for colorimetric detection. A positive reaction was defined as a threshold value greater than 0.1. Turbidity data were analyzed using the LA-320c software package that reports when the change in turbidity over time (dT/dt) reaches a value of 0.1, which we then assigned to be the threshold time (Tt). For determination of amplification measured by color change (purple to sky blue), 0.15 µL of 120 µM hydroxy naphthol blue (HNB, Sigma-Aldrich Inc, St. Louis, MO, USA) was added to the reaction mixture. All experiments were performed in duplicate at least 3 times.

PCR assay

LAMP primers B3 and F3 were used to PCR amplify *OvGST1a* in 25 µL reactions containing 3 µL DNA template, 0.2 µM of each primer, and 1.25 U of *Taq* DNA polymerase in 1× standard buffer (New England Biolabs) containing 3.5 mM $MgCl_2$, 0.2 mM and 0.2 mM dNTP each. All reactions were denatured once at 94°C for 5 min followed by 35 cycles of the following cycling conditions: 30 s at 94°C, 1 min at 53°C, 1 min at 72°C, and a final extension for 5 min at 72°C using a Gene Amp PCR system 9700 (Applied Biosystems). PCR products were visualized by UV transillumination in a 1.5% agarose gel after electrophoresis and staining with ethidium bromide. As a positive control for the presence of intact DNA, a 244 bp actin fragment was PCR amplified as described [40].

```
              950        960        970              2360       2370       2380       2390       2400       2410       2420
             ·|···|···|···|···|···|···|                ·|···|···|···|···|···|···|···|···|···|···|···|···|···|···|···|···|···|···|···|···|
O.Ochengi scaffold 04163  CTC                  TCT      ATTTATCTCTCAAGTAGCGAATT                                                      TAT
    O.volvulus GST1b       CTC                  TCT      ATT                    T                                                    TAT
    O.volvulus GST1a       CTCAAAATTACAATTTATCTCTTCT    ATTTATCTCTCAAGTAGC      AATTTATCTCTCAAGTAGCAAATTTATCTCTCAAGTAGCGAATTTTAT
```

```
          ...0         688          96                    1639                         143   87    185    141    145   3870...
                        1            2                      3                            4     5     6      7      8
                              I    II                                                   III   IV    V     VI    VII
                              55   76                                                   146   91   114   108   156
```

```
                1040       1050
               ·|···|···|···|···|···|
O.ochengi scaffold 04163  CCT              AAA
    O.volvulus GST1b       CCT              AAA
    O.volvulus GST1a       CCTTCTTTACCTGTAACATTCAAA
```

Figure 2. Diagrammatic view of the similarity of *Onchocerca* sigma-class GST gene models for *O. volvulus* GSTs 1a and 1b and the homologous *O. ochengi* sigma-class GST t09064. Gene models were aligned over the full-length sequence (total distance, 3,870 bp). Numbers associated with gene model exons (*I–VII shaded blocks*) and introns (*1–8 non-shaded blocks*) display the number of base-pairs within those sections over which the alignment is spaced. The three major differences between the genes (all insertions in *O. volvulus GST1a* intron 3) are highlighted in the diagram.

A

```
                                                                                    F3
OvGST1a  ATAACTTCGGAAAACTCTATTAAGCCCAAAGGAAAGGTAATTTATAGAATGCAATTATGCAATAATTCTCAAAATTACAA 955
OvGST1b  ATAACTTCGGAAAACTCTATTAAGCCCAAAGAAAAGGTAATTTATAGAATGCAATTATGCAATGATTCTC---------- 948
OchGST   ATAACTTCGGAAAACTCTATTAAGCCCAAAGAAAAGGTAATTTATAGAATGCAATTATGCAATGATTCTC---------- 264

                                       F2                              LF
OvGST1a  TTTATCTCTTCTTTAGTAAATTTGGATATAAACGATGATTTTTCCATAAAAATAGAATTCTTTCATAGATGCCTTCTTTAC 1035
OvGST1b  ---------TCTTCAGTAAATTTGGAT--AAACGATGATTTTTCCATAAAAATAGAATTCTTTCATAGATGCCT------- 1010
OchGST   ---------TCTTCAGTAAATTTGGATATAAACGATGATTTTTCCATAAAAATAGAATTCTTTCATAGATGCCT------- 328

            F1c                  B1                         LB
OvGST1a  CTGTAACATTCAAAAATATCAAGCATAAATGGCCTATTAG--CGAGCAAAAATAGAAA-TGCATCTTTGCGCTATAATTT 1112
OvGST1b  ----------AAAAATTTCAAGCATAAATGGCCTATTAGGCCGAGCAAAAATAGAAAATGCATCTTTGCGCTATAATTT 1079
OchGST   ----------AAAAATATCAAGCATAAATGGCCTATTAGGCCGAGCAAAAATAGAAAATGCATCTTTGCGCTATAATTT 397

           B2c                  B3
OvGST1a  GTTTCATTTTATTTTAATCCATTCATTGGCAAATGTTTATTCTAATTTTTACACTTCAAATATATGGAATGGTTAAAATT 1192
OvGST1b  GTTTCATTTTATTTTAATCCATTCATTGGCAAATGTTTATTCCAATTTTTACACTTCAAATATATGGAATGGTTAAAATT 1159
OchGST   GTTTCATTTTATTTTAATCCATTCATTGGCAAATGTTTATTCCAATTTTTACACTTCAAATATATGGAATGGTTAAAATT 477
```

B

PRIMER	SEQUENCE (5' to 3')
FIP (F1c+F2)	AATGTTACAGGTAAAGAAGGCATCT-TTTGGATATAAACGATGATTTTTCC
BIP (B1+B2c)	ATCAAGCATAAATGGCCTATTAGCG-ATGAAACAAATTATAGCGCAAAG
F3	CTCAAAATTACAATTTATCTCTTC
B3	TTTGCCAATGAATGGATT
LF	ATGAAAGAATTCTATTTTAT
LB	GCAAAAATAGAAATGCAT

Figure 3. Alignment of partial gene sequences of glutathione *S*-transferases (GSTs) from *O. volvulus* (*OvGST1a*, *OvGST1b*) and *O. ochengi (OoGST1)* (A) and primer sets targeting *OvGST1a* (B). Primers are indicated by solid black arrows and dash arrows represent the binding regions of the loop forward (LFP) and loop back (LBP) primers respectively.

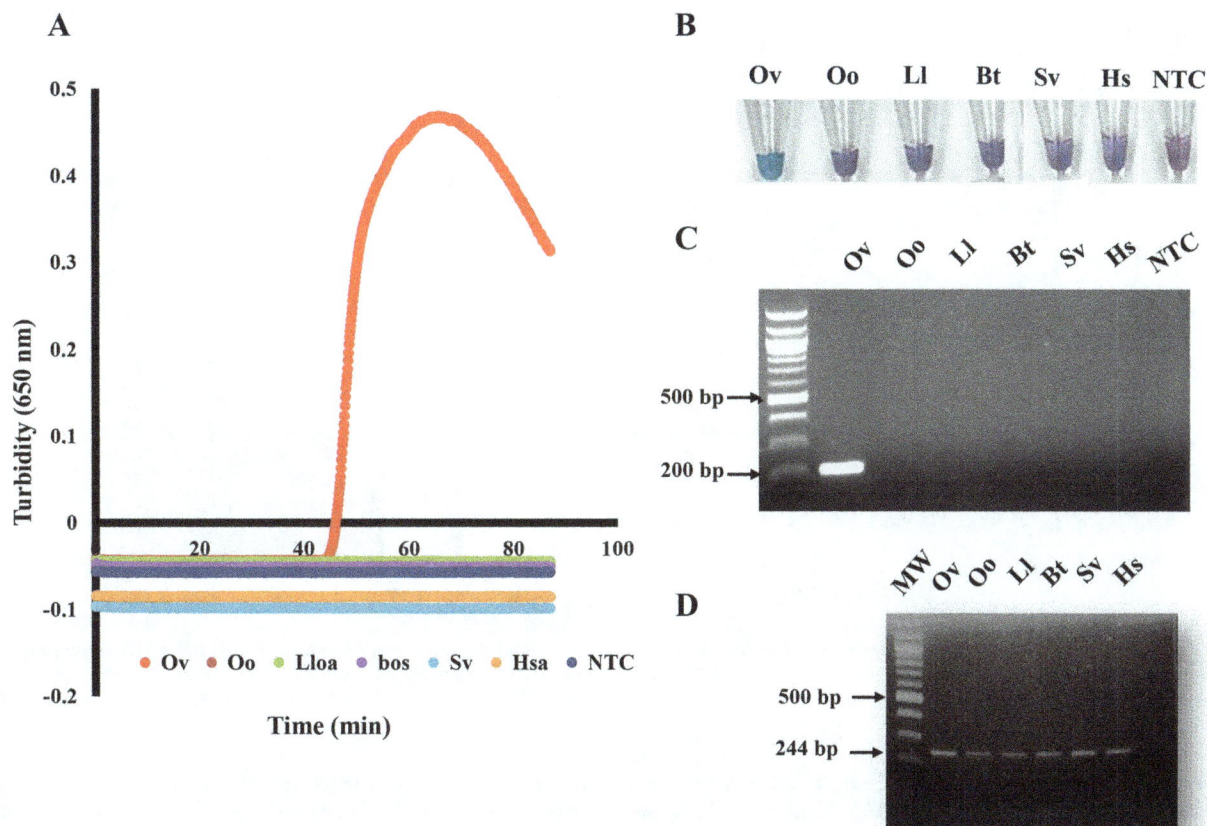

Figure 4. Species-specific LAMP assay targeting *OvGST1a.* Genomic DNAs from *O. volvulus* (Ov), *O. ochengi* (Oo), *L. loa* (Lloa), *Bos taurus* (Bos), *Simulium vitattum* (Sv) and *Homo sapiens* (Hsa) were used as template in the LAMP assay. Detection using turbidity (**A**). Each curve represents the calculated average of triplicate turbidity curves generated with various genomic DNAs (1 ng) using *Bst* 2.0 DNA polymerase. Turbidity was observed only using *O. volvulus* genomic DNA as template. Detection using hydroxy naphthol blue (**B**). Genomic DNAs from *O. volvulus* (Ov), *O. ochengi* (Oo), *L. loa* (Ll), Bovine (Bt), *Simulium vitattum* (Sv) and human (Hs) were used as template in a PCR assay (**C**). Amplification product (~200 bp) using LAMP primers F3 and B3 was obtained when *O. volvulus* genomic DNA was used (indicated by arrow). As a positive control, an actin gene fragment was PCR amplified from (Ov), (Oo), (Ll), (Bt), (Sv) and Hs DNAs using degenerate primers (**D**). Agarose gel showing amplification of a 244 bp fragment of the actin gene. Water was used in a non-template control (NTC) in all experiments. Molecular weight marker (MW) is indicated.

Results

During manual curation of gene predictions in the *O. ochengi* genome (http://www.nematodes.org/genomes/onchocerca_ochengi), it was noted that this species has one copy of the glutathione *S*-transferase-1 gene (*OoGST1*), whereas *O. volvulus* has two copies [56]. Phylogenetic analysis using protein sequences demonstrated that although two additional gene models containing GST sigma-like domains are present in the *O. ochengi* genome, these are unrelated to the two OvGST1 paralogues and cluster at different branches of the tree (**Fig. 1**). Indeed, the "GST1" group [comprising OvGST1a, OvGST1b and OoGST1 (CDS t09064)] form a highly distinctive clade, which is distant not only from insect and mammalian sigma GSTs, but also from those of other nematodes, including filarial representatives and *Ascaris suum* (an additional clade III nematode) (**Fig. 1**). Intron/exon sequence and gene structure were found to be highly conserved within the "GST1" group (**Fig. 2**). Overall nucleotide identity was>90% for all exons and introns between *OoGST1* and both of the *O. volvulus* GST1 genes. However, *OvGST1b* is most similar to *OoGST1* at 98% overall identity, in comparison to *OvGST1a* at 96% identity (**Fig. 1 and Fig. 2**). The three major differences between the genes comprised insertions in intron 3 of *OvGST1a*.

Based on the phylogenetic tree and comparative sequence analyses, several primer sets targeting *OvGST1a* and/or *OvGST1b* were evaluated (data not shown). Assays were performed in the temperature range 60–65°C for up to 90 minutes using various concentrations of $MgSO_4$ (4, 6, 8, and 10 mM) and primers (0.1, 0.2, and 0.4 µM F3 and B3; 1, 1.5, 2, and 4 µM FIP and BIP; and 0.5, 1, and 2 µM FLP and BLP), as well as varying the primer sequences. The optimum incubation condition was established as 63°C for 60 min in a buffer containing 4 mM $MgSO_4$, followed by heating at 80°C for 2 min to terminate the reaction. In accordance with the sequence analysis, *OvGST1a* was revealed as the best target (data not shown). Primer sets (**Fig. 3A and Fig. 3B**) targeting *OvGST1a* were designed after optimization and used for specificity and sensitivity studies.

Specificity of this primer set was determined in LAMP, using a real time turbidimeter (**Fig. 4A**) and colorimetric detection (**Fig. 4B**), to monitor amplification of genomic DNA from *O. volvulus*, *O. ochengi*, or a related human filarial parasite, *Loa loa*. Bovine, human, and black fly genomic DNAs, and non-template controls were also included for comparison. Turbidity reached a threshold value of 0.1 in approximately 45 minutes when 1 ng *O. volvulus* DNA was added to the reaction, whereas no turbidity was observed within the time interval examined (90 minutes) when the

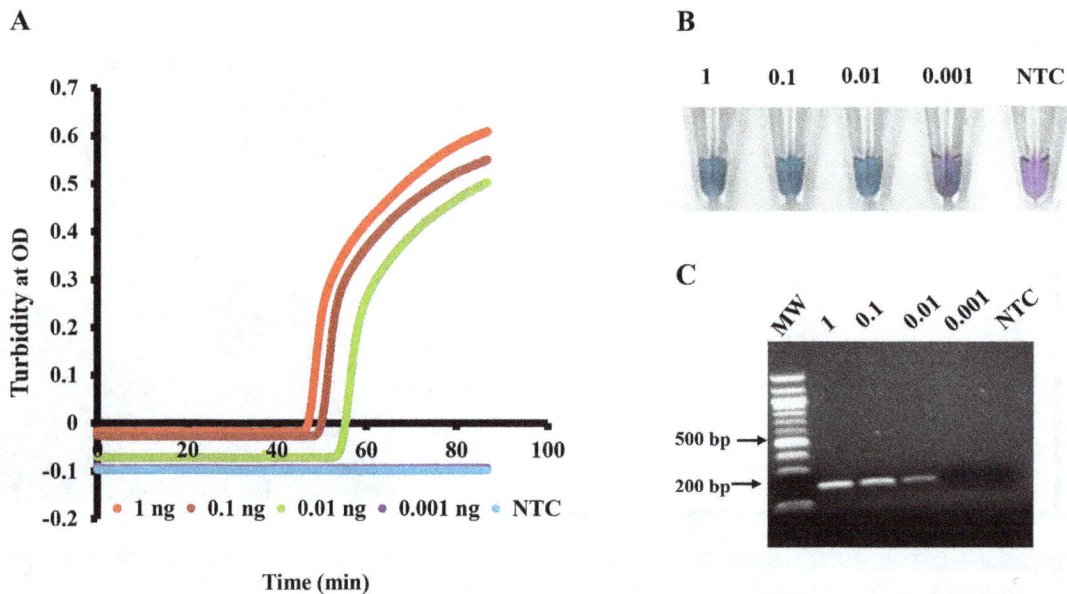

Figure 5. Sensitivity of LAMP and PCR methods for the detection of *O. volvulus* **using ten-fold serial dilutions of** *O. volvulus* **genomic DNA ranging from 0.001–1.0 ng.** Detection of LAMP product using turbidity (**A**) or hydroxy napthol blue (**B**). PCR amplification of a ~200 bp product using LAMP primers F3 and B3 was obtained when *O. volvulus* genomic DNA was used (**C**). Molecular weight marker (MW) is indicated.

same amount of heterologous DNAs from *O. ochengi*, *L. loa*, mammal or black fly was used (**Fig. 4A**). Similar results were observed using the more simplified colorimetric detection method, where a color change (purple to blue) was only evident when *O. volvulus* genomic DNA was present (**Fig. 4B**). Conversely, in the absence of template or primers, no reactions were observed when using either turbidity or color change as the readout (**Fig. 4A and 4B**).

Specificity studies were also performed by PCR amplification of *OvGST1a* using primers F3 and B3 (**Fig. 4C**). A 200 bp fragment of the expected size was obtained when *O. volvulus* genomic DNA was used as a template, whereas no product was observed from samples containing heterologous DNA or no template. The integrity of the various DNAs was confirmed in PCR experiments using primers designed to amplify a conserved actin gene. A single amplification product of the correct size (244 bp) was observed in all cases (**Fig. 4D**).

To determine and compare the detection limits of LAMP and PCR, ten-fold serial dilutions of *O. volvulus* genomic DNA ranging from 0.001–1.0 ng were amplified (**Fig. 5A–C**). Both amplification methods were able to detect levels as low as 0.01 ng, which is equivalent to $^1/_{10}$th of a single microfilaria. In the case of LAMP a positive result was evident within one hour (**Fig. 5A**).

Since the goal is to use the LAMP assay to evaluate infection in the vector, pools of uninfected, laboratory-reared black flies were spiked with 0.001–1.0 ng *O. volvulus* genomic DNA, and total genomic DNA was then isolated using a commercially available DNA extraction kit or by boiling. Samples from each pool and extraction method were then used as templates for amplification of *OvGST1a* in LAMP and PCR reactions (**Table 1**). Consistent with previous results using highly purified DNA as template, LAMP was positive in samples prepared from an insect pool containing 50–200 black flies spiked with 0.1 ng *O. volvulus* DNA (equivalent to a single microfilaria) when DNA was purified using a commercially available kit, or extracted in a more crude fashion by boiling. PCR was less effective following crude extraction with a pool size limit of 150 black flies. At the 0.01 ng level using kit

purified material, LAMP efficiently amplified *OvGST1a* in pool sizes up to 150 black flies, whereas for PCR the pool size limit was 50 insects. When boiling was used to extract DNA, a positive signal was obtained for LAMP at a ratio of 0.01 ng target DNA in 100 insects, while the limit for PCR was 0.01 ng DNA in 50 insects. These results demonstrate the ability of the LAMP assay to withstand the inhibitory effects of components present in the purified or crude black fly extracts without severely affecting sensitivity.

Discussion

In recent years there has been significant progress in the control of onchocerciasis by treating whole populations with repeated, semi-annual (Latin America) or yearly (most African foci) cycles of ivermectin [57]. Several agencies are involved in these activities for example, the African Programme for Onchocerciasis Control (APOC), and the Onchocerciasis Elimination Program for the Americas (OEPA). Surveys of *Simulium* vectors are recommended by WHO to determine if transmission has been interrupted and to certify that elimination of the parasite has been achieved [7]. Previous studies have shown the value of molecular xenodiagnosis(detection of parasite DNA in insects by DNA amplification methodologies) as a tool for assessing changes in parasite prevalence rates in endemic populations after MDA [12,17,21,23,58]. This method requires collection of representative samples of insects, isolation of total DNA from insect pools, amplification of parasite-specific DNA sequences, and detection of the amplified product. Currently, PCR pool screening of large numbers of flies is employed since infection levels are likely to be low or non-existent in treated areas. There is a limit to the number of flies in each pool, since the DNA polymerases used in PCR reactions are highly sensitive to inhibitors present in insect extracts. Currently, either silica-purified DNA or oligonucleotide capture of *O. volvulus* genomic DNA from homogenates of insects is used to reduce the amount of inhibitors carried over into the reaction [23]. Another approach involves reducing the insect

Table 1. A comparison of LAMP and PCR methods to detect varying amounts of genomic DNA isolated from pools of black flies using different methods.

Pool size	LAMP/PCR Kit purified (ng/reaction)				LAMP/PCR Boiled (ng/reaction)			
	1	0.1	0.01	0.001	1	0.1	0.01	0.001
50	+/+	+/+	+/+	-/-	+/+	+/+	+/+	-/-
100	+/+	+/+	+/-	-/-	+/+	+/+	+/-	-/-
150	+/+	+/+	+/-	-/-	+/+	+/+	-/-	-/-
200	+/+	+/+	-/-	-/-	+/+	+/-	-/-	-/-

biomass by limiting the analysis to insect heads alone. This will also reveal the prevalence of flies carrying infective-stage larvae (L3) and therefore provide an accurate assessment of transmission, and high-throughput methods for collecting black fly heads have been developed for this purpose [22,25]. Current OEPA guidelines require that the prevalence of flies carrying L3s be less than 1/2000 in every sentinel community for transmission to be interrupted [59], which necessitates surveying approximately 6000 flies from each area to state with 95% confidence that the prevalence of infective flies is in this range [23].

In sub-Saharan Africa where cattle-biting *S. damnosum s.l.* flies and zebu cattle are present, *O. ochengi* infections are common in the vector population [60,61]. Based on the presence of microfilariae, the prevalence in cattle is as high as 66–71% in some areas [62]. The parasite is extremely closely related to *O. volvulus*, as determined by phylogenetic distance [63] and natural history [64]. Indeed, it has been hypothesized that *O. volvulus* diverged from *O. ochengi* as recently as 5,000 years ago during the domestication of cattle in sub-Saharan Africa [65]. The routinely used O-150 diagnostic marker for *O. volvulus* clusters with other *Onchocerca* species, thereby hampering species discrimination [66].

In the present study we identified a gene (*OvGST1a*), encoding a glutathione *S*-transferase, as an alternative biomarker for *O. volvulus* infection. GSTs (EC 2.5.1.18) are an ancient and diverse superfamily of multifunctional proteins. Three different classes of GST (*OvGST*1-3) have been isolated and characterized from *O. volvulus* [67,68]. The *OvGST*1a and *OvGST*1b isoforms (differing in only 10 amino acids) [56,69] are unique sigma-class GSTs that encode an extracellular enzyme located in the outer zone of the hypodermis at the host-parasite interface, where they are thought to influence host inflammatory and immune cells due to their GSH-dependent prostaglandin D Synthase activity [56,67,70]. GSTs are present in all the developmental stages of the parasite and have been pursued as potential vaccine/drug targets [70]. The presence of two GST1 paralogues in *O. volvulus* suggests that the GST1 gene underwent a duplication event following the speciation of the human parasite from its bovine-specific sister. We evaluated the suitability of *OvGST1b* (data not shown) and *OvGST1a* for diagnosis of *O. volvulus* infection using both LAMP and PCR methods. High levels of specificity were achieved in *OvGST1a*-based LAMP and PCR assays. LAMP primers amplified *O. volvulus* DNA but not DNA isolated from the closely related filarial parasites *O. ochengi* or *L. loa*, or from human, bovine or black fly. LAMP primers F3 and B3 showed a similar specificity profile when used in PCR reactions, highlighting the versatility of this target for molecular diagnostic studies.

High levels of specificity and sensitivity can be achieved in LAMP because the amplification reaction involves four specific oligonucleotide primers that anneal to six distinct regions within the target sequence [32]. The addition of loop primers may further improve performance [34]. We observed comparable levels of sensitivity (0.01 ng), equivalent to $1/10^{th}$ of a single microfilaria [71], using either LAMP or PCR to amplify *OvGST1a* when highly purified DNA was used as template. We would therefore predict that the assays would permit detection of a single infective stage larva given that they are considerably larger in size. However, LAMP was more efficient than PCR in detecting *O. volvulus* DNA recovered from black fly material (0.01 ng in 150 insects within 60 minutes). This is likely due to the fact that black flies contain a number of biological substances that inhibit the polymerases used in PCR which cannot be removed completely during classical extraction protocols. The most efficient method used to circumvent this problem involves paramagnetic bead purification, but it is expensive [25]. Other studies have also shown superior tolerance of LAMP tests for biological substances [72–74]. Furthermore unlike PCR, LAMP proved effective even when DNA was extracted using a simple boiling method, rather than using commercially available kits that add a significant cost to the process (as well as time and effort). This is a significant finding representing an important technical advance, and emphasizes the usefulness of the LAMP technique as a surveillance tool for mass screening of infected vectors. In addition, recent estimates suggest that diagnostic LAMP tests are significantly cheaper than PCR. The estimated cost of a *W. bancrofti* LAMP test is $0.82 compared with more than $2.20 for PCR [40]. Other distinct advantages of LAMP over PCR include its operational simplicity and isothermal nature. In PCR, thermal cycling is required to denature the template, anneal primers and extend the amplicon. LAMP employs *Bst* DNA polymerase, which provides both strand displacement and target amplification at a single temperature in a simple heat block or water bath at 60–65°C [32]. Rapidity and versatility in readout options also make LAMP a particularly appealing technology. In the present study, real-time turbidity was used for assay design and optimization yielding positive results within 60 minutes, and results were confirmed using the more field-friendly hydroxy naphthol blue [75,76].

All the data on detecting *O. volvulus*-specific *OvGSTa* DNA were derived from pools of laboratory reared *S. vittatum* spiked with purified *O. volvulus* gDNA. Further work is required to demonstrate that the extraction techniques employed are able to release sufficient template for detection from at least one infected fly in a pool of insects. The current recommendation for the number of flies in a pool, limited by the DNA purification process, is 50 flies for Latin American vectors and 100 flies for African

vectors [23]. We anticipate that the *OvGSTa* LAMP assay will accommodate these pool sizes since the data from DNA-seeded pools (up to 200 insects) indicates that the method is robust and the extraction protocol employed will likely suffice to release measurable DNA target from a single infected black fly.

In summary, we describe a simple *OvGST1a*-based LAMP diagnostic assay for *O. volvulus* infection that generates a robust read-out within 60 minutes. The assay has considerable potential as a new field tool for implementation and management of MDA programs for onchocerciasis.

Acknowledgments

We gratefully acknowledge support from Don Comb and Jim Ellard. We thank Germanus Bah and Vincent Tanya (Institut de Recherche Agricole pour le Développement, Ngaoundéré, Cameroon) for providing *O. ochengi* material, Samuel Wanji (Research Foundation in Tropical Diseases and the Environment, Buea, Cameroon) for provision of *L. loa* L3, and Catherine Hartley (University of Liverpool, UK) for performing the DNA extractions on these samples. We are grateful to Gaganjot Kaur, Alex Marshall and Mark Blaxter (University of Edinburgh) for assembly, annotation and public release of the *O. ochengi* genome, without which this study would not have been possible. We also thank Catherine Poole, Liz Li, Nathan Tanner and Yinhua Zhang for useful discussions. We are grateful to Bill Jack, Barton Slatko, and Jeremy Foster for critical reading of this manuscript.

Author Contributions

Conceived and designed the experiments: AA BLM EJL CKSC. Performed the experiments: AA BLM EJL. Analyzed the data: AA BLM EJL CKSC. Contributed reagents/materials/analysis tools: BLM MYOA. Wrote the paper: AA BLM EJL MYOA.

References

1. Hotez PJ, Kamath A (2009) Neglected tropical diseases in sub-saharan Africa: review of their prevalence, distribution, and disease burden. PLoS Negl Trop Dis 3: e412.

2. Coffeng LE, Stolk WA, Zoure HG, Veerman JL, Agblewonu KB, et al. (2014) African programme for onchocerciasis control 1995–2015: updated health impact estimates based on new disability weights. PLoS Negl Trop Dis 8: e2759.

3. World Health Organization (WHO) (2010) Report "Working to overcome the global impact of neglected tropical diseases". Available: http://www.who.int/neglected_diseases/2010report/en/

4. African Programme for Onchocerciasis Control APOC (2009) Informal Consultation on elimination of onchocerciasis transmission with current tools in Africa "Shrinking the map"; 2009 25–27; Ouagadougou, Burkina Faso: African Programme for Onchocerciasis Control.

5. Diawara L, Traore MO, Badji A, Bissan Y, Doumbia K, et al. (2009) Feasibility of onchocerciasis elimination with ivermectin treatment in endemic foci in Africa: first evidence from studies in Mali and Senegal. PLoS Negl Trop Dis 3: e497.

6. Traore MO, Sarr MD, Badji A, Bissan Y, Diawara L, et al. (2012) Proof-of-principle of onchocerciasis elimination with ivermectin treatment in endemic foci in Africa: final results of a study in Mali and Senegal. PLoS Negl Trop Dis 6: e1825.

7. World Health Organization (WHO) (2001) Certification of elimination of human onchocerciasis: criteria and procedures. Available: http://apps.who.int/iris/handle/10665/66889

8. Chandrashekar R, Ogunrinade AF, Weil GJ (1996) Use of recombinant *Onchocerca volvulus* antigens for diagnosis and surveillance of human onchocerciasis. Trop Med Int Health 1: 575–580.

9. Weil GJ, Steel C, Liftis F, Li BW, Mearns G, et al. (2000) A rapid-format antibody card test for diagnosis of onchocerciasis. J Infect Dis 182: 1796–1799.

10. Rodriguez-Perez MA, Dominguez-Vazquez A, Mendez-Galvan J, Sifuentes-Rincon AM, Larralde-Corona P, et al. (2003) Antibody detection tests for *Onchocerca volvulus*: comparison of the sensitivity of a cocktail of recombinant antigens used in the indirect enzyme-linked immunosorbent assay with a rapid-format antibody card test. Trans R Soc Trop Med Hyg 97: 539–541.

11. Golden A, Steel C, Yokobe L, Jackson E, Barney R, et al. (2013) Extended result reading window in lateral flow tests detecting exposure to *Onchocerca volvulus*: a new technology to improve epidemiological surveillance tools. PLoS One 8: e69231.

12. Toe L, Boatin BA, Adjami A, Back C, Merriweather A, et al. (1998) Detection of *Onchocerca volvulus* infection by O-150 polymerase chain reaction analysis of skin scratches. J Infect Dis 178: 282–285.

13. Fink DL, Fahle GA, Fischer S, Fedorko DF, Nutman TB (2011) Toward molecular parasitologic diagnosis: enhanced diagnostic sensitivity for filarial infections in mobile populations. J Clin Microbiol 49: 42–47.

14. Boatin BA, Toe L, Alley ES, Nagelkerke NJ, Borsboom G, et al. (2002) Detection of *Onchocerca volvulus* infection in low prevalence areas: a comparison of three diagnostic methods. Parasitology 125: 545–552.

15. Bradley JE, Unnasch TR (1996) Molecular approaches to the diagnosis of onchocerciasis. Adv Parasitol 37: 57–106.

16. Boatin BA, Toe L, Alley ES, Dembele N, Weiss N, et al. (1998) Diagnostics in onchocerciasis: future challenges. Ann Trop Med Parasitol 92 Suppl 1: S41–45.

17. Meredith SE, Lando G, Gbakima AA, Zimmerman PA, Unnasch TR (1991) *Onchocerca volvulus*: application of the polymerase chain reaction to identification and strain differentiation of the parasite. Exp Parasitol 73: 335–344.

18. Zimmerman PA, Katholi CR, Wooten MC, Lang-Unnasch N, Unnasch TR (1994) Recent evolutionary history of American *Onchocerca volvulus*, based on analysis of a tandemly repeated DNA sequence family. Mol Biol Evol 11: 384–392.

19. Merriweather A, Unnasch TR (1996) Onchocerca volvulus: development of a species specific polymerase chain reaction-based assay. Exp Parasitol 83: 164–166.

20. Unnasch TR, Meredith SE (1996) The use of degenerate primers in conjunction with strain and species oligonucleotides to classify *Onchocerca volvulus*. Methods Mol Biol 50: 293–303.

21. Katholi CR, Toe L, Merriweather A, Unnasch TR (1995) Determining the prevalence of *Onchocerca volvulus* infection in vector populations by polymerase chain reaction screening of pools of black flies. J Infect Dis 172: 1414–1417.

22. Yameogo L, Toe L, Hougard JM, Boatin BA, Unnasch TR (1999) Pool screen polymerase chain reaction for estimating the prevalence of *Onchocerca volvulus* infection in *Simulium damnosum* sensu lato: results of a field trial in an area subject to successful vector control. Am J Trop Med Hyg 60: 124–128.

23. Gopal H, Hassan HK, Rodriguez-Perez MA, Toe LD, Lustigman S, et al. (2012) Oligonucleotide based magnetic bead capture of *Onchocerca volvulus* DNA for PCR pool screening of vector black flies. PLoS Negl Trop Dis 6: e1712.

24. Guevara AG, Vieira JC, Lilley BG, Lopez A, Vieira N, et al. (2003) Entomological evaluation by pool screen polymerase chain reaction of

Onchocerca volvulus transmission in Ecuador following mass Mectizan distribution. Am J Trop Med Hyg 68: 222–227.

25. Rodriguez-Perez MA, Gopal H, Adeleke MA, De Luna-Santillana EJ, Gurrola-Reyes JN, et al. (2013) Detection of *Onchocerca volvulus* in Latin American black flies for pool screening PCR using high-throughput automated DNA isolation for transmission surveillance. Parasitol Res 112: 3925–3931.

26. Rodriguez-Perez MA, Lilley BG, Dominguez-Vazquez A, Segura-Arenas R, Lizarazo-Ortega C, et al. (2004) Polymerase chain reaction monitoring of transmission of *Onchocerca volvulus* in two endemic states in Mexico. Am J Trop Med Hyg 70: 38–45.

27. Wahl G, Ekale D, Schmitz A (1998) *Onchocerca ochengi*: assessment of the *Simulium* vectors in north Cameroon. Parasitology 116 (Pt 4): 327–336.

28. Toe L, Merriweather A, Unnasch TR (1994) DNA probe-based classification of *Simulium damnosum s. l.*-borne and human-derived filarial parasites in the onchocerciasis control program area. Am J Trop Med Hyg 51: 676–683.

29. Zimmerman PA, Toe L, Unnasch TR (1993) Design of *Onchocerca* DNA probes based upon analysis of a repeated sequence family. Mol Biochem Parasitol 58: 259–267.

30. Pischke S, Buttner DW, Liebau E, Fischer P (2002) An internal control for the detection of *Onchocerca volvulus* DNA by PCR-ELISA and rapid detection of specific PCR products by DNA Detection Test Strips. Trop Med Int Health 7: 526–531.

31. McCarthy JS, Lustigman S, Yang GJ, Barakat RM, Garcia HH, et al. (2012) A research agenda for helminth diseases of humans: diagnostics for control and elimination programmes. PLoS Negl Trop Dis 6: e1601.

32. Notomi T, Okayama H, Masubuchi H, Yonekawa T, Watanabe K, et al. (2000) Loop-mediated isothermal amplification of DNA. Nucleic Acids Res 28: E63.

33. Nagamine K, Hase T, Notomi T (2002) Accelerated reaction by loop-mediated isothermal amplification using loop primers. Mol Cell Probes 16: 223–229.

34. Nagamine K, Watanabe K, Ohtsuka K, Hase T, Notomi T (2001) Loop-mediated isothermal amplification reaction using a nondenatured template. Clin Chem 47: 1742–1743.

35. Han ET, Watanabe R, Sattabongkot J, Khuntirat B, Sirichaisinthop J, et al. (2007) Detection of four *Plasmodium* species by genus- and species-specific loop-mediated isothermal amplification for clinical diagnosis. J Clin Microbiol 45: 2521–2528.

36. Iseki H, Alhassan A, Ohta N, Thekisoe OM, Yokoyama N, et al. (2007) Development of a multiplex loop-mediated isothermal amplification (mLAMP) method for the simultaneous detection of bovine *Babesia* parasites. J Microbiol Methods 71: 281–287.

37. Alhassan A, Thekisoe OM, Yokoyama N, Inoue N, Motloang MY, et al. (2007) Development of loop-mediated isothermal amplification (LAMP) method for diagnosis of equine piroplasmosis. Vet Parasitol 143: 155–160.

38. Hopkins H, Gonzalez IJ, Polley SD, Angutoko P, Ategeka J, et al. (2013) Highly sensitive detection of malaria parasitemia in a malaria-endemic setting: performance of a new loop-mediated isothermal amplification kit in a remote clinic in Uganda. J Infect Dis 208: 645–652.

39. Poole CB, Tanner NA, Zhang Y, Evans TC Jr., Carlow CK (2012) Diagnosis of brugian filariasis by loop-mediated isothermal amplification. PLoS Negl Trop Dis 6: e1948.

40. Takagi H, Itoh M, Kasai S, Yahathugoda TC, Weerasooriya MV, et al. (2011) Development of loop-mediated isothermal amplification method for detecting *Wuchereria bancrofti* DNA in human blood and vector mosquitoes. Parasitol Int 60: 493–497.

41. Drame PM, Fink DL, Kamgno J, Herrick JA, Nutman TB (2014) Loop-mediated isothermal amplification for rapid and semiquantitative detection of *Loa loa* infection. J Clin Microbiol 52: 2071–2077.

42. Fernandez-Soto P, Mvoulouga PO, Akue JP, Aban JL, Santiago BV, et al. (2014) Development of a highly sensitive loop-mediated isothermal amplification (LAMP) method for the detection of *Loa loa*. PLoS One 9: e94664.

43. Boehme CC, Nabeta P, Henostroza G, Raqib R, Rahim Z, et al. (2007) Operational feasibility of using loop-mediated isothermal amplification for diagnosis of pulmonary tuberculosis in microscopy centers of developing countries. J Clin Microbiol 45: 1936–1940.

44. Mitarai S, Okumura M, Toyota E, Yoshiyama T, Aono A, et al. (2011) Evaluation of a simple loop-mediated isothermal amplification test kit for the diagnosis of tuberculosis. Int J Tuberc Lung Dis 15: 1211–1217, i.

45. Mitashi P, Hasker E, Ngoyi DM, Pyana PP, Lejon V, et al. (2013) Diagnostic accuracy of loopamp *Trypanosoma brucei* detection kit for diagnosis of human African trypanosomiasis in clinical samples. PLoS Negl Trop Dis 7: e2504.

46. Osei-Atweneboana MY, Boakye DA, Awadzi K, Gyapong JO, Prichard RK (2012) Genotypic analysis of beta-tubulin in *Onchocerca volvulus* from communities and individuals showing poor parasitological response to ivermectin treatment. Int J Parasitol Drugs Drug Resist 2: 20–28.

47. Marchler-Bauer A, Lu S, Anderson JB, Chitsaz F, Derbyshire MK, et al. (2011) CDD: a Conserved Domain Database for the functional annotation of proteins. Nucleic Acids Res 39: D225–229.

48. Altschul SF, Lipman DJ (1990) Protein database searches for multiple alignments. Proc Natl Acad Sci U S A 87: 5509–5513.

49. Altschul SF, Wootton JC, Gertz EM, Agarwala R, Morgulis A, et al. (2005) Protein database searches using compositionally adjusted substitution matrices. FEBS J 272: 5101–5109.

50. Thompson JD, Gibson TJ, Plewniak F, Jeanmougin F, Higgins DG (1997) The CLUSTAL_X windows interface: flexible strategies for multiple sequence alignment aided by quality analysis tools. Nucleic Acids Res 25: 4876–4882.

51. Larkin MA, Blackshields G, Brown NP, Chenna R, McGettigan PA, et al. (2007) Clustal W and Clustal X version 2.0. Bioinformatics 23: 2947–2948.

52. Saitou N, Nei M (1987) The neighbor-joining method: a new method for reconstructing phylogenetic trees. Mol Biol Evol 4: 406–425.

53. Page RD (1996) TreeView: an application to display phylogenetic trees on personal computers. Comput Appl Biosci 12: 357–358.

54. Lassmann T, Sonnhammer EL (2005) Kalign–an accurate and fast multiple sequence alignment algorithm. BMC Bioinformatics 6: 298.

55. McWilliam H, Li W, Uludag M, Squizzato S, Park YM, et al. (2013) Analysis Tool Web Services from the EMBL-EBI. Nucleic Acids Res 41: W597–600.

56. Krause S, Sommer A, Fischer P, Brophy PM, Walter RD, et al. (2001) Gene structure of the extracellular glutathione S-transferase from *Onchocerca volvulus* and its overexpression and promoter analysis in transgenic *Caenorhabditis elegans*. Mol Biochem Parasitol 117: 145–154.

57. Crump A, Morel CM, Omura S (2012) The onchocerciasis chronicle: from the beginning to the end? Trends Parasitol 28: 280–288.

58. Rodriguez-Perez MA, Katholi CR, Hassan HK, Unnasch TR (2006) Large-scale entomologic assessment of *Onchocerca volvulus* transmission by poolscreen PCR in Mexico. Am J Trop Med Hyg 74: 1026–1033.

59. Lindblade KA, Arana B, Zea-Flores G, Rizzo N, Porter CH, et al. (2007) Elimination of *Onchocercia volvulus* transmission in the Santa Rosa focus of Guatemala. Am J Trop Med Hyg 77: 334–341.

60. Bwangamoi O (1969) *Onchocerca ochengi* new species, an intradermal parasite of cattle in East Africa. Bull Epizoot Dis Afr 17: 321–335.

61. Trees AJ (1992) *Onchocerca ochengi*: Mimic, model or modulator of *O. volvulus*? Parasitol Today. pp. 337–339.

62. Trees AJ, Wahl G, Klager S, Renz A (1992) Age-related differences in parasitosis may indicate acquired immunity against microfilariae in cattle naturally infected with *Onchocerca ochengi*. Parasitology 104 (Pt 2): 247–252.

63. Morales-Hojas R, Cheke RA, Post RJ (2006) Molecular systematics of five *Onchocerca* species (Nematoda: Filarioidea) including the human parasite, *O. volvulus*, suggest sympatric speciation. J Helminthol 80: 281–290.

64. Wahl G, Achu-Kwi MD, Mbah D, Dawa O, Renz A (1994) Bovine onchocercosis in north Cameroon. Vet Parasitol 52: 297–311.

65. Bain O (1981) [Species of the genus *Onchocerca* and primarily *O. volvulus*, considered from an epidemiologic and phylogenetic point of view]. Ann Soc Belg Med Trop 61: 225–231.

66. Krueger A, Fischer P, Morales-Hojas R (2007) Molecular phylogeny of the filaria genus *Onchocerca* with special emphasis on Afrotropical human and bovine parasites. Acta Trop 101: 1–14.

67. Perbandt M, Hoppner J, Betzel C, Walter RD, Liebau E (2005) Structure of the major cytosolic glutathione S-transferase from the parasitic nematode *Onchocerca volvulus*. J Biol Chem 280: 12630–12636.

68. Liebau E, Eschbach ML, Tawe W, Sommer A, Fischer P, et al. (2000) Identification of a stress-responsive *Onchocerca volvulus* glutathione S-transferase (Ov-GST-3) by RT-PCR differential display. Mol Biochem Parasitol 109: 101–110.

69. Sommer A, Nimtz M, Conradt HS, Brattig N, Boettcher K, et al. (2001) Structural analysis and antibody response to the extracellular glutathione S-transferases from *Onchocerca volvulus*. Infect Immun 69: 7718–7728.

70. Perbandt M, Hoppner J, Burmeister C, Luersen K, Betzel C, et al. (2008) Structure of the extracellular glutathione S-transferase OvGST1 from the human pathogenic parasite *Onchocerca volvulus*. J Mol Biol 377: 501–511.

71. Lizotte MR, Supali T, Partono F, Williams SA (1994) A polymerase chain reaction assay for the detection of *Brugia malayi* in blood. Am J Trop Med Hyg 51: 314–321.

72. Enomoto Y, Yoshikawa T, Ihira M, Akimoto S, Miyake F, et al. (2005) Rapid diagnosis of *herpes simplex* virus infection by a loop-mediated isothermal amplification method. J Clin Microbiol 43: 951–955.

73. Poon LL, Wong BW, Ma EH, Chan KH, Chow LM, et al. (2006) Sensitive and inexpensive molecular test for falciparum malaria: detecting *Plasmodium falciparum* DNA directly from heat-treated blood by loop-mediated isothermal amplification. Clin Chem 52: 303–306.

74. Kaneko H, Kawana T, Fukushima E, Suzutani T (2007) Tolerance of loop-mediated isothermal amplification to a culture medium and biological substances. J Biochem Biophys Methods 70: 499–501.

75. Goto M, Honda E, Ogura A, Nomoto A, Hanaki K (2009) Colorimetric detection of loop-mediated isothermal amplification reaction by using hydroxy naphthol blue. Biotechniques 46: 167–172.

76. Yang BY, Liu XL, Wei YM, Wang JQ, He XQ, et al. (2014) Rapid and sensitive detection of human astrovirus in water samples by loop-mediated isothermal amplification with hydroxynaphthol blue dye. BMC Microbiol 14: 38.

18

A New Method to Predict the Epidemiology of Fungal Keratitis by Monitoring the Sales Distribution of Antifungal Eye Drops

Marlon Moraes Ibrahim[1], Rafael de Angelis[1], Acacio Souza Lima[2,3], Glauco Dreyer Viana de Carvalho[3], Fuad Moraes Ibrahim[1], Leonardo Tannus Malki[1], Marina de Paula Bichuete[1], Wellington de Paula Martins[4,5,6], Eduardo Melani Rocha[1]*

1 Department of Ophthalmology, Faculty of Medicine of Ribeirão Preto, University of São Paulo, Ribeirão Preto, Brazil, 2 Department of Ophthalmology, São Paulo Federal University, São Paulo, Brazil, 3 Ophthalmos Industria Farmacêutica, São Paulo, Brazil, 4 Departamento de Ginecologia e Obstetrícia da Faculdade de Medicina de Ribeirão Preto, Universidade de São Paulo, Ribeirão Preto, Brazil, 5 Escola de Ultra-sonografia e Reciclagem Médica de Ribeirão Preto, Ribeirão Preto, Brazil, 6 Instituto Nacional de Ciência e Tecnologia de Hormônios e Saúde da Mulher, Ribeirão Preto, Brazil

Abstract

Purpose: Fungi are a major cause of keratitis, although few medications are licensed for their treatment. The aim of this study is to observe the variation in commercialisation of antifungal eye drops, and to predict the seasonal distribution of fungal keratitis in Brazil.

Methods: Data from a retrospective study of antifungal eye drops sales from the only pharmaceutical ophthalmologic laboratory, authorized to dispense them in Brazil (Opthalmos) were gathered. These data were correlated with geographic and seasonal distribution of fungal keratitis in Brazil between July 2002 and June 2008.

Results: A total of 26,087 antifungal eye drop units were sold, with a mean of 2.3 per patient. There was significant variation in antifungal sales during the year ($p < 0.01$). A linear regression model displayed a significant association between reduced relative humidity and antifungal drug sales ($R2 = 0.17, p < 0.01$).

Conclusions: Antifungal eye drops sales suggest that there is a seasonal distribution of fungal keratitis. A possible interpretation is that the third quarter of the year (a period when the climate is drier), when agricultural activity is more intense in Brazil, suggests a correlation with a higher incidence of fungal keratitis. A similar model could be applied to other diseases, that are managed with unique, or few, and monitorable medications to predict epidemiological aspects.

Editor: Abdisalan Mohamed Noor, Kenya Medical Research Institute - Wellcome Trust Research Programme, Kenya

Funding: This study was supported by grants of the following Brazilian governmental institutions: Conselho Nacional de Desenvolvimento Científico e Tecnológico (302005/2009-9)and Fundação de Apoio ao Ensino, Pesquisa e Assistência do Hospital das Clinicas da Faculdade de Medicina de Ribeirão Preto da Universidade de São Paulo. The funders had no role in study design, data collection and analysis, decision to publish, or preparation of the manuscript.

Competing Interests: ASL and GDVC are employees of Ophthalmos Industria Farmaceutica Ltda.

* E-mail: emrocha@fmrp.usp.br

Introduction

Fungal keratitis is a common and important cause of corneal morbidity in tropical regions of the world. Perhaps because it is less common among industrialized countries located in more temperate climates, research into the risk factors and treatment options of this orphan disease has sometimes been lower than expected [1,2].

In tropical and developing countries, fungal ulcers represent from 4% to 60% of infectious corneal ulcers [1,3–5]. This distribution is believed to result from socioeconomic conditions, environmental characteristics, and geographical variations, such as latitude and climatic differences, especially humidity [1,6–8]. Previous works has revealed a significant increase in the number of reported cases of fungal keratitis during the harvest period [1,2,8,9].

Brazil is a developing tropical country with extensive dimensions and various environmental, climatic, and socio-economic characteristics along its length. According to the Köppen system [10], Brazil hosts five major climatic subtypes: equatorial, tropical, semiarid, highland tropical, and temperate. Biomes range from equatorial rainforests in the north and semiarid in the northeast, to temperate coniferous forests in the south and tropical savannas in central Brazil, but the largest part of the country is tropical.

Fusarium species of fungi are commonly associated with fungal keratitis in Brazil [3,11,12,13], where natamycin and amphotericin B eye drops are available for the management of fungal keratitis. Indeed, these drops are widely prescribed [12]. Natamycin is the only topical ophthalmic antifungal agent approved by the US Food and Drug Administration, and is the drug of choice for filamentous fungal keratitis worldwide [14]. The commercialisation of antifungal eye drops is tightly regulated in Brazil; these drugs are not available in drugstores and must be exclusively formulated for each patient. Ophtalmos was the first and major laboratory authorised by ANVISA (National Health Surveillance Agency) to produce, market and distribute eye drops, that are not manufactured by the pharmaceutical industry. Therefore, the company provides most of the eye drops used by patients. The alternative is the manipulation (dilution) of a commercial presentation for systemic (intravenous) use by the physician or someone from his/her staff.

Kaiserman et al [15] previously used drug prescriptions to predict the prevalence of eye disease in diabetic patients, however, a similar approach to identify the geographical distribution and correlation with potential risk factors has not been used in ophthalmology.

The current study aims to examine the commercialisation of formulated antifungal eye drops, by the only pharmaceutical company formally able to distribute them in this country, and to predict the distribution and seasonality of fungal keratitis in Brazil.

Methods

The Research Ethics Committee of the Faculty of Medicine of Ribeirão Preto, University of São Paulo approved this study, and it was conducted in accordance with the guidelines for confidentiality of medical records and the Declaration of Helsinki.

Antifungal eye drops are not commercially available in drugstores in Brazil. Rather, these drugs must be exclusively formulated for each patient and are sold directly by the laboratory, either through a call-in prescription or by postal delivery.

Antifungal eye drops are commercialised mainly by Ophtalmos Labs, in Brazil and dispensed only with the retention of prescription. We retrospectively analysed sales of natamycin and amphotericin B from this laboratory between July 2002 and June 2008. The company data bank of antifungal eye drops was analyzed and the distribution of dispensed units was registered by number of units/month for each drug and for each state of the federation. Population data were obtained from IBGE (Brazilian Institute of Geography and Statistics) at www.ibge.gov.br. The antifungal prescription was not necessarily made after microbiological confirmation of the aetiological agent and the clinical judgment to initiate or to continue antibiotic concomitant treatment was not evaluated.

We evaluated the data regarding units of antifungal eye drops sold during 72 months (6 years) for each one of the 27 Brazilian States. The total of units sold in each month was divided by the State population to reduce heterogeneity caused by different population size between States by using the following formula: antifungal eye drop units sold per million inhabitants = total units sold in one month/population of the State ×1,000,000. For each of the 72 months, data regarding total rain precipitation (mm), average relative humidity (%) and average temperature (°C) were also acquired for all 27 States. Climatic characteristics of each region were obtained from INMET (National Institute of Weather) at www.inmet.gov.br.

Statistical analysis was performed by using GraphPad Prism 5.0 (GraphPad Inc., San Diego, CA, USA) and SPSS 16.0 for Windows (SPSS Inc. Chicago, IL, USA). We evaluated the linear regression (R^2 and p-value) between the antifungal eye drop sales per million inhabitants and total rain precipitation (mm), average relative humidity (%) and average temperature (°C) considering all 1,944 State-months. Additionally we performed multiple linear regression (stepwise model) between the same parameters.

When comparing antifungal eye drop sales differences between months, we performed one-way analysis of variance (ANOVA)

considering the total units sold in the whole country for each month averaging for the 6-year period the outcome variable (dependent) and the months of the year the predictor (independent) variable. The Huber-White variance correction was applied in order to determine the robust estimator using each state as a subject and each of 72 months as repetition (12 months of 6 years). This analysis was performed using the Generalized Linear Models.

Results

The antifungal eye drops sold were categorised into types: natamycin or amphotericin. There were more than five times as many sales of natamycin as there were sales of amphotericin throughout the study period and a total of 26,087 antifungal eye drop units were sold during the study period. In addition, the units per patient was almost double for natamycin compared to amphotericin (**Table 1**).

Along of the 6 years evaluated there was no significant increase of antifungal eye drops sale.

The total number of individuals was 10175, dividing this number by the six years and the average Brazilian population in the period (188,298,099 inhabitants in 2006), it was estimated that the incidence of cases of fungal keratitis was 9.01/million of inhabitants per year [16].

When analysing the plots and the linear regression of the units of antifungal eye drop sold per million inhabitants with relative humidity, total rain precipitation and average temperature, we observed a significant association between the amount of antifungal eye drops units sold per inhabitant with both relative humidity and rain precipitation, but not with the temperature (**Figure 1**). When performing multiple linear regression, we observed that only relative humidity was associated with the amount of antifungal eye drops units sold per inhabitant (Beta = −0.41, p<0.01); after correction for humidity, there was no association of the amount of units sold per inhabitant and rain (Beta = −0.03, p = 0.17) or temperature (Beta = 0.04, p = 0.06).

We observed significant differences in the total of units of antifungal eye drop sold in Brazil between months during the 6-year period (p<0.01; ANOVA; **Figure 2**): the month with the highest sales was August (478±50 units; mean±SD); while the month with the lowest sales was April (289 ± 28 units; mean±SD). In **Figure 2** we also report the relative humidity in Brazil averaged in the 6-year period, demonstrating that the months with highest sales were also those with lowest relative humidity. Using Huber-White variance correction (robust estimator), there was significant correlation between sales and humidity (p<0.01), but not with temperature (p = 0.10) or rain precipitation (p = 0.23).

Discussion

The estimated incidence of fungal keratitis n Brazil is much higher than reported in United Kingdom (UK) (9.01 versus 0.32 cases/million per year) [17]. However, the present study is

Table 1. Units of each antifungal eye drop sold between July 2002 and June 2008 in Brazil by Ophtalmos Labs.

Antifungal	Total Units	Total Patients	Units/Patient
Natamycin	21.707	7.688	2,82
Amphotericin B	4.380	2.487	1,76

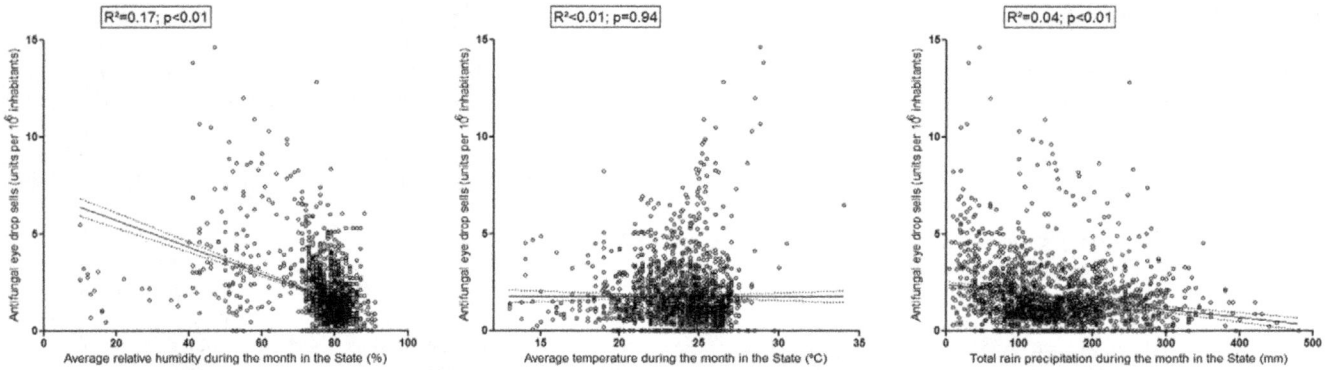

Figure 1. Plots of and the linear regression of the units of antifungal eye drop sold per million inhabitants with relative humidity, total rain precipitation and average temperature. The solid line represents the best fit curve and the dotted lines the 95% confidence interval.

probably overestimating the number of cases, since the survey here was based on number of individuals to whom the drugs were prescribed, and in UK, the numbers were related to microbiological confirmed cases. By now, it is not possible to make a similar survey, because there is not a national database for fungal keratitis and most of cases are treated based on clinical presentation. A recent study in Brazil estimated that 48% of clinically predicted fungal keratitis were confirmed by microbiological exam [18]. Even with those numbers, the incidence of fungal keratitis in Brazil would be more than 10 times higher than in UK. Moreover, the present work reveals that antifungal sales correlate with the driest season of the year.

Location and weather may play a major role in the epidemiology of eye diseases [19]. For instance, in more temperate climate areas, fungal corneal ulcers are more frequently caused by *Candida spp.* than by filamentous fungi [20]. However, this pattern is reversed in the tropics, where keratitis is predominantly caused by filamentous fungi. These geographic differences could be influenced by several factors, including climate, ecology, behavior, and socio-economics. In this study, we show that climate seems to play a substantial role for fungal keratitis, with humidity accounting for 17% of the variability in antifungal prescriptions in Brazil. [2,12,20,21].

Studies have shown that areas where the climate is warm and humid, especially near the Equator, have more cases of fungal keratitis; in these areas, filamentous fungi are the dominant fungal corneal pathogen [12,22]. Temperature and humidity have a major role in determining the microorganisms found in the environment; for example, *Fusaisum spp.* predominates in tropical areas [23,24]. However, the specific seasonal behaviour was not previously documented. Observing that other important risk factors for fungal keratitis are agricultural activity and ocular vegetal injury and individuals have been shown to be more vulnerable to ocular trauma when harvesting or collecting, our findings agree with the hypothesis that in tropical region the driest season, when those activities are more frequent, present the highest frequency of antifungal eye drops sales [2].

Our study shows an increase in antifungal sales during the third trimester of the year in Brazil. This period coincides with the collection and harvest season for many crops, such as corn, soybeans, sugar cane, coffee, rice and oranges, however any correlation among our data and agricultural activity in Brazil is still speculative. Some researchers have shown that the incidence of fungal keratitis is higher during harvesting and also during other times of the year when agricultural activity is higher, thus correlating the disease with harvesting crops such as rice [25] and onion [7]. In Brazil, harvest time is a period when there is a low precipitation index, dry air and a lower mean temperature than at other times of the year. The peak incidence of fungal keratitis has already been correlated with windy and dry weather in other countries, where the principal fungus isolated from patients was *Fusarium* [2,26]. However, studies in India have shown inverse disease seasonality, with disease incidence increasing during humid months [25], or even during the winter and monsoon (rainy) season [26,27]. This discrepancy could be explained by a variety of factors. The causative organisms could be different in the 2 countries, with some Indian studies reporting high numbers of *Curvalaria* or *Aspergillus*, whereas Brazilian studies have reported mostly *Fusarium*. Though both are tropical countries, there are nonetheless ecological differences. For example, India has 6 major climatic subtypes, ranging from desert to glacial, whereas Brazil has only 5 major subtypes, and does not have either the desert or glacial subtype, according to the Köppen system [3,8,10,27].

Although all five regions presented similar levels of antifungal topical eye drops sales and also comparable levels of humidity and rain precipitation, we saw high sales in Piaui, a state in the Northeast region, compared to the other states. It is one of the driest Brazilian states with a mean humidity of 70 ± 10.9%, while

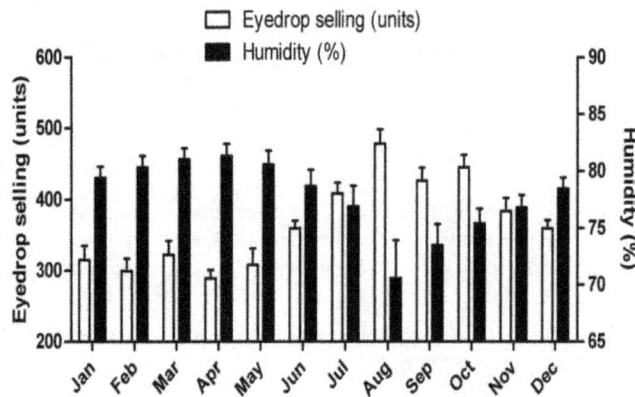

Figure 2. Antifungal eye drop units sold in Brazil (white columns) and the average relative humidity (black columns) separated by month averaged in 6-year period (from July 2002 to June 2008; white columns). Bars represent means and errors the 95% confidence interval.

the national mean is 77.9 ± 7.4%. We did not see many sales of eye drops in the Amazon area, a place that is hot and wet, even though it is similar to places where a high incidence of fungal keratitis cases are seen. This low incidence may be explained by the low population density and predominant forest vegetation, both of which contribute to low levels of agricultural activity. In addition, a lower number of health care professionals in the region may explain the lower number of antifungal prescribed.

Combining these findings with the high incidence of filamentary fungal keratitis in males enrolled in agricultural work, it appears that fungal keratitis is a major labour–related disease [2].

Another relevant aspect in fungal keratitis is the paucity of therapeutical options and providers. In Brazil, this study was only possible because no industry commercializes antifungal eye drops and the only registered company dispenses them by prescriptions. It is possible that non-registered formulations, or patients treated with systemic drugs are a source of bias in the present work. However, the severity of fungal keratitis and the difficulty in resolving the infection generally leads patients to referral centers that comply with broadly accepted treatments.

Our results are consistent with other studies of fungal keratitis conducted in Brazil [12,18] In previous studies, patients with fungal keratitis have on average been younger than patients with bacterial keratitis, which would be expected if younger agricultural

workers are especially at risk for fungal keratitis. Moreover, previous studies have specifically identified ocular trauma and male gender as risk factors, which is consistent with the theory that agricultural work is the primary risk factor for fungal keratitis.

The observed trend in drug sales is a useful method to study seasonal distribution of filamentary fungal keratitis. The present data, combined with previous observations of a higher risk in individuals involved in agricultural work in Brazil, suggests relationship of this infection with agricultural routines, as well as the need to improve preventive methods, such as the use of protective glasses [12,18]. This information should support the implementation of such strategies in vulnerable populations.

Acknowledgments

The authors also acknowledge the NIH Fellows Editorial Board for editorial assistance with the present manuscript and Geraldo Cassio dos Reis for assistance with statistics.

Author Contributions

Conceived and designed the experiments: MMI EMR. Performed the experiments: RD ASL GDVC FMI LTM MPB. Analyzed the data: MMI WPM EMR. Contributed reagents/materials/analysis tools: ASL GDVC WPM. Wrote the paper: MMI ASL EMR.

References

1. Leck AK, Thomas PA, Hagan M, Kaliamurthy J, Ackuaku E, et al. (2002) Aetiology of suppurative corneal ulcers in Ghana and south India, and epidemiology of fungal keratitis. Br J Ophthalmol 86: 1211–1215.
2. Bharathi MJ, Ramakrishnan R, Meenakshi R, Padmavathy S, Shivakumar C, et al. (2007) Microbial keratitis in South India: influence of risk factors, climate, and geographical variation. Ophthalmic Epidemiol 14: 61–69.
3. Hofling-Lima AL, Forseto A, Duprat JP, Andrade A, Souza LB, et al. (2005) [Laboratory study of the mycotic infectious eye diseases and factors associated with keratitis]. Arq Bras Oftalmol 68: 21–27.
4. Laspina F, Samudio M, Cibils D, Ta CN, Farina N, et al. (2004) Epidemiological characteristics of microbiological results on patients with infectious corneal ulcers: a 13-year survey in Paraguay. Graefes Arch Clin Exp Ophthalmol 242: 204–209.
5. Xie L, Zhong W, Shi W, Sun S (2006) Spectrum of fungal keratitis in north China. Ophthalmology 113: 1943–1948.
6. Ou JI, Acharya NR (2007) Epidemiology and treatment of fungal corneal ulcers. Int Ophthalmol Clin 47: 7–16.
7. Lin SH, Lin CP, Wang HZ, Tsai RK, Ho CK (1999) Fungal corneal ulcers of onion harvesters in southern Taiwan. Occup Environ Med 56: 423–425.
8. Wilhelmus KR (2005) Climatology of dematiaceous fungal keratitis. Am J Ophthalmol 140: 1156–1157.
9. Yilmaz S, Ozturk I, Maden A (2007) Microbial keratitis in West Anatolia, Turkey: a retrospective review. Int Ophthalmol 27: 261–268.
10. Peel MC, Finlayson BL, McMahon TA (2007) Updated world map of the Köppen-Geiger climate classification. Hydrol Earth Syst Sci 11: 1633–1644.
11. Carvalho M, Bordignon GP, Queiroz-Telles F (2001) Ceratite fúngica no estado do Paraná - Brasil: aspectos epidemiológicos, etiológicos e diagnósticos. Revista Iberoamericana de Micologia. pp 76–78.
12. Ibrahim MM, Vanini R, Ibrahim FM, Fioriti LS, Furlan EM, et al. (2009) Epidemiologic aspects and clinical outcome of fungal keratitis in southeastern Brazil. Eur J Ophthalmol 19: 355–361.
13. Passos RM, Cariello AJ, Yu MC, Höfling-Lima AL (2010) Microbial keratitis in the elderly: a 32-year review. Arq Bras Oftalmol 73: 315–319.
14. O'Day DM (1987) Selection of appropriate antifungal therapy. Cornea 6: 238–245.
15. Kaiserman I, Kaiserman N, Nakar S, Vinker S (2005) Dry eye in diabetic patients. Am J Ophthalmol 139: 498–503.
16. IBGE website (2006) http://www.ibge.gov.br/home/estatistica/populacao/estimativa2006/estimativa.shtm. Accessed 2011, Dec 17.
17. Tuft SJ, Tullo AB (2009) Fungal keratitis in the United Kingdom 2003–2005. Eye (Lond) 23: 1308–1313.
18. Ibrahim MM, Vanini R, Ibrahim FM, Martins WeP, Carvalho RT, et al. (2011) Epidemiology and medical prediction of microbial keratitis in southeast Brazil. Arq Bras Oftalmol 74: 7–12.
19. Johnson GJ (2004) The environment and the eye. Eye (Lond) 18: 1235–1250.
20. Galarreta DJ, Tuft SJ, Ramsay A, Dart JK (2007) Fungal keratitis in London: microbiological and clinical evaluation. Cornea 26: 1082–1086.
21. Jurkunas U, Behlau I, Colby K (2009) Fungal keratitis: changing pathogens and risk factors. Cornea 28: 638–643.
22. Saha R, Das S (2006) Mycological profile of infectious Keratitis from Delhi. Indian J Med Res 123: 159–164.
23. Rosa RH, Jr., Miller D, Alfonso EC (1994) The changing spectrum of fungal keratitis in south Florida. Ophthalmology 101: 1005–1013.
24. Mino de Kaspar H, Zoulek G, Paredes ME, Alborno R, Medina D, et al. (1991) Mycotic keratitis in Paraguay. Mycoses 34: 251–254.
25. Dunlop AA, Wright ED, Howlader SA, Nazrul I, Husain R, et al. (1994) Suppurative corneal ulceration in Bangladesh. A study of 142 cases examining the microbiological diagnosis, clinical and epidemiological features of bacterial and fungal keratitis. Aust N Z J Ophthalmol 22: 105–110.
26. Gopinathan U, Garg P, Fernandes M, Sharma S, Athmanathan S, et al. (2002) The epidemiological features and laboratory results of fungal keratitis: a 10-year review at a referral eye care center in South India. Cornea 21: 555–559.
27. Kotigadde S, Ballal M, Jyothirlatha, Kumar A, Srinivasa R, et al. (1992) Mycotic keratitis: a study in coastal Karnataka. Indian J Ophthalmol 40: 31–33.

19

Oleanolic Acid Controls Allergic and Inflammatory Responses in Experimental Allergic Conjunctivitis

Claudia Córdova[1◑], **Beatriz Gutiérrez**[1◑], **Carmen Martínez-García**[2], **Rubén Martín**[3], **Patricia Gallego-Muñoz**[2], **Marita Hernández**[1], **María L. Nieto**[1]*

1 Instituto de Biología y Genética Molecular, Consejo Superior de Investigaciones Científicas-Universidad de Valladolid, Valladolid, Spain, 2 Departamento de Biología Celular, Histología y Farmacología, Universidad de Valladolid, Valladolid, Spain, 3 Instituto de Ciencias del Corazón. Hospital Clínico Universitario, Valladolid, Spain

Abstract

Pollen is the most common aeroallergen to cause seasonal conjunctivitis. The result of allergen exposure is a strong Th2-mediated response along with conjunctival mast cell degranulation and eosinophilic infiltration. Oleanolic acid (OA) is natural a triterpene that displays strong anti-inflammatory and immunomodulatory properties being an active anti-allergic molecule on hypersensitivity reaction models. However, its effect on inflammatory ocular disorders including conjunctivits, has not yet been addressed. Hence, using a Ragweed pollen (RWP)-specific allergic conjunctivitis (EAC) mouse model we study here whether OA could modify responses associated to allergic processes. We found that OA treatment restricted mast cell degranulation and infiltration of eosinophils in conjunctival tissue and decreased allergen-specific Igs levels in EAC mice. Th2-type cytokines, secreted phospholipase A2 type-IIA (sPLA2-IIA), and chemokines levels were also significantly diminished in the conjunctiva and serum of OA-treated EAC mice. Moreover, OA treatment also suppressed RWP-specific T-cell proliferation. In vitro studies, on relevant cells of the allergic process, revealed that OA reduced the proliferative and migratory response, as well as the synthesis of proinflammatory mediators on EoL-1 eosinophils and RBL-2H3 mast cells exposed to allergic and/or crucial inflammatory stimuli such as RWP, sPLA2-IIA or eotaxin. Taken together, these findings demonstrate the beneficial activity of OA in ocular allergic processes and may provide a new intervention strategy and potential therapy for allergic diseases.

Editor: Hua Zhou, Macau University of Science and Technology, Macau

Funding: The study was supported by grants from the Spanish MINECO (reference SAF2009-08407). Patricia Gallego-Muñoz and Claudia Cordova were funded by the FPI Program from the Government of Castilla y León (co-funded by FSE). Rubén Martín was supported by the Sara Borrell Program from the Spanish MINECO. The funders had no role in study design, data collection and analysis, decision to publish, or preparation of the manuscript.

Competing Interests: The authors have declared that no competing interests exist.

* E-mail: mlnieto@ibgm.uva.es

◑ These authors contributed equally to this work.

Introduction

Allergic conjunctivitis (AC) is one of the most common ocular surface diseases. The disease encompasses a variety of pathological conditions, and based on immunopathological mechanisms, it can be subdivided into seasonal and perennial allergic conjunctivitis [1]. AC is an abnormal immune-hypersensitivity response to allergens mainly pollen, animal dander and house dust mites, although some food substances may also trigger it. They have common immunopathogenic mechanisms characterized by IgE-mediated mast cell degranulation and/or T-lymphocyte-mediated immune response. Allergen-specific Th2-type lymphocytes play important roles in the immunopathophysiology of allergic disorders because of their ability to produce IL-4, IL-5 and IL-13, which are involved in IgE production and eosinophil activation [2].

Medications for AC include drug treatment (anti-histamines, mast cell stabilizers, corticosteroids, non-steroidal anti-inflammatories, immunomodulatories), and allergen-specific immunotherapy. However, its effectiveness can be endangered by adherence problems related to factors, such as discomfort associated with treatment administration, complexity of administration guidelines, perception of a lack of efficacy at treatment initiation, and/or adverse effects. Therefore, the development of new therapeutic strategies will be a valuable tool to achieve better control of the disease and, thus, will improve healthcare outcome for patients with allergic conjunctivitis.

Because alternative treatments are needed, plants and other natural materials may prove to be valuable sources of useful new anti-allergic agents [3]. Research groups have conducted clinical trials with remedies from complementary and alternative medicine [4–7]. Plant formulations have demonstrated, in general, to be safe, revealing additional effects along with Western medicines such as synergism and modulation of the immune system. Triterpenes, including oleanolic acid (OA) are compounds that widely exist in the human diet, medicinal herbs and plants. OA has been identified in more than 120 plant species, including *olea europaea*, a plant that has gained more and more interest because of its multiple bioactive components [8]. Among the numerous beneficial effects, OA has been shown to have cardioprotective, antihypertensive, antiatherosclerotic, antihyperlipidemic and antioxidant activities, among other, as well as anti-inflammatory and immunomodulatory properties, being active on hypersensitivity reactions, such as the delayed-type hypersensitivity reaction, or allergic asthma, and in Th1-mediated diseases, including experimental colitis and multiple sclerosis [9–16]. However, the effectiveness of OA in the treatment of ocular diseases such as allergic conjunctivitis is still unknown.

The IgE-mediated conjunctival allergic reaction can be reproduced easily in mice by using RWP as antigen [17]. The result is an early reaction followed by a predominant infiltration of eosinophilic inflammatory cells, which are the hallmark of allergic disease, and mast cell activation. This experimental allergic conjunctivitis (EAC) model mimics the pathological symptoms of AC in human, being a valuable tool to understand the pathogenesis of the disease, as well as for new drugs evaluation. The aim of this study was, therefore, to evaluate the effectiveness of OA using this well-characterized EAC model induced by RWP in BALB/c mice.

Materials and Methods

Disease Induction and Treatment

Animal care and experimental protocols were reviewed and approved by the Animal Ethics Committee of the University of Valladolid and complied the standards in the ARVO Statement. Mice (Charles River Laboratories, Barcelona, Spain) were housed in the animal facilities of the University of Valladolid and provided food and water ad libitum.

Immunization. EAC was induced in 6- to 7-week-old females BALB/c mice by intraperitoneal (i.p.) sensitization with 200 µl from a mixture of 50 µg RWP (Polyscience, Warrington, PA) in 0.25 ml Imject Alum (Thermo Scienctific, Rockford, IL). Then, on day 10, mice were topically instilled into each eye with 1.25 mg of RWP in powder form [3,18]. Twenty-four hours later, eyes, blood and spleens were collected.

Treatment. Oleanolic acid (Extrasynthese, Genay Cedex, France) was dissolved in 2% w/v DMSO. Then, this stock solution was 10 times diluted to a working concentration of 2 mg/ml (0.2%, w/v DMSO final concentration), using a sterile saline solution (pre-warmed to 37°C) with mild shaking. Always, OA working solution was prepared fresh the day of the injection and sterile-filtered through a 0.22 µm filter. OA (50 mg/kg body weight/day) was administered i.p. once a day from sensitization day (OA_{10}) or 5 days after sensitization (OA_5) as shown in Figure 1B (n = 10 per group). The molecular structure of OA is shown in Fig. 1A (OA molecular formula: $C_{30}H_{48}O_3$, molecular weight: 456.70).

Evaluation of Cell Infiltration

Eyes including eyelids and conjunctiva were exenterated and fixed in 4% paraformaldehyde for 24 h. Then, they were cut into cross sections 3-µm thick and stained with toluidine blue and hematoxylin-eosine for detection of mast cells and eosinophils, respectively. In each section, infiltrating cells in the lamina propria mucosae of the palpebral and bulbar conjunctivas were counted by two masked observers. Palpebral zone: connective tissue between the epithelium and the Meibomio gland in the centre of the lid. Bulbar conjunctiva: near the cornea in reflection zone that form the conjunctival sac. In each slide there were two non-consecutive sections and three slides per eye and per stain were counted. An Olympus B–H (Olympus optical Co. LTD, Tokio, Japan) microscope and a micrometer ocular grid were used to evaluate the slides (magnification x400). Data are presented as mean ± SD per mm^2.

Cytokines, Chemokines and RWP-specific Igs Quantitation

Serum was aliquoted and stored at $-80°C$. Immunoplates (Nalge Nunc International, Naperville, IL) were coated with RWP (5 mg/ml) overnight at 4°C. After blocking with 1% BSA-PBS for 2 h, serum samples diluted 1:60 were added and incubated for 3 h. After washing, plates were incubated for 1 h with horseradish peroxidase-conjugated rat anti-mouse IgE, IgG, IgG1 or IgG2a antibodies (1:2000) from Serotec (Sigma-Aldrich, St Louis, MO). Color reaction was developed with 3,3',5,5'-tetramethyl-benzidine and stopped with 0.1N HCl. Data are expressed as mean optical density (OD) at 450 nm.

For cytokine and chemokine quantification - IL-10, IL-13, IL-33, monocyte chemoattractant protein-1 (MCP-1) and eotaxin - cell culture medium, serum and conjunctival tissue were analyzed by ELISA according to the manufacturer's protocols (eBioscience, San Diego, CA). Secreted phospholipase A_2-typeIIA ($sPLA_2$-IIA) levels were determined by commercial ELISA (USCNK Life Science Inc, Houston, TX). Conjunctival tissue was homogenized by using a tissue homogenizer (Cole-Parmer Instrument, Vernon Hills, IL) in an ice bath in 0.5 ml ice-cold PBS supplemented with 0.4 M NaCl, 0.05% Tween-20 and a protease inhibitor cocktail: 20 mg/ml of leupeptin, 20 KI units of aprotinin, 0.1 mM phenylmethylsulphonyl fluoride, and centrifuged for 10 min at 4°C. Supernatant were stored at $-80°C$ until cytokine assays were performed. Total protein was assayed using the Bradford method.

Ex vivo Lymphoid Cell Culture and Analysis of Proliferation and Cytokine Production

To prepared single cell suspension, spleens were pressed though a wire mesh and then washed with ice-cold PBS. Red blood cells-depleted splenocytes (10×10^6 cells/ml) were cultured in triplicate in 96-well plates, and stimulated with medium alone or with 50 µg/ml of RWP in presence or absence of different doses of OA. After 24 h, supernatants were harvested and concentrations of IL-33, IL-13 and MCP-1 were measured. Cells were prepared for proliferation analyses using the Promega kit, Cell Titer 96RAqueous One Solution Cell Proliferation Assay (Promega Corporation, Madison, WI), according to the manufacturer's recommendations. Formazan product formation was determined by measuring the absorbance at 490 nm. Results were expressed as OD values, as an assessment of the number of metabolically active cells.

In vitro Studies

Cell culture. The rat basophilic leukemia (RBL) mast cell line RBL-2H3 (kindly provided by Dr. Ruiz; Hospital Universitario Puerta del Mar, Facultad de Medicina, Universidad de Cádiz, Spain) was grown in EMEM supplemented with 15% heat-inactivated FCS, 0.1 mM nonessential amino acids, 50 U/ml penicillin, and 50 µg/ml streptomycin [19].

The human eosinophilic cell line EoL-1 (kindly provided by Dr. Wicklein, University Medical-Center Hamburg-Eppendorf, Hamburg, Germany) was grown in RPMI 1640 medium, supplemented with 10% heat-inactivated FCS, 2 mM L-glutamine, 100 U/ml penicillin, and 100 µg/ml streptomycin [20,21].

Both cell lines were cultured in standard conditions (37°C and 5% CO2).

Proliferation assay. The proliferative activity of EoL-1 and RBL-2H3 cells was quantified using the Promega kit, Cell Titer 96RAqueous One Solution Cell Proliferation Assay, as described for the ex vivo proliferation assay. In brief, cells (1×10^5 cells/ml) were serum-starved for 24 h, incubated as indicated and measured. Results were expressed as OD values.

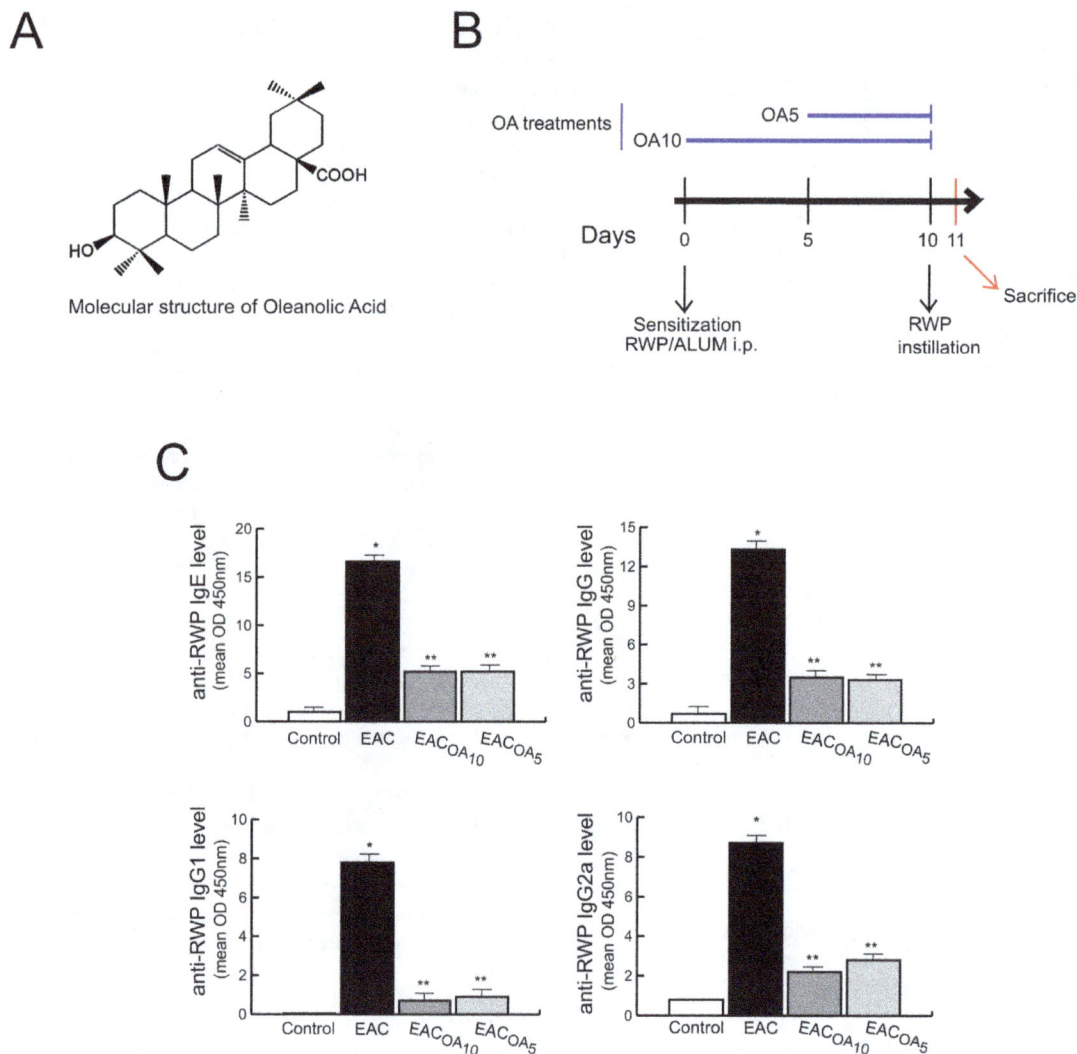

Figure 1. Reduction of circulating anti-RWP antibodies in OA-treated mice. Molecular structure of OA (A). Experimental protocol (B). BALB/c mice were sensitized on day 0 via i.p. injection with RWP emulsified in aluminum hydroxide. 10 days latter, individual mice were challenged through ocular instillation with RWP. OA was administered i.p. at the sensitization day (OA$_{10}$) or 5 days after sensitization (OA$_5$). Animals were sacrificed 24 h after the challenge. (C) Titers of RWP-specific immunoglobulins in serum samples. *P<0.001 versus control, and **P<0.001 versus untreated EAC-mice.

Chemotaxis assay. Cell migration was assayed using 24-well Transwell chambers with 8 μm-pore polycarbonate filters. Lower wells were filled with medium containing eotaxin, sPLA$_2$-IIA or vehicle, as indicated. Cells (1×10^6 cells/ml) were added to the upper chamber. When indicated, cells were treated with sPLA$_2$-IIA, RWP or OA for 20 min at 37°C before seeding. Migration was allowed for 3–4 h at 37°C in 5% CO$_2$. Migrated RHL-2H3 cells were fixed with 4% paraformaldehyde and stained with 0.1% Crystal Violet in 20% methanol-PBS for 3 minutes. The stain was solubilized and absorbance measured at 590 nm. Migrated EoL-1 cells were quantified by flow cytometry analysis. Chemotactic index was calculated from the number of cells migrating towards chemoatractant/number of cells migrating towards vehicle control.

Flow cytometry of intracellular major basic protein (MBP). EoL-1 cells were treated with butyric acid, or the stimuli eotaxin, RWP, sPLA$_2$-IIA or combinations for 7 days. Then, cells were washed with 0.5% BSA-PBS, fixed with 4% paraformaldehyde for 30 min and permeabilized with 0.2%

Triton-X 100 in PBS for 10 min. Non-specific antibody binding was blocked by incubating cells with normal mouse IgG for 30 min. Then, cells were stained with an anti-MBP antibody (1:200) for 2 h. After washing, they were incubated with FITC-labeled goat anti-mouse IgG for 1 h at 4°C. Baseline fluorescence values were obtained by incubation with isotype mouse IgG antibody. After washing, the stained cells were analyzed using a Gallios Flow cytometer (Beckman Coulter), and acquisition and analysis were performed using CellQuest software. The data are presented as an average of mean intensity fluorescence (MIF).

Statistical Analysis

Statistical significance between groups was examined by one-way ANOVA using the GraphPad Prism Version 4 software (San Diego, CA). A post hoc analysis was made by the Bonferroni's multiple comparison test. P<0.05 was considered statistically significant.

Results

OA Treatment Inhibits RWP-specific Antibody Production in EAC Mice

To investigate whether OA treatment modulates adaptive immune response to conjunctival allergens, as well as the influence of the pre-treatment period in its effectiveness, EAC mice were treated with OA from sensitization day (OA_{10}) or 5 days after sensitization (OA_5) as shown in Figure 1B. The severity of EAC was elucidated by assessing RWP-specific IgE antibody levels in serum. The combination of systemic sensitization and local boosting with RWP resulted in significantly higher levels of Ag-specific IgE antibody secretion (Fig. 1C) compared with those in normal mice. However, the administration of OA, both under OA_{10} and OA_5 protocols, led to a dramatic and similar reduction of Ag-specific IgE antibody levels (Fig. 1C). To address overall immunosuppression by OA, we also assessed levels of RWP-specific IgG, IgG1 and IgG2a antibodies in serum, finding similar results to those obtained for RWP-specific IgE antibodies. Taken together, these data suggest that oleanolic acid suppressed both allergen specific IgE production and overall immune responses.

OA Treatment Attenuates Cellular Infiltration into Conjunctiva in EAC Mice

Histological findings demonstrated by toluidine blue staining the presence of numerous mast cells infiltrating lamina propria and stroma of conjunctiva in EAC mice, being most of them degranulated mast cells (Fig. 2A and C). In contrast, in the OA-treated EAC groups infiltrating mast cells were mainly granulated and the number of degranulated mast cells was significant lower, compared to untreated ones.

In the same way, hematoxylin-eosine staining revealed a significant infiltration of eosinophils in the conjunctiva of RWP-challenged mice 24 h after systemic priming (Fig. 2B and D). Interestingly, the number of eosinophils infiltrating the conjunctiva after allergen challenge was minimal in mice treated with OA.

Mast cell and eosinophil counts were not significantly different between EAC mice injected with either oleanolic acid regimens (OA_{10} or OA_5).

OA Treatment Reduces the Release of EAC-associated Cytokines and Chemokines

Th2-associated cytokines and chemokines are typically secreted in allergic reactions. To evaluate the effect of OA on cytokine secretion, levels of IL-13 and IL-33 were investigated in serum and conjunctival tissue by commercial ELISAs. As shown in Figure 3 A and B, IL-33 and IL-13 were remarkably up-regulated in the allergic state and OA treatment diminished their expression levels.

We also evaluated the presence of IL-10, a known suppressive cytokine of T-cell proliferation and cytokine production, in normal, allergic and OA-treated allergic mice. We found that IL-10 levels in serum and tissue were significantly diminished in the allergic state, but were up-regulated reaching values of the normal state, in OA-treated EAC mice.

Production and build up of $sPLA_2$-IIA, an acute-phase reactant associated with a number of inflammatory, autoimmune, and allergic diseases, was also evaluated [22]. $sPLA_2$-IIA was augmented in serum and conjunctivas of mice from the untreated-EAC group, compared with the healthy-control group (Fig. 3 A and B). However, and according to Th2-type cytokines data, we found that this inflammatory protein was significantly lower in OA-treated EAC mice, at both systemic and local level.

Moreover, we also measured the concentration of two chemokines: eotaxin, given its critical role in eosinophil recruitment, Th2-related cytokines production and mast cell priming; and MCP-1, which is essential for mast cell-mediated acute inflammatory responses [23]. Again, we observed that OA treatment suppressed the high levels of eotaxin and MCP-1 found in sera and conjunctivas of allergic mice (Fig. 3 C and D).

There was no difference in regulating these conjunctivitis-associated markers between the two treatment protocols: EAC_{OA5} and EAC_{OA10}.

OA Treatment Regulates T Cell Responses in EAC

Next, to investigate whether OA treatment inhibits EAC by modifying/affecting systemic immune responses, we evaluated the function of splenocytes harvested from mice of the four experimental groups.

Spleen cells were assessed for antigen-specific proliferation and cytokine secretion after in vitro stimulation with RWP in the presence or absence of different doses of OA. RWP-specific proliferative response, as well as IL-13, IL-33 and MCP-1 production were significantly increased in spleen cells from mice with EAC, and addition of OA markedly suppressed, in a dose-dependent manner, these ex-vivo responses to the allergen (Fig. 4, A and C). In contrast, splenocytes isolated from healthy-control mice did not respond to in vitro RWP challenge, and no major responses were detected in spleen cells from EAC_{OA10} and EAC_{OA5} mice (Fig. 4, B and D).

OA Inhibits in vitro Functional Activation of Allergy-related Cells

We next investigated whether the anti-inflammatory effect found in vivo, in OA-treated EAC mice, comprises also direct in vitro actions on cells particularly important for the development of allergic disorders. Therefore, the well-characterized eosinophil cell line EoL-1 and RBL-2H3 mast cells were used to mimic responses activated on ocular allergic reactions.

Proliferation and survival. EoL-1 eosinophils and RBL-2H3 mast cells were treated with different concentrations of RWP or eotaxin in presence or absence of either 5 or 10 μM of OA for 24 h. As shown in Figure 5A and B, the presence of OA significantly reduced, the proliferative response induced by the agonists, in a dose-dependent manner. The presence of OA had no significant influence on the viability of either resting or activated cells.

Chemotactic migration. The capacity of OA to modulate EoL-1 eosinophils and RBL-2H3 mast cells migration was assessed using Transwell chambers. As shown in Fig. 5 C and D, cell pretreatment with OA reduced in a dose-dependent manner the chemotactic activity of eotaxin in both cell lines.

We also assessed the capacity of $sPLA_2$-IIA, found up-regulated in EAC mice, and RWP to elicit and/or modify chemotactic migration. As schematically colored-indicated in Figure 6, $sPLA_2$-IIA added in the lower compartment of transwell chamber induced a significant increase in EoL-1 eosinophils (Fig. 6A) and RBL-2H3 mast cells (Fig. 6B) migration over controls. In addition, both $sPLA_2$-IIA- and RWP-cell pretreatment potently stimulated both spontaneous and chemoattractant-induced cell migration.

Then, we investigated the effects of OA, and we observed that cell migration was potently inhibited when cells were pre-incubated with OA. Addition of OA to the lower chamber had no detectable effect on cell motility (data not shown).

EoL-1 eosinophils differentiation. Differentiation of EoL-1 cells was triggered chemically with butyric acid, or with stimuli such as eotaxin, RWP and $sPLA_2$-IIA, and the expression of MBP,

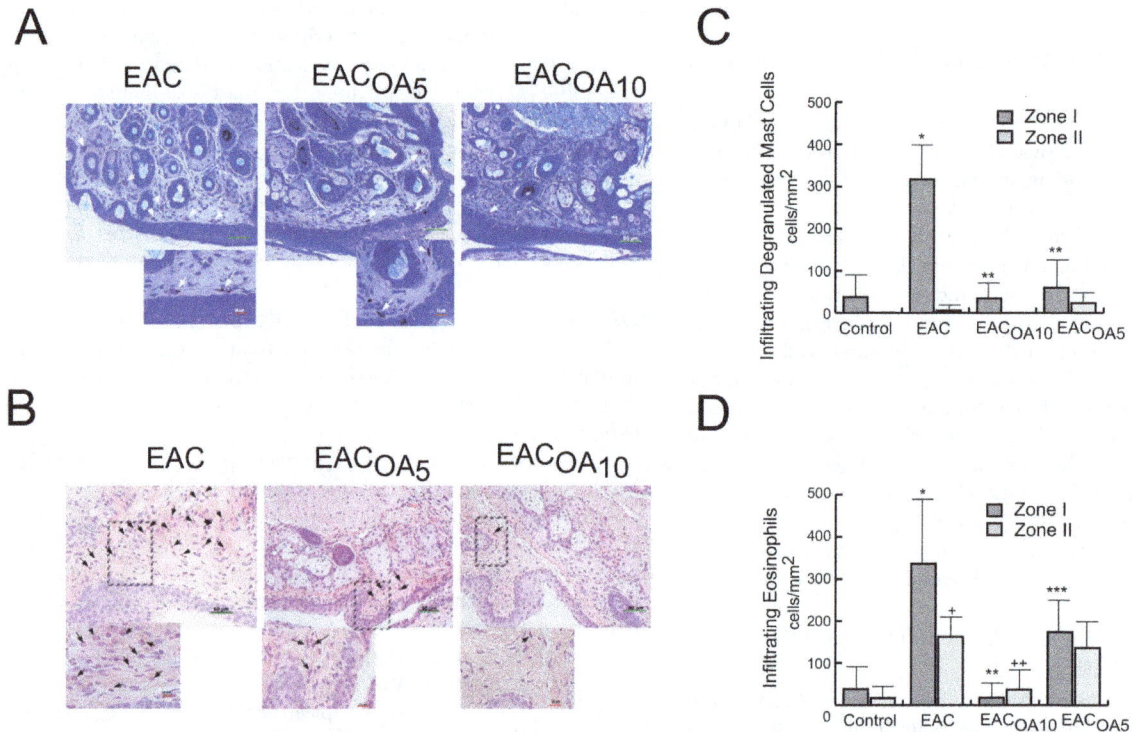

Figure 2. OA administration prevents development of allergic conjunctival inflammation. Light micrograph of conjunctival sections in mice from allergic untreated, OA5-treated and OA10-treated groups. Representative toluidine (A) and H-E (B) stained sections showed infiltration in palpebral conjunctiva of mast cells and eosinophils, respectively. (C, D) Number of degranulated mast cells/mm² and eosinophils/mm², respectively. In images, green bars = 50 μm. In inserts, red bars = 10 μm. * and **P<0.01 (n = 10, three independent experiments). Zone I: conjunctiva palpebral. Zone II: conjunctiva bulbar. * and +P<0.001 versus control zone I and zone II, respectively; ** and ++P<0.001 versus untreated EAC-mice zone I and zone II, respectively; and ***P<0.01 versus untreated EAC-mice zone I.

a mature eosinophil marker, was evaluated by flow cytometry. As shown in Figure 7A all the agonists on their own promoted the upregulation of MBP at day 7 after treatment. Interestingly, when the agonists eotaxin, RWP, or sPLA$_2$-IIA were added in combination with butyric acid, the differentiation process was significantly increased over butyric acid alone. As expected, the presence of OA before incubation the cells with the agonists, abrogated the differentiation process (Fig. 7B).

Discussion

OA is a powerful anti-inflammatory agent, whose activity in ocular inflammatory disorders has never been investigated. Here, we examined the effect of OA on allergic conjunctivitis in a RWP-induced EAC model as well as its effects in vitro on eosinophils and mast cells functions. We focused on these cells since they are important mediators in the development of allergic diseases and inflammatory processes.

Intraperitoneal administration of OA, either on the sensitization day or 5 days after sensitization to an EAC model, provided strong evidence of its anti-allergic effects; while, its administration to healthy BALB/c mice did not induce signs of any pro-inflammatory response (data not sown), as found in other experimental mice models [14,15]. The main pathophysiological changes in conjunctival allergic reactions include preferential generation of IgE antibodies in serum, as well as IgE-dependent mast cell degranulation and infiltration of eosinophils into the conjunctiva [24]. Our mouse model displayed these pathological hallmarks, and OA treatment effectively reduced the number of eosinophils and degranulated mast cells in the conjunctival tissue,

and suppressed the presence of allergen-specific Igs titers in serum, showing no remarkable difference in the degree of suppression of these features between the two OA administration protocols. These findings were consistent with the decreased levels of inflammatory mediators and Th2 cytokine found in the OA-treated mice (EAC$_{OA10}$ and EAC$_{OA5}$).

The pathological processes of an allergic reaction are thought to be mediated by Th2-type cells which release interleukins such as IL-5 and IL-13. These cytokines are responsible for a cascade of events necessary for allergic inflammation: IgE production by B-cells, eosinophil activation and recruitment, and mast cell activation. IL-13 is a crucial mediator of hypersensivity reactions [25–29]. Different studies in murine models of allergen challenge have shown that IL-13 is a critical factor to induce responses that have a striking resemblance to human diseases. IL-13 regulates synthesis of IgE and coordinates the inflammatory process due to its ability to stimulate expression of adhesion molecules, chemokines and metalloproteinases, which influence the recruitment, trafficking and activation of many inflammatory cells. Meanwhile, IL-33 is another powerful inducer of allergic inflammation which has been found highly expressed in Th2-associated diseases including asthma, allergic conjunctivitis and rhinitis [30,31]. IL-33 promotes responses which include activation and migration of Th2 lymphocytes, eosinophils, mast cells and basophiles.

Our data clearly demonstrated that the expected increased levels of IL-13, and IL-33 in the conjunctival tissue and serum of EAC mice were markedly suppressed by OA treatment. Likewise, we did see an allergen-induced increase in the release of these cytokines in splenocytes cultures after allergen challenge. Treat-

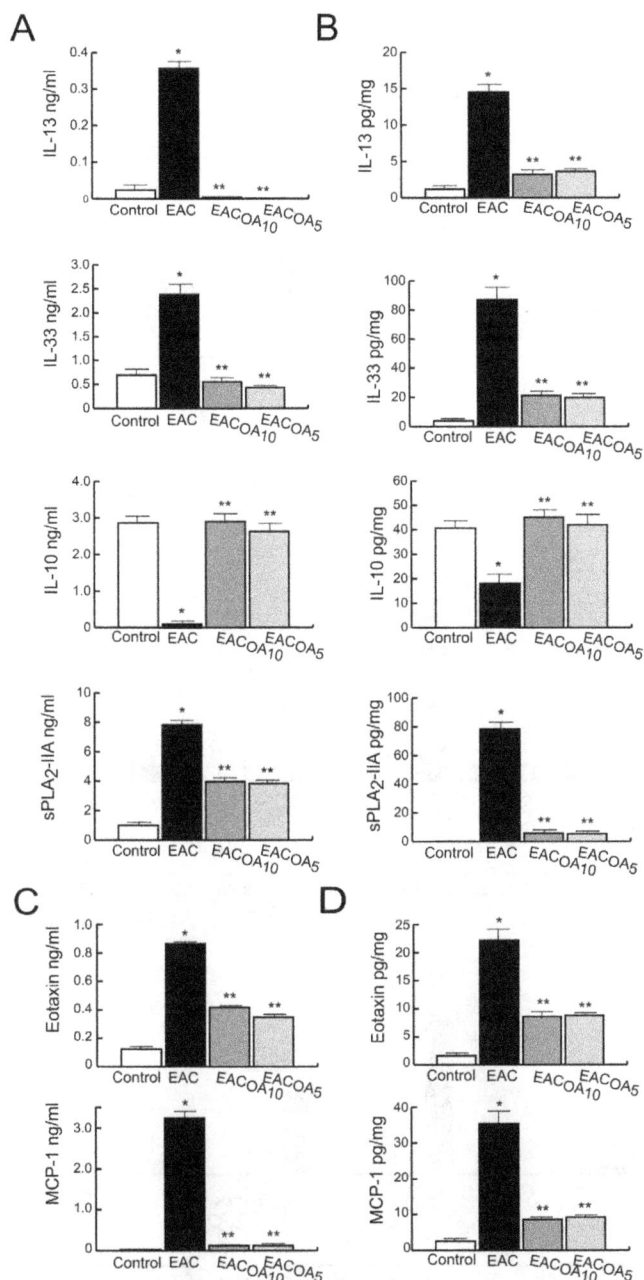

Figure 3. Effect of OA on cytokine and chemokine levels in EAC mice. The cytokines IL-13, IL-33, IL-10 and sPLA$_2$-IIA (A,B), as well as the chemokines eotaxin and MCP-1 (C,D) were quantified in serum samples (A,C) and ocular conjunctiva extracts (B,D) from mice of the indicated groups 24 h after challenge. Results were expressed as the mean ± SD (n = 7/group). *$P<0.001$ vs control, and **$P<0.001$ vs untreated-EAC mice.

ment with OA, both in vivo and in vitro, significantly reduced IL-13 and IL-33 cytokine production. Additionally, examination of chemokine induction revealed that the upregulated levels of eotaxin and MCP-1, in both serum and the conjunctiva of sensitized mice after allergen challenge, were substantially decreased in OA-treated mice. Similar results were found in vitro: splenocytes from the different experimental groups also showed a substantial reduction in the allergen-induced eotaxin and MCP-1 by the action of OA, along with a minimization of the proliferative

response of these T-cell cultures. All of this suggests that OA was able not only to down-modulate both the systemic and local allergen-induced inflammatory response, but also to impair allergen-induced T cell responses in vivo and in vitro.

IL-13 has been shown to regulate the expression of MCP-1 and eotaxin in the respiratory and gastrointestinal mucosa, and exogenous application of IL-33 to an EAC model strongly induces local production of the chemoattractant eotaxin, and potentiates the capacity of Th2 cells to produce cytokines including IL-13 [30,32–36]. At the same time, eotaxin-1 is considered as the most relevant chemokine in the pathophysiology of allergic conditions, because of its contribution to eosinophil homing or allergen-dependent chemoattraction and its regulatory function in mast cells at the ocular tissue regulating both IgE-induced degranulation and presumably maturation [30]. Therefore, the reduced presence of eosinophils and degranulated mast cells, in the conjunctiva of the OA-treated EAC mice treated, might be closely linked to the decreased expression of IL-13, IL-33 and eotaxin, all of which were clearly down-modulated by OA. Similarly, the improvement of allergic conjunctivitis in mice subjected to treatment with natural products such as curcumin or thymoquinine, an anti-oxidant and anti-inflammatory active component of *Nigella sativa*, has also been linked to its capacity to suppress Th2-driven immune responses [37,38].

Another finding was that treatment of EAC mice with OA prevented the diminished secretion of IL-10 observed in untreated-EAC mice. In fact, the expression levels in serum and conjunctival tissue of this Treg-type cytokine involved in the Th1/Th2 homeostasis were similar in OA-treated EAC mice and in healthy control mice. It is noteworthy that in addition to its anti-inflammatory properties on human mast cells, IL-10 has recently been shown to stabilize murine mast cells and reduce their degranulation in vitro [39,40]. Data which are in accordance with an in vivo study in a rodent model, which report that IL-10 attenuates allergic conjunctivitis by protecting from mast cell activation/degranulation, instead of affecting its numbers in the conjunctiva [40]. Similarly, our study neither revealed significant differences in the number of mast cells in the conjunctiva between untreated- and OA-treated-EAC mice (data not shown), but rather OA treatment prevented from mast cells degranulation.

In addition, we found an increased presence of sPLA$_2$-IIA in serum and conjunctiva of allergic mice as compared to control healthy mice, and the administration of OA again abrogated this augmented expression. High concentrations of sPLA$_2$-IIA have already been found in the tears of patients with AC both seasonal and perennial, dry eye disease, chronic blepharitis and contact lens intolerance, when compared to tears of age-matched normal controls [41–43]. Recently, a dry eye experimental model in mice has revealed increased expression of sPLA$_2$-IIA in the goblet, as well as in epithelial cells associated with the signs and symptoms of the diseases [22]. sPLA$_2$-IIA in the normal ocular surface was shown to be an innate immune barrier of the ocular surface against microbial infection, but when the ocular surface is compromised, it amplifies the inflammatory process [22,43]. These findings might support the hypothesis that the elevated levels of sPLA$_2$-IIA on conjunctiva of our EAC model might play an important role triggering ocular inflammation by affecting to the conjunctiva epithelial cells. Consequently, lowering its presence by the administration of OA should result in a diminished, or abrogated, ocular surface inflammation.

In our study we also demonstrated sPLA$_2$-IIA- and allergen-specific signals in eosinophils and mast cells, which are abolished by the presence of OA. We focused on these cell-types because of its significant contribution to the development of AC due to its

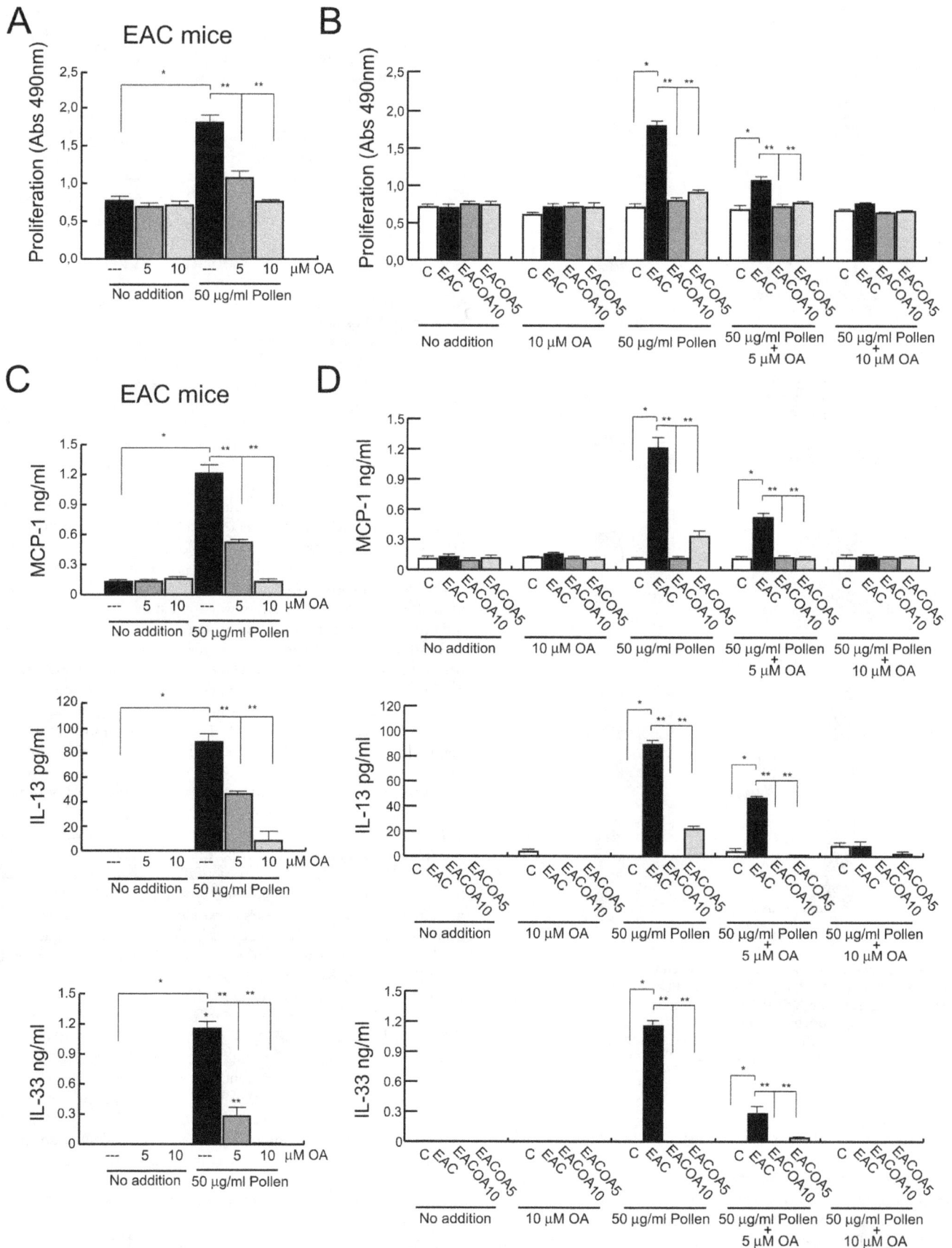

Figure 4. Effect of OA on splenocyte functions. RWP-specific proliferative responses of splenic cells from untreated-EAC mice (A), and from mice of the indicated groups (B). Cells were treated for 24 h with 50 μg/ml of RWP in presence or absence of the indicated doses of OA, and proliferation

was measured. Each bar represents the mean ± SD. (C and D) Quantification of IL-13, IL-33, and MCP-1 in supernatants from (A) and (B). Bars represents means ± SD. (n = 5). * and **P<0.001.

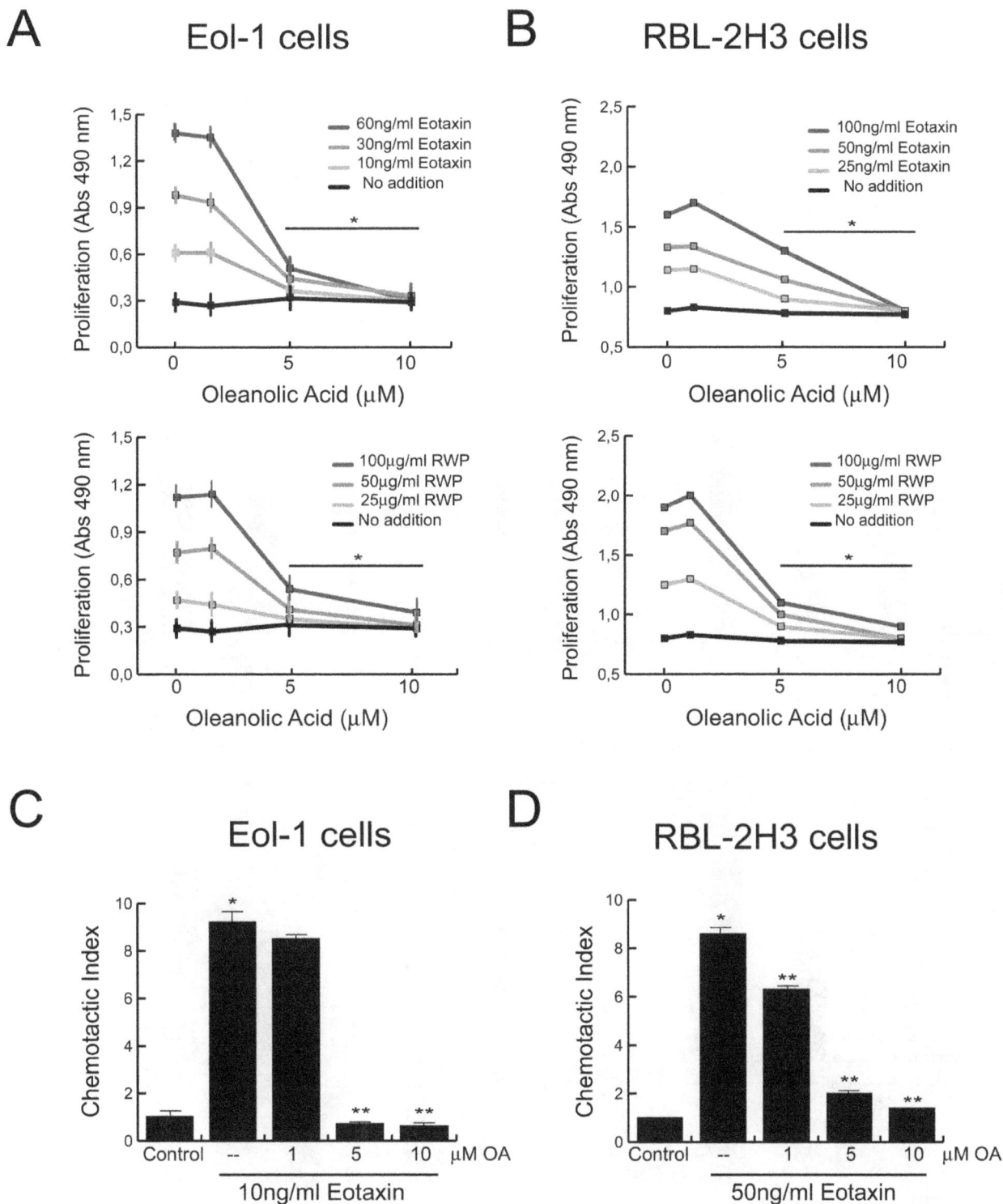

Figure 5. OA abrogated *in vitro* biological functions on EoL-1 and RBL-2H3 cells. EoL-1 (A,C) and RBL-2H3 (B,D) cells were incubated with the indicated stimuli in presence or absence of different concentrations of OA. (A,B) Cell proliferation was assayed 24 h after stimulation. (C,D) Cell migration was measured as described in Materials and Methods. Bars represent means ± SD. (*P<0.001 vs unstimulated cells; **P<0.001 vs stimuli without triterpene; n = 3).

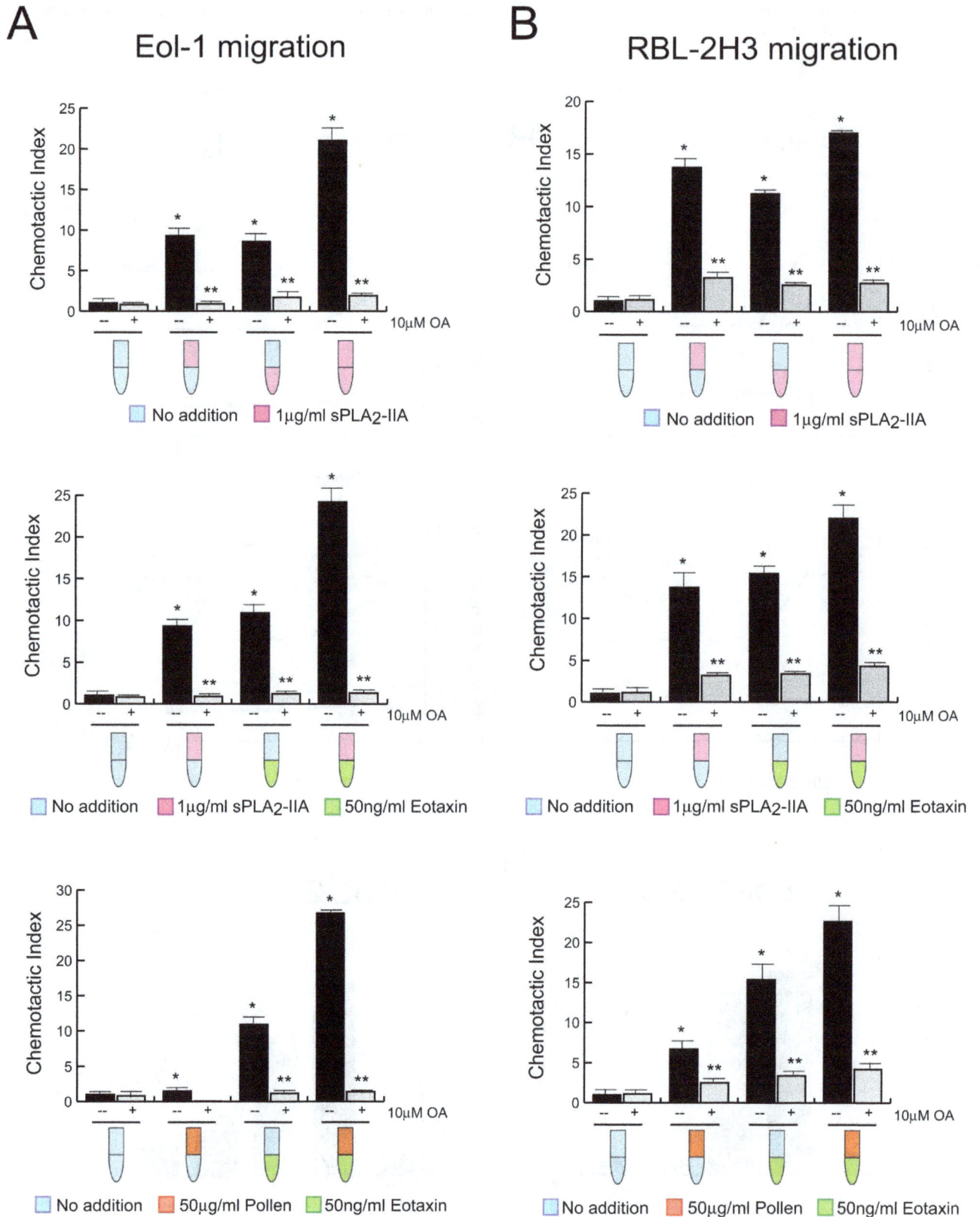

Figure 6. OA inhibits cell migration. EoL-1 (A) and RBL-2H3 (B) cells treated, or not, with 10 µM of OA for 30 min, were allowed to migrate as described in Materials and Methods. Cell migration was assayed using eotaxin, RWP and sPLA2-IIA as schematically indicated by the green, red and pink color, respectively. Bars represent means ± SD. (*P<0.001 vs untreated control condition, and **P<0.001 vs stimuli without triterpene; n = 3).

A

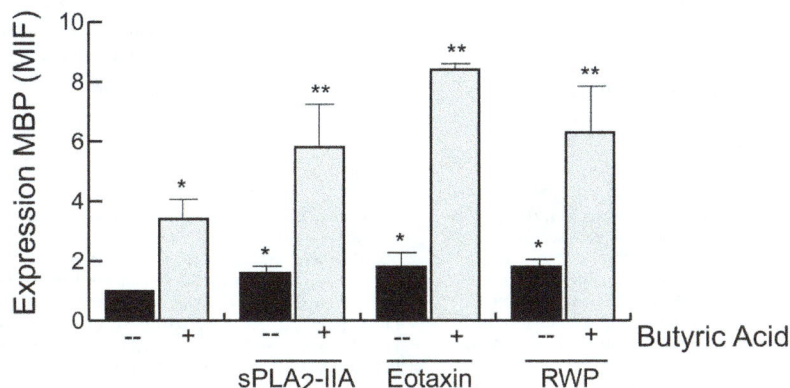

B

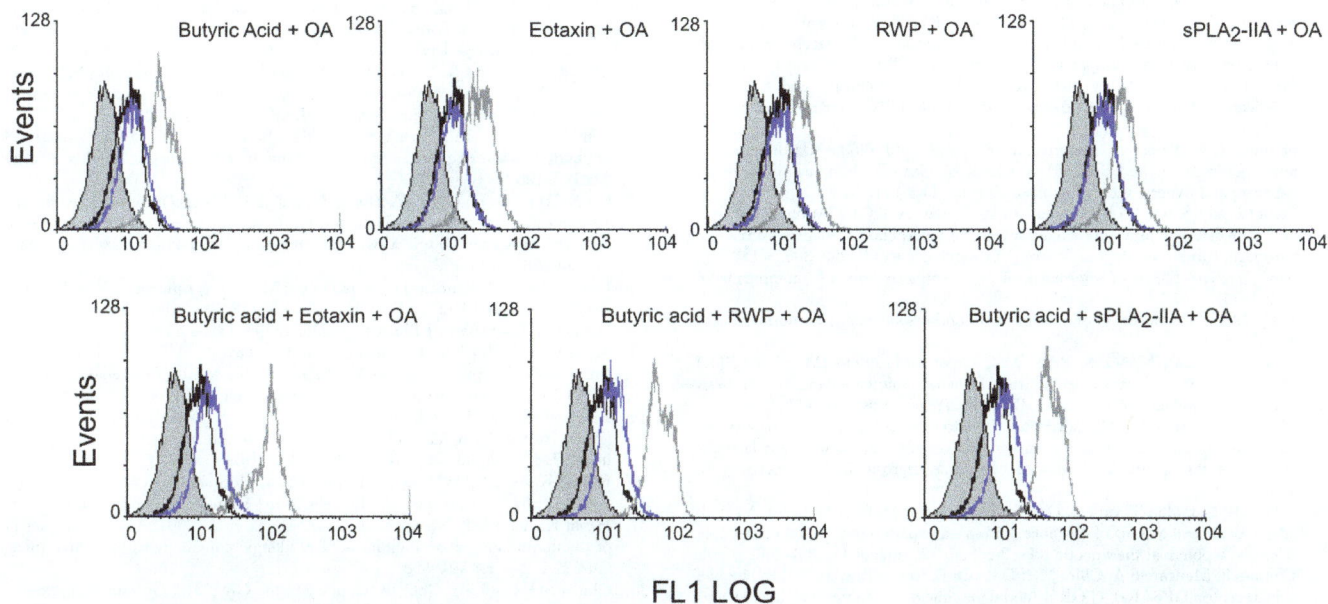

Figure 7. Effect OA on EoL-1 cell differentiation. EoL-1 cells were treated without and with 0.5 mM butyric acid, and 30 ng/ml of eotaxin, or 1 μg/ml sPLA$_2$-IIA or 50 μg/ml RWP for 7 days, in absence (A) or presence of 5 μM OA (B). MBP expression was analyzed by Flow cytometry. In A, data are expressed as the means of MFI ± SD. *P<0.001 vs control cells, and **P<0.01 vs butyric acid-treated cells; n=3. In B, histograms are representative of three independent experiments: untreated (open black curves), stimulated (open dark grey curves) and OA+stimulated (open blue curves). EoL-1 cells are compared with isotype controls (solid grey curves).

cytotoxic and inflammatory effects by the release of their granule proteins and the production of crucial inflammatory mediators. We showed that sPLA$_2$-IIA behaves as a chemoattractant for EoL-1 eosinophils and RBL-2H3 mast cells as potent as eotaxin, and amplifies eotaxin-induced chemotaxis similarly to what is observed with direct interaction of cells with RWP. These results are inline with previous studies demonstrating cooperative chemotactic responses between eotaxin and the cytokine IL-5 [44]. Thus, suggesting that diverse inflammatory mediators, including sPLA$_2$-IIA, may act cooperatively to potentiate local chemotactic responses. In addition, the phospholipase has been shown to effectively trigger mast cell degranulation, and here we found that it enhanced EoL-1 cells to undergo morphological differentiation

into mature eosinophil-like cells [45]. Interestingly, all the studied responses were abolished in cells pretreated with OA. Therefore, our data point to a critical role for sPLA$_2$-IIA in the activity and migratory capability into tissues of eosinophils and mast cells, and a regulatory role for the triterpene OA in the prevention of cell recruitment and activation. However, signaling pathways involved in these events remain obscure and deserve a further and deeper investigation.

In conclusion, OA seems to be a promising candidate for the treatment of allergic eye disorders in addition to the conventional therapies. It provided an effective treatment against the allergic and immune-inflammatory responses in the EAC model. Thus, the therapeutic potential for the treatment of allergic inflammatory diseases such as allergic rhinitis and asthma should be also considered. Further studies should also be directed to explore its activity when administered topically.

Acknowledgments

We gratefully acknowledge Roberto Cantalapiedra Rodríguez by his technical assistance.

References

1. Leonardo A, Bogacka E, Fauquert JL, Kowalski ML, Groblewska A, et al. (2012) Ocular allergy: recognizing and diagnosing hypersensitivity disorders of the ocular surface. Allergy 67: 1327–1337.
2. Sánchez MC, Fernández Parra B, Matheu V, Navarro A, Ibáñez MD, et al. (2011) Allergic Conjunctivitis. J Investig Allergol Clin Immunol. 21: 1–19.
3. Cota BB, Bertollo CM, de Oliveira DM (2013) Anti-allergic potential of herbs and herbal natural products - activities and patents. Recent Pat Endocr Metab Immune Drug Discov 7: 26–56.
4. Mainardi T, Kapoor S, Bielory L (2009) Complementary and alternative medicine: herbs, phytochemicals and vitamins and their immunologic effects. J Allergy Clin Immunol 123: 283–294.
5. Bielory L, Heimall J (2003) Review of complementary and alternative medicine in treatment of ocular allergies. Curr Opin Allergy Clin Immunol 3: 395–399.
6. Lee DK, Carstair IJ, Haggart K, Jackson CM, Currie GP, et al. (2003) Butterbur, a herbal remedy, attenuates adenosine monophosphate induced nasal responsiveness in seasonal allergic rhinitis. Clin Exp Allergy 3: 882–886.
7. Schempp CM, Windeck T, Hezel S, Simon JC (2003) Topical treatment of atopic dermatitis with St. John's wort cream–a randomized, placebo controlled, double blind half-side comparison. Phytomedicine 1031–37.
8. Price KR, Johnson IT, Fenwick RR (1987) The chemistry and biological significance of saponins in foods and feeding stuffs. CRC Cr Rev Food Sci 26: 27–135.
9. Somova LO, Nadar A, Rammanan P, Shode FO (2003) Cardiovascular, antihyperlipidemic and antioxidant effects of oleanolic and ursolic acids in experimental hypertension. Phytomedicine 10: 115–121.
10. Somova LI, Shode FO, Ramnanan P, Nadar A (2003) Antihypertensive, antiatherosclerotic and antioxidant activity of triterpenoids isolated from Olea europaea, subspecies africana leaves. J Ethnopharmacol 84299–305.
11. Ríos JL (2010) Effects of triterpenes on the immune system. J Ethnopharmacol 128: 1–14.
12. Liu J (1995) Pharmacology of oleanolic acid and ursolic acid. J Ethnopharmacol 49: 57–68.
13. Giner-Larza EM, Máñez S, Recio MC, Giner RM, Prieto JM, et al. (2001) Oleanonic acid, a 3-oxotriterpene from Pistacia, inhibits leukotriene synthesis and has anti-inflammatory activity. Eur J Pharmacol 428: 137–143.
14. Martín R, Hernández M, Córdova C, Nieto ML (2012) Natural triterpenes modulate immune-inflammatory markers of experimental autoimmune encephalomyelitis: therapeutic implications for multiple sclerosis. Br J Pharmacol 166: 1708–1723.
15. Martín R, Carvalho-Tavares J, Hernández M, Arnés M, Ruiz-Gutiérrez V, et al. (2010) Beneficial actions of oleanolic acid in an experimental model of multiple sclerosis: a potential therapeutic role. Biochem Pharmacol 15: 198–208.
16. Cipriani S, Mencarelli A, Chini MG, Distrutti E, Renga B, et al. (2011) The bile acid receptor GPBAR-1 (TGR5) modulates integrity of intestinal barrier and immune response to experimental colitis. PLoS One 6: e25637.
17. Magone MT, Chan CC, Rizzo LV, Kozhich AT, Whitcup SM (1998) A novel murine model of allergic conjunctivitis. Clin Immunol Immunopathol 87: 75–84.
18. Fukushima A, Yamaguchi T, Ishida W, Fukata K, Ueno H (2006) TLR2 agonist ameliorates murine experimental allergic conjunctivitis by inducing CD4 positive T-cell apoptosis rather than by affecting the Th1/Th2 balance. Biochem Biophys Res Commun 339: 1048–1055.
19. Barsumian EL, Isersky C, Petrino MG, Siraganian RP (1981) IgE-induced histamine release from rat basophilic leukemia cell lines: isolation of releasing and nonreleasing clones. Eur J Immunol 11: 317–323.
20. Mayumi M (1992) EoL-1, a human eosinophilic cell line. Leuk Lymphoma 7: 243–250.
21. Saito H, Bourinbaiar A, Ginsburg M, Minato K, Ceresi E, et al. (1985). Establishment and characterization of a new human eosinophilic leukemia cell line. Blood. 66: 1233–1240.
22. Wei Y, Epstein SP, Fukuoka S, Birmingham NP, Li XM, et al. (2011) sPLA2-IIa amplifies ocular surface inflammation in the experimental dry eye (DE) BALB/c mouse model. Invest Ophthalmol Vis Sci 52: 4780–4788.
23. Tominaga T, Miyazaki D, Sasaki S, Mihara S, Komatsu N, et al. (2009) Blocking mast cell-mediated type I hypersensitivity in experimental allergic conjunctivitis by monocyte chemoattractant protein-1/CCR2. Invest Ophthalmol Vis Sci 50: 5181–5188.
24. Hingoran M, Calder V, Jolly G, Buckley RJ, Lightman SL (1998) Eosinophil surface antigen expression and cytokine production vary in different ocular allergic diseases. J Allergy Clin Immunol 102: 821–830.
25. Ingram JL, Kraft M (2012) IL-13 in asthma and allergic disease: asthma phenotypes and targeted therapies. J Allergy Clin Immunol 130: 829–842.
26. Miyahara S, Miyahara N, Matsubara S, Takeda K, Koya T, et al. (2006) IL-13 is essential to the late-phase response in allergic rhinitis. J Allergy Clin Immunol 118: 1110–1116.
27. Mannon P, Reinisch W (2012) Interleukin 13 and its role in gut defense and inflammation. Gut 61: 1765–1773.
28. Oh MH, Oh SY, Yu J, Myers AC, Leonard WJ, et al. (2011) IL-13 induces skin fibrosis in atopic dermatitis by thymic stromal lymphopoietin. J Immunol 186: 7232–7242.
29. Zheng T, Oh MH, Oh SY, Schroeder JT, Glick AB, et al. (2009) Transgenic expression of interleukin-13 in the skin induces a pruritic dermatitis and skin remodeling. J Invest Dermatol 129: 742–751.
30. Matsuba-Kitamura S, Yoshimoto T, Yasuda K, Futatsugi-Yumikura S, Taki Y, et al. (2010) Contribution of IL-33 to induction and augmentation of experimental allergic conjunctivitis. Int Immunol 22: 479–489.
31. Kim YH, Yang TY, Park CS, Ahn SH, Son BK, et al. (2012) Anti-IL-33 antibody has a therapeutic effect in a murine model of allergic rhinitis. Allergy 67: 183–190.
32. Gu N, Kang G, Jin C, Xu Y, Zhang Z, et al. (2010) Intelectin is required for IL-13-induced monocyte chemotactic protein-1 and -3 expression in lung epithelial cells and promotes allergic airway inflammation. Am J Physiol Lung Cell Mol Physiol 298: L290–296.
33. Lim EJ, Lu TX, Blanchard C, Rothenberg ME (2011) Epigenetic Regulation of the IL-13-induced Human Eotaxin-3 Gene by CREB-binding Protein-mediated Histone 3 Acetylation. J Biol Chem 286: 13193–13204.
34. Matsukura S, Stellato C, Georas SN, Casolaro V, Plitt JR, et al. (2001) Interleukin-13 Upregulates Eotaxin Expression in Airway Epithelial Cells by a STAT6-Dependent Mechanism. Am J Respir Cell Mol Biol 24: 755–761.
35. Pecaric-Petkovic T, Didichenko SA, Kaempfer S, Spiegl N, Dahinden CA (2009) Human basophils and eosinophils are the direct target leukocytes of the novel IL-1 family member IL-33. Blood 113: 1526–1534.
36. Komai-Koma M, Xu D, Li Y, McKenzie AN, McInnes IB, et al. (2007) IL-33 is a chemoattractant for human Th2 cells. Eur J Immunol 7: 2779–2786.
37. Hayat K, Asim MB, Nawaz M, Li M, Zhang L, et al. (2001) Ameliorative effect of thymoquinone on ovalbumin-induced allergic conjunctivitis in Balb/c mice. Curr Eye Res 36: 591–598.
38. Chung SH, Choi SH, Choi JA, Chuck RS, Joo CK (2012) Curcumin suppresses ovalbumin-induced allergic conjunctivitis. Mol Vis 18: 966–972.
39. Bundoc VG, Keane-Myers A (2007) IL-10 confers protection from mast cell degranulation in a mouse model of allergic conjunctivitis. Exp Eye Res 85: 575–579.
40. Royer B, Varadaradjalou S, Saas P, Guillosson JJ, Kantelip JP, et al. (2001) Inhibition of IgE-induced activation of human mast cells by IL-10. Clin Exp Allergy 31: 694–704.
41. Li K, Liu X, Chen Z, Huang Q, Wu K (2010) Quantification of tear proteins and sPLA2-IIa alteration in patients with allergic conjunctivitis. Mol Vision 16: 2084–2091.
42. Aho VV, Nevalainen TJ, Saari KM (2002) Group IIA phospholipase A2 content of tears in patients with keratoconjunctivitis sicca. Graefes. Arch Clin Exp Ophthalmol 240: 521–523.
43. Chen D, Wei Y, Li X, Epstein S, Wolosin JM, et al. (2009) sPLA2-IIa is an inflammatory mediator when the ocular surface is compromised. Exp Eye Res 88: 880–888.
44. Mould AW, Matthaei KI, Young IG, Foster PS (1997) Relationship between interleukin-5 and eotaxin in regulating blood and tissue eosinophilia in mice. J Clin Invest 99: 1064–1071.
45. Murakami M, Hara N, Kudo I., Inoue K (1993) Triggering of degranulation in mast cells by exogenous type II phospholipase A2. J Immunol 151: 5675–5684.

Author Contributions

Conceived and designed the experiments: MLN CM-G MH. Performed the experiments: CC BG RM PG-M. Analyzed the data: MLN CM-G MH CC BG RM PG-M. Contributed reagents/materials/analysis tools: MLN CM-G. Wrote the paper: MLN CM-G MH.

20

Evaluation of a Prednisolone Acetate-Loaded Subconjunctival Implant for the Treatment of Recurrent Uveitis in a Rabbit Model

Marcus Ang[1,2,9], **Xuwen Ng**[3,9], **Cheewai Wong**[1,2], **Peng Yan**[3], **Soon-Phaik Chee**[1,2], **Subbu S. Venkatraman**[3]*, **Tina T. Wong**[1,2,3]*

1 Singapore National Eye Centre, Singapore, Singapore, 2 Singapore Eye Research Institute, Singapore, Singapore, 3 Materials Science and Engineering, Nanyang Technological University, Singapore, Singapore

Abstract

Aim: To assess the efficacy of a biodegradable, prednisolone acetate implant in a rabbit uveitis model.

Methods: Randomized, controlled study of biodegradable microfilms preloaded with prednisolone acetate (PA) in a rabbit uveitis model. Experimental uveitis was induced by unilateral intravitreal injection of *Mycobacterium tuberculosis* H37Ra antigen (50 ug; 1 ug/uL) in preimmunized rabbits. PA-loaded poly[d,l-lactide-co-ε-caprolactone] (PLC) microfilms (n = 10) and blank microfilms (n = 6) were implanted subconjunctivally. An estimate of PA release *in vivo* was calculated from measured residual PA amounts in microfilms after the rabbits were sacrificed. The eyes were clinically monitored for ocular inflammation for 28 days. Histopathological examination of the enucleated eyes was performed at the end of the study period.

Results: In vitro studies revealed that sandwich PA-loaded microfilm formulations exhibited higher release kinetic compared to homogenous PA-loaded microfilms. The 60–40–60% microfilm released an average of 0.034 mg/day of PA over the period of 60 days *in vitro*; and we found that approximately 0.12 mg/day PA was released *in vivo*. Animals implanted with the PA-loaded microfilms exhibited significantly lowered median inflammatory scores when compared against the control group in this model for recurrent uveitis (P<0.001). The implants were clinically well tolerated by all the animals. Histology results showed no significant scarring or inflammation around the PA-loaded microfilms.

Conclusion: Our pilot study demonstrated that a subconjunctival PA-loaded implant is effective in suppressing inflammation in the rabbit model of uveitis, by providing therapeutic levels of PA that attenuated the inflammatory response even after a rechallenge. Longer term studies are now needed to establish the therapeutic potential of such a delivery system for treatment of ocular inflammation.

Editor: James T. Rosenbaum, Oregon Health & Science University, United States of America

Funding: The authors report funding from the National Medical Research Council/Early Development Grant/ 0064/2010 (Singapore). The funders had no role in study design, data collection and analysis, decision to publish, or preparation of the manuscript.

Competing Interests: Co-authors Tina Wong and Subbu Venkatraman are named patent holders for the material investigated in the manuscript, "A biodegradable ocular implant, PCT/SG2011/000282." There are no further patents, products in development or marketed products to declare.

* E-mail: ASSubbu@ntu.edu.sg (SSV); tina.wong.t.l@snec.com.sg (TTW)

9 These authors contributed equally to this work.

Introduction

Uveitis is an inflammatory disorder affecting the iris, ciliary body or choroid, which is a relatively common eye disorder, with an estimated incidence rate of 17 and 22.6 per 100,000 person years[1,2]. Inadequate diagnosis and treatment in severe or prolonged ocular inflammation may lead to sight threatening complications [1]. Currently, the mainstay of treatment is corticosteroids, which may be administered topically or as a periocular/intravitreal injection, with or without the concurrent use of oral steroids [2]. There are, however, problems associated with these routes of administration. Topical steroids have poor ocular penetration and rapid clearance from the eye necessitating

frequent application. Patients who require a higher intraocular concentration of steroid than topical steroids can provide may be given periocular injections - but the drug is rapidly cleared within 2 weeks of administration[3] and frequent injections are associated with risks of globe perforation and retrobulbar haemorrhage. In patients with posterior uveitis, topical steroids are often unable to control inflammation due to poor ocular penetration to the posterior segment. In these patients, intravitreal administration delivers the highest concentration of steroid and sustained release intravitreal implants can provide therapeutic drug levels for up to 6 months[4]. The disadvantages of this route of administration are the increased risk of raised intraocular pressure, endophthalmitis and retinal detachment. Moreover, should these corticosteroid-related complications such as raised intraocular pressure leading to glaucoma occur, removal of the steroid implant from the posterior segment would be difficult.

A subconjunctival implant may circumvent the risks involved with intravitreal administration; and due to its anatomical siting, may be removed relatively easily if necessary. Prednisolone acetate achieves the highest aqueous concentration within 2 hours and maintains higher levels for 24 hours, compared to dexamethasone and other commonly used corticosteroids[5]. We have demonstrated in previous studies the anti-fibrotic and anti-inflammatory properties of a subconjunctivally implanted prednisolone acetate (PA)-preloaded microfilm in the rabbit model of subconjunctival scarring following glaucoma filtration surgery [6] and rat keratoplasty model[7]. Our *in vivo* studies have shown that PA-loaded poly[d,l-lactide-co-ε-caprolactone] (PLC) microfilms display good biocompatibility, feasibility, and desirable sustained drug release profiles, maintaining high anterior chamber PA levels at 76.7±5.9, 70.3±2.3, and 42.7±4.1 ng/mL at 2, 4, and 12 weeks, respectively[8,9].

Thus, in this study, we sought to determine whether the biodegradable PA-loaded microfilm is able to deliver sustained therapeutic levels of corticosteroid to effectively reduce ocular inflammation and attenuate the intensity of recurrence uveitis following a rechallenge in the rabbit model of uveitis.

Methods

In Vitro Study

Polymeric films were prepared using a previously described solution casting method, using biomedical grade of copolymer poly(d-, l-lactide-co-ε-caprolactone) or PLC70/30 (l-lactide to ε-caprolactone molar ratio = 70/30, with intrinsic viscosity of 1.6 dl/g) (Purac Far East, Singapore) and prednisolone 21-acetate (≥97%) (Sigma-Aldrich, Singapore)[10]. High performance liquid chromatography (HPLC) grade dichloromethane (DCM) and acetone nitrile (ACN) were used as received. Phosphate buffer saline pellets were purchased from Sigma-Aldrich and prepared in accordance to the manufacturer's protocol. PLC70/30 with predetermined PA drug-loading percentage of 40, 50 and 60 wt % were dissolved in DCM to form a polymer-drug solution - **Table 1.** For the single layer film formulation, the films were prepared by solution casting a single drug-polymer solution on the glass plate using an automatic film applicator. For the tri-layer film formulations, drug layers were cast layer by layer with a 10 minutes interval between each cast. **Figure 1** depicts the respective drug loading and thickness of each film.

Subsequently, all the films were dried in room-temperature ambience for 1 day, followed by drying in the 37°C vacuum oven for 1 week. The residual solvent was measured using a thermogravimetric analyzer (TGA, TA instruments Q500) and verified to be less than 1% before use. After drying, all samples were cut to the desired dimensions (4.0×8.0×0.2 mm) with their

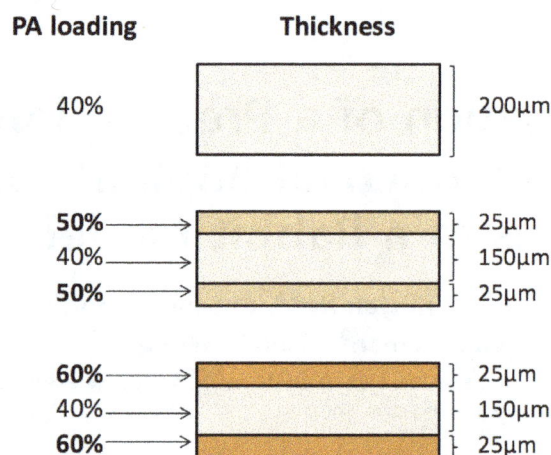

Figure 1. Figure depicting the single layer and tri-layer matrices with their respective drug loading and thickness.

edges rounded for *in vitro* and *in vivo* studies. All the samples were sterilized by room temperature-ethylene oxide (RT-ETO) prior *in vivo* implantation. For the *in vitro* drug release study, three PA-loaded microfilms of the single and tri-layered formulations were studied *in vitro* to determine the rate of drug release. All samples were immersed in PBS in the 37°C incubator throughout the study and the amount of PA released in PBS over time was quantified using the HPLC. The PA-loaded microfilm with the optimal PA release was selected for the *in vivo* study.

In Vivo Study

This is a double armed, parallel designed, randomized, placebo controlled study to assess the efficacy of a subconjunctivally implanted biodegradable PA-loaded microfilm in attenuating the inflammation in an animal model of experimental uveitis. **Figure 2** shows a summary of our study design.

Animals

Approval was obtained from the SingHealth Institute Animal Care and Use Committee (IACUC Singhealth Approval Number 2012/SHS/730) and all procedures were performed in accordance with the ARVO Statement for the Use of Animals in Ophthalmic and Vision Research. 16 Adult male New Zealand White rabbits, weighing 2-2.5 kg were used in this study. All rabbits were examined with a slit lamp and only rabbits with no ocular pathology were included in the study. In the placebo arm of the study, rabbits received subconjunctival implantation of a blank microfilm containing no PA. In the treatment arm, rabbits received subconjunctival implantation of the PA-loaded microfilm.

Table 1. Various microfilm formulations analyzed during *in vitro* study.

Formulation combination	Type	First Layer	Second Layer	Third Layer
40%	Single layer	PLC with 40 wt% PA; 200 μm	Nil	Nil
50–40–50%	Sandwich	PLC with 50 wt% PA; 25 μm	PLC with 40 wt% PA; 150 μm	PLC with 50 wt% PA; 25 μm
60–40–60%	Sandwich	PLC with 60 wt% PA; 25 μm	PLC with 40 wt% PA; 150 μm	PLC with 60 wt% PA; 25 μm
PLC= poly[d,l-lactide-co-ε-caprolactone]; PA= prednisolone acetate; wt%= weight percentage				

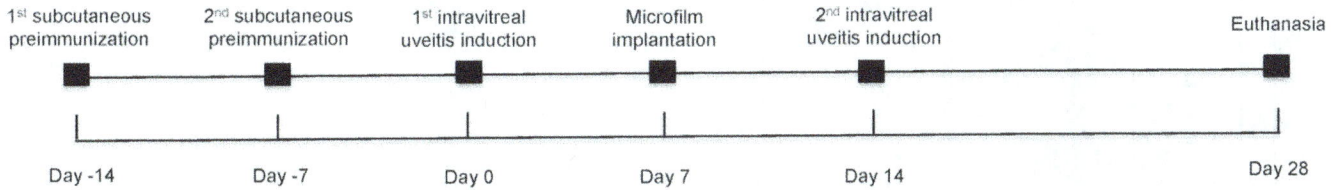

Figure 2. Flow chart to describe our study design. Days -14 to Day 0 is the preimmunization phase. The first intravitreal uveitis induction was performed on Day 0. The 2nd intravitreal uveitis induction on Day 14 simulates a recurrence of uveitis.

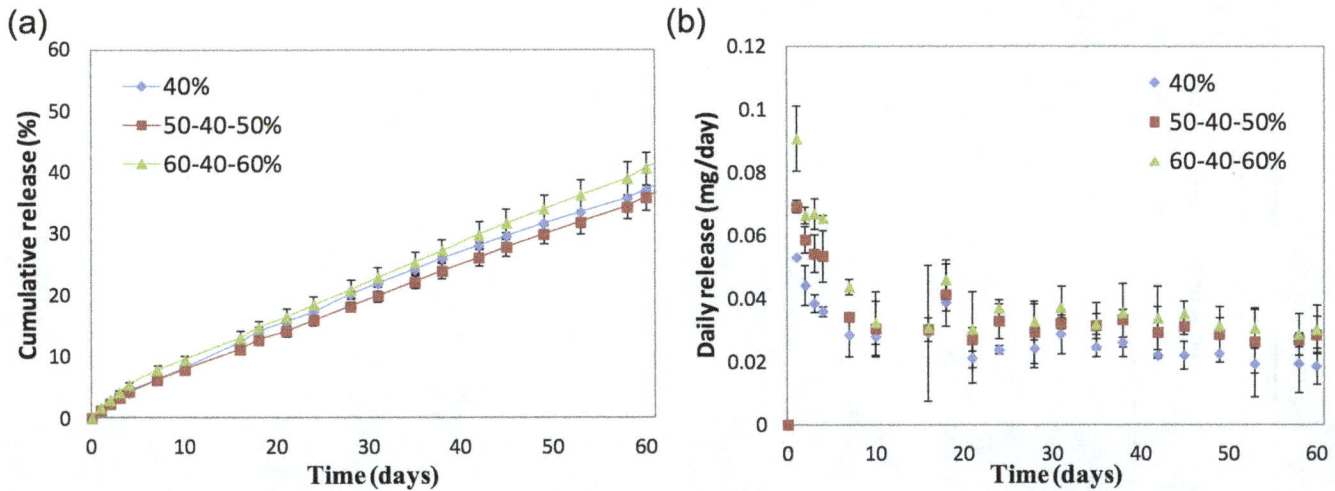

Figure 3. In vitro and In vivo release profiles depicting (a) cumulative release of prednisolone acetate (%) and (b) daily release of prednisolone acetate (mg/day) amount from three formulations of poly(d-, l-lactide-co-ε-caprolactone) films loaded with prednisolone acetate.

Six rabbits were randomized into the placebo arm and 10 into the treatment arm.

Induction of experimental uveitis

A subcutaneous injection of *Mycobacterium tuberculosis* H37Ra antigen (10 mg; Difco, Detroit, MI) suspended in mineral oil (500 uL) was given as preimmunization.[11] Successful preimmu-

nization was confirmed after one week by the presence of a visible skin nodule at the injection site. Uveitis was induced on Days 0 and 14 of the study – **Figure 2**. The rabbits were anesthetized with intraperitoneal injection of ketamine hydrochloride (5 mg/kg) and xylazine hydrochloride (2 mg/kg). Following topical anaesthesia (Minims Tetracaine Hydrochloride 0.5%; Bausch and Lomb, UK) the right eye of each rabbit was disinfected with 5% povidone iodine. An intravitreal injection of *Mycobacterium*

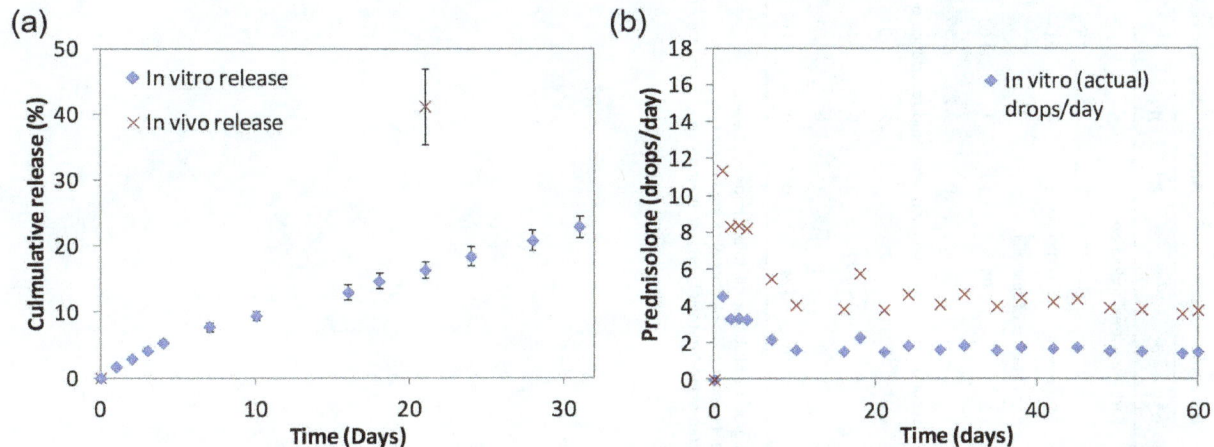

Figure 4. In vitro and in vivo of (a) cumulative release of prednisolone acetate and (b) daily estimated number of prednisolone acetate 1% eye drops per day, from the 60–40–60% prednisolone acetate loaded poly(d-, l-lactide-co-ε-caprolactone) films.

Table 2. Median and combined inflammatory scores of control and prednisolone implant groups over study period.

Day	Iris congestion			Anterior chamber cells			Anterior chamber flare			Vitreous haze			Intraocular pressure			Combined inflammatory score			Remarks
	A*	B†	P‡	A*	B†	P‡	A*	B†	P‡	A*	B†	P‡	A*	B†	P‡	A*	B†	P‡	
0	First intravitreal induction																		
1	3	1	<0.001	3	2.5	1.00	2	1	<0.001	1	0.5	0.48	8	15.5	<0.001	5	3.5	0.16	
4	2.5	1	<0.001	3	4	0.04	1	2	0.04	3	2	0.24	9	10.5	1.00	3.5	2.25	1.00	
7	Implantation of microfilms																		
8	1.5	1	0.96	1	3	1.00	1	1	1.00	2	1	0.72	9	14	0.72	2	3.5	1.00	
13	1	1	1.00	1	0.3	0.96	0	0	1.00	1	0	0.06	8	11.5	0.16	0	0.25	0.96	Actual baseline
14	Second intravitreal induction Simulated recurrence of uveitis																		
15	2.5	1	<0.001	3.5	2	0.08	2.5	1	0.06	3.5	2	0.02	7.5	11.5	0.08	6	3	0.04	
19	3	1	<0.001	2.5	0	0.08	2	0	0.008	4	0	<0.001	8	10.5	1.00	4.5	1	<0.001	
22	2	0	0.02	1	0	0.04	1	0.5	0.96	2.5	0	<0.001	7	16.5	<0.001	2	0.50	0.04	
28	1	0	0.24	0	0	1.00	0	0	1.00	0	0	1.00	7.5	13.5	0.60	0	0	1.00	

*A: Control group with blank microfilm implanted eyes.
†B: Treatment group with PA-microfilm implanted eyes.
‡p values from Mann Whitney U test, comparing control and treatment group at each time point, adjusted with Bonferroni correction.

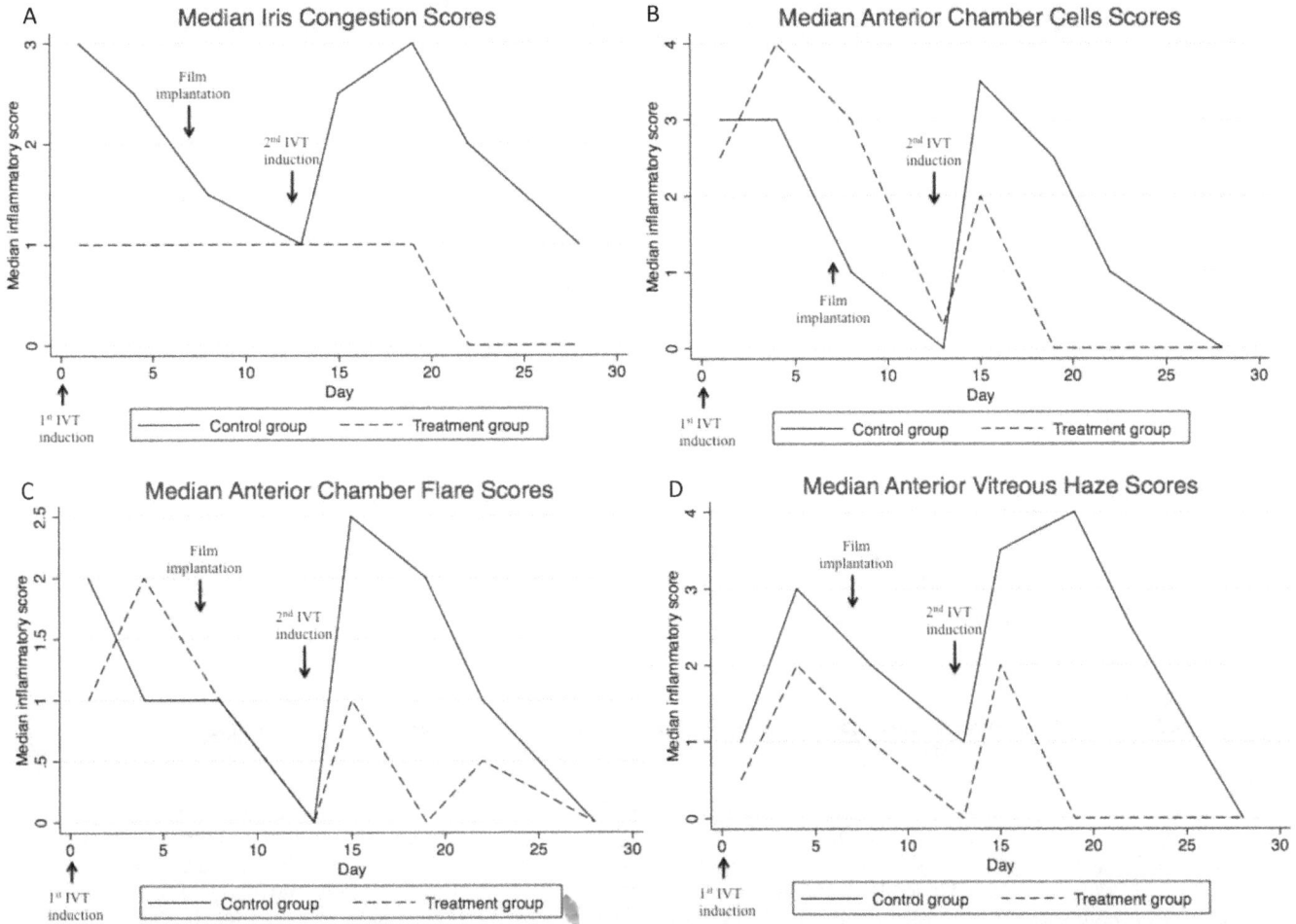

Figure 5. Median inflammatory scores for iris congestion (a), anterior chamber cells (b), anterior chamber flare (c), and vitreous haze (d) - comparing control group and treatment group.

tuberculosis H37Ra antigen suspended in sterile saline (50 ug; 1 ug/uL) using a Hamilton syringe with a 31-gauge needle was given through the superotemporal sclera, 1.5 mm from the limbus. One drop of tobramycin 0.3% ophthalmic solution (Alcon Lab. USA) was instilled at the end of the procedure.

Implantation of microfilms

Implantation of microfilms was performed on Day 7 i.e. 7 days after the first uveitis intravitreal induction, by 2 masked independent investigators (MA, CW). Each rabbit was anesthetized with intraperitoneal injection of ketamine hydrochloride (5 mg/kg) and xylazine hydrochloride (2 mg/kg). After the animal had been adequately anaesthetized, the eye was cleaned with povidone–iodine (10%) and draped with sterile cloth. A subconjunctival pocket was created via blunt dissection just at the limbus with a 5–6 mm incision in the superior-temporal aspect of the eye. Microfilms were sterilized in ethyl alcohol and chlorhexidine before soaking in sterile normal saline. The microfilm was then inserted into the subconjunctival pocket 1 mm from the limbus using a conjunctival forceps. Closure with 10-0 nylon sutures was performed to secure implantation of each microfilm to the sclera. Topical tobramycin 0.3% ophthalmic solution (Alcon Lab. USA) was administered in each eye 4 times a day for 5 days.

Clinical Examination

Daily visual inspection of the operated eyes following surgery was conducted to document any changes at the implant site, gross appearance of the microfilm implants and for evidence of local erosion of the implant or infection by 1 masked independent investigator (CW). Slit-lamp biomicroscopy, photography of the anterior segment and dilated fundal examination with binocular indirect ophthalmoscopy using a 20 D lens was performed prior to uveitis induction and at 8 defined time points thereafter (Days 1, 4, 8, 13, 15, 19, 22 and 28). Clinical severity of uveitis was scored using anterior chamber cells/flares, vitreous haze, and iris vessels as described in previous literature[12,13].

Enucleation, euthanasia & pathology procedures

All rabbits were euthanized at the end of the study period of 28 days. Euthanasia was carried out with intraperitoneal pentobarbitone (60–150 mg/kg) followed by enucleation and immersing the eyes in a mixture of 4% paraformaldehyde and 2.5% neutral buffered formalin for 24 hours. The globes were dehydrated, embedded in paraffin and sent for microtome sectioning and staining (Sirius red F3BA; Sigma, St. Louis, MO). We used polarization microscopy of stained collagen fibers to reveal gross collagen bundling patterns to assess fibrosis and scarring. Next, sectioned slides were heated, deparaffinized, and rehydrated before antigen retrieval, by incubating in citrate buffer at 95–100°C.

Combined inflammatory score

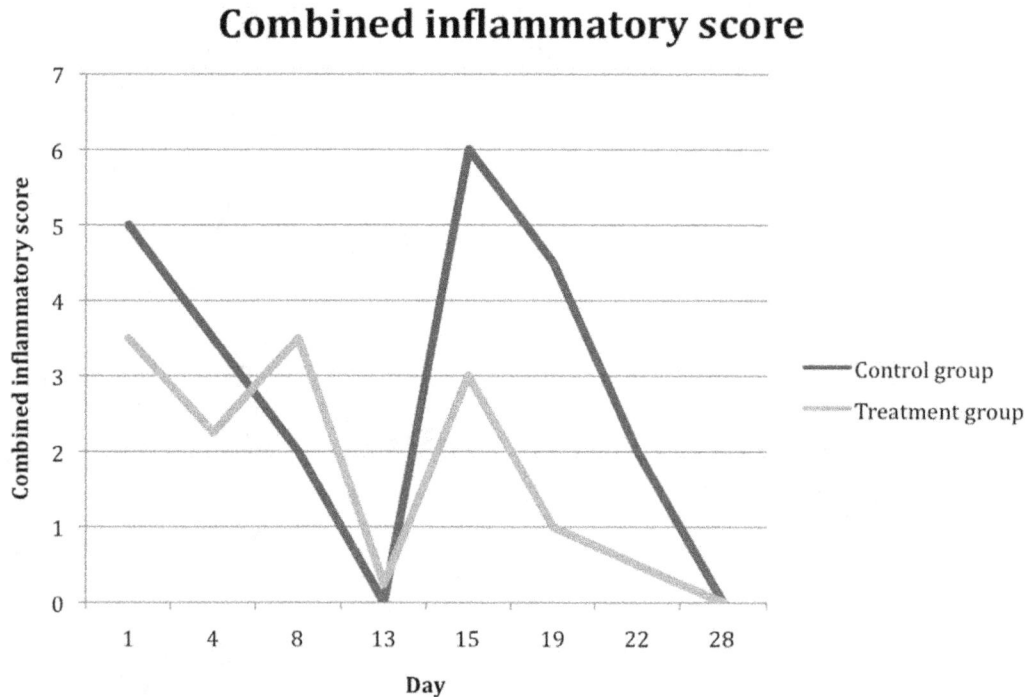

Figure 6. Median combined inflammatory score, as compared between control group and treatment group.

Sections were then washed and incubated with a mouse CD45 monoclonal IgG (Santa Cruz Biotechnology Inc., Europe) for detection of CD45 on all leukocytes of rabbit origin, then detection of the primary antibodies with Alexa Fluor 488 Goat antimouse IgG (H+C) secondary antibodies 1:100 dilution (Invitrogen Molecular Probes, USA).

For the *in vivo* drug release study, microfilms were retrieved on Day 28 (n = 11). The retrieved samples were rinsed with deionized water and dried in the 37°C vacuum oven for a week. Subsequently, the dried samples were dissolved in ACN and the released amounts were quantified using the HPLC. The amounts of PA released were determined by calculating the difference in the initial drug loaded and the residual drug detected. The cumulative percentage of drug released was also derived accordingly.

Statistical Analysis

The main outcome measures were the clinical scores for 1) iris vessels, 2) anterior chamber cells, 3) anterior chamber flare, 4) vitreous haze and the combined inflammatory score, defined as the sum of the scores for anterior chamber cells and flare. Statistical Package for the Social Sciences version 17.0 (SPSS Inc., Chicago, IL) was used to analyze the data. Ordinal variables were described with medians and analyzed using Mann Whitney U test for independent samples. All p-values are 2 sided with appropriate significance of $p < 0.05$.

Results

Prednisolone acetate release from microfilm

Figure 3a depicts the cumulative release profile of PA from all three formulations of microfilms over 60 days *in vitro*. All three formulations, regardless of single layer or tri-layer formulations showed an initial burst release followed by steady sustained release of PA. On Day 60, the 40%, 50–40–50% and 60–40–60% loaded microfilms released approximately 37%, 36% and 40% of the

initial drug loading, respectively. **Figure 3b** demonstrates the daily release rates of PA from all three formulations of microfilms over 60 days *in vitro*. For the first 4 days, the 60–40–60% formulation displayed highest average release amounts of 0.072 mg/ day, while the 40% and 50–40–50% formulations achieved 0.043 mg/ day and 0.059 mg/ day respectively. The 60–40–60% formulation continued to show relatively higher release amounts throughout the 60 days. For the drug release that followed until day 60, the 40%, 50–40–50% and 60–40–60% displayed average release amounts of 0.025 mg/ day, 0.031 mg/ day and 0.034 mg/ day respectively. From these observations, it appears that although the cumulative release does not differentiate between the 3 formulations, the drug loading percentage affects the daily release.

Figure 4a plots the *in vitro* and an estimate of *in vivo* cumulative release of the 60–40–60% PA-loaded PLC microfilm formulation. The *in vivo* release was obtained by measuring the residual PA in the microfilms retrieved from the eyes after the animals were sacrificed. At 3 weeks, approximately 16% of PA was released in the *in vitro* study compared to 41% of PA released *in vivo*. **Figure 4b** demonstrates the estimated equivalent number of PA eye drops per day over time. When we correlate the *in vitro* and *in vivo* release, the *in vivo* release rate was calculated to be approximately 2.5 times faster than the *in vitro* release. In clinical practice, prednisolone acetate 1% ophthalmic suspension is used topically. From the estimated rate of release *in vivo*, a corresponding dose to approximately 11.3 drops/day was observed in the first day and 8.3 drops/ day was observed between Days 2 to 4. Subsequently, an estimation of a dose of approximately 4.3 drops per/ day was observed to Day 60.

Inflammatory scores

Table 2 shows the overall inflammatory scores and median scores for iris vessels, anterior chamber cells, anterior chamber flare and vitreous haze during the study period. Just before the

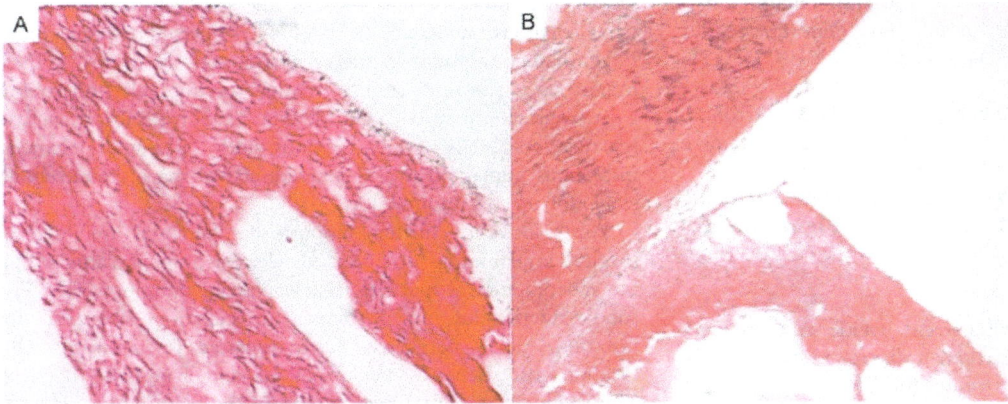

Figure 7. Histology images of the iris and ciliary body stained with Picosirius red. (A) Eye implanted with blank microfilm. (B) Eye implanted with prednisolone acetate loaded microfilm.

second intravitreal induction that simulates a recurrence of uveitis (Day 13), there was no significant baseline difference in the overall inflammatory score (control group: 0 versus treatment group: 0.25, P = 0.96). Following the induction of recurrent uveitis, an increase in scores for all parameters was observed. However, this increase was significantly reduced in the PA-loaded microfilm implanted eyes for all parameters on Day 15 (1 day after the second intravitreal induction, P = 0.04) and Day 19 (5 days after the second intravitreal induction, P<0.001). The difference in iris vessel score remained significantly less in the treatment arm on Day 22. Anterior chamber cells and vitreous haze scores were similarly less in the PA-loaded microfilm implanted eyes on Day

22 but not significantly different by Day 28. Anterior chamber flare was not significantly different between the 2 groups by Day 22. **Figures 5a–d** show the median scores for each parameter in the placebo and treatment arms respectively. The median combined inflammatory scores (**Figure 6**) were significantly lower in the treatment arm on Days 15, 19 and 22 (1, 5 and 8 days after the second intravitreal induction, P = 0.04).

Histopathology

Eyes implanted with the blank microfilm demonstrated a greater intensity in Sirius red staining in the iris and ciliary body than eyes implanted with PA-loaded microfilms (**Figure 7a–b**),

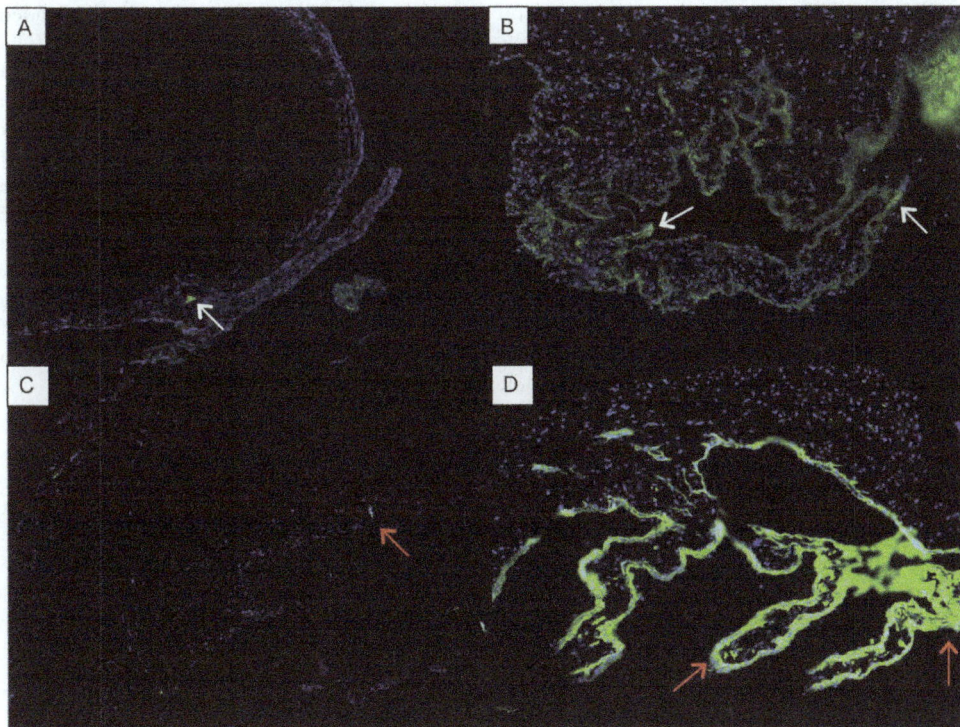

Figure 8. Histology images of the iris and ciliary body with immunohistochemistry stain. (A and C) Eye implanted with prednisolone acetate loaded microfilm. (B and D) Eye implanted with blank microfilm. White arrows: Positive stain for CD45+ leukocytes. Red arrows: Positive stain for CD4+ T cells.

indicating the presence of a more significant inflammatory response in the control group. Immunohistochemistry results revealed minimal infiltration of CD45+ leukocytes and CD 4+ T cells in the iris and ciliary body of eyes implanted with PA-loaded microfilms compared to eyes implanted with blank microfilm (mean number of cells from 10 immunohistochemistry stained slides:

Control group = 14.36±7.57 versus PA-loaded microfilm implant treatment group: 5.66±3.59; P = 0.004 - **Figure 8a–d**).

Discussion

Visual impairment caused by recurrent uveitis or prolonged ocular inflammation may be prevented if diagnosed and treated adequately[14]. However, current routes for administering corticosteroids to the eyes to treat chronic uveitis have several disadvantages [15]. For example, the current mainstay of topical administration faces the problems of patient complicance and poor intravitreal penetration. Although both periocular or intravitreal injections can provide higher doses of corticosteroids locally, frequent injections may increase the risk of sight threatening complications such as endophthalmitis. Thus, a new treatment option to deliver local therapeutic levels of corticosteroids over a sustained treatment period would be a welcome addition to the clinician's armamentarium against ocular inflammation. Thus, we sought to develop a sustained release PA-loaded microfilm that could be safely implanted in the subconjunctival space, demonstrating its efficacy in a recurrent uveitis animal model in this pilot study.[11] From our in vivo studies, an estimated sustained release of 0.12 mg/day PA was achieved over a period of 60 days. This is comparable to the dosing provided by a single drop of Predforte (prednisolone acetate ophthalmic suspension, USP) 1% every 2–3 hours used for treating acute uveitis. Although both the treatment and control groups demonstrated 2 episodes of ocular inflammation which mimics the normal cycle seen with 'recurrent uveitis', the treatment group demonstrated a significant attenuation in the magnitude of inflammatory response compared to the control group (P = 0.005).

Currently, topical application of corticosteroids remains the most common route for treating ocular inflammation and uveitis[16]. Thus, our initial in vitro and in vivo studies sought to demonstrate that the subconjunctival implant provided levels of PA-release similar to therapeutic levels from topical application. First, our in vitro studies found that all formulations demonstrated a favourable an initial burst followed by steady subsequent release of PA. However, we found that the 60–40–60% sandwich formulation was the most optimal, releasing 0.065–0.090 mg of PA in the initial release followed by 0.034 mg/day of PA over the period of 60 days. This formulation provides approximately 8 drops per day for the first 4 days followed by approximately 4 drops per day up to 60 days. Similar to our clinical practice, patients with moderate to severe uveitis are prescribed topical corticosteroids such as Predforte (prednisolone acetate ophthalmic suspension, USP) 1% every 1–2 hours for the initial 2–4 days during the awaking hours of the patient; and the dose is subsequently tapered to 4 times a day if ocular inflammation deceases. Thus, this 60–40–60%

sandwich formulation was used for the subsequent in vivo study, which demonstrated that the PA-loaded microfilms reduced the inflammatory response in the second episode of uveitis. Futhermore, our in vivo study confirmed that the implanted microfilms were well tolerated without inciting excessive subconjunctival scarring, consistent with a previous study of similar polymeric microfilms implanted in the subconjunctival space could remain stable for up to 6 months [9].

This pilot study further supports the potential usefulness of surgical implantation of sustained-released drug implants within the subconjunctival space to treat ocular inflammation.[6,7] The subconjunctival location provides a surgically accessible place for insertion and if necessary, easily accessed for removal. This location also bypasses ocular blood and lymphatic barriers. Moreover, the eventual degradation of the poly (d,l-lactide-co-ε-caprolactone) microfilm to harmless by-products allows for repeated implantations without any further surgery (if removal is not needed). In addition to the formulation that was used in the animal study, we also discovered other formulations that may be useful for eyes with less severe ocular inflammation. In particular, the non-sandwich formulation consisting of 40% PA throughout the entire thickness of the microfilm resulted in a release of approximately 5 drops for the first 4 days followed by 3 drops consistently up to 60 days. This profile might be suitable for use in treatment of mild anterior uveitis, which may be recurrent or chronic. However, the efficacy of different drug release profiles needs to be evaluated in further studies comparing mild and severe anterior uveitis models. We recognize the information derived from this pilot study with small numbers and a short duration of study, due to the limited duration of ocular inflammation in the animal model. However, this animal model is the most appropriate for demonstrating chronic and recurrent ocular inflammation available to us currently. Nonetheless, we believe this preliminary experiment provides the needed evidence to study this PA-loaded implant further for the treatment of ocular inflammation. The potential clinical use may not only be isolated to treating recurrent uveitis,[17] but also be useful for macular edema associated with uveitis,[18] and post-operative ocular inflammation such as after glaucoma filtration surgery, corneal graft and cataract surgery.[19]

In conclusion, in this pilot study we have demonstrated that the use of a sustained releasing PA-loaded microfilm implanted in the subconjunctival is effective in suppressing induced inflammation in uveitis model in rabbits. The implantation of such a system may be able to provide an alternative treatment option to current eyedrops that can deliver a consistent and clinically therapeutic amount of PA to the eye without depending on patient compliance to correctly administer their topical medication.

Author Contributions

Conceived and designed the experiments: MA XN CW PY SPC TW SV. Performed the experiments: MA XN CW TW SV. Analyzed the data: MA XN CW PY SPC TW SV. Contributed reagents/materials/analysis tools: MA XN CW PY SPC TW SV. Wrote the paper: MA XN CW PY SPC TW SV.

References

1. Paivonsalo-Hietanen T, Tuominen J, Vaahtoranta-Lehtonen H, Saari KM (1997) Incidence and prevalence of different uveitis entities in Finland. Acta Ophthalmol Scand 75: 76–81.
2. Dandona L, Dandona R, John RK, McCarty CA, Rao GN (2000) Population based assessment of uveitis in an urban population in southern India. Br J Ophthalmol 84: 706–709.
3. Hyndiuk RA (1969) Radioactive depot-corticosteroid penetration into monkey ocular tissue. II. Subconjunctival administration. Arch Ophthalmol 82: 259–263.
4. Chang-Lin JE, Attar M, Acheampong AA, Robinson MR, Whitcup SM, et al. (2011) Pharmacokinetics and pharmacodynamics of a sustained-release dexamethasone intravitreal implant. Invest Ophthalmol Vis Sci 52: 80–86.

5. Awan MA, Agarwal PK, Watson DG, McGhee CN, Dutton GN (2009) Penetration of topical and subconjunctival corticosteroids into human aqueous humour and its therapeutic significance. Br J Ophthalmol 93: 708–713.

6. Ang M, Yan P, Zhen M, Foo S, Venkatraman SS, et al. (2011) Evaluation of sustained release of PLC-loaded prednisolone acetate microfilm on postoperative inflammation in an experimental model of glaucoma filtration surgery. Curr Eye Res 36: 1123–1128.

7. Liu YC, Peng Y, Lwin NC, Venkatraman SS, Wong TT, et al. (2013) A biodegradable, sustained-released, prednisolone acetate microfilm drug delivery system effectively prolongs corneal allograft survival in the rat keratoplasty model. PLoS One 8: e70419.

8. Liu YC, Peng Y, Lwin NC, Wong TT, Venkatraman SS, et al. (2013) Optimization of subconjunctival biodegradable microfilms for sustained drug delivery to the anterior segment in a small animal model. Invest Ophthalmol Vis Sci 54: 2607–2615.

9. Peng Y, Ang M, Foo S, Lee WS, Ma Z, et al. (2011) Biocompatibility and biodegradation studies of subconjunctival implants in rabbit eyes. PLoS One 6: e22507.

10. Lao LL, Venkatraman SS, Peppas NA (2008) Modeling of drug release from biodegradable polymer blends. Eur J Pharm Biopharm 70: 796–803.

11. Ghosn CR, Li Y, Orilla WC, Lin T, Wheeler L, et al. (2011) Treatment of experimental anterior and intermediate uveitis by a dexamethasone intravitreal implant. Invest Ophthalmol Vis Sci 52: 2917–2923.

12. Nussenblatt RB, Palestine AG, Chan CC, Roberge F (1985) Standardization of vitreal inflammatory activity in intermediate and posterior uveitis. Ophthalmology 92: 467–471.

13. Bloch-Michel E, Nussenblatt RB (1987) International Uveitis Study Group recommendations for the evaluation of intraocular inflammatory disease. Am J Ophthalmol 103: 234–235.

14. Cheng CK, Berger AS, Pearson PA, Ashton P, Jaffe GJ (1995) Intravitreal sustained-release dexamethasone device in the treatment of experimental uveitis. Invest Ophthalmol Vis Sci 36: 442–453.

15. Haghjou N, Soheilian M, Abdekhodaie MJ (2011) Sustained release intraocular drug delivery devices for treatment of uveitis. Invest Ophthalmol Vis Sci 6: 317–329.

16. Gutteridge IF, Hall AJ (2007) Acute anterior uveitis in primary care. Clinical and Experimental Optometry 90: 70–82.

17. Siddique SS, Shah R, Suelves AM, Foster CS (2011) Road to remission: a comprehensive review of therapy in uveitis. Expert Opin Investig Drugs 20: 1497–1515.

18. Lowder C, Belfort R, Jr., Lightman S, Foster CS, Robinson MR, et al. (2011) Dexamethasone intravitreal implant for noninfectious intermediate or posterior uveitis. Arch Ophthalmol 129: 545–553.

19. Eperon S, Rodriguez-Aller M, Balaskas K, Gurny R, Guex-Crosier Y (2013) A new drug delivery system inhibits uveitis in an animal model after cataract surgery. Int J Pharm 443: 254–261.

21

Sustainable Control of Onchocerciasis: Ocular Pathology in Onchocerciasis Patients Treated Annually with Ivermectin for 23 Years

Méba Banla[1,2], Solim Tchalim[1,2], Potochoziou K. Karabou[3], Richard G. Gantin[1,4], Aide I. Agba[2], Abiba Kére-Banla[1], Gertrud Helling-Giese[1,4], Christoph Heuschkel[1,4], Hartwig Schulz-Key[1,4], Peter T. Soboslay[1,4]*

1 Onchocerciasis Reference Laboratory, Institut National d'Hygiène, Sokodé, Togo, 2 Centre Hospitalier Universitaire Campus, Université de Lomé, Lomé, Togo, 3 National Onchocerciasis Control Programme, Kara, Togo, 4 Institute for Tropical Medicine, University Clinics of Tübingen, Tübingen, Germany

Abstract

The evolution and persistence of ocular pathology was assessed in a cohort of *Onchocerca volvulus* infected patients treated annually with ivermectin for 23 years. Patients were resident in rural Central and Kara Region of Togo and ocular examinations included testing of visual acuity, slit lamp examination of the anterior eye segment and the eye fundus by ophthalmoscopy. Before ivermectin treatment, vivid *O.volvulus* microfilariae (MF) were observed in the right and left anterior eye chamber in 52% and 42% of patients (n = 82), and dead MF were seen in the right and left cornea in 24% and 15% of cases, respectively. At 23 years post initial treatment (PIT), none of the patients (n = 82) presented with MF in the anterior chamber and cornea. A complete resolution of punctate keratitis (PK) lesions without observable corneal scars was present at 23 years PIT (p<0.0001), and sclerosing keratitits (SK) lessened by half, but mainly in patients with lesions at early stage of evolution. Early-stage iridocyclitis diminished from 42%(rE) and 40%(IE) to 13% (rE+IE)(p<0.0001), but advanced iridocyclitis augmented (p<0.001) at 23 years PIT compared to before ivermectin. Advanced-stage papillitis and chorioretinitis did not regress, while early-stage papillitis present in 28%(rE) and 27%(IE) of patients at before ivermectin regressed to 17%(rE) and 18%(IE), and early-stage chorioretinitis present in 51%(rE+IE) of cases at before ivermectin was observed in 12%(rE) and 13%(IE) at 23 years PIT (p<0.0001). Thus, regular annual ivermectin treatment eliminated and prevented the migration of *O. volvulus* microfilariae into the anterior eye chamber and cornea; keratitis punctata lesions resolved completely and early-stage sclerosing keratitits and iridocyclitis regressed, whilst advanced lesions of the anterior and posterior eye segment remained progressive. In conclusion, annual ivermectin treatments may prevent the emergence of ocular pathology in those populations still exposed to *O.volvulus* infection.

Editor: Philip Bejon, Kenya Medical Research Institute (KEMRI), Kenya

Funding: This work was supported by WHO/TDR (ID 930543), Gesellschaft für Internationale Zusammenarbeit (giz), Deutsche Forschungsgemeinschaft (DFG grant no. 367/1–2), Commission of the European Community (CEC-TS*-CT92-0057 and FP6-INCO-SCOOTT contract no. 032321) and the Togolese Ministry of Health (Autorisation no. 0407/2007/MS/CAB/DGS). The funders had no role in study design, data collection and analysis, decision to publish, or preparation of the manuscript.

Competing Interests: The authors have declared that no competing interests exist.

* E-mail: peter.soboslay@uni-tuebingen.de

Introduction

In West Africa, onchocerciasis is successfully controlled by the African Program for Onchocerciasis Control (APOC) and in large parts the disease is no longer considered a public health problem [1], and in certain onchocerciasis endemic foci in Mali and Senegal elimination is considered achievable [2,3]. Complete control or elimination of onchocerciasis in the near future may be attainable with high rates of ivermectin treatment coverage (> 85%) administered twice annually, and applied for more than 15 years which is expected to exceed the reproductive life span and natural life expectancy of adult *Onchocerca volvulus* [1,4]. However, onchocerciasis is considered as not eradicable in Africa using the currently available tools [5]. Ivermectin treatment will reduce within a few days *O. volvulus* microfilaria (MF) numbers in patients' skin by more than 70% [6,7], and progressively during the

following months MF will decline in the anterior chamber and cornea of the patients' eyes [8,9], but until 12 month post initial treatment (PIT) MF numbers may increase again [10,11]. Ivermectin therapy is associated with mild systemic adverse responses [6] and repeated treatments will alleviate hyper-reactive skin manifestations in patients and prevent the progression to chronic dermal pathology [12,13]. In onchocerciasis endemic foci in Cameroon and Nigeria, recent works have shown that community directed treatment with ivermectin (CDTI) will not interrupted *O. volvulus* transmission [13], and CDTI did not prevent evolution of ocular onchocerciasis [14,15], respectively. Despite repeated ivermectin treatments for years female adult *O. volvulus* remain reproductive [16], and unresponsiveness of *O. volvulus* to ivermectin treatment in some areas of West Africa might have emerged as a further problem for onchocerciasis control [17].

Replicated longitudinal surveys are required to determine the impact of ivermectin on dermal and ocular pathology in the APOC area, notably in the risk zones of the former Onchocerciasis Control Programme (OCP) where low level parasite transmission and few active *O. volvulus* infections still persist [18]; here the risk for recurrence of onchocerciasis may threaten the success of disease control.

The present ophthalmological study examined the evolution and changes of ocular pathology in a cohort of onchocerciasis patients permanently resident in central Togo and treated annually with ivermectin for 23 years. Patients were initially enrolled in a phase III double-blind placebo-controlled dose finding study of ivermectin, and from month 18 post initial treatment (PIT) onwards all patients received annual ivermectin treatment with 150 ug/kg as a single dose. Ocular onchocerciasis manifestations in ivermectin treatment groups evolved, persisted or regressed similarly in the patient groups [7], and ivermectin treatments applied annually for more than 2 decades permanently eliminated ocular *O.volvulus* microfilaria, and such regular interventions may prevent the emergence of ocular pathology in those populations still exposed to *O.volvulus* infection.

Methods

Ethics Statement

The protocol of the study was reviewed and approved by the Advisory Council of the Ministry of Health in Togo, the Committee on Research Involving Human subjects of the World Health Organization Ethics Commission and the Medical Board at University Clinics of Tübingen. The study has been registered at the Pan African Clinical Trial Registry and the WHO clinical trial registry platform (PACTR201303000464219: Onchocerciasis Ocular Pathology post Ivermectin; date of registry: 25/11/2012). Authorization and approval granted by the Ministry of Health in Togo were re-approved every 4–5 years (no. 2824/87/MSP-ASCF; no. 292//MS/CAB; no. 261//MSP/ DGSP/DRSP-RC, no. 0407/2007/MS/CAB/DGS, no. 0129/2011/MS/CAB/ DGS/ DPLET/CBRS). The protocol for this trial and supporting CONSORT checklist are available as supporting information; see Checklist S1 and Protocol S1. At beginning (in 1985), this study was a phase III double-blind placebo-controlled dose finding study of ivermectin for treatment of onchocerciasis. The aims of the work, risks, procedures of examination and follow up intervals were explained thoroughly to the respective village population, the village authorities and honourables, notably the village chief council. Before the very beginning of the phase III double-blind placebo-controlled dose finding study of ivermectin, all patients gave their consent for participation. The consent from each study participant was documented and confirmed by signature in the study protocol by the responsible physicians and/or their medical assistants. Consent for study participation by those less than 18 years of age was given verbally by each participant, and approval for participation was always obtained by the parents or the accompanying responsible adults. Written consent was not obligatory requested and such accepted by the national Togolese Health Authorities, i.e. the Ministry of Health, and approval for participation for those less than 18 years of age was always recorded by the responsible physician of the study in the study protocol. In 1985, the beginning of the phase III double-blind placebo-controlled dose finding study of ivermectin, the responsible authority for ethical approval of clinical trials was the Ministry of Health in Togo, which has approved this protocol. Until 54 months post initial treatment (PIT), and at each time patients were examined, patients' consent, absence or refusals were documented in the study protocol. For correct and complete understanding explanations were always given in the local language. Before each follow up survey, approval was obtained from the appropriate regional (Direction Regional de la Santé de la Population) and district-level (Direction Prefectural de la Santé) health authorities. At each follow up examination, all participants gave their informed oral consent; as such it was approved by the Review Boards owing to the low risk and routine nature of the ophthalmological examination procedures. Each patient's participation, absence or refusal was recorded in the individual study protocol sheets (MSD-Nr519: Ivermectin (MK933) versus placebo in onchocerciasis ophthalmologic examinations (OE).

Patients

Patients were enrolled in the phase III double-blind placebo-controlled dose finding study of ivermectin for treatment of onchocerciasis. All patients from this study originated from villages in the Central and Kara Region of Togo, where *O. volvulus* infection was hyper- to meso-endemic. Patients were resident in the villages Bougabou, Bouzalo, Kemeni, Mo, Tabalo, Tchapossi, Sagbadai and Sirka. Patients were apparently healthy males and non-pregnant women with a body weight over 30 kg, without history of multiple allergies or drug intolerance, with normal laboratory parameters except for the clinical features of onchocerciasis, with skin biopsies positive for microfilaria of *O. volvulus* and with palpable nodules (onchocercomata). Criteria for exclusion were allergies or drug intolerance, concomitant infection with *Loa loa* or *Wuchereria bancrofti*, haematocrit below 30%, renal or hepatic disease, convulsions or other central nervous system disease, clinical signs suggestive of meningitis, pregnant females or nursing mothers and patients who had received microfilaricidal drugs during the preceding year. The protocol of the study was reviewed and approved by the Ethics Commission of the Medical Board at University of Tübingen, the Advisory Council of the Ministry of Health in Togo and the Committee on Research Involving Human subjects of the World Health Organization.

Patient groups and examination during and after chemotherapy

In patients, the densities of microfilaria of *O. volvulus* (MF/mg) in the skin were determined at the right and left iliac crest and the right and left calf by means of corneascleral punch (Holth- or Walser-type) before ivermectin treatment and at day 3, at month 3, month 6 and at 1 year post treatment. Skin biopsies were immediately weighed and then immersed in 0.1 ml physiological saline in a well in a flat bottomed micro titre plate, and stored at room temperature in a high-humidity atmosphere. Microfilariae were counted after overnight incubation. Patients were randomly assigned to receive either 0(placebo), 100, 150, or 200 μg/kg of ivermectin. Patients were examined physically and intensity of signs and symptoms following ivermectin or placebo were scored, as described in detail previously by Greene and co-workers [5]. All onchocerciasis patients participated in regular surveys conducted by the Onchocerciasis Reference Laboratory (ORL) and the National Onchocerciasis Control Program (NOCP). Clinical data of all patients were gathered in a double-blind fashion, those of the ivermectin and placebo patients during the first 12 months after therapy. From months 18 post initial treatment (PIT) onwards all patients received annual ivermectin treatment (150 μg/kg) as a single dose distributed by the ORL and the NOCP in Togo. At regular intervals thorough physical, parasitological and ophthalmological examinations were conducted and the density of *O. volvulus* microfilariae (MF) was determined in skin biopsies (MF/ mg skin) taken from the right and left hip.

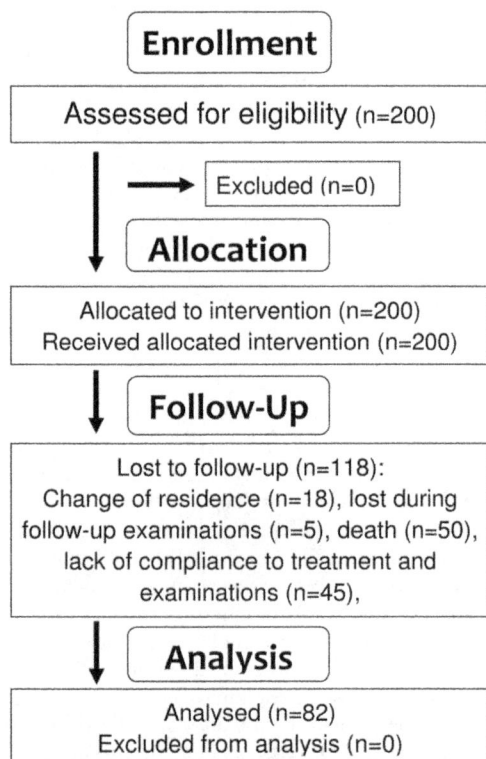

Figure 1. Flowchart showing the recruitment, allocation and follow up of study participants.

Table 1. Onchocerciasis patients' age and their profession at 23 years post initial ivermectin treatment.

Patients		n
Age (in groups)	35 y–45 y	20
	46 y–55 y	28
	56 y–65 y	19
	>65 y	15
Profession	Farmer	65
	House wife	5
	Administrator/Teacher	6
	Others (Trader, Retired)	6

Ophthalmologic Examinations

Visual Acuity. The ocular examinations included the testing of visual acuity eye by eye with an illiterate E chart (SNELEN) placed 6 meters away from the patient's seat, and visual acuity was graded according to WHO/OCP criteria; blind were those with a visual acuity on one or both eyes of less than 1/20 (3/60 or unable to count fingers at 3 meters); impaired vision had those with a visual acuity on one or both eyes between 1/20 and less than 3/10 (6/18) and good vision had those with a visual acuity equal or greater than 3/10 (6/18). Note: Pin hole was used when visual acuity was less than 3/10 (6/18).

Slit Lamp Examination. The ophthalmology examinations until 36 months PIT were conducted by M.Banla together with other ophthalmologists, and thereafter, all follow-up examinations were conducted by one examiner (M. Banla). The anterior chamber and cornea were examined with a HAAG STREIT Slit Lamp 900 after the patients were placed in the head down position for at least two minutes. The microfilaria in the cornea and the anterior chamber of each eye were counted. Limbitis was diagnosed by the presence of limbal vessel dilatation, limbal oedema, and white globular opacities, and each sign was graded as absent, mild, moderate, or severe. Iridocyclitis in evolution was diagnosed by the presence of anterior chamber cells and flare with or without iris atrophy, anterior or posterior synechiae and secondary cataract due to iridocyclitis. The classification of iridocyclitis was according to the criteria applied by the Onchocerciasis Control Program (OCP) iridocyclitis was graded as: absent, early stage iridocyclitis was without synechiae and or secondary cataract. Advanced iridocyclitis was with synechiae and/or secondary cataract. Sclerosing keratitis was graded

according to the presence of limbal haze, the extent of characteristic corneal involvement starting in the nasal and or temporal periphery, being confluent inferiorly, or covering the pupil.

Posterior Eye Segment Examinations. Examinations until 36 months PIT were conducted by M.Banla together with other ophthalmologists, and thereafter, all follow-up examinations were conducted by one examiner (M. Banla). The fundus was examined by direct and indirect ophthalmoscopy after pupil dilatation with 1% tropicamide and 10% epinephrine hydrochloride. The classification of lesions was according to the criteria applied by the Onchocerciasis Control Program (OCP). Early stage chorio-retinitis due to onchocerciasis was with patchy non confluent atrophies of the retinal pigmented epithelium (RPE). Advanced chorioretinitis due to onchocerciasis were at least confluent atrophies of the RPE of any grade alone or associated with other lesions as choroïdo retinitis atrophy of any grade or sub retinal fibrosis. Early stage papillitis due to onchocerciasis was patchy papillary bleeding with pale, atrophic papilla or papilla abnormally pink associated with other ocular onchocerciasis lesions. Advanced stage papillitis was post neuritis optical atrophy with vessel sheathing, with or without papillary or peri-papillary haemorrhages associated with other ocular onchocerciasis lesions. The presence and extent of intraretinal deposits, intraretinal pigment hypertrophy as well as any other abnormalities were noted. After initial treatment the ocular examinations were repeated at day 3 PIT and at three, six, and twelve and 48 months PIT. Thereafter, the physical, parasitological and ocular examinations were repeated in 3-5 year intervals by the ORL and NOCP.

Statistical data analysis

JMP software (versions 9.0.0; SAS Institute) was used for statistical analysis of data. Due to multiple comparisons, the level of significance was adjusted according to Bonferroni–Holm (alpha = 0.0025). The manifestations of ocular pathologies at different time points post treatment and between groups were evaluated by contingency analyses using Pearson's chi-square test, and unpaired data of patients were compared using Wilcoxon's rank sum test. Multivariate correlation analysis was applied to show relationships between pairs of variables, e.g. patients' age, treatment groups, Years post treatment, ocular manifestation of onchocerciasis.

Table 2. Visual acuity in the onchocerciasis patients' cohort (n = 82) before ivermectin treatment, and at 4 years and 23 years post initial treatment (PIT).

Visual acuity	before ivermectin* (in %)			4 years PIT* (in %)			23 years PIT* (in %)		
	RE	LE	RLE	RE	LE	RLE	RE	LE	RLE
<1/20	2.4	2.4	0	4.9	7.3	1.2	2.4	7.3	17.1
≥1/20 and <3/10	2.4	1.2	6.1	1.2	2.4	9.7	10.9	3.6	11.7
≥3/10	3.6	4.9	87.7	7.5	3.6	80.4	1.2	4.9	58.5

For visual acuity an illiterate E chart (SNELEN) was used placed 6 meters away from the patient's seat. The patients' visual acuity was graded according to WHO criteria; blind were those with a visual acuity on the right (RE) or left eye (LE) or both eyes (RLE) of less than 1/20 (3/60 or unable to count fingers at 3 meters); impaired vision had those with a visual acuity between 1/20 (3/60) and less than 3/10 (6/18); good vision had those with a visual acuity equal or greater than 3/10. *Note: At before treatment and at 4 and 23 years PIT, visual acuity was not possible to determine in 11% (n = 9), 13% (11) and 17% (19) of the patients due to lack of comprehension, respectively.

Results

O. volvulus skin microfilaria in patients post ivermectin treatments

From the two hundred patients initially included in this longitudinal study, eighty two patients attended all follow-up examinations (Fig. 1). At 23 years post initial ivermectin treatment (PIT), the patient cohort consisted of 76 males and 5 females with a mean age of 54.3 years (min 36, max 77) (Table 1). Patients were initially enrolled in a phase III double-blind placebo-controlled dose finding study of ivermectin and were treated either with 100, 150 or 200 ug/kg ivermectin or received placebo; from months 18 post initial treatment (PIT) onwards, all patients received annual ivermectin treatment with 150 μg/kg as a single dose. In the ivermectin-treated patients' cohort, the density of *O. volvulus* microfilariae (MF) per mg skin (before: mean 73 MF/mg) decreased by 85% (11 MF/mg), 95% (4 MF/mg), 97% (3 MF/mg), 89% (8 MF/mg) and 59% (30 MF/mg) on day 3, month 3, month 6, month 12 and month 18 PIT, respectively. In the initial placebo group patients, the density of mf was reduced following ivermectin treatment by 75% to 17 MF/mg at 22 months PIT. At 4 years PIT, the mean mf density in n = 82 patients was 17 MF/mg and following ivermectin treatment it lessened to 2 Mf/mg at 3 days later. Thereafter, ivermectin treatments (150 μg/kg) were applied annually by the National Program for Onchocerciasis Control (PNLO/APOC) i.e. by community-directed ivermectin distribution. At 7 years PIT, all onchocerciasis patients were negative for mf in skin biopsies, and remained such during all the following re-examinations.

Visual Acuity

Despite annually repeated ivermectin treatments the visual acuity degraded gradually in the patients' cohort (Table 2). At the beginning of study, none of the patients presented with bilateral blindness. Good vision, as present in 88% of the patients at study begin, was observable only in 59% of the patients at 23 years PIT. At 23 years PIT, 17% of the treated patients were classified as bilaterally blind (Table 3). Noteworthy, this degradation cannot unequivocally be attributed to onchocerciasis as other ocular anomalies (Table 4), i.e. vascular retinopathy (18%), pterigium conjunctivae (20%) and band-shaped keratopathy (7%), emerged in the onchocerciasis patients cohort.

Microfilaria and lesions of the anterior eye segment

At the beginning of study, more than half of the onchocerciasis patients had living MF in their eyes' anterior chamber (AC) (Table 5). Living MF of *O.volvulus* in the AC (MFAC) regressed considerably in the patients from 52%(rE) and 42%(lE) at before ivermectin to 29%(rE) and 19%(lE) at 4 years and to 0% (rE+lE) at 23 years PIT, respectively. Similarly, dead MF of *O.volvulus* in the cornea (DMFC) diminished from 24%/15% (rE/lE) at before to 10%/7% (rE/lE) at 4 years PIT and to 0% (rE+lE) at 23 years PIT. Thus, regular annual treatment with ivermectin has achieved a complete elimination of MF from the AC and cornea of the patients' eyes.

While MFAC and DMFC diminished by half in patients until 4 years PIT, the number of puctate keratitis (PK) lesions did not regress at 4 years PIT (Table 5). At 23 years PIT, PK lesions were resolved completely without leaving residual corneal scars. Sclerosing keratitis (SK) was present before ivermectin in 9%/11% (rE/lE), at 4 years PIT in 27%/26% (rE/lE) and at 23 years PIT, in 5%/4% (rE/lE) of the patients. The early evolving SK regressed in 80% of the patients, whilst the advanced-stage SK

Table 3. Causes of bilateral visual impairment and blindness in the onchocerciasis patients' cohort (n = 82) before ivermectin treatment, and at 4 years and 23 years post initial treatment (PIT).

Bilateral visual impairment and blindness	before ivermectin	4 years PIT	23 years PIT
Visual Acuity: ≥1/20 and <3/10	n (%)	n (%)	n (%)
Impaired by non onchocerciasis cataract	2 (2.4)	1 (1.2)	2 (2.4)
Impaired by onchocerciasis	3 (3.6)	4 (4.8)	5 (6.0)
Impaired by glaucoma	0	0	2 (2.4)
Impaired by other causes	0	3 (3.6)	1 (1.2)
Total with impaired vision	**5 (6.0)**	**8 (9.6)**	**10 (12.0)**
Visual Acuity: (<1/20 or <3/60)			
Blindness by non onchocerciasis cataract	0	1 (1.2)	2 (2.4)
Blindness by onchocerciasis	0	0	6 (7.3)
Blindness by onchocerciasis & other causes	0	0	3 (3.6)
Blindness by glaucoma	0	0	1 (1.2)
Blindness by other causes	0	0	2 (2.4)
Total of blindness	**0**	**1 (1.2)**	**14 (16.9)**

The patients' visual acuity was graded according to WHO criteria; blind were those with a visual acuity on the right (RE) or left eye (LE) or both eyes (RLE) of less than 1/20 (3/60 or unable to count fingers at 3 meters); impaired vision had those with a visual acuity between 1/20 (3/60) and less than 3/10 (6/18); good vision had those with a visual acuity equal or greater than 3/10.

lesions did not resolve until 23 years PIT; only in one patient advanced SK reduced to early stage.

Iridocyclitis early-stage lesions regressed slightly from 42%/40% (rE/lE) to 26%/23% at 4 years PIT, but advanced stage lesions were detected more often (Table 6). At 23 years PIT, iridocyclitis early lesions were observed in 13% (rE+lE) with none occurring to be in evolution, advanced iridocyclitis lesions were present in 9%/10% (rE/lE) and none appeared as progressive. Thus, anterior eye segment lesions in an early stage of evolution disappeared completely, i.e. MFAC, DMFC and PK, and early-stage iridocyclitis diminished by 67% and 68%, but advanced-stage iridocyclitis as observed in 1–2% of the patients at before was present in 9–10% at 23 years PIT. Notably, cataract (44%) emerged in the onchocerciasis patients' cohort (Table 6).

Lesions of the posterior eye segment

Papillitis and chorioretinitis were present in 27%/28% (rE/lE) and 69%/73% (rE/lE) of the patients, respectively (Table 6). Until 4 years PIT, both early and advanced stage papillitis lessened to 5%/6% (rE/lE) and chorioretinitis to 63%(rE) and 66%(lE). At 23 years PIT, papillitis was present in 24%/23% (rE/lE) of the patients and chorioretinitis was observed in 33%/37% (rE/lE) of

the patients; this regression is due to the fact that only in 77/78 (rE/lE) patients the fundus was accessible for examination because of anterior segment lesions. Only early-stage papillitis and chorioretinitis regressed, whilst advanced stage papillitis enhanced from 0% to 7%/5% (rE/lE) while severe chorioretinitis present in 18%/22% (rE/lE) of the patients at before treatment was found enhanced by 2–3% at 23 years PIT.

Multivariate correlations analysis of patients, groups, treatment and ocular pathology

Cataract and visual impairment correlated positively (p< 0.0001) with the patients' age and the years PIT such disclosing the age-related decline of visual functions in the patient cohort (Table 7). A negative correlation with age and the years PIT was present for MFAC, DMFC, PK (for each p<0.0001) and iridocyclitis (p = 0.0002), and this highlighted the positive effect of the repeatedly applied ivermectin treatments. The visual acuity impairment throughout the duration of study was observed to have a strong positive correlation with papillitis, chorioretinitis, iridocyclitis, SK and cataract (for each p = 0.0001 or less) such disclosing the progression of ocular pathology and visual impairment in onchocerciasis patients despite treatment. The

Table 4. Ocular anomalies not caused by *Onchocerca volvulus* infection in patients (n = 82) examined before ivermectin treatment, and at 4 and 23 years post initial ivermectin treatment (PIT).

	before ivermectin (in %)	4 years PIT (in %)	23 years PIT (in %)
Band-shaped keratopathy	6.1	7.3	7.3
Glaucoma	4.9	4.9	4.9
Vascular retinopathy	2.4	4.9	18.2
Pterygium conjunctivae	2.4	4.8	19.5
Suspected glaucoma by Cup/disc ≥0.5	2.4	2.4	4.9
POA (primary optic atrophy)	1.2	1.2	1.2

Table 5. Microfilaria in the anterior chamber of the eye, the cornea, and puctate and sclerosing keratitis in onchocerciasis patients (n = 82) post ivermectin treatment. Differences were evaluated using Pearson's chi-square test.

	right EYE			left EYE		
	before ivermectin	4 years PIT[$]	23 years PIT	before ivermectin	4 years PIT	23 years PIT
Microfilaria (MF) in the anterior chamber of the eye (MFAC)						
MF Absent (in %)	37 (45)	54 (66)	78 (95)**	47 (57)	64 (78)	80 (98)**
Impossible to examine (in %)	2 (2)	4 (5)	4 (5)	1 (1)	2 (2)	2 (2)
MFAC >20 (in %)	1 (1)	1 (1)	0	1 (1)	1 (1)	0
MFAC 1–10 (in %)	40 (49)	20 (24)	0***	30 (37)	14 (17)	0***
MFAC 11–20 (in %)	2 (2)	3 (4)	0	3 (4)	1 (1)	0
Dead microfilaria (MF) in the cornea (DMFC)						
MF Absent (in %)	60 (73)	71 (87)	79 (96)	69 (84)	74 (90)	80 (98)
Impossible to examine (in %)	2 (2)	3 (4)	3 (4)	1 (1)	2 (2)	2 (2)
DMFC 1–10 (in %)	20 (24)	8 (10)	0**	12 (15)	6 (7)	0**
Punctate Keratitis						
Absent (in %)	44 (54)	20 (24)	80 (98)***	47(57)	26 (32)	80 (98)***
Impossible to examine (in %)	1(1)	2 (2)	2 (2)	1 (1)	1 (1)	2 (2)
Number of Lesions 1–10 (in %)	36 (44)	59 (72)	0***	33 (40)	50 (61)	0***
Number of Lesions 11–20 (%)	1 (1)	1 (1)	0	1 (1)	5 (6)	0
Sclerosing Keratitis (SK)						
Absent (in %)	74 (90)	58 (71)	75 (92)	73 (89)	60 (73)	77(94)
Impossible to examine (in %)	0	2 (2)	2 (2)	0	1 (1)	2 (2)
SK advanced (in %)	2 (2)	1 (1)	1 (1)	1 (1)	0	0
SK in evolution (in %)	6 (7)	21 (26)	4 (5)*	8 (10)	21 (26)	3 (4)*

[$]PIT = post initial treatment.
*p<0.001 compared to 4 years PIT;
**p<0.001 compared to before ivermectin;
***p<0.0001 compared to before ivermectin and 4 years PIT.

highest positive correlations for ocular pathologies were for papillitis and chorioretinitis (r = 0.40), iridocyclitis and chorioretinitis (r = 0.38), iridocyclitis and MFAC (r = 0.37), and MFAC and DMFC (r = 0.35) (for each p<0.0001).

Discussion

Repeated ivermectin treatments for more than two decades have persistently eliminated microfilaria (MF) of *O. volvulus* from the patients' anterior eye chamber and cornea. The regression of punctate keratitis, early-stage iridocyclitis and chorioretinitis and to some extent scelorosing keratitis confirm ivermectin as an effective long term control means against ocular pathology in human *O. volvulus* infection [9,10,19], and the efficacy of annually repeated treatments extends to disease prevention, as it may halt migration of MF of *O. volvulus* into the eye and evolution of onchocerciasis-related ocular lesions. Previous studies accomplished in Africa have similarly observed that annual treatments for 2 to 8 years strongly reduced prevalence of ocular MF [10,20,21,22,23]. In the Americas, a complete reduction of disease of the anterior eye segment has been achieved with semi annual ivermectin dosing for 14 years [24,25]. In African onchocerciasis cohorts, ivermectin therapy applied bi-annually or annually for up to eight years lessened the number of ocular MF and significantly improved anterior eye segment lesions, despite persisting skin MF [22,23].

Punctate keratitis (PK) lesions did not disappear or regress in our patients' cohort until 4 years PIT, and PK may persist even after 10 years of ivermectin [25]. At 23 years PIT, PK lesions were completely resolved. Such long duration for complete clearance of MF and resolution of punctuate opacities is most likely due to the low physiologic activity and turnover of corneal epithelia and endothelia. Earlier clinical studies which have followed ivermectin-treated onchocerciasis patients for several years found clear indications that early lesions of the anterior eye segment will regress including sclerosing keratitis and iridocyclitis [9,19,23]. In our patients, only early-stage sclerosing keratitis regressed and this occurred in half of the effected individuals only, and similarly, only early-stage iridocyclitis ameliorated significantly. Previous observations have found similar regression of iridocyclitis within shorter intervention times [10,23], and from our observations we may conclude that advanced anterior eye segment lesions may not regress despite repeated annual ivermectin treatments for two decades. However, none of the patients presented at 23 years PIT with new or evolving iridocyclitis suggesting that inflammatory processes induced by MF or circulating filarial antigens may not have occurred.

Despite two decades of treatment with ivermectin, posterior eye segment lesion did not evolve favourably, only early-stage papillitis lesions and early-stage chorioretinitis cases were reduced by one third at 23 years PIT whilst advanced-stage papillitis and chorioretinitis cases augmented. Such unfavourable development

Table 6. Iridocyclitis, cataract, papillitis and chorioretinitis in onchocerciasis patients (n = 82) post ivermectin treatment. Differences were evaluated using Pearson's chi-square test.

	right EYE			left EYE		
	before ivermectin	4 years PIT$^\$$	23 years PIT	before ivermectin	4 years PIT	23 years PIT
Iridocyclitis						
1/2 Mydriase (in %)	1 (1)	1(1)	1 (1)	1 (1)	1 (1)	1 (1)
Iris Normal (in %)	36 (44)	45 (55)	63 (77)**	34 (42)	46 (56)	62 (76)**
Other Lesions (in %)$^{\$\$}$	1(1)	1 (1)	0	3 (4)	3 (4)	0
Iridocyclitis (advanced stage)	1 (1)	2 (2)	7 (9)**	2 (2)	3 (4)	8 (10)**
Iridocyclitis (early stage) (in %)	34 (42)	21 (26)	11 (13)**	33 (40)	19 (23)	11(13)**
Iridocyclitis (torpide, in evolution)(in %)	9 (11)	12 (15)	0*	9 (11)	10 (12)	0*
Lens (Cataract)						
Other Lesions non Cataract (in %) $^{\$\$}$	3 (4)	3 (4)	3 (4)	5 (6)	5 (6)	4 (5)
Cataract (early stage; PES clearly visible) (%)	13 (16)	14 (17)	18 (22)	13 (16)	15 (18)	18 (22)
Cataract (in evolution; PES difficult to examine) (in %)	1 (1)	4 (5)	10 (12)**	1 (1)	4 (5)	8 (10)**
Cataract (mature; PES not visible) (in %)	2 (2)	2 (2)	9 (11)	2 (2)	0	10 (12)**
Lens Normal (in %)	63 (77)	59 (72)	42 (51)	61 (74)	58 (71)	42 (51)
Papillitis						
Optic Disc Atrophy (secondary) (%)	7 (8)	10 (12)	0*	7 (9)	11 (13)	0*
Other Lesions (in %)$^{\&\&}$	1 (1)	1 (1)	12 (15)**	0	1 (1)	14 (17)**
Excavation (in %)	2 (2)	4 (5)	4 (5)	3 (4)	3 (4)	4 (5)
Impossible to examine (in %)	0	3 (4)	0	1 (1)	3 (4)	0
Papille normal (in %)	49 (60)	60 (73)$^\&$	46 (56)	49 (60)	59 (72)$^\&$	45 (55)
Papillitis (avanced stage) (%)	0	0	6 (7)	0	0	4 (5)
Papillitis (early stage) (in %)	23 (28)	4 (5)$^\&$	14 (17)**	22 (27)	5 (6)$^\&$	15 (18)**
Chorioretinitis						
Other Lesions (in %) $^{\$\$\$}$	1 (1)	4 (5)	5 (6)	3 (4)	4 (5)	4 (5)
Chorioretinitis (advanced) (in %)	15 (18)	14 (17)	17 (21)	18 (22)	19 (23)	20 (24)
Chorioretinitis (early stage) (%)	42 (51)	38 (46)	10 (12)**	42 (51)	35 (43)	11 (13)**
Chorion Normal (in %)	24 (30)	26 (32)	50 (61)**	19 (23)	24 (29)	47 (57)**

$^\$$PIT = post initial treatment.
PES = Posterior Eye Segment.
$^{\$\$}$Other Lesions: Phtyse, Pupille scleroatrophic, Synechie post trauma, Pigments on posterior Capsule.
$^{\$\$}$Other Lesions: Phtyse, dead O.volvulus microfilariae on posterior capsule.
$^{\&\&}$Other Lesions: optic cup/disc >0.5.
$^{\$\$\$}$Other Lesions = retina detachment from the retinal pigment epithelium, drusen.
*p<0.001 compared to 4 years PIT;
**p<0.001 compared to before ivermectin;
***p<0.0001 compared to before ivermectin and 4 years PIT.
$^\&$p<0.01 compared to before ivermectin.

has been described previously in onchocerciasis patients studied for 3 years [26] indicating that immune pathologic processes, i.e. destruction of cells and adjacent tissues of the retina, continued despite the ivermectin-facilitated clearance of MF from skin and eyes. Certain advanced retinal lesions may regress by secondary revascularisation [19], but such changes we could not observe. All our patients were resident in the rural Central and Kara Regions of Togo where the risk for onchocercal blindness was medium to high [27], and this area was one of the special intervention zones [19] where ongoing parasite transmission required extended vector control and intensified ivermectin distribution. The onchocerciasis control measures as applied during the past decades prevented re-emergence of patent *O. volvulus* infections in our patients and halted the dispersion and migration of MF into the anterior eye segment. An evolution of new lesions of the cornea was not observed, but already existent advanced ocular pathology did not resolve.

The degradation of visual acuity in our patients is mainly due to the persistence of advanced *O.volvulus*–induced posterior eye segment lesions and secondary anomalies, mostly the evolution of cataract - the main cause for visual impairment worldwide [28] and in sub-Saharan Africa total blindness due to cataract ranges between 21% and 67% [29]. In urban Togo, the main ocular blinding disease was also found to be cataract with 8.3% prevalence [30], while in our patients, resident in rural central and northern Togo, the prevalence and incidence of cataract was higher and rising with age. Cataract correlated positively with years' post initiation of treatment thus not supporting a causal preventive effect of ivermectin on its evolution. In Uganda, the impact of community-directed treatment with ivermectin (CDTI)

Table 7. Multivariate correlation analyses of ocular pathology and visual impairment in onchocerciasis patients treated annually with ivermectin for 23 years.

Variable	Variable	Spearman ρ	p value
Age	Cataract	0,2949	<0.0001
Age	Punctate Keratitis	−0,2934	<0.0001
Age	Visual Impairment	0,2696	<0.0001
Age	MF in the AC of the eye	−0,2461	0,0001
Years PIT	MF in the AC of the eye	−0,4103	<0.0001
Years PIT	Punctate Keratitis	−0,3425	<0.0001
Years PIT	MF in the cornea	−0,2639	<0.0001
Years PIT	Iridocyclitis	−0,2379	0,0002
Years PIT	Cataract	0,2331	0,0002
Years PIT	Visual Impairment	0,2188	0,0005
Visual Acuity	Cataract	0,5379	<0.0001
Visual Acuity	Papillitis	0,4351	<0.0001
Visual Acuity	Chorioretinitis	0,3747	<0.0001
Visual Acuity	Sclerosing Keratitis	0,2541	0,0001
Visual Acuity	Iridocyclitis	0,2511	0,0001
Cataract	Papillitis	0,2800	<0.0001
Cataract	Chorioretinitis	0,1950	0,0020
Iridocyclitis	Chorioretinitis	0,3792	<0.0001
Iridocyclitis	Cataract	0,2593	<0.0001
Iridocyclitis	Papillitis	0,2202	0,0005
Punctate Keratitis	Sclerosing Keratitis	0,2793	<0.0001
Punctate Keratitis	Chorioretinitis	0,1991	0,0016
Sclerosing Keratitis	Cataract	0,2567	<0.0001
Sclerosing Keratitis	Chorioretinitis	0,2553	<0.0001
Sclerosing Keratitis	Iridocyclitis	0,2149	0,0007
Dead MF in the cornea	Sclerosing Keratitis	0,2818	<0.0001
Dead MF in the cornea	Iridocyclitis	0,2282	0,0003
Dead MF in the cornea	Punctate Keratitis	0,2276	0,0003
MF in the AC of the eye	Iridocyclitis	0,3726	<0.0001
MF in the AC of the eye	Dead MF in the cornea	0,3511	<0.0001
MF in the AC of the eye	Sclerosing Keratitis	0,3162	<0.0001
MF in the AC of the eye	Punctate Keratitis	0,2583	<0.0001
MF in the AC of the eye	Chorioretinitis	0,2552	<0.0001
Papillitis	Chorioretinitis	0,4057	<0.0001

Significant correlations of p<0.0025 are shown. (MF = microfilariae; AC = anterior chamber; Years PIT = Years post initial treatment).

on ocular manifestations showed a paucity of acute ocular onchocerciasis-related lesions but a significant presence of irreversible onchocerciasis-related ocular lesions - not only cataract but also optic atrophy and chorioretinitis [31]. In elderly members (>60 years) of a rural community in West Africa, more than 30% were with blindness and low vision, and age-related macular degeneration and glaucoma dominated next to cataract. These studies highlighted the substantial increases of blindness due to posterior eye segment anomalies and low vision in rural dwellers [32,33]. In our cohort, none of the early-stage onchocercal posterior eye lesions became a primary cause for blindness and recent data analysis did not find evidence that ivermectin will prevent visual acuity loss [34]. Thus, in addition to the advanced non-resolving anterior and posterior eye segment onchocercal pathologies, age-related cataract and further ocular anomalies have to be considered as contributors to the observed visual deterioration in our patients' cohort.

This longitudinal cohort study disclosed that repeated ivermectin therapy will persistently eliminate MF of *O.volvulus* from the AC and cornea, achieve complete regression of PK, and advanced sclerosing keratitis will stabilize. These results endorse observations from previous studies of shorter duration [11,20,23], and also suggest, that the regression of certain ocular manifestations is achievable within a decade of CDTI activities. Annual ivermectin treatments for 23 years did not significantly improve existing advanced posterior eye segment lesions, and visual acuity in patient gradually lessened, and this aggravation developed together with other ocular age-related anomalies. Irreversible posterior onchocerciasis-related ocular lesions which were already present in patients before the initial ivermectin treatment, did not resolve, and this has similarly been observed in earlier investigations of shorter duration [26,32]. The long term application of ivermectin has the potential to stop the evolution of ocular onchocerciasis, but parasite eradication in Africa may require control activities associated with a macrofilaricidal drug. The depletion of Wolbachia endosymbionts in adult *O. volvulus* by doxycycline antibiotics will accelerate the death of MF and adult *O. Volvulus* [35], and the rapid disappearance of MF from the eye anterior chamber and cornea when ivermectin is combined with doxycycline [36] may provide an additional measure for prevention and elimination of *O. volvulus* infection-associated ocular pathologies; such combined therapeutic approaches may supplement the available means for onchocerciasis elimination.

Supporting Information

Protocol S1   Onchocerciasis Ivermectin Study Examination Sheet Ophthalmology: 1985-1989. Study protocol sheets (MSD-Nr519: Ivermectin (MK933) versus placebo in onchocerciasis ophthalmologic examinations (OE).

Checklist S1   CONSORT 2010 checklist. Checklist of information reporting a clinical trial.

Author Contributions

Conceived and designed the experiments: MB GHG CH HSK PTS. Performed the experiments: MB ST GHG CH RGG HSK PTS. Analyzed the data: MB ST GHG CH HSK PTS. Contributed reagents/materials/analysis tools: MB GHG CH AKB HSK PTS. Wrote the paper: MB ST HSK PTS. Patient recruitment, clinical examination and treatment: GHG CH HSK RGG MB ST AIA AKB PKK PTS.

References

1. Sékétéli A, Adeoye G, Eyamba A, Nnoruka E, Drameh P, et al. (2002) The achievements and challenges of the African Programme for Onchocerciasis Control (APOC). Ann Trop Med Parasitol (Suppl 1): S15–S28.
2. Diawara L, Traoré MO, Badji A, Bissan Y, Doumbia K, et al. (2009) Feasibility of onchocerciasis elimination with ivermectin treatment in endemic foci in Africa: first evidence from studies in Mali and Senegal. PLoS Negl Trop Dis 3: e497.
3. Tekle AH, Elhassan E, Isiyaku S, Amazigo UV, Bush S, et al. (2012) Impact of long-term treatment of onchocerciasis with ivermectin in Kaduna State, Nigeria: first evidence of the potential for elimination in the operational area of the African Programme for Onchocerciasis Control. Parasit Vectors 7: 5–28.
4. Boatin B (2008) The Onchocerciasis Control Programme in West Africa (OCP). Ann Trop Med Parasitol. 102 (Suppl 1): 13–17.
5. Dadzie Y, Neira M, Hopkins D (2003) Final report of the Conference on the eradicability of Onchocerciasis. Filaria J 2: 1–134.
6. Greene BM, Taylor HR, Cupp EW, Murphy RP, White AT, et al. (1985) Comparison of ivermectin and diethylcarbamazine in the treatment of onchocerciasis. N Engl J Med 313: 133–138.
7. Newland HS, White AT, Greene BM, D'Anna SA, Keyvan-Larijani E, et al. (1988) Effect of single-dose ivermectin therapy on human Onchocerca volvulus infection with onchocercal ocular involvement. Br J Ophthalmol 72: 561–569.
8. Larivière M, Vingtain P, Aziz M, Beauvais B, Weimann D (1985) Double blind study of ivermectin and diethylcarbamazine in african onchocerciasis patients with ocular involvement. Lancet 1: 174–177
9. Taylor HR, Murphy RP, Newland HS, White AT, D'Anna SA, et al. (1986) Treatment of onchocerciasis. The ocular effects of ivermectin and diethylcarbamazine. Arch Ophthalmol 104: 863–870.
10. Dadzie KY, Awadzi K, Bird AC, Schulz-Key H (1989) Ophthalmological results from a placebo controlled comparative 3-dose ivermectin study in the treatment of onchocerciasis. Trop Med Parasitol 40: 355–360.
11. Dadzie KY, Remme J, De Sole G (1991) Changes in ocular onchocerciasis after two rounds of community-based ivermectin treatment in a holo-endemic onchocerciasis focus. Trans R Soc Trop Med Hyg 85: 267–271
12. Baraka OZ, Mahmoud BM, Ali MM, Ali MH, el Sheikh EA, et al. (1995) Ivermectin treatment in severe asymmetric reactive onchodermatitis (sowda) in Sudan. Trans R Soc Trop Med Hyg 89: 312–315.
13. Darge K, Büttner DW (1995) Ivermectin treatment of hyperreactive onchodermatitis (sowda) in Liberia. Trop Med Parasitol 46: 206–212.
14. Katabarwa MN, Eyamba A, Nwane P, Enyong P, Yaya S, et al. (2011) Seventeen years of annual distribution of ivermectin has not interrupted onchocerciasis transmission in North Region, Cameroon. Am J Trop Med Hyg. 85: 1041–1049.
15. Umeh RE, Mahmoud AO, Hagan M, Wilson M, Okoye OI, et al. (2010) Prevalence and distribution of ocular onchocerciasis in three ecological zones in Nigeria. Afr J Med Sci. 39: 267–275.
16. Kläger SL, Whitworth JA, Downham MD (1996) Viability and fertility of adult *Onchocerca volvulus* after 6 years of treatment with ivermectin. Trop Med Int Health 1: 581–589.
17. Osei-Atweneboana MY, Eng JK, Boakye DA, Gyapong JO, Prichard RK (2007) Prevalence and intensity of Onchocerca volvulus infection and efficacy of ivermectin in endemic communities in Ghana: a two-phase epidemiological study. Lancet 369: 2021–2029
18. Yaméogo L (2008) Special intervention zones. Ann Trop Med Parasitol. (Suppl 1): 23–24.
19. Abiose A (1998) Onchocercal eye disease and the impact of Mectizan treatment. Ann Trop Med Parasitol (Suppl 1): S11–S22.
20. Whitworth JA, Gilbert CE, Mabey DM, Maude GH, Morgan D, et al. (1991) Effects of repeated doses of ivermectin on ocular onchocerciasis: community-based trial in Sierra Leone. Lancet 338: 1000–1003.
21. Abiose A, Jones BR, Cousens SN, Murdoch I, Cassels-Brown A, et al. (1993) Reduction in incidence of optic nerve disease with annual ivermectin to control onchocerciasis. Lancet 341: 130–134.
22. Mabey DM, Whitworth JA, Eckstein M, Gilbert CE, Maude GH, et al. (1996) The effects of multiples doses of ivermectin on ocular onchocerciasis. Ophthalmology 103: 1001–1008.
23. Chippaux JP, Boussinesq M, Fobi G, Lafleur C, Audugé A, et al. (1999) Effect of repeated ivermectin treatments on ocular onchocerciasis: evaluation after six to eight doses. Ophthalmic Epidemiol 6: 229–246.
24. Rodriguez-Perez MA, Rodriguez MH, Margeli-Pperez HM, Rivas-Alcala AR (1995) Effects of semianual treatments of Ivermectin on the prevalence and intensity of *Onchocerca volvulus* skin infection, ocular lesions, and intensity of *Simulium ochraceum* populations in southern Mexico. Am J Trop Medicine Hyg 52: 429–434.
25. Vieira JC, Cooper PJ, Lovato R, Mancero T, Rivera J, et al. (2007) Impact of long-term treatment of onchocerciasis with ivermectin in Ecuador: potential for elimination of infection. BMC Med 5: 9.
26. Semba RD, Murphy RP, Newland HS, Awadzi K, Greene BM, et al. (1990) Longitudinal study of lesions of the posterior segment in onchocerciasis. Ophthalmol 97: 1334–41.
27. De Sole G, Accorsi S, Cresveaux H, Remme J, Walsh F, et al. (1992) Distribution and severity of onchocerciasis in southern Benin, Ghana and Togo. Acta Trop 52: 87–97.
28. Resnikoff S, Pascolini D, Etya'ale D, Kocur I, Pararajasegaram R, et al. (2004) Global data on visual impairment in the year 2002. Bull World Health Organ 82: 844–851.
29. Bastawrous A, Dean WH, Sherwin JC (2013) Blindness and visual impairment due to age-related cataract in sub-Saharan Africa: a systematic review of recent population-based studies. Br J Ophthalmol 97: 1237–1243.
30. Balo PK, Wabagira J, Banla M, Kuaovi RK (2000) Specific causes of blindness and vision impairment in a rural area of Southern Togo. J Fr Ophthalmol. 23: 459–464.
31. Ejere H, Schwartz E, Wormald R (2001) Ivermectin for onchocercal eye disease (river blindness). Cochrane Database Systemic Reviews 1:CD002219.
32. Babalola OE, Ogbuagu FK, Maegga BT, Braide EI, Magimbi C, et al. (2011) African programme for Onchocerciasis control: ophthalmological findings in Bushenyi, Uganda. West Afr J Med. 30: 104–109.
33. Fafowora OF, Osuntokun OO (1997) Age-related eye disease in the elderly members of rural African community. East Afr Med J. 74: 435–437.
34. Adegbehingbe BO, Majengbasan TO (2007) Ocular health status of rural dwellers in south-western Nigeria. Aust J Rural Health. 15: 269–272.
35. Hoerauf A, Specht S, Büttner M, Pfarr K, Mand S, et al. (2008) Wolbachia endobacteria depletion by doxycycline as antifilarial therapy has macrofilaricidal activity in onchocerciasis: a randomized placebo-controlled study. Med Microbio Immunol 197: 295–311.
36. Masud H, Qureshi TQ, Dukley M (2009) Effects of Ivermectin with and without doxycycline on clinical symptoms of onchocerciasis. J Coll Physicians Surg Pak 19: 34–38.

Permissions

The contributors of this book come from diverse backgrounds, making this book a truly international effort. This book will bring forth new frontiers with its revolutionizing research information and detailed analysis of the nascent developments around the world.

We would like to thank all the contributing authors for lending their expertise to make the book truly unique. They have played a crucial role in the development of this book. Without their invaluable contributions this book wouldn't have been possible. They have made vital efforts to compile up to date information on the varied aspects of this subject to make this book a valuable addition to the collection of many professionals and students.

This book was conceptualized with the vision of imparting up-to-date information and advanced data in this field. To ensure the same, a matchless editorial board was set up. Every individual on the board went through rigorous rounds of assessment to prove their worth. After which they invested a large part of their time researching and compiling the most relevant data for our readers.

The editorial board has been involved in producing this book since its inception. They have spent rigorous hours researching and exploring the diverse topics which have resulted in the successful publishing of this book. They have passed on their knowledge of decades through this book. To expedite this challenging task, the publisher supported the team at every step. A small team of assistant editors was also appointed to further simplify the editing procedure and attain best results for the readers.

Apart from the editorial board, the designing team has also invested a significant amount of their time in understanding the subject and creating the most relevant covers. They scrutinized every image to scout for the most suitable representation of the subject and create an appropriate cover for the book.

The publishing team has been an ardent support to the editorial, designing and production team. Their endless efforts to recruit the best for this project, has resulted in the accomplishment of this book. They are a veteran in the field of academics and their pool of knowledge is as vast as their experience in printing. Their expertise and guidance has proved useful at every step. Their uncompromising quality standards have made this book an exceptional effort. Their encouragement from time to time has been an inspiration for everyone.

The publisher and the editorial board hope that this book will prove to be a valuable piece of knowledge for researchers, students, practitioners and scholars across the globe.

List of Contributors

Mandana Zandian, Kevin R. Mott, Sariah J. Allen and Homayon Ghiasi
Department of Surgery, Center for Neurobiology and Vaccine Development, Ophthalmology Research, Cedars-Sinai Medical Center, Los Angeles, California, United States of America

Shuang Chen
Division of Pediatric Infectious Diseases and Immunology, Cedars-Sinai Medical Center, Los Angeles, California, United States of America

Moshe Arditi
Division of Pediatric Infectious Diseases and Immunology, Cedars-Sinai Medical Center, Los Angeles, California, United States of America
Department of Medicine, David Geffen School of Medicine at UCLA, Los Angeles, California, United States of America

Hyun Su Kim, Ho Chun Choi and Belong Cho
Department of Family Medicine, Seoul National University Hospital, Seoul, Republic of Korea

Joon Yong Lee
Department of Family Medicine, Korea University Guro Hospital, Seoul, Republic of Korea

Min Jeong Kwon
Division of Infectious Disease Surveillance, Korea Centers for Disease Control and Prevention, Chungcheongbuk-Do, Republic of Korea

Ken Fukuda, Waka Ishida, Tamaki Sumi and Atsuki Fukushima
Department of Ophthalmology and Visual Science, Kochi Medical School, Kochi, Japan

Jumpei Uchiyama, Mohammad Rashel, Shigenobu Matsuzaki and Masanori Daibata
Department of Microbiology and Infection, Kochi Medical School, Kochi, Japan

Shin-ichiro Kato
Research Institute of Molecular Genetics, Kochi University, Kochi, Japan

Tamae Morita
Kochi Medical School Hospital, Kochi, Japan

Asako Muraoka
Kochi Gakuen Junior College, Kochi, Japan

María Cruz Arnal, Miguel Revilla, David Martínez-Durán and Daniel Fernández de Luco
Departamento de Patología Animal, Facultad de Veterinaria, Universidad de Zaragoza, Zaragoza, Spain

Juan Herrero
Área de Ecología, Departamento de Ciencias Agrarias y Medio Natural, Escuela Politécnica Superior de Huesca, Universidad de Zaragoza, Huesca, Spain

Christian de la Fe, Ángel Gómez-Martín, Joaquín Amores and Antonio Contreras
Departamento de Sanidad Animal, Facultad de Veterinaria, Universidad de Murcia, Murcia, Spain

Carlos Prada, Olatz Fernández-Arberas and Alicia García-Serrano
Ega Wildlife Consultants, Zaragoza, Spain

Helen Mi
Yong Loo Lin School of Medicine, National University of Singapore, Singapore, Singapore

Su L. Ho and Elizabeth P. Y. Wong
National Healthcare Group Eye Institute, Tan Tock Seng Hospital, Singapore, Singapore

Wee K. Lim and Stephen C. Teoh
National Healthcare Group Eye Institute, Tan Tock Seng Hospital, Singapore, Singapore
Eagle Eye Centre, Singapore, Singapore

Yong Jie Qin, Kai On Chu, Yolanda Wong Ying Yip, Wai Ying Li, Ya Ping Yang, Kwok Ping Chan and Chi Pui Pang
Department of Ophthalmology and Visual Sciences, The Chinese University of Hong Kong, Hong Kong

Jia Lin Ren and Sun On Chan
School of Biomedical Sciences, The Chinese University of Hong Kong, Hong Kong, China

Lung-Chang Chien
Division of Biostatistics, University of Texas School of Public Health at San Antonio Regional Campus, San Antonio, Texas, United States of America

Yi-Jen Lien and Hwa-Lung Yu
Department of Bioenvironmental Systems Engineering, National Taiwan University, Taipei, Taiwan

Chiang-Hsin Yang
Department of Health Care Management, National Taipei University of Nursing and Health Sciences, Taipei, Taiwan

Richard L. Thompson and Malak Kotb
Department of Molecular Genetics, Microbiology, and Biochemistry, University of Cincinnati College of Medicine, Cincinnati, Ohio, United States of America

Robert W. Williams
Center of Genomics and Bioinformatics and Department of Anatomy and Neurobiology, University of Tennessee Health Science Center, Memphis, Tennessee, United States of America

Nancy M. Sawtell
Division of Infectious Diseases, Cincinnati Children's Hospital Medical Center, Cincinnati, Ohio, United States of America

Chih-Chun Chuang
Department of Ophthalmology, Chang Gung Memorial Hospital, Linkou, Taiwan
Department of Ophthalmology, Changhua Christian Hospital, Changhua, Taiwan
Department of Ophthalmology, Yuan-Sheng Hospital, Changhua, Taiwan

Ching-Hsi Hsiao, Hsin-Yuan Tan, David Hui-Kang Ma and Ken-Kuo Lin
Department of Ophthalmology, Chang Gung Memorial Hospital, Linkou, Taiwan
College of Medicine, Chang Gung University, Taoyuan, Taiwan

Chee-Jen Chang
Graduate Institute of Clinical Medical Science, Chang Gung University, Taoyuan, Taiwan
Clinical Informatics and Medical Statistics Research Center, Chang Gung University, Taoyuan, Taiwan

Yhu-Chering Huang
College of Medicine, Chang Gung University, Taoyuan, Taiwan
Division of Pediatric Infectious Diseases, Department of Pediatrics, Chang Gung Memorial Hospital Linkou, Taiwan

Bin Wu, Xian Qi, Ke Xu, Hong Ji, Yefei Zhu, Fenyang Tang and Minghao Zhou
Department of Acute Infectious Disease Control and Prevention, Jiangsu Province Center for Disease Control and Prevention, Nanjing, Jiangsu, China

Sivagnanam Ananthi and Murugesan Valarnila
Dr. G. Venkataswamy Eye Research Institute, Aravind Medical Research Foundation, Aravind Eye Care System, Madurai, India

Namperumalsamy Venkatesh Prajna
Cornea Clinic, Aravind Eye Hospital, Aravind Eye Care System, Madurai, India

Prajna Lalitha
Department of Microbiology, Aravind Eye Hospital, Aravind Eye Care System, Madurai, India

Kuppamuthu Dharmalingam
School of Biotechnology, Madurai Kamaraj University, Madurai, India

Lisette Hoeksema and Leonoor I. Los
Department of Ophthalmology, University Medical Center Groningen, University of Groningen, Groningen, the Netherlands
W.J. Kolff Institute, Graduate School of Medical Sciences, University of Groningen, Groningen, the Netherlands

Radhika Susarla, Lei Liu, Jawaher Alsalem, Geraint P. Williams, Sreekanth Sreekantam, Mohammad Tallouzi, H. Susan Southworth, Philip I. Murray, Graham R. Wallace and Saaeha Rauz
Academic Unit of Ophthalmology, Centre for Translational Inflammation Research, College of Medical and Dental Sciences, University of Birmingham, Birmingham, United Kingdom

Elizabeth A. Walker, Iwona J. Bujalska and Angela E. Taylor
Centre for Endocrinology, Diabetes and Metabolism, College of Medical and Dental Sciences, University of Birmingham, Birmingham, United Kingdom

Hanjuan Shao and Sherri-Gae Scott
Department of Medicine, Johns Hopkins School of Medicine, Baltimore, Maryland, United States of America

Chiaki Nakata and Abdel R. Hamad
Department of Pathology, Johns Hopkins School of Medicine, Baltimore, Maryland, United States of America,

Shukti Chakravarti
Department of Medicine, Johns Hopkins School of Medicine, Baltimore, Maryland, United States of America
Department of Cell Biology, Johns Hopkins School of Medicine, Baltimore, Maryland, United States of America
Department of Ophthalmology, Johns Hopkins School of Medicine, Baltimore, Maryland, United States of America

Mari Narumi, Hiroyuki Namba and Hidetoshi Yamashita
Department of Ophthalmology and Visual Sciences, Yamagata University Faculty of Medicine, Yamagata, Japan

Yoshiko Kashiwagi
Department of Health and Nutrition, Yamagata Prefectural Yonezawa Women's Junior College, Yamagata, Japan

Rintaro Ohe and Mitsunori Yamakawa
Department of Pathological Diagnostics, Yamagata University Faculty of Medicine, Yamagata, Japan

Hsin-Chiung Lin, Hui-Kang Ma and Hung-Chi Chen
Department of Ophthalmology, Chang Gung Memorial Hospital, Chang Gung University College of Medicine, Taoyuan, Taiwan

Ja-Liang Lin and Dan-Tzu Lin-Tan
Department of Internal Medicine, Chang Gung Memorial Hospital, Chang Gung University College of Medicine, Taoyuan, Taiwan

Andy Alhassan and Clotilde K. S. Carlow
Division of Genome Biology, New England Biolabs, Ipswich, Massachusetts, United States of America

Benjamin L. Makepeace
Institute of Infection and Global Health, University of Liverpool, Liverpool, United Kingdom

Elwyn James La Course
Liverpool School of Tropical Medicine, Liverpool, United Kingdom

Mike Y. Osei-Atweneboana
Council for Scientific and Industrial Research, Water Research Institute, Accra, Ghana

Marlon Moraes Ibrahim, Rafael de Angelis, Fuad Moraes Ibrahim, Leonardo Tannus Malki, MarinadePaulaBichuete and Eduardo Melani Rocha
Department of Ophthalmology, Faculty of Medicine of Ribeirão Preto, University of São Paulo, Ribeirão Preto, Brazil

Acacio Souza Lima
Department of Ophthalmology, São Paulo Federal University, São Paulo, Brazil
Ophthalmos Industria Farmacêutica, São Paulo, Brazil

Glauco Dreyer Viana de Carvalho
Ophthalmos Industria Farmacêutica, São Paulo, Brazil

Wellington de Paula Martins
Departamento de Ginecologia e Obstetrıcia da Faculdade de Medicina de Ribeirão Preto, Universidade de São Paulo, Ribeirão Preto, Brazil

Escola de Ultra-sonografia e Reciclagem Médica de Ribeirão Preto, Ribeirão Preto, Brazil
Instituto Nacional de Ciência e Tecnologia de Hormônios e Saúde da Mulher, Ribeirão Preto, Brazil

Claudia Córdova, Beatriz Gutiérrez, Marita Hernández and María L. Nieto
Instituto de Biología y Genética Molecular, Consejo Superior de Investigaciones Científicas-Universidad de Valladolid, Valladolid, Spain

Carmen Martínez-García and Patricia Gallego-Muñoz
Departamento de Biología Celular, Histología y Farmacología, Universidad de Valladolid, Valladolid, Spain

Rubén Martín
Instituto de Ciencias del Corazón. Hospital Clínico Universitario, Valladolid, Spain

Marcus Ang, Cheewai Wong and Soon-Phaik Chee
Singapore National Eye Centre, Singapore, Singapore
Singapore Eye Research Institute, Singapore, Singapore

Tina T. Wong
Singapore National Eye Centre, Singapore, Singapore
Singapore Eye Research Institute, Singapore, Singapore
Materials Science and Engineering, Nanyang Technological University, Singapore, Singapore

Xuwen Ng, Peng Yan and Subbu S. Venkatraman
Materials Science and Engineering, Nanyang Technological University, Singapore, Singapore

Abiba Kére-Banla
Onchocerciasis Reference Laboratory, Institut National d'Hygiéne, Sokodé, Togo

Méba Banla and Solim Tchalim
Onchocerciasis Reference Laboratory, Institut National d'Hygiéne, Sokodé, Togo
Centre Hospitalier Universitaire Campus, Université de Lomé, Lomé, Togo

Richard G. Gantin, Gertrud Helling-Giese, Christoph Heuschke, Hartwig Schulz-Key and Peter T. Soboslay
Onchocerciasis Reference Laboratory, Institut National d'Hygiéne, Sokodé, Togo
Institute for Tropical Medicine, University Clinics of Tübingen, Tübingen, Germany

Aide I. Agba
Centre Hospitalier Universitaire Campus, Université de Lomé, Lomé, Togo

Potochoziou K. Karabou
National Onchocerciasis Control Programme, Kara, Togo

Index